W9-BSC-647

Mucosal Biopsy of the Gastrointestinal Tract

MPP

3

RICHARD WHITEHEAD
M.D., Ch.B., F.R.C. Path., F.R.C.P.A.
Emeritus Professor of Pathology
Flinders University of South Australia
Consultant Pathologist
ClinPath Laboratories
South Australia

Mucosal Biopsy of the Gastrointestinal Tract

Volume 3 in the Series

MAJOR PROBLEMS IN PATHOLOGY

fifth edition

W.B. SAUNDERS COMPANY
A Division of Harcourt Brace & Company
PHILADELPHIA LONDON TORONTO MONTREAL SYDNEY TOKYO

W.B. SAUNDERS COMPANY

A Division of Harcourt Brace & Company

The Curtis Center
Independence Square West
Philadelphia, Pennsylvania 19106

Library of Congress Cataloging-in-Publication Data

Whitehead, Richard.

  Mucosal biopsy of the gastrointestinal tract / Richard Whitehead.—5th ed.

    p. cm.—(Major problems in pathology; v. 3)

Includes bibliographical references and index.

ISBN 0–7216–6192–0

1. Gastric mucosa—Biopsy.   2. Gastrointestinal system—Diseases—Diagnosis.   I. Title.
II. Series.   [DNLM: 1. Gastric Mucosa—pathology.   2. Intestinal
Mucosa—pathology.   3. Biopsy.   W1 MA492X v.3 1997 / WI 141 W592m 1997]

RC804.B5W47   1997

616.3'30758—dc20
DNLM/DLC   96-20545

Mucosal Biopsy of the Gastrointestinal Tract   ISBN 0–7216–6192–0

Printed in the United States of America.

Last digit is the print number: 9   8   7   6   5   4   3   2   1

Preface

The sheer volume of biopsies being produced by today's gastroenterologists, who are virtually all practicing endoscopists, makes it almost mandatory that the general histopathologist have skill in their interpretation. Numerically, these biopsies are a major component of the general hospital or private laboratory workload. On the broad front, in the 6 years that have elapsed since the last edition of this book, there has been steady progress in the diagnostic information that endoscopic biopsy interpretation provides. In particular, there has been an increasing awareness of the subtleties involved in the interpretation of these biopsies in non overtly malignant conditions. This awareness is in many ways comparable to the fine-tuning of diagnostic parameters that occurred in dermatopathology, in which for so much longer easy access to biopsy tissue has been available. There does not seem to be any reason to suppose that the mucosa of the gastrointestinal tract would manifest any more or any less a series of pathological responses or entities, exposed as it is to a similar range of noxious circumstances both external and internal.

Certainly, there have been remarkable revelations in several different areas. The impact of the putative role of *Helicobacter pylori* has caused shock waves rather than mere ripples through the whole of the gastroenterological fraternity. There has been considerable fine-tuning in the classification and diagnosis of chronic gastritis generally.

Our understanding of the range of abnormalities in malabsorption states has improved dramatically, and what is and what is not meant by gluten-sensitive enteropathy is somewhat different from the dogma of years gone by. Allergic enteropathies and a new group of forms of colitis, although still incompletely understood, have emerged, and there has been the impact of the AIDS virus.

As with previous editions, it is not the aim of this work to present a comprehensive text in gastroenterology; it is an attempt to guide the practising histopathologist. At the same time, this volume is intended to be a guide to gastroenterologists as to what and what not information their biopsies might be expected to reveal.

I am again indebted to Mrs. Eugenie Efinger for her dedication and meticulous effort in performing literature searches and in preparing the manuscript. ClinPath Laboratories have given me great encouragement and ready access to case material and photographic facilities. I would like to thank the technical staff and especially Mrs. Debbie Dyer for her skill in producing excellent tissue sections. I know I can rely upon W.B. Saunders Co. to deliver a professionally produced fifth edition with the shortest possible delay. My wife and family have given me great support, and I dedicate this book to them.

Contents

Oesophageal Biopsy

1

NORMAL APPEARANCES IN OESOPHAGEAL BIOPSY SPECIMENS

Fibreoptic endoscopy and biopsy are fast becoming the usual diagnostic procedures in the investigation of oesophageal disorders. The tissue samples are small and superficial, only rarely including the muscularis mucosa. The normal epithelium is stratified and squamous (Fig. 1–1) and, despite assertions to the contrary (Hendrix and Yardley 1976), is the nonkeratinising type; although it occasionally exhibits a few keratohyalin granules, it lacks granular and keratin layers. It consists of a basal proliferative compartment that, for all except the last 2 or 3 cm, constitutes 10%–15% of the whole thickness of the mucosa. This layer contains both reserve cells, which

Figure 1–1. Normal oesophageal epithelium. Note the height of the papillae and the thickness of the basal layer; the clarity of cells in the upper layers is due to glucogen. Arrows indicate interepithelial lymphocytes (H&E ×150).

Figure 1–2. Low-power view of Figure 1–1 shows the lamina propria, which contains relatively few lymphocytes (H&E ×75).

Figure 1–3. Lower oesophageal biopsy shows oesophageal cardiac-type glands in the lamina propria; glycogenic vacuolation of the squamous cells is not a feature (H&E ×150).

remain basal, and cells that eventually lose mitotic ability and become progressively superficial before desquamating at the surface. During this process the cells acquire glycogen, which can be demonstrated in periodic acid–Schiff (PAS) preparations. The width of the zone of unstained basal cells, although it does not necessarily correspond accurately with the population of cells still capable of division, is a useful indicator of that population and of value in the diagnosis of reflux oesophagitis. The increased thickness of the basal layer in the distal 2 cm probably reflects a response to the normal physiological reflux of gastric contents (Kaye 1977). It is also known that the interpapillary basal cells have a faster cell cycle time than the papillary basal cells (Jankowski et al 1992), and the latter may well represent the functional stem cell component. The melanoblasts and putative endocrine polypeptide argyrophil cells can on occasion be scattered among the cells of the basal layer. Tateishi et al (1974) found melanocytes in 4 and argyrophil cells in 14 of 50 oesophageal specimens obtained at autopsy. Oesophageal melanocytes have also been studied at the ultrastructural level (Ohashi et al 1990, Yamazaki et al 1991). Intraepithelial lymphocytes and Langerhans's cells similar to those present in the skin have also been described (Al Yassin and Toner 1976). Neutrophil granulocytes, although said to occur rarely in the normal oesophagus (Seefeld et al 1977), are for all practical purposes absent, and certainly the presence of macrophages and eosinophils is always abnormal.

Extending into the epithelium from below are the subepithelial papillae of the lamina propria consisting of delicate vascular connective tissue. The number of papillae per unit length of epithelium has not been accurately determined; in height papillae usually do not extend above halfway to the surface. The lamina propria of the oesophageal epithelium is composed of loose connective tissue (Fig. 1–2) that contains scattered lymphocytes and plasma cells or small lymphoid aggregates that are mainly located around the ducts of the oesophageal glands and are obviously only ever seen in deep forceps biopsies of the type usually performed through rigid endoscopes. The ducts are lined with cuboidal cells as they leave the oesophageal glands and become a stratified squamous type after passing through the muscularis mucosa. The glands vary quite markedly in number from patient to patient. They occupy the submucosa and are of mixed salivary type, being either purely mucinous, purely serous, or mucinous with serous crescents. At the lower end of the oesophagus, however, it is not rare to see in more superficial biopsies a few simple mucinous glands in the lamina propria. These are similar to the gastric cardiac mucous glands (Fig. 1–3) and are referred to as oesophageal cardiac glands.

In premature infants, less commonly in term babies, and rarely in adults, scattered islands of ciliated epithelium may occur in patches throughout the oesophageal lining. This represents persistence of a developmental stage in the oesophageal mucosa and a simple variation from normal that is without significance (Raeburn 1951).

2

GASTRO-OESOPHAGEAL REFLUX AND OESOPHAGITIS, BARRETT'S OESOPHAGUS, AND ECTOPIC GASTRIC MUCOSA

GASTRO-OESOPHAGEAL REFLUX AND OESOPHAGITIS

In geographical areas of low incidence for squamous carcinoma of the oesophagus, by far the most common diagnostic problem posed by oesophageal biopsy interpretation relates to the consequence of reflux of gastric contents. In the absence of ulceration or a Barrett's columnar lining, there is debate as to what constitutes the histological grounds for the diagnosis of gastric reflux. It has long been held that a poor correlation exists between symptoms of reflux and inflammatory change of the oesophageal mucosa (Siegel and Hendrix 1963). Ismail-Beigi, Horton and Pope (1970), however, drew attention to basal cell hyperplasia and elongation of the papillae as indications of reflux, whether or not inflammatory cells were present in the epithelium. Weinstein, Bogoch and Bowes (1975) showed that these changes are present in 57% of asymptomatic volunteers in biopsies from the lower 2.5 cm of the oesophagus and 19% above this level. Using an automated image analyser Adami, Eckardt and Paulini (1979) demonstrated an inter- and intraobserver error in excess of 20% in the estimation of these parameters and concluded that assessment of basal cell thickness and papillary height as an index of gastro-oesophageal reflux was of limited value. This study was performed on autopsy material, but Seefeld et al (1977) had reached similar conclusions using biopsy tissues.

Central to this controversy is the fact that reflux is a normal phenomenon, and the likelihood is that the same degree of reflux will stimulate different levels of symptoms in different individuals. In addition there is the fact that the effect of reflux depends on its composition, volume, and frequency, the effectiveness of the peristaltic clearance mechanism, the inherent resistance to damage due to the nature of the oesophageal epithelium, the neutralising effect of swallowed saliva, and the protection afforded by the secretions of the oesophageal mucous glands. Given that the cause of oesophageal pain is not fully understood, it is hardly surprising that correlation of the histological consequences of reflux with symptoms is poor. Indeed it is well recognized that patients with oesophagitis and stricture may have few or no reflux symptoms before dysphagia develops (Volpicelli, Yardley and Hendrix 1975).

The concern of the tissue pathologist, however, is the recognition of changes in oesophageal biopsies due to significant reflux of gastric contents (Figs. 2–1 to 2–4).

Figure 2–1. Epithelium shows elongation of the papillae, basal cell hyperplasia, and loss of glycogenic vacuolation in all except the superficial layers (H&E ×100).

Figure 2–2. Marked basal cell hyperplasia is maximum between the papillae, and there is an obvious increase in intraepithelial lymphocytes (H&E ×175).

Figure 2–3. Features as in Figures 2–1 and 2–2, but the papillae are cross-cut. The intraepithelial inflammatory cell infiltration contains polymorphonuclear leukocytes, and there is obvious increased cellularity of the lamina propria (H&E ×150).

Figure 2–4. Reflux oesophagitis with impending erosion at left (H&E ×75).

Because reflux is a normal event, minor degrees of histological variations could be regarded as part of the normal spectrum of oesophageal histology, especially at its distal end. If the pathophysiology of oesophageal damage due to reflux is considered, it is possible to predict the morphological changes that might ensue regardless of whether or not they are related to symptoms, and the histological assessment of biopsies does provide evidence for the evaluation of reflux disease (Funch-Jensen et al 1986). There is ample evidence for a damaging effect of acid, pepsin, and bile on the oesophageal mucosa in humans (Hopwood et al 1981) and experimental animals (Carney et al 1981, Dodds et al 1981, Salo, Lehto and Kivilaakso 1983). More recently there have been claims that the role of bile as an irritant may be greater than previously thought, so that "alkaline" reflux may be as important as acid reflux as a damaging agent (Bremner and Mason 1993). This cell damage results in a shortened cell life and increased surface exfoliation. There is evidence from scanning and transmission electron microscope studies that detectable cellular lesions due to reflux precede light microscope abnormalities and in particular any inflammatory cell infiltrates (Sbarbati et al 1993). In association with minor degrees of damage, the response of the oesophageal epithelium is to counteract the increased cell loss with increased production. Evidence for increased cell turnover in biopsies with proven reflux was provided by a morphometric analysis of various nuclear parameters in the different layers of the oesophageal epithelium (Jarvis, Dent and Whitehead 1985). The increased cell turnover results in a thickening of the basally situated proliferative component. This thickening tends to occur principally in the areas between subepithelial papillae. Damage to the basal cells due to diffusion of gastric contents across the oesophageal epithelium would be expected to be least marked in the cells farthest from the lumen, those lying between the subepithelial papillae. As stated in Chapter 1, this thickness, which is normally 10%–15% of the whole mucosa, can be readily assessed in periodic acid–Schiff (PAS)-stained sections. Another method is to define its upper extent arbitrarily as that level at which the distance between nuclei equals the average nuclear diameter, but this only achieves the same purpose and is more time-consuming.

In association with basal cell hyperplasia, elongation of the subepithelial papillae occurs, and these papillae tend to approach the surface. This is also a consequence of the mechanism of damage due to back diffusion. The lower cell turnover of damaged basal cells over the papillae and a uniform surface loss tend to bring the papillae nearer to the surface. Clearly, when the damage is such that exfoliation exceeds the rate of cell renewal, erosions appear first over the papillae and then extend to the areas between. The tendency, with increased severity of damage, is for the epithelium as a whole to reduce in thickness. When ulceration occurs, a mixed inflammatory infiltration is seen in the related submucosa, and gradually a layer of granulation tissue is formed at its base. When ulceration is recurrent it is followed by subepithelial scarring, and a stricture may result (Fig. 2–5).

Neutrophil polymorphonuclear leukocytes are a prominent component of the infiltrate and can also be seen in the neighbouring oesophageal epithelium. There has been a debate as to the importance of polymorph infiltration of the nonulcerated oesophageal epithelium as an indication of reflux damage, although in approximately 20% of cases showing the epithelial changes of basal cell hyperplasia and elongation of papillae they are seen in the lamina propria below the epithelium. When polymorph infiltration of the lamina propria is prominent, it is usually also seen in small numbers within the epithelium. This phenomenon is more obvious evidence of increasing damage and progressive thinning before ulceration occurs. As lymphocytes occur in the lamina propria in normal circumstances, their presence is of no diagnostic significance, although their numbers do tend to increase along with polymorphs and plasma cells in severe oesophagitis with ulceration.

Attention has also been drawn to the presence of intraepithelial eosinophils as a sensitive indicator of reflux in both children and adults (Winter et al 1982, Brown, Goldman and Antonioli 1984). The infiltrate, it is claimed, may occur before other histological evidence develops. The recognition of eosinophils is facilitated by exam-

Figure 2-5. Thickened oesophageal epithelium and subepithelial scarring characteristic of stricture (H&E ×150).

ining Chromotrope 2R preparations in which eosinophils stand out brightly red against the weakly stained pale blue background of the epithelium (Figs. 2–6 and 2–7).

Certainly cases with a pronounced eosinophil infiltrate do occur in younger patients, but in cases seen by the author there has been no correlation with peripheral blood eosinophilia and no evidence that the phenomenon is related to eosinophilic gastroenteritis, although involvement of the oesophagus in this condition apparently does occur. The claim that eosinophil infiltration is a good indication of reflux has been challenged in studies showing they have no diagnostic importance (Janisch et al 1984, Tummala et al 1987). Thus in the majority of cases that satisfy the histological criteria for reflux based on basal cell hyperplasia, papillary elongation, and the other features already mentioned, distinct eosinophil infiltration does not appear to be a feature, and it is possible that cases characterised by eosinophils represent a subgroup in which a different aetiological mechanism operates. On rare occasions apparently it is a manifestation of eosinophilic gastroenteropathy and is associated with a peripheral eosinophilia and infiltrates in other parts of the bowel (Dobbins, Sheahan and Behar 1977, Lee 1985). This is discussed in greater detail in Chapter 9.

Intraepithelial cell nuclei other than those of the epithelium itself are certainly often observed in oesophageal biopsies. In ordinary haematoxylin and eosin–stained slides these nuclei are small, variable in shape, and are seemingly being moulded between the epithelial cells themselves. Most of these nuclei are probably intraepithelial lymphocytes, but it is possible that some represent eosinophils or neutrophils that are degranulated. Certainly these irregular-shaped nuclear forms appear to

Figure 2–6. Oesophageal mucosa with a pronounced eosinophil polymorph infiltration. Arrows indicate nuclei (H&E ×175).

Figure 2–7. Oesophageal mucosa with a pronounced eosinophil leukocyte infiltration. The eosinophils stand out against the pale background; compare with Figure 2–5 (Chromotrope 2R ×400).

increase in number in oesophagitis. Geboes et al (1983) in a study using monoclonal antibodies have shown that in reflux oesophagitis Langerhans's cells and cytotoxic T lymphocytes are present in increased numbers within the epithelium. Lewis blood group antigen expression correlates with oesophagitis, and the flow cytometry technique can be used for Lewis blood group antigen demonstration (Jankowski et al 1991, Hopwood and Jankowski 1992). Epidermal growth factor receptors are also increased in number (Jankowski et al 1992), and the demonstration of nucleolar organiser regions by a silver technique can differentiate normal from inflamed mucosa (Jankowski et al 1992).

In summary, oesophageal biopsy appearances can indicate gastric reflux. A basal cell thickness in excess of 10%–15% and papillae extending into the upper half of the epithelium are the important features of minimal reflux and are seen in very distal biopsies in approximately half of a normal asymptomatic population. As some reflux is a normal phenomenon, this is to be expected. Abnormal reflux is associated with more severe alterations, thinning, and eventual ulceration and secondary inflammatory changes. Whereas in a younger age group eosinophil infiltration may signify reflux, in most other patients this does not seem to be the case. It can now be stated that the morphological assessment of reflux oesophagitis by subjective histology and in particular by sophisticated image analysis, although criticised by some workers (Collins et al 1989), is still the best means available.

BARRETT'S OESOPHAGUS (COLUMNAR LINED OESOPHAGUS)

Although there have been claims for a congenital origin for the columnar lined oesophagus (Haque and Merkel 1981, Stadelmann, Elster and Kuhn 1981), the consensus of opinion is that when limited to the distal oesophagus or extending to involve most of its length, the condition is acquired and the end result of severe longstanding reflux. A congenital susceptibility to the acquisition of Barrett's oesophagus deserves consideration, because it is not entirely clear why some individuals with reflux develop squamous oesophagitis and others develop Barrett's metaplasia (Hassall 1993a and b) (see the next section on ectopic gastric mucosa).

The evidence for the acquisition of Barrett's mucosa following oesophagogastrectomy (Naef et al 1975, Hamilton and Yardley 1977) as a late complication of anastomotic operations for oesophageal atresia complicated by reflux (Lindahl, Rintala and Sariola 1993) following cardiomyotomy for achalasia (Goldblum 1994, Jaakkola et al 1994), the healing of canine oesophageal lesions by columnar epithelium after destruction of the "anti-reflux" mechanism (Bremner, Lynch and Ellis 1970), the observation of orad migration of the squamocolumnar junction with time (Naef et al 1975), and the partial regression of Barrett's epithelium after antireflux operations (Brand et al 1980) or omeprazole therapy (Gore et al 1992) all point to an acquired aetiology.

It would appear therefore that reflux of gastric or even intestinal contents following total gastrectomy (Meyer, Vollmar and Bär 1979) can lead to severe epithelial damage and erosion, with a tendency to early healing by gastric-type mucosa. It is most usual for the reflux to persist and possibly increase in severity, and there is increasing evidence that Barrett's oesophagus is more common than is generally appreciated (Cooper and Barbezat 1987). The metaplastic change associated with recurrent ulceration and healing comes to occupy more and more of the oesophageal lining. The ulceration in Barrett's oesophagus is therefore found where expected, at the junction of squamous and columnar mucosa where attendant fibrosis may also produce a stricture. Barrett's oesophagus is occasionally familial (Prior and Whorwell 1986, Eng et al 1993, Fahmy and King 1993) and has been described in children following chemotherapy for leukaemia, apparently associated with reflux (Dahms et al 1987). There is increasing evidence from studies in children that aggressive antireflux therapy biopsy evaluation of dysplasia and early surgical intervention are mandatory if malignant transformation is to be avoided (Cheu et al 1992, Hassall 1993).

There has been some controversy with respect to the type of mucosa that constitutes a Barrett's oesophagus; this is the result of the simple fact that the morphological features are variable not only from case to case but also in the same case. At the lower gastric end it has been described as of fundic gastric type (Fig. 2–8) in that the mucosa contains both parietal and chief cells. The mucosa is, however, commonly gastritic and may be atrophic. In the author's experience this type of mucosa is never extensive and usually located distally, although very rarely at a higher level, but it can occur as is shown in the examination of surgical excision specimens performed in cases complicated by malignancy. When distal it is clearly responsible for difficulty in determining the precise gastro-oesophageal junction, and thus there is a case for arguing that in biopsy specimens this type of mucosa is not acceptable as part of the spectrum of Barrett's columnar mucosa unless accompanied by an element of intestinal metaplasia (Hassall 1993). A second type of columnar mucosa, which approximates gastric cardiac mucosa, is also seen (Fig. 2–9). A few parietal cells may occur among the cells forming the simple coiled mucinous glands (Fig. 2–10) that empty into the short crypts dipping down from the lumenal epithelium of gastric superficial type. This type of mucosa can exhibit a variety of intermediate appearances as it undergoes progressive metaplastic change into a more or less fully intestinalised mucosa.

These appearances are due to the acquisition of a variety of cell types. First, there is the appearance of intestinal goblet cells (Figs. 2–11 and 2–12); second, there

Figure 2–8. Barrett's oesophagus. Fundic (body)-type mucosa. Note the mixed mucinous and body-type glands and the inflammation (H&E ×150).

Figure 2–9. Barrett's oesophagus. Cardiac-type mucosa (H&E ×150).

Figure 2–10. Barrett's oesophagus. Cardiac-type mucosa with occasional parietal cells *(arrows)* (H&E ×500).

Figure 2–11. Barrett's oesophagus. A few goblet cells are beginning to appear, but most of the surface cells are gastric (H&E ×500).

Figure 2–12. Barrett's oesophagus. Goblet cells are numerous, and the remaining cells are difficult to identify (H&E ×250).

are cells with superficial cytoplasmic mucous droplets, but also with a lumenal border equipped with microvilli (Fig. 2–13). These cells were described in electron microscope preparations by Trier (1970), who regarded them as unlike any other type of cell seen in the gastrointestinal tract. In fact, they are similar to gastric surface cells showing partial intestinalisation (Ming, Goldman and Freiman 1967) and to the intermediate stages of metaplastic gastric superficial cells in the duodenum (Patrick, Denham and Forrest 1974). Apparently, however, they do not possess the capacity to absorb lipid and do not have the fully developed histochemical characteristics of absorptive enterocytes. In the author's experience with Barrett's oesophagus in paraffin sections, some cells have the appearance of enterocytes (Fig. 2–14), but the majority are best described as in a stage halfway between an enterocyte and a gastric superficial epithelial cell.

These mucus-secreting cells in Barrett's oesophagus have been investigated by histochemical procedures (Jass 1981), and it is claimed that whereas the goblet cells secrete mainly acid sialomucins, the other mucus-secreting cells contain predominantly either neutral or acid sulphomucins. This form of intestinalisation is said to correspond to the incomplete metaplasia type IIA and IIB of Jass and Filipe (1981), but in fact the mucin pattern based on the use of the PAS Alcian blue and high iron diamine Alcian blue methods is extremely variable in Barrett's oesophagus, showing a variety of combinations of mucins in the goblet cells and the columnar mucinous cells. The real value of using these stains is the easier recognition of the intermediate type of Barrett's epithelium.

It has been shown by others, however, that there is a poor correlation between mucin type and cancer risk in Barrett's oesophagus, and that its demonstration has

Figure 2–13. Barrett's oesophagus. Obvious goblet cells and intervening cells with mucous droplets and a brush border (H&E ×500).

Figure 2–14. Barrett's oesophagus. Goblet cells and cells that cannot be differentiated from enterocytes *(arrows)* (H&E ×500).

no value in managing patients. Flow cytometry abnormalities of DNA content seemed to offer a better prospect in this regard (Reid et al 1987, Haggitt et al 1988), but this has not been proved. The neoplastic progression in Barrett's oesophagus is also associated with cell cycle abnormalities (Reid et al 1993), the expression of intestinal brush-border–associated aminopeptidase N (Moore et al 1994), and alteration in the overexpression of the tumour suppressor protein p53 (Flejou et al 1993, Hardwick et al 1994, Neshat et al 1994). The use of these as biomarkers for predicting the development of cancer in Barrett's oesophagus is, however, still controversial, and there are conflicting reports in particular of the usefulness of the application of p53 measurements in this regard (Flejou et al 1994, Jones et al 1994). Other cells that also appear in the metaplastic process are enterochromaffin cells of intestinal type. In immunohistochemical studies these have been shown to contain 5-hydroxytryptamine, somatostatin, motilin, pancreatic polypeptide, glucose-dependent insulinotropic polypeptide, gastrin, glucagon, peptide tyrosine-tyrosine, secretin, and neurotensin (Rindi et al 1987). Paneth's cells often easily recognized only in specially stained preparations also occur. They are seen predominantly in areas where the mucosa most closely approximates to the small intestine (Fig. 2–15), even to the extent of exhibiting finger-like villous processes (Thompson, Zinsser and Enterline 1983). Pepsinogens A and C have also been demonstrated (Meuwissen et al 1988).

It is also worth noting that the junction of the squamous and columnar epithelium is often irregular. Sometimes squamous islands are left behind by the advancing edge of columnar epithelium. This may exhibit quite long tongue-shaped extensions upward from the main columnar-lined area. Small squamous islands also tend to persist at the mouths of the ducts of the oesophageal glands (Fig. 2–16). In rare instances squamous epithelium can overlie Barrett's mucosa over quite extensive areas (Sampliner et al 1988).

The metaplastic gastric epithelium in Barrett's oesophagus occasionally gives rise to hyperplastic polyps with appearances essentially similar to the same lesions arising in the stomach. As in the stomach, they probably represent a mucosal reaction to erosion or ulceration.

In longstanding cases of Barrett's oesophagus, it is not unusual to see the additional features of dysplasia (Fig. 2–17). The range of dysplastic appearances is essentially similar to that which occurs in the stomach in atrophic gastritis with intestinal metaplasia, and all stages of severity up to carcinoma in situ can be recognized (Hamilton and Smith 1987, Reid et al 1988a). Levine et al (1989) have shown, however, that the recognition of these dysplastic changes can be greatly facilitated by the use of electron microscopy and flow cytometry. Neoplastic progression is characterized by abnormalities in the cytoplasmic organelles concerned with mucin production and by aneuploid or G_2/tetraploid nuclei, in addition to the other abnormalities previously mentioned. The assessment of dysplasia subjectively as elsewhere in the bowel is prone to significant observer variation (Reid et al 1988b). Nevertheless it is still arguably the most reliable parameter on which therapy can be based in endoscopic surveillance programmes aimed at treating and curing malignancy complicating Barrett's oesophagus (Li 1993, Streitz, Andrews and Ellis 1993, Levine et al 1994, Streitz 1994). The importance of this lies in the fact that antireflux surgical procedures have no effect on the acquisition of dysplasia in Barrett's patients (Moghissi, Sharpe and Pender 1993). Sometimes the dysplastic epithelium occurs in the form of adenomatous polyps (McDonald, Brand and Thorning 1977, Thompson, Zinsser and Enterline 1983, Keeffe, Hisken and Schubert 1986). The invasive carcinoma that occurs in Barrett's oesophagus arises therefore from the partially or incompletely intestinalised epithelium and has as its counterpart in the stomach the intestinal type of carcinoma. Occasionally mucoepidermoid carcinoma (Pascal and Clearfield 1987) and carcinosarcoma (Dworak and Koerfgen 1993) are reported.

There is a difficulty in the interpretation of biopsy specimens from patients with longstanding Barrett's oesophagus. In some cases fibrosis or fibromuscular

Figure 2–15. Barrett's oesophagus. Villous process mimics small intestine (H&E ×250).

Figure 2–16. Barrett's oesophagus. Squamous island at the site of the opening of the duct of an oesophageal gland (H&E ×200).

Figure 2–17. Barrett's oesophagus. Severe dysplasia. Note the mitotic figures (H&E ×500).

Figure 2–18. Inlet patch of heterotopic gastric mucosa (H&E ×200).

Figure 2–19. Detail of Figure 2–18 shows chief and parietal cells (H&E ×400).

proliferation entraps normal or dysplastic glands, and these can easily be mistaken for invasive adenocarcinoma (Rubio and Riddell 1988).

ECTOPIC GASTRIC MUCOSA

Heterotopia of ectopic gastric mucosa is known to occur in a variety of sites in the gastrointestinal tract. Nevertheless its presence in the oesophagus has been the subject of some controversy. There are two reasons for this. First, some confusion has arisen between gastric ectopia proper and the presence of columnar epithelium, which is ciliated (see Chapter 1). Second, the condition of gastric mucosal ectopia as a developmental defect has been discussed in the context of Barrett's mucosa, but it is an entirely separate entity.

Early autopsy studies (Rector and Connerley 1941) revealed microscopic evidence of gastric mucosa in 7.8% of 1,000 infant and child subjects, and in more than half the abnormality was present in the upper one third. With the increasing practice of endoscopy, evidence is now firm that heterotopic gastric mucosa, which is usually of body type but sometimes simply mucinous as seen in the cardia or antrum (Figs. 2–18 to 2–20), can be found in up to 4% of cases, including adults (Jabbari et al 1985). This mucosa is sometimes called the "inlet patch" and can

Figure 2–20. Inlet patch of cardio pyloric simple mucinous gastric mucosa (H&E ×200).

show gastritis or ulceration and be associated with dysphagia or other symptoms and may lead to stricture (Raine 1983, Shah, DeRidder and Shah 1986, Truong, Stroehlein and McKechnie 1986, Wang, Spear and McGrew 1986, Schroeder, Myer and Schechter 1987, Steadman et al 1988, Borhan-Manesh and Farnum 1991). This is no doubt related to the secretory capacity of the gastric mucosa, which has been demonstrated by Nakajima et al (1993). It is rarely reported as a cause of an oesophageal web (Buse, Zuckerman and Balfe 1993) and may be colonised by *Helicobacter pylori* (Borhan-Manesh and Farnum 1993).

NONREFLUX OESOPHAGITIS AND ULCERATION

NONSPECIFIC OESOPHAGITIS

This form of oesophagitis forms part of the spectrum of oesophageal injury due to the ingestion of strong acids or alkalis, physical agents and radiation, and an increasing list of drugs. The injury usually results in a localised oesophageal ulceration with or without subsequent fibrosis and stricture. Histologically it is normally nonspecific, and biopsy specimens reveal only the range of appearances seen in reflux oesophagitis with or without ulceration. In the early stages of acid/alkali injury, however, more tissue necrosis is evident, and in ulcers secondary to radiotherapy deep biopsies show the characteristic hyalinisation of vessels and bizarre fibroblasts. There also may be epithelial nuclear abnormalities in more superficial biopsies that, in the absence of a clinical history, can cause difficulties in interpretation because there may be changes similar to those in primary premalignant dysplasia (Figs. 3–1 and 3–2). This is sometimes a problem in oesophageal lesions that may complicate chemotherapy for malignancies in other parts of the body (Fig. 3–3). Collins et al (1979), who reviewed drug-induced oesophageal ulceration, listed evidence for the implication of the following agents: emepronium bromide, Slow-K, doxycycline, tetracycline, clindamycin, phenylbutazone, as well as prednisone, fluorouracil, and carbachol. This list has been substantially lengthened to include nonsteroidal anti-inflammatory drugs (NSAIDs), and the most detailed list of drugs involved is given by Becouarn, Lamouliatte and Quinton (1983). There is evidence (Wilkins, Ridley and Pozniak 1984, Levine et al 1994) for an association between the use of NSAIDs and benign oesophageal stricture. Oesophageal injury due to ingested chemicals or drugs tends to occur at sites of anatomical narrowing, e.g., at the level of the aortic arch or where there is pathological narrowing due to, for example, an enlarged left atrium. It is more likely to occur if there is any disorder of oesophageal motility.

Necrotising lesions with secondary inflammatory changes have also been described in chronic graft versus host disease, particularly in the upper oesophagus (McDonald et al 1981). Ulceration of the oesophagus (Korula 1985) and the development of mucosal bridges presumably due to healing of ulceration such as occurs in other ulcerative lesions of the bowel have also been described (Gottfried and Goldberg 1985).

SPECIFIC FORMS OF OESOPHAGITIS

Specific forms of oesophagitis with or without ulceration and stricture are due to a variety of infective agents.

Figure 3–1. Oesophageal biopsy following irradiation of the mediastinum, resulting in ulceration and dysphagia. Note irregular epithelial maturation and degenerative nuclear changes (H&E ×75).

Figure 3–2. Detail of Figure 3–1. Nuclear abnormalities simulate neoplastic dysplasia (H&E ×500).

Figure 3–3. Dysplastic change in oesophageal epithelium due to chemotherapy (H&E ×300)

It is now well recognized that a wide range of gram-positive and gram-negative organisms can cause oesophagitis in the immunocompromised person, and this can be diagnosed in biopsy specimens (Walsh, Belitsos and Hamilton 1986, Laso, Cordero and Garcia-Sanchez 1994, Radhi and Schweiger 1994). Staphylococcal oesophagitis has been described in association with giant ulcer formation (Miller, Slywka and Ellis 1993).

In tuberculosis the oesophagus is usually involved by extension of adjacent bone, lymph node, or lung disease. Consequently oesophageal mucosal biopsies may or may not reveal diagnostic information (Dow 1981). Primary tuberculous oesophagitis actually diagnosed by endoscopic biopsy on the basis of granulomas and the demonstration of acid-fast organisms is on record (Scivewright, Feehally and Wicks 1984, Chase et al 1986, Catinella and Kittle 1988, Mokoena et al 1992). In two of these cases the disease eroded an atherosclerotic aortic aneurysm and caused death. Sometimes primary oesophageal tuberculosis can present as a tumour (Laajam 1984), contrary to what might be expected when the diagnosis is established antemortem; with appropriate therapy oesophageal tuberculosis has a favourable outcome. Syphilitic gummas of the oesophagus are extremely rare and their diagnosis on mucosal biopsy has not been described. Involvement by actinomyces, blastomyces, aspergillus, and *Histoplasma* is also uncommon, but distinctive histological appearances due to the presence of these agents have been described (Barrett 1950, Lee, Neumann and Welsh 1977, Hull 1979, Miller and Everett 1979, Knohe and Bernhardt 1980, McKenzie and Khakoo 1985). The same is true of candidal or monilial oesophagitis (Mathieson and Dutta 1983, Boylston et al 1987). Although commonly an acute complication in patients with acquired immunodeficiency syndrome (AIDS) (Porro, Parente and Cernuschi 1989) and in other immunodeficient hosts, in those with severe debilitating disease or diabetes, and in postoperative patients, especially after liver or renal transplantation (Alexander et al 1988), it has been recognized in a subacute or chronic form as a primary cause of oesophageal ulceration, tracheo-oesophageal fistula, and stenosis (Kodsi et al 1976, Orringer and Sloan 1978, Agha 1984, Obrecht et al 1984). Occasionally it presents as an oesophageal polypoidal lesion (Ho, Cullen and Gray 1977). It is also described in neonates (Petru and Azimi 1984), although immaturity of the immune response may be implicated. The oval yeasts and hyphal forms can be easily recognized in biopsy tissue, especially if a PAS stain is examined (Fig. 3–4). Moniliasis also occurs as a secondary phenomenon in oesophageal ulcers due to other causes such as in Barrett's oesophagus (Scott and Jenkins 1982, Kalogeropoulos and Whitehead 1988).

Viruses may also cause oesophageal ulceration. Cytomegalovirus infection is well recognized as a complication in immunosuppressed individuals and those with AIDS (Freeman et al 1977, Allen et al 1981, Weller 1985), but occasionally it causes erosive oesophagitis in healthy young adults (Villar, Massanari and Mitros 1984). The large intranuclear inclusions may be seen in fibroblasts and capillary endothelial cells in the ulcer base, but usually not in the squamous epithelium. Herpes simplex type 1 may also occur in the same type of patient or one with severe debilitating disease (Agha, Lee and Nostrant 1986), but it has been described as a cause of dysphagia due to ulceration in previously healthy individuals (Depew et al 1977, DiPalma and Brady 1984, Desigan and Schneider 1985). Furthermore, the great variability of both the clinical and endoscopic findings is being realised (Byard, Champion and Orizaga 1987). Apart from evidence of ulceration, the characteristic features in biopsies include multinucleate giant cells with their typical ground-glass nuclei.

Cells in the ulcer margin less frequently contain intranuclear inclusions (Fig. 3–5). These are characteristically eosinophilic and are surrounded by a clear zone with the nuclear chromatin condensed to a peripheral membranous ring (Cowdry type A cells). The endoscopic, light microscopic, and electron microscopic appearances have been described in detail (McKay and Day 1983, Burrig et al 1984, Feiden et al 1984). Oesophagitis can also occur in patients who have concurrent cutaneous herpes zoster; biopsy tissues show diffuse eosinophilic intranuclear inclusions (Gill et al 1984).

OTHER FORMS OF OESOPHAGITIS

Another cause of oesophageal ulceration is Behçet's syndrome. This has been reviewed by Kikuchi et al (1982). The pathology is not distinctive.

In systemic sclerosis the vascular changes and fibrosis affect the muscle layers and are not normally seen in biopsy tissues. However, the functional alteration of the cardio-oesophageal junction allows excessive reflux, and reflux oesophagitis is

Figure 3–4. Oesophageal biopsy shows yeast and hyphal forms of *Candida* organisms among squamous epithelial debris (PAS ×500).

Figure 3–5. Herpes oesophagitis. Ulcer margin with multinucleated giant cells *(arrows)* and Cowdry type A inclusions *(arrowheads)* (H&F. ×500).

common (Zamost et al 1987). This may progress to the acquisition of a Barrett's columnar lining (Cameron and Payne 1978). A similar range of pathological lesions is described as a less common complication of other collagen diseases, e.g., rheumatoid arthritis (Nishikai, Asaba and Homma 1977, Schneider et al 1984), systemic lupus erythematosus (Saladin et al 1966), and dermatomyositis (Greamer, Andersen and Code 1956). Similar basically reflux mucosal changes are seen in the neuromuscular disorder secondary to Chagas's disease and in visceral myopathy and neuropathy (Schuffler and Pope 1976, Cohen 1979, McDonald et al 1981). The oesophagus can also be involved in the Stevens-Johnson syndrome precipitated by an immunological response to certain drugs (Stoschus and Allescher 1993).

That involvement of the oesophagus in Crohn's disease occurs is well recognized. Freson, Kottler and Wright (1984) describe a case with granulomas in an oesophageal biopsy, and the author has experience of a similar case (Fig. 3–6), but in most instances the appearances are nonspecific. This is true of most of the cases that have been reported in the literature, and the diagnosis is presumptive because of documented Crohn's disease in other parts of the gastrointestinal tract (Davidson and Sawyers 1983, Tishler and Helman 1984, Pepe et al 1985). Huchzermeyer et al (1976), however, who reported five cases, make the point that an exact diagnosis requires histological examination of a resection specimen. LiVolsi and Jaretzki (1973) describe the occurrence of oesophageal Crohn's disease in the absence of gastrointestinal involvement proved at subsequent autopsy. A similar case was reported more recently by Howden, Mills and Rubin (1994). Successful treatment by oesophageal resection is also recorded (Zhang et al 1994).

Sometimes endoscopists see oesophageal rings or webs, and the appearances of

Figure 3–6. Crohn's disease of oesophagus with typical giant cell granulomatous reaction (H& E ×300).

the mucosa vary between normal and severe reflux oesophagitis with ulceration (Eastridge, Pate and Mann 1984). The biopsy appearances are also similar and are reviewed by Janisch and Eckardt (1982), who reported two patients with multiple webs. Endoscopic biopsy has also been used in the diagnosis of idiopathic acute oesophageal necrosis, and although it frequently accompanies preexistent serious illness, it is not necessarily a terminal event, some cases being successfully treated (Moreto et al 1993). Goodman et al (1994) have reported the radiological, endoscopic, and pathological findings of a spontaneous mucocele of the oesophagus.

4

OESOPHAGEAL PLAQUES AND MISCELLANEOUS CONDITIONS

There are several histological entities that, in the gross, at endoscopy appear as discrete surface white or yellow plaques. Some are due to fungal infections previously mentioned.

GLYCOGENIC ACANTHOSIS

This is the most common cause of oesophageal plaques (Bender et al 1973, Stern et al 1980). They are seen most commonly in the lower third of the oesophagus, are usually a few millimetres and rarely up to a centimetre in size, and occur predominantly on the crests of the longitudinal folds. Histologically, the epithelium is thickened due to an obvious increase in the glycogen-filled layer above the basal zone, which itself does not usually show hyperplasia, nor is there any nuclear atypia or keratinization (Fig. 4–1). The condition probably has no malignant potential or clinical significance, but it has been suggested that it may be part of the spectrum of human papillomavirus (HPV) infection (Morris and Price 1986). Others have claimed that it may be related to reflux, although antireflux therapy usually fails to eradicate the lesions (Vadva and Triadafilopoulos 1993). Glycogenic acanthosis has also been described in association with Cowden's disease (Hizawa et al 1994).

LIPID ISLANDS

Lipid islands similar to so-called xanthelasma of stomach and intestine are occasionally reported and on biopsy show the same histological appearance of collections of typical foam cells (Remmele and Engelsing 1984).

WHITE SPONGE NAEVI

Although primarily oral lesions, white sponge naevi also occur in the oesophagus (Haye and Whitehead 1968, Krajewska, Moore and Brown 1992). A rare, usually inherited disorder, they present as white nonpainful plaques. The plaques show a thickened epithelium composed of cells bloated with PAS-positive glycogen that occupy the full depth of the mucosa from the base up to the surface. This helps to differentiate the lesions from glycogenic acanthosis.

Figure 4–1. Oesophageal biopsy shows a pronounced glycogen-rich zone above the basal layer (PAS ×400).

OESOPHAGEAL LEUKOPLAKIA

Despite claims to the contrary (Rotterdam and Sommers 1981) it is the experience of most pathologists dealing with large numbers of biopsies that leukoplakia of the oesophagus comparable to the oral lesion is somewhat rare. The oral lesion is white because of keratinisation of a normally nonkeratinised epithelium. The latter may be either hyperplastic or somewhat atrophic. Its importance lies in the fact that it can exhibit a range of cellular atypia up to carcinoma in situ and is regarded as premalignant, some 10% of oral cases developing squamous carcinoma (King 1964). There are undoubted examples of oesophageal leukoplakia due to hyperkeratosis reported in the literature (Herschman et al 1978), but histological dysplasia has not been described. Hyperkeratotic white plaques may sometimes occur following acid or alkali burns and ulceration or in association with achalasia, scleroderma, or severe reflux disease (Fig. 4–2). Although the malignant potential of this variety of oesophageal plaque has yet to be determined in view of the increased incidence of squamous cell carcinoma in achalasia (Meijssen et al 1992), it does seem likely, however, that leukoplakia is premalignant.

OESOPHAGEAL PAPILLOMAS

In the past single or multiple oesophageal papillomas were often reported as rarities, usually being diagnosed because they had produced symptoms due to their size (Walker 1978, Waterfall, Somers and Desa 1978, Colina, Solis and Munoz 1980, Al-Rashed 1992). However, single or multiple small symptomless papillomas or polyps, sometimes described as low-domed plaques endoscopically, occur with an incidence of up to 0.45% in upper gastrointestinal endoscopy examinations, and there are increasing numbers of reports of quite large series of cases (Javdan and Pitman 1984, Toet et al 1985, Fernandez-Rodriguez et al 1986, Sablich et al 1988, Odze et al 1993, Carr et al 1994, Carr, Mohihan and Sobin 1994). A single case of multiple oesophageal papillomas occurring in association with Goltz's syndrome has been recorded (Brinson et al 1987). Goltz's syndrome is a congenital disease characterised by focal dermal hypoplasia; dysplasia of the skeleton, teeth, and other

Figure 4–2. Oesophageal epithelium in prolonged achalasia has acquired a granular layer and has been keratinised (H&E ×100).

structures of mesodermal and ectodermal origin; linear hyperpigmentation; and sclerodactyly. Oesophageal papillomas are usually benign histologically (Figs. 4–3 and 4–4) and show the usual features of squamous papillomas in other sites with irregular acanthosis and sometimes perinuclear cytoplasmic vacuolation of the superficial cells. Occasionally keratinisation may occur and the papillary stromal component may show an increase of lymphocytes and plasma cells. Although a relationship to HPV was not demonstrated in early studies (Colina, Solis and Munoz 1980), there is more recent evidence, based on immunohistochemical methods, that HPV infection may be implicated in some cases (Winkler et al 1985). The use of more sophisticated in situ hybridisation and polymerase chain reaction techniques, how-

Figure 4–3. Oesophageal squamous epithelial papilloma removed endoscopically (H&E ×25).

Figure 4–4. A higher power of one of the papillomas in Figure 4–3. Note the stromal inflammatory infiltrate and lack of epithelial atypia (H&E ×150).

ever, indicates that only a minority of papillomas contain HPV antigen (Carr et al 1994). The incidence of HPV in squamous carcinomas, however, is greater (Van-Rensburg, Venter and Simson 1993). Thus it seems that only some of these lesions proceed through stages of increasing atypia and dysplasia to invasive squamous carcinoma (Hille et al 1986). Morris and Price (1986) have drawn a comparison with the role of HPV infection in squamous carcinomas in other epithelial surfaces such as the uterine cervix. It is likely that a combination of factors causes squamous papillomas and carcinomas and that the presence of HPV infection is only one of them. It is of interest in this respect that in the uncommon genetic disorder tylosis (Marger and Marger 1993), which predisposes to oesophageal squamous carcinoma, HPV does not appear to be involved (Ashworth et al 1993).

SEBACEOUS GLANDS IN THE OESOPHAGUS

Rarely has this lesion been diagnosed by endoscopy and biopsy (Salgado et al 1980, Bambirra et al 1983). They appear as yellow raised plaques anywhere in the oesophagus and are composed histologically of mature sebaceous glands. They are presumably a developmental defect. Reconstructive surgery of the oesophagus, which requires the use of skin flaps, sometimes results in the condition known as hairy or hirsute oesophagus (Agha and Wimbish 1984, Llaneza, Menendez and Dunn 1987).

DYSPLASIA AND EARLY SQUAMOUS CARCINOMA OF THE OESOPHAGUS

In areas of low incidence squamous carcinoma is usually diagnosed late in the course of the disease when the patient presents with dysphagia. Workers in areas of high incidence have delineated the early stages of oesophageal squamous cancer (Figs. 4–5 to 4–7) (Crespi et al 1979, Dreyer 1980, Barge et al 1981, Munoz et al 1982, Crespi et al 1984, Mandard et al 1984). Wang (1981) described four endoscopic appearances in a group of 117 Chinese patients with early oesophageal cancer. The

Figure 4–5. Dysplasia of the oesophageal epithelium, which also is thickened and shows inflammatory cell infiltration (H&E ×150).

most common, occurring in 53%, was a friable irregular erosion; 25.6% presented with a raised polypoidal lesion with or without erosions; 12.8% showed a hyperaemic roughening that bled easily; and 8.6% showed one or more white plaques. In all cases the oesophagus exhibited a normal elasticity and peristaltic movement. It has become clear that squamous carcinoma of the oesophagus emerges mainly through a sequence of chronic oesophagitis, progressive dysplasia, carcinoma in situ, and finally invasive carcinoma (Munoz et al 1982, Benasco et al 1985, Oettle et al 1986, Ohta et al 1986). There is also the evidence that the situation is comparable to the

Figure 4–6. More severe dysplasia than in Figure 4–5. There is a marked variation in the nuclear size, shape, and polarity in the widened basal zone (H&E ×250).

Figure 4–7. Severe dysplasia in a rather atrophic epithelium. Note the mitotic figures, one of them very near to the surface (H&E ×250).

same tumour arising in the uterine cervix, and that at least in a proportion of cases HPV infection may play a role.

Carcinoma in situ and early squamous carcinoma of the oesophagus have also been reported in low-incidence areas (Seifert et al 1973), and it becomes increasingly likely that these curable lesions will be diagnosed more frequently outside China, South Africa, the Caspian littoral, and parts of France and other areas where the incidence is high. It could well be that in these areas HPV plays a relatively more important role than other factors. Certainly in France alcohol intake, tobacco smoking, and a high butter intake appear to be the most important factors (Jacob et al 1993). The histological changes documented in high-risk populations include parabasal clear cell hyperplasia, which is PAS negative, acanthosis, and lymphocyte–plasma cell infiltrations. Sometimes the abnormal epithelium is thin and atrophic, but the important features are the dysplastic nuclear changes and keratohyaline granules in the superficial cells (Jacob et al 1993, Dawsey et al 1994). More severe dysplasia, amounting to carcinoma in situ in either a thick or thin epithelium, is also seen as a precursor of invasion. Similar dysplasia and carcinoma in situ is described in mucosa adjacent to invasive squamous carcinomas of the oesophagus (Mandard et al 1980). Those cases associated with HPV in addition to dysplasia exhibit typical koilocytosis with perinuclear halos and sometimes either pyknosis of the nuclei or a ground-glass appearance.

Investigation of the overexpression of the P53 tumour suppressor gene, DNA ploidy, and the role of HPV, although giving variable results, continues to raise hope for a better understanding of the dysplasia cancer sequence in oesophageal squamous carcinoma (Chang et al 1993, Odze et al 1993, Chang et al 1994, Gao et al 1994, Goukon et al 1994, Lewensohn-Fuchs et al 1994). These precancerous changes appear to be identical in some cases to the postcricoid abnormalities that precede squamous carcinoma in patients with the Patterson-Kelly syndrome (Entwistle and Jacobs 1965). This entity occurs in women and combines dysplasia, iron deficiency anaemia, and gastric achlorhydria. It is rare except in Northern Europe, and it is particularly common in Scandinavia. Because iron deficiency is worldwide, these changes are clearly not due simply to lack of iron, and it is of interest that postcricoid carcinoma may also complicate pernicious anaemia (Jacobs 1962). In rare examples of biopsy material the author has seen from patients with pernicious anaemia, mild nuclear enlargement occurs in association with a chronic inflammatory infiltrate of the lamina propria (Fig. 4–8). Chronic oesophagitis, which may prove to be premalig-

Figure 4–8. Oesophageal mucosa in pernicious anaemia. There is increased basal layer thickness and slight irregular nuclear enlargement most noticeable in the middle layer. A lymphoid infiltrate of the lamina propria is prominent (H&E ×250).

nant, could well be more common than previously held. Cheli et al (1982) found chronic inflammation in biopsies of approximately 26% of asymptomatic Hungarian and Italian subjects. The incidence was highest in the fifth and sixth decades of the subjects' age.

RADIATION-INDUCED OESOPHAGEAL CARCINOMA

With the increasingly successful use of radiation therapy for mediastinal malignancy and the resulting prolonged patient survival, there have been increasingly common reports of subsequent oesophageal radiation effect and subsequent malignancy (Morichau-Beauchant et al 1983, O'Connell, Seaman and Ghahremani 1984, Sherrill et al 1984, Ohta et al 1986). The evidence to date indicates that this postirradiation invasive carcinoma also develops through a progressively dysplastic phase.

DERMATOLOGICAL CONDITIONS

Although the oesophagus is affected by certain primarily dermatological entities, e.g., epidermolysis bullosa dystrophica, pemphigoid, pemphigus, bullous pemphigoid, and toxic epidermal necrolysis, in the past reports of diagnosis based on oesophageal biopsy were few; only rarely was this made necessary when the oesophagus was affected in the absence of skin lesions (Wood, Patterson and Orlando 1982). Reports of endoscopic biopsy diagnosis have been increasingly more common in cases of lichen planus (Lefer 1982), pemphigus vulgaris (Yamamoto et al 1983, Goldin and Lijovetzky 1985, Mobacken et al 1988), benign mucous membrane pemphigoid (Al-Kutoubi and Eliot 1984), cicatricial pemphigoid (Anstey et al 1991), Behçet's disease (Mori et al 1983, Anti et al 1986), Stevens-Johnson syndrome (Zweiban, Cohen and Chandrasoma 1986), lichen ruber (Van Maercke et al 1988), bullous lesions associated with co-trimoxazole therapy (Heer et al 1985), and epidermolysis bullosa (Ergun et al 1992). Oesophageal acanthosis nigricans has been described in association with metastatic adenocarcinoma (Kozlowski and Nigra 1992).

INTRAMURAL PSEUDODIVERTICULOSIS

This is a rare condition of unknown aetiology and is commonly diagnosed radiologically (Foxworthy 1985, Stephens et al 1986). The ostia may be visible endoscopically, and biopsy may reveal the dilated excretory ducts of the oesophageal submucous glands that are the basic pathological lesion in this condition (Hover et al 1982, Lax, Haroutiounian and Attia 1986). In a detailed autopsy study (Medeiros, Doos and Balogh 1988) chronic inflammatory changes around submucous glands and early pseudodiverticula formation were common findings, which suggest that chronic inflammation plays an aetiological role in this condition.

FOCAL LYMPHOID HYPERPLASIA

An obstructive exophytic lesion of the mid oesophagus due to a hyperplastic lymphoid proliferation was described by Gervaz et al (1992), a similar case having previously been reported by Sheahan and West (1985). The former authors drew attention to some likeness with Castleman's disease (Frizzera 1988).

OESOPHAGEAL EOSINOPHILIA WITH DYSPHAGIA

Attwood et al (1993) described 12 cases of very dense eosinophil leukocyte infiltration (> 20 per high power field) in oesophageal biopsies from adult patients presenting with dysphagia but no mechanical obstruction. There was associated squamous hyperplasia but no evidence of increased acid exposure on 24-hour pH monitoring. Attwood et al claim that this is a distinct clinicopathological condition. This condition does at first sight seem to be different from reflux oesophagitis with an intraepithelial eosinophil component and also distinct from eosinophilic gastroenteritis with oesophageal involvement such as has been described (Olson and Fukui-Miner 1994).

LEUKAEMIC INFILTRATION OF THE OESOPHAGUS

Endoscopic examination and biopsy have facilitated the histological diagnosis of leukaemic infiltration of the oesophagus, a condition usually recognized only at autopsy (Fulp et al 1993).

REFERENCES—SECTION ONE: OESOPHAGEAL BIOPSY

Adami B., Eckardt V. F. and Paulini K. (1979) Sampling error and observer variation in the interpretation of esophageal biopsies. Digestion 19:404–410.

Agha F. P. (1984) Candidiasis-induced esophageal strictures. Gastrointestinal Radiology 9:283–286.

Agha F. P., Lee H. H. and Nostrant T. T. (1986) Herpetic esophagitis: a diagnostic challenge in immunocompromised patients. American Journal of Gastroenterology 81:246–253.

Agha F. P. and Wimbish K. J. (1984) Hirsute esophagus: clinical and roentgen features. Gastrointestinal Radiology 9:297–300.

Alexander J. A., Brouillette D. E., Chien M-C., Yoo Y-K., Tarter R. E., Gavaler J. S. and Van Thiel D. H. (1988) Infectious esophagitis following liver and renal transplantation. Digestive Diseases and Sciences 33:1121–1126.

Al-Kutoubi M. A. and Eliot C. (1984) Oesophageal involvement in benign mucous membrane pemphigoid. Clinical Radiology 35:131–135.

Allen J. I., Silvis S. E., Sumner H. W. and McClain C. J. (1981) Cytomegalic inclusion disease diagnosed endoscopically. Digestive Diseases and Sciences 26:133–135.

Al-Rashed R. S. (1992) Squamous papilloma of the esophagus: a case report and review of the literature. Annals of Saudi Medicine 12:313–315.

Al Yassin T. M. and Toner P. G. (1976) Langerhans cells in the human oesophagus. Journal of Anatomy 122:435–445.

Anstey A., Wojnarowska F., Whitehead P., Leigh I. M. and Rutty G. N. (1991) Oesophageal webs preceding carcinoma and rupture of the oesophagus in cicatricial pemphigoid. Clinical and Experimental Dermatology 16:395–398.

Anti M., Marra G., Rapaccini G. L., Barone C., Manna R., Bochicchio G. B. and Fedeli G. (1986) Esophageal involvement in Behcet's syndrome. Journal of Clinical Gastroenterology 8:514–519.

Ashworth M. T., McDicken I. W., Southern S. A. and Nash J. R. (1993) Human papillomavirus in squamous cell carcinoma of the oesophagus associated with tylosis. Journal of Clinical Pathology 46:573–575.

Attwood S. E., Smyrk T. C., Demeester T. R. and Jones J. B. (1993) Esophageal eosinophilia with dysphagia. A distinct clinicopathologic syndrome. Digestive Diseases and Sciences 38:109–116.

Bambirra E. A., de Souza Andrade J., de Souza L. A. H., Savi A., Lima G. F. and de Oliveira C. A. (1983) Sebaceous glands in the esophagus. Gastrointestinal Endoscopy 29:251–252.

Barge J., Molas G., Maillard J. N., Fekete F., Bogomoletz W. V. and Potet F. (1981) Superficial oesophageal carcinoma: an oesophageal counterpart of early gastric cancer. Histopathology 5:499–510.

Barrett N. R. (1950) Chronic peptic ulcer of the oesophagus and "oesophagitis." British Journal of Surgery 38:175–182.

Becouarn Y., Lamouliatte H. and Quinton A. (1983) Drug induced acute esophageal lesions. Gastroenterologie Clinique et Biologique 7:868–876.

Benasco C., Combalia N., Pou J. M. and Miquel J. M. (1985) Superficial esophageal carcinoma: a report of 12 cases. Gastrointestinal Endoscopy 31:64–67.

Bender M. D., Allison J., Cuartas F. and Montgomery C. (1973). Glycogenic acanthosis of the esophagus: a form of benign epithelial hyperplasia. Gastroenterology 65:373–380.

Borhan-Manesh F. and Farnum J. B. (1991) Incidence of heterotopic gastric mucosa in the upper oesophagus. Gut 32:968–972.

Borhan-Manesh F. and Farnum J. B. (1993) Study of *Helicobacter pylori* colonization of patches of heterotopic gastric mucosa (HGM) at the upper esophagus. Digestive Diseases and Sciences 38:142–146.

Boylston A. W., Cook H. T., Francis N. D. and Goldin R. D. (1987) Biopsy pathology of acquired immune deficiency syndrome (AIDS). Journal of Clinical Pathology 40:1–8.

Brand D. L., Ylvisaker J. T., Gelfand M. and Pope C. E. (1980) Regression of columnar esophageal (Barrett's) epithelium after anti-reflux surgery. The New England Journal of Medicine 302:844–848.

Bremner C. G., Lynch V. P. and Ellis F. H. Jr (1970) Barrett's esophagus: congenital or acquired? An experimental study of esophageal mucosal regeneration in the dog. Surgery 68:209–216.

Bremner C. G. and Mason R. J. (1993). Bile in the oesophagus. British Journal of Surgery 80:1374–1376.

Brinson R. R., Schuman B. M., Mills L. R., Thigpen S. and Freedman S. (1987) Multiple squamous papillomas of the esophagus associated with Goltz syndrome. American Journal of Gastroenterology 82:1177–1179.

Brown L. F., Goldman H. and Antonioli D. A. (1984) Intraepithelial eosinophils in endoscopic biopsies of adults with reflux esophagitis. American Journal of Surgical Pathology 8:899–905.

Burrig K-F., Borchard F., Feiden W. and Pfitzer P. (1984) Herpes oesophagitis II: electron microscopical findings. Virchows Archiv (A) 404:177–185.

Buse P. E., Zuckerman G. R. and Balfe D. M. (1993) Cervical esophageal web associated with a patch of heterotopic gastric mucosa. Abdominal Imaging 18:227–228.

Byard R. W., Champion M. C. and Orizaga M. (1987) Variability in the clinical presentation and endoscopic findings of herpetic esophagitis. Endoscopy 19:153–155.

Cameron A. J. and Payne W. S. (1978) Barrett's esophagus occurring as a complication of scleroderma. Mayo Clinic Proceedings 53:612–615.

Carney C. N., Orlando R. C., Powell D. W. and Dotson M. M. (1981) Morphologic alterations in early acid-induced epithelial injury of the rabbit esophagus. Laboratory Investigation 45:198–208.

Carr N. J., Bratthauer G. L., Lichy J. H., Taubenberger J. K., Monihan J. M. and Sobin L. H. (1994)

Squamous cell papillomas of the esophagus: a study of 23 lesions for human papillomavirus by in situ hybridization and polymerase chain reaction. Human Pathology 25:536–540.

Carr N. J., Monihan J. M. and Sobin L. H. (1994) Squamous cell papilloma of the esophagus: a clinicopathologic and follow-up study of 25 cases. American Journal of Gastroenterology 89:245–248.

Catinella F. P. and Kittle C. F. (1988) Tuberculous esophagitis with aortic aneurysm fistula. Annals of Thoracic Surgery 45:87–88.

Chang F., Syrjanen S., Shen Q., Wang L. and Syrjanen K. (1993) Screening for human papillomavirus infections in esophageal squamous cell carcinomas by in situ hybridization. Cancer 72:2525–2530.

Chang F., Syrjanen S., Tervahauta A., Kurvinen K. and Wang L. (1994) Frequent mutations of p53 gene in oesophageal squamous cell carcinomas with and without human papillomavirus (HPV) involvement suggest the dominant role of environmental carcinogens in oesophageal carcinogenesis. British Journal of Cancer 70:346–351.

Chase R. A., Haber M. H., Pottage J. C., Schaffner J. A., Miller C. and Levin S. (1986) Tuberculous esophagitis with erosion into aortic aneurysm. Archives of Pathology and Laboratory Medicine 110:965–966.

Cheli R., Simon L., Elster K. and Bocchini R. (1982) Oesophagitis in Italian and Hungarian asymptomatic subjects. Endoscopy 14:1–3.

Cheu H. W., Grosfeld J. L., Heifetz S. A., Fitzgerald J., Rescorla F. and West K. (1992) Persistence of Barrett's esophagus in children after antireflux surgery: influence on follow-up care. Journal of Pediatric Surgery 27:26–28.

Cohen S. (1979) Motor disorders of the esophagus. The New England Journal of Medicine 301:184–192.

Colina F., Solis J. A. and Munoz M. T. (1980) Squamous papilloma of the esophagus. American Journal of Gastroenterology 74:410–414.

Collins F. J., Matthews H. R., Baker S. E. and Strakova J. M. (1979) Drug-induced oesophageal injury. British Medical Journal 1:1673–1676.

Collins J. S. A., Watt P. C. H., Hamilton P. W., Collins B. J., Sloan J. M., Elliott H. and Love A. H. G. (1989) Assessment of oesophagitis by histology and morphometry. Histopathology 14:381–389.

Cooper B. T. and Barbezat G. O. (1987) Barrett's oesophagus: a clinical study of 52 patients. Quarterly Journal of Medicine 62:97–108.

Crespi M., Grassi A., Munoz N., Guo-Quing W. and Guanrei Y. (1984) Endoscopic features of suspected precancerous lesions in high-risk areas for esophageal cancer. Endoscopy 16:85–91.

Crespi M., Munoz N., Grassi A., Aramesh B., Amiri G., Mojtabai A. and Casale V. (1979) Oesophageal lesions in northern Iran: a premalignant condition? Lancet 2:217–221.

Dahms B. B., Greco M. A., Strandjord S. E. and Rothstein F. C. (1987) Barrett's esophagus in three children after antileukemia chemotherapy. Cancer 60:2896–2900.

Davidson J. T. and Sawyers J. L. (1983) Crohn's disease of the esophagus. The American Surgeon 49:168–172.

Dawsey S. M., Lewin K. J., Wang G. Q., Liu F. S., Nieberg R. K., Yu Y., Li J. Y., Blot W. J., Li B. and Taylor P. R. (1994) Squamous esophageal histology and subsequent risk of squamous cell carcinoma of the esophagus. A prospective follow-up study from Linxian, China. Cancer 74:1686–1692.

Depew W. T., Prentice R. S. A., Beck I. T., Blakeman J. M. and Da Costa L. R. (1977) Herpes simplex ulcerative esophagitis in a healthy subject. American Journal of Gastroenterology 68:381–385.

Desigan G. and Schneider R. P. (1985) Herpes simplex esophagitis in healthy adults. Southern Medical Journal 78:1135–1137.

DiPalma J. A. and Brady C. E. (1984) Herpes simplex esophagitis in a nonimmunosuppressed host with gastroesophageal reflux. Gastrointestinal Endoscopy 30:24–25.

Dobbins J. W., Sheahan D. G. and Behar J. (1977) Eosinophilic gastroenteritis with oesophageal involvement. Gastroenterology 72:1312–1316.

Dodds W. J., Hogan W. J., Helm J. F. and Dent J. (1981) Pathogenesis of reflux esophagitis. Gastroenterology 81:376–394.

Dow C. J. (1981) Oesophageal tuberculosis: four cases. Gut 22:234–236.

Dreyer L. (1980) The incidence of dysplasia and associated epithelial lesions in the oesophageal mucosa of South African blacks. South African Medical Journal 58:406–408.

Dworak O. and Koerfgen H. P. (1993) Carcinosarcoma in Barrett's oesophagus: a case report with immunohistological examination. Virchows Archiv (A) 422:423–426.

Eastridge C. E., Pate J. W. and Mann J. A. (1984) Lower esophageal ring: experience in treatment of 88 patients. Annals of Thoracic Surgery 37:103–107.

Eng C., Spechler S. J., Ruben R. and Li F. P. (1993) Familial Barrett's esophagus and adenocarcinoma of the gastroesophageal junction. Cancer Epidemiology, Biomarkers and Prevention 2:397–399.

Entwistle C. C. and Jacobs A. (1965) Histological findings in the Paterson-Kelly syndrome. Journal of Clinical Pathology 18:408–413.

Ergun G. A., Lin A. N., Dannenberg A. J. and Carter D. M. (1992) Gastrointestinal manifestations of epidermolysis bullosa: a study of 101 patients. Medicine (Baltimore) 71:121–127.

Fahmy N. and King J. F. (1993) Barrett's esophagus: an acquired condition with genetic predisposition. American Journal of Gastroenterology 88:1262–1265.

Feiden W., Borchard F., Burrig K-F. and Pfitzer P. (1984) Herpes oesophagitis I: light microscopical and immunohistochemical investigations. Virchows Archiv (A) 404:167–176.

Fernandez-Rodriguez C. M., Badia-Figuerola N., del Arbol L. R., Fernandez-Seara J., Dominguez F. and Aviles-Ruiz J. F. (1986) Squamous papilloma of the esophagus: report of 6 cases with long-term follow-up in 4 patients. American Journal of Gastroenterology 81:1059–1062.

Flejou J. F., Paraf F., Potet F., Museau F., Fekete F. and Henin D. (1994) P53 protein expression in Barrett's adenocarcinoma: a frequent event with no prognostic significance. Histopathology 24:487–489.

Flejou J. F., Potet F., Muzeau F., Le Pelletier F., Fekete F. and Henin D. (1993) Overexpression of p53 protein in Barrett's syndrome with malignant transformation. Journal of Clinical Pathology 46:330–333.

Foxworthy V. (1985) Diffuse intramural pseudodiverticulosis of the oesophagus. British Journal of Clinical Practice 39:449–450.

Freeman H. J., Shnitzka T. K., Piercey J. R. A. and Weinstein W. M. (1977) Cytomegalovirus infection of the gastrointestinal tract in a patient with late onset immunodeficiency syndrome. Gastroenterology 73:1397–1403.

Freson M., Kottler R. E. and Wright J. P. (1984) Crohn's disease of the oesophagus. South African Medical Journal 66:417–418.

Frizzera G. (1988) Castleman's disease and related disorders. Seminars of Diagnostic Pathology 5:346–364.

Fulp S. R., Nestok B. R., Powell B. L., Evans J. K., Geisinger K. R. and Gilliam J. H. (1993) Leukemic infiltration of the esophagus. Cancer 71:112–116.

Gao H., Wang L. D., Zhou Q., Hong J. Y., Huang T. Y. and Yang C. S. (1994) P53 tumor suppressor gene mutation in early esophageal populations in Hunan, China. Cancer Research 54:4342–4346.

Geboes K., De Wolf-Peeters C., Rutgeerts P., Janssens J., Vantrappen G. and Desmet V. (1983) Lymphocytes and Langerhans cells in the human oesophageal epithelium. Virchows Archiv (A) 401:45–55.

Gervaz E., Potet F., Mahe R. and Lemasson G. (1992) Focal lymphoid hyperplasia of the oesophagus: report of a case. Histopathology 21:187–189.

Gill R. A., Gebhard R. L., Dozeman R. L. and Sumner H. W. (1984) Shingles esophagitis: endoscopic diagnosis in two patients. Gastrointestinal Endoscopy 30:26–27.

Goldblum J. R., Whyte R. I., Orringer M. B. and Appelman H. D. (1994) Achalasia: a morphologic study of 42 resected specimens. American Journal of Surgical Pathology 18:327–337.

Goldin E. and Lijovetzky G. (1985) Esophageal involvement by pemphigus vulgaris. American Journal of Gastroenterology 80:828–830.

Goodman P., Kalangi S. S., Kumar D. and Balachandran S. (1994) Spontaneous mucocele of the upper esophagus: radiologic demonstration. Dysphagia 9:199–201.

Gore S., Healey C. J., Sutton R., Shepherd N. A. and Wilkinson S. P. (1992) Regression of columnar lined Barrett's oesophagus with continuous omeprazole therapy. Gut 33 (suppl) I532, T127.

Gottfried E. B. and Goldberg H. J. (1985) Mucosal bridge of the distal esophagus after esophageal variceal sclerotherapy. Gastrointestinal Endoscopy 31:267–269.

Goukon Y., Sasano H., Nishihira T., Nagura H. and Mori S. (1994) P53 overexpression in human esophageal carcinoma: a correlation with tumor DNA ploidy and two parameter flow cytometric study. Anticancer Research 14:1305–1312.

Greamer B., Andersen H. A. and Code C. F. (1956) Esophageal motility in patients with scleroderma and related diseases. Gastroenterologia 86:763–775.

Haggitt R. C., Reid B. J., Rabinovitch P. S. and Rubin C. E. (1988) Barrett's esophagus. American Journal of Pathology 131:53–61.

Hamilton S. R. and Smith R. R. L. (1987) The relationship between columnar epithelial dysplasia and invasive adenocarcinoma arising in Barrett's esophagus. American Journal of Clinical Pathology 87:301–312.

Hamilton S. R. and Yardley J. II. (1977) Regeneration of cardiac type mucosa and acquisition of Barrett mucosa after esophagogastrostomy. Gastroenterology 72:669–675.

Haque A. K. and Merkel M. (1981) Total columnar-lined esophagus. Archives of Pathology and Laboratory Medicine 105:546–548.

Hardwick R. H., Shepherd N. A., Moorghen M., Newcomb P. V. and Alderson D. (1994) Adenocarcinoma arising in Barrett's oesophagus: evidence for the participation of p53 dysfunction in the dysplasia/carcinoma sequence. Gut 35:764–768.

Hassall E. (1993a) Barrett's esophagus: congenital or acquired? American Journal of Gastroenterology 88:819–824.

Hassall E. (1993b) Barrett's esophagus: new definitions and approaches in children. Journal of Pediatric Gastroenterology and Nutrition 16:345–364.

Haye K. R. and Whitehead F. I. H. (1968). Hereditary leukokeratosis of the mucous membrane. British Journal of Dermatology 80:529–533.

Heer M., Altorfer J., Burger H-R. and Walti M. (1985) Bullous esophageal lesions due to co-trimoxazole: an immune-mediated process? Gastroenterology 88:1954–1957.

Hendrix T. R. and Yardley J. H. (1976) Consequences of gastro-oesophageal reflux. Clinics in Gastroenterology 5:155–174.

Herschman B. R., Uppaputhangkule V., Maas L. and Gelzayd E. (1978) Esophageal leukoplakia: a rare entity. Journal of the American Medical Association 239:2021.

Hille J. J., Margolius K. A., Markowitz S. and Isaacson C. (1986) Human papillomavirus infection related to oesophageal carcinoma in black South Africans. South African Medical Journal 69:417–420.

Hizawa K., Iida M., Matsumoto T., Kohrogi N., Suekane H., Yao T. and Fujishima M. (1994) Gastrointestinal manifestations of Cowden's disease: report of four cases. Journal of Clinical Gastroenterology 18:13–18.

Ho C-S., Cullen J. B. and Gray R. R. (1977) An unusual manifestation of esophageal moniliasis. Radiology 123:287–288.

Hopwood D., Bateson M. C., Milne G. and Bouchier I. A. D. (1981) Effects of bile acids and hydrogen ion on the fine structure of oesophageal epithelium. Gut 22:306–311.

Hopwood D. and Jankowski J. (1992) Flow cytometry of oesophageal mucosal biopsies. Journal of Pathology 167:321–326.

Hover A. R., Brady C. E., Williams J. R., Stewart D. L. and Christian C. (1982) Multiple retention cysts of the lower esophagus. Journal of Clinical Gastroenterology 4:209–212.

Howden F. M., Mills I. R. and Rubin J. W. (1994) Crohn's disease of the esophagus. American Surgeon 60:656–660.

Huchzermeyer H., Paul F., Seifert E., Froehlich H. and Rasmussen Ch. W. (1976). Endoscopic results in five patients with Crohn's disease of the oesophagus. Endoscopy 8:75–81.

Hull P. R. (1979) Systemic histoplasmosis with oesophageal obstruction due to histoplasma granulomas. South African Medical Journal 55:639–640.

Ismail-Beigi F., Horton P. F. and Pope C. E. (1970) Histological consequences of gastroesophageal reflux in man. Gastroenterology 58:163–174.

Jaakkola A., Reinikainen P., Ovaska J. and Isolauri J. (1994) Barrett's esophagus after cardiomyotomy for esophageal achalasia. American Journal of Gastroenterology 89:165–169.

Jabbari M., Goresky C. A., Lough J., Yaffe C., Daly D. and Cote C. (1985) The inlet patch: heterotopic gastric mucosa in the upper esophagus. Gastroenterology 89:352–356.

Jacob J. H., Riviere A., Mandard A. M., Munoz N., Crespi M., Etienne Y., Castellsague X., Marnay J., Lebigot G. and Qiu S. L. (1993) Prevalence survey of precancerous lesions of the oesophagus in a high-risk population for oesophageal cancer in France. European Journal Cancer Prevention 2:53–59.

Jacobs A. (1962) Post-cricoid carcinoma in patients with pernicious anaemia. British Medical Journal 3:91–92.

Janisch H. D. and Eckardt V. F. (1982) Histological abnormalities in patients with multiple esophageal webs. Digestive Diseases and Sciences 27:503–506.

Janisch H. D., Pfannkuch F., von Kleist D., Degenhardt U., Bauer E. and Hampel K. E. (1984) Histologic abnormalities in routine biopsies of patients with esophagitis and different gastric acid secretion. Applied Pathology 2:272–276.

Jankowski J., Austin W., Howat K., Coghill G., Hopwood D., Dover R. and Wormsley K. G. (1992) Proliferating cell nuclear antigen in oesophageal mucosa: comparison with autoradiology. European Journal of Gastroenterology and Hepatology 4:579–584.

Jankowski J., Coghill G., Murphy S., Hopwood D., Kerr M. and Wormsley K. G. (1992) Epidermal growth factor receptors in the oesophagus. Gut 33:439–443.

Jankowski J., Sanders D. S. A., Coghill G., Wormsley K. G., Hopwood D. and Kerr M. (1991) The expression of Lewis blood group antigens in the oesophagus. Journal of Pathology 163:173A.

Jankowski J., Tregaskis B., Grant A., Correll C., Hopwood D., Kerr M. and Wormsley K. G. (1992) Nucleolar organiser regions in oesophageal diseases. Gullet 2:85–90.

Jarvis L. R., Dent J. and Whitehead R. (1985) Morphometric assessment of reflux oesophagitis in fibreoptic biopsy specimens. Journal of Clinical Pathology 38:44–48.

Jass J. R. (1981) Mucin histochemistry of the columnar epithelium of the oesophagus: a retrospective study. Journal of Clinical Pathology 34:866–870.

Jass J. R. and Filipe M. I. (1981) The mucin profiles of normal gastric mucosa, intestinal metaplasia and its variants and gastric carcinoma. Histochemical Journal 13:931–939.

Javdan P. and Pitman E. R. (1984) Squamous papilloma of esophagus. Digestive Diseases and Sciences 29:317–320.

Jones D. R., Davidson A. G., Summers C. L., Murray G. F. and Quinlan D. C. (1994) Potential application of p53 as an intermediate biomarker in Barrett's esophagus. Annals of Thoracic Surgery 57:598–603.

Kalogeropoulos N. K. and Whitehead R. (1988) *Campylobacter*-like organisms and *Candida* in peptic ulcers and similar lesions of the upper gastrointestinal tract: a study of 247 cases. Journal of Clinical Pathology 41:1093–1098.

Kaye M. D. (1977) Postprandial gastro-oesophageal reflux in healthy people. Gut 18:709–712.

Keeffe E. B., Hisken E. C. and Schubert F. (1986) Adenomatous polyp arising in Barrett's esophagus. Journal of Clinical Gastroenterology 8:271–274.

Kikuchi K., Suga T., Senoue I., Nomiyama T., Miwa M. and Miwa T. (1982). Esophageal ulceration in a patient with Behçet's syndrome. Tokai Journal of Experimental and Clinical Medicine 7:135–143.

King D. H. (1964) Intraoral leukoplakia? Cancer 17:131–136.

Knohe M. and Bernhardt H. (1980) Endoscopic aspects of mycosis in the upper digestive tract. Endoscopy 12:295–298.

Kodsi B. E., Wickremesinghe P. C., Kozinn P. J., Iswara K. and Goldberg P. K. (1976) Candida esophagitis. Gastroenterology 71:715–719.

Korula J. (1985) Pseudotumor of the esophagus: an unusual complication of esophageal variceal sclerotherapy. American Journal of Gastroenterology 80:954–956.

Kozlowski L. M. and Nigra T. P. (1992) Esophageal acanthosis nigricans in association with adenocarcinoma from an unknown site. Journal of American Academy of Dermatology 26:348–351.

Krajewska I. A., Moore L. and Brown J. H. (1992) White sponge nevus presenting in the esophagus: case report and literature review. Pathology 24:112–115.

Laajam M. A. (1984) Primary tuberculosis of the esophagus: pseudotumoral presentation. American Journal of Gastroenterology 79:839–841.

Laso F. J., Cordero M. and Garcia-Sanchez J. E. (1994) Esophageal brucellosis: a new location of *Brucella* infection. Clinical Investigations 72:393–395.

Lax J. D., Haroutiounian G. and Attia A. (1986) An unusual case of dysphagia: esophageal intramural pseudodiverticulosis. American Journal of Gastroenterology 81:1002–1004.

Lee J-H., Neumann D. A. and Welsh J. D. (1977) Disseminated histoplasmosis presenting with esophageal symptomatology. The American Journal of Digestive Diseases 22:831–834.

Lee R. G. (1985) Marked eosinophilia in esophageal mucosal biopsies. American Journal of Surgical Pathology 9:475–479.

Lefer L. G. (1982) Lichen planus of the esophagus. The American Journal of Dermatopathology 4:267–269.

Levine D. S., Haggitt R. C., Blount P. L., Rabinovitch P. S., Rusch V. W. and Reid B. J. (1994) An endoscopic biopsy protocol can differentiate high-grade dysplasia from early adenocarcinoma in Barrett's esophagus. Gastroenterology 105:40–50.

Levine D. S., Reid B. J., Haggitt R. C., Rubin C. E. and Rabinovitch P. S. (1989) Correlation of ultrastructural aberrations with dysplasia and flow cytometric abnormalities in Barrett's epithelium. Gastroenterology 96:355–367.

Levine M. S., Borislow S. M., Rubesin S. E. and O'Brien C. (1994) Esophageal stricture caused by a Motrin tablet (ibuprofen). Abdominal Imaging 19:6–7.

Lewensohn-Fuchs I., Munck-Wikland E., Berke Z., Magnusson K. P., Pallesen G., Auer G., Lindholm J., Linde A., Aberg B., Rubio C. et al. (1994) Involvement of aberrant p53 expression and human papillomavirus in carcinoma of the head, neck and oesophagus. Anticancer Research 14:1281–1285.

Li H. (1993) Malignant Barrett's oesophagus. European Journal of Cancer Prevention 2:47–52.

Lindahl H., Rintala R. and Sariola H. (1993) Chronic esophagitis and gastric metaplasia are frequent late complications of esophageal atresia. Journal of Pediatric Surgery 28:1178–1180.

LiVolsi V. A. and Jaretzki A. (1973) Granulomatous oesophagitis: a case of Crohn's disease limited to the oesophagus. Gastroenterology 64:313–319.

Llaneza P. P., Menendez A. M. and Dunn G. D. (1987) Hairy esophagus contributing to dysphagia. Gastrointestinal Endoscopy 33:331–332.

McDonald G. B., Brand D. L. and Thorning D. R. (1977) Multiple adenomatous neoplasms arising in columnar-lined (Barrett's) esophagus. Gastroenterology 72:1317–1321.

McDonald G. B., Sullivan K. M., Schuffler M. D., Shulman H. M. and Thomas E. D. (1981) Esophageal abnormalities in chronic graft-vs-host disease in humans. Gastroenterology 80:914–921.

McKay J. S. and Day D. W. (1983) Herpes simplex oesophagitis. Histopathology 7:409–420.

McKenzie R. and Khakoo R. (1985) Blastomycosis of the esophagus presenting with gastrointestinal bleeding. Gastroenterology 88:1271–1273.

Mandard A. M., Marnay J., Gignoux M., Segol P., Blanc L., Ollivier J. M., Borel B. and Mandard J. C. (1984) Cancer of the esophagus and associated lesions. Human Pathology 15:660–669.

Mandard A. M., Tourneux J., Gignoux M., Blanc L., Segol P. and Mandard J. C. (1980) In situ carcinoma of the esophagus: macroscopic study with particular reference to the Lugol test. Endoscopy 12:51–57.

Marger R. S. and Marger D. (1993) Carcinoma of the esophagus and tylosis: a lethal genetic combination. Cancer 72:17–19.

Mathieson R. and Dutta S. K. (1983) *Candida* esophagitis. Digestive Diseases and Sciences 28:365–370.

Medeiros L. J., Doos W. G. and Balogh K. (1988) Esophageal intramural pseudodiverticulosis. Human Pathology 19:928–931.

Meijssen M. A. C., Tilanus H. W., van Blankenstein M., Hop W. C. J. and Ong G. L. (1992) Achalasia complicated by oesophageal squamous cell carcinoma: a prospective study in 195 patients. Gut 33:155–158.

Meuwissen S. G. M., Bosma A., van Donk E., Waalewijn R., Pals G., Pronk J. C., Eriksson A. W., Mullink H. and Meijer C. J. L. M. (1988) Immunohistochemical localization of pepsinogen A and C containing cells in Barrett's oesophagus. Virchows Archiv (A) 413:11–16.

Meyer W., Vollmar F. and Bär W. (1979) Barrett-esophagus following total gastrectomy. Endoscopy 2:121–126.

Miller D. P. and Everett E. D. (1979) Gastrointestinal histoplasmosis. Journal of Clinical Gastroenterology 1:233–236.

Miller J. T., Slywka S. W. and Ellis J. H. (1993) Staphylococcal esophagitis causing giant ulcers. Abdominal Imaging 18:225–226.

Ming S. C., Goldman H. and Freiman D. G. (1967) Intestinal metaplasia and histogenesis of carcinoma of the human stomach. Cancer 20:1418–1429.

Mobacken H., Al Karawi M., Mohamed A. and Coode P. (1988) Oesophageal pemphigus vulgaris. Dermatologica 176:266–269.

Moghissi K., Sharpe D. A. and Pender D. (1993) Adenocarcinoma and Barrett's oesophagus: a clinico-pathological study. European Journal of Cardiothoracic Surgery 7:126–131.

Mokoena T., Shama D. M., Ngakane H. and Bryer J. V. (1992) Oesophageal tuberculosis: a review of eleven cases. Postgraduate Medical Journal 68:110–115.

Moore J. H., Lesser E. J., Erdody D. H., Natale R. B., Orringer M. B. and Beer D. G. (1994) Intestinal differentiation and p53 gene alterations in Barrett's esophagus and esophageal adenocarcinoma. International Journal of Cancer 56:487–493.

Moreto M., Ojembarrena E., Zaballa M., Tanago J. G. and Ibanez S. (1993) Idiopathic acute esophageal necrosis: not necessarily a terminal event. Endoscopy 25:534–538.

Mori S., Yoshihira A., Kawamura H., Takeuchi A., Hashimoto T. and Inaba G. (1983) Esophageal involvement in Behçet's disease. American Journal of Gastroenterology 78:548–553.

Morichau-Beauchant M., Touchard G., Battandier D., Maire P., Fontanel J-P., Daban A., Babin P. and Matuchansky C. (1983) Chronic radiation esophagitis after treatment of carcinoma of the oropharynx: a poorly recognized entity. Gastroenterologie Clinique et Biologique 7:843–850.

Morris H. and Price S. (1986) Langerhans' cells, papillomaviruses and oesophageal carcinoma. South African Medical Journal 69:413–417.

Munoz N., Crespi M., Grassi A., Qing W. G., Qiong S. and Cai L. Z. (1982) Precursor lesions of oesophageal cancer in high-risk populations in Iran and China. Lancet 1:876–879.

Naef A. P., Savary M., Ozzello L. and Pearson F. G. (1975) Columnar-lined lower esophagus: an acquired lesion with malignant predisposition. Journal of Thoracic Cardiovascular Surgery 70:826–835.

Nakajima H., Munakata A., Sasaki Y. and Yoshida Y. (1993) pH profile of esophagus in patients with inlet patch of heterotopic gastric mucosa after tetragastrin stimulation: an endoscopic approach. Digestive Diseases and Sciences 38:1915–1919.

Neshat K., Sanchez C. A., Galipeau P. C., Blount P. L., Levine D. S., Joslyn G. and Reid B. J. (1994) P53 mutations in Barrett's adenocarcinoma and high-grade dysplasia. Gastroenterology 106:1589–1595.

Nishikai M., Asaba G. and Homma M. (1977) Rheumatoid esophageal disease. American Journal of Gastroenterology 67:29–33.

Obrecht W. F., Richter J. E., Olympio G. A. and Gelfand D. W. (1984) Tracheoesophageal fistula: a serious complication of infectious esophagitis. Gastroenterology 87:1174–1179.

O'Connell E. W., Seaman W. B. and Ghahremani G. G. (1984) Radiation-induced esophageal carcinoma. Gastrointestinal Radiology 9:287–291.

Odze R., Antonioli D., Shocket D., Noble-Topham S., Goldman H. and Upton M. (1993) Esophageal squamous papillomas. American Journal of Surgical Pathology 17:803–812.

Oettle G. J., Paterson A. C., Leiman G. and Segal I. (1986) Esophagitis in a population at risk for esophageal carcinoma. Cancer 57:2222–2229.

Ohashi K., Kato Y., Kanno J. and Kasuga T. (1990) Melanocytes and melanosis of the oesophagus in Japanese subjects: analysis of factors affecting their increase. Virchows Archiv (A) 417:137–143.

Ohta H., Nakazawa S., Segawa K., and Yoshino J. (1986) Distribution of epithelial dysplasia in the cancerous esophagus. Scandinavian Journal of Gastroenterology 21:392–398.

Olson A. D. and Fukui-Miner K. (1994) Eosinophilic mucosal infiltrate in infants with congenital gastrointestinal obstruction. American Journal of Gastroenterology 89:934–936.

Orringer M. B. and Sloan H. (1978) Monilial esophagitis: an increasingly frequent cause of esophageal stenosis? Annals of Thoracic Surgery 26:364–374.

Pascal R. R. and Clearfield H. R. (1987) Mucoepidermoid (adenosquamous) carcinoma arising in Barrett's esophagus. Digestive Diseases and Sciences 32:428–432.

Patrick W. J. A., Denham D. and Forrest A. P. M. (1974) Mucous change in the human duodenum: a light and electron microscopic study and correlation with disease and gastric acid secretion. Gut 15:767–776.

Pepe G., Pepe F., Cali V., Sanfilippo G. and Pecorella G. (1985). Crohn's disease of the esophagus: a case report. The Italian Journal of Surgical Sciences 15:369–371.

Petru A. and Azimi P. H. (1984) Esophagitis associated with Candida infection in a neonate. Clinical Pediatrics 23:179–181.

Porro G. B., Parente F. and Cernuschi M. (1989) The diagnosis of esophageal candidiasis in patients with acquired immune deficiency syndrome: is endoscopy always necessary? American Journal of Gastroenterology 84:143–146.

Prior A. and Whorwell P. J. (1986) Familial Barrett's oesophagus? Hepato-gastroenterology 33:86–87.

Radhi J. M. and Schweiger F. (1994) Bacterial oesophagitis in an immunocompromised patient. Postgraduate Medical Journal 70:233–234.

Raeburn C. (1951) Columnar ciliated epithelium in the adult oesophagus. Journal of Pathology and Bacteriology 63:157–159.

Raine C. H. (1983) Ectopic gastric mucosa in the upper esophagus as a cause of dysphagia. Annals of Otology, Rhinology and Laryngology 92:65–66.

Rector L. E. and Connerley M. I. (1941) Aberrant mucosa in the esophagus in infants and children. Archives of Pathology and Laboratory Medicine 31:285–294.

Reid B. J., Haggitt R. C., Rubin C. E. and Rabinovitch P. S. (1987) Barrett's esophagus. Gastroenterology 93:1–11.

Reid B. J., Weinstein W. M., Lewin K. L., Haggitt R. C., Van Deventer G., Den Besten L. and Rubin C. E. (1988a) Endoscopic biopsy can detect high-grade dysplasia or early adenocarcinoma in Barrett's esophagus without grossly recognizable neoplastic lesions. Gastroenterology 94:81–90.

Reid B. J., Haggitt R. C., Rubin C. E., Roth G., Surawicz C. M., Van Belle G., Lewin K., Weinstein W. M., Antonioli D. A., Goldman H., MacDonald W. and Owen D. (1988b) Observer variation in the diagnosis of dysplasia in Barrett's esophagus. Human Pathology 19:166–178.

Reid B. J., Sanchez C. A., Blount P. L., and Levine D. S. (1993) Barrett's esophagus: cell cycle abnormalities in advancing stages of neoplastic progression. Gastroenterology 105:119–129.

Remmele W. and Engelsing B. (1984) Lipid island of the esophagus. Endoscopy 16:240–241.

Rindi G., Bishop A. E., Daly M. J., Isaacs P., Lee F. I. and Polak J. M. (1987) A mixed pattern of endocrine cells in metaplastic Barrett's oesophagus. Histochemistry 87:377–383.

Rotterdam H. and Sommers S. C. (1981). In: Biopsy Diagnosis of the Digestive Tract. New York: Raven Press, p 13.

Rubio C. A. and Riddell R. (1988) Musculo-fibrous anomaly in Barrett's mucosa with dysplasia. American Journal of Surgical Pathology 12:885–889.

Sablich R., Benedetti G., Bignucolo S. and Serraino D. (1988) Squamous cell papilloma of the esophagus. Endoscopy 20:5–7.

Saladin T. A., French A. B., Zarafonetis C. J. D. and Pollard H. M. (1966) Esophageal motor abnormalities in scleroderma and related diseases. American Journal of Digestive Diseases 11:522–535.

Salgado J. A., Filho J. de S. A., Lima G. F. Jr, Savi A., Fonseca L. M. A. and de Oliveira C. A. (1980) Sebaceous glands in the esophagus. Gastrointestinal Endoscopy 26:150.

Salo J. A., Lehto V-P. and Kivilaakso E. (1983) Morphological alterations in experimental esophagitis: light microscopic and scanning and transmission electron microscopic study. Digestive Diseases and Sciences 28:440–448.

Sampliner R. E., Steinbronn K., Garewal H. S. and Riddell R. H. (1988) Squamous mucosa overlying columnar epithelium in Barrett's esophagus in the absence of anti-reflux surgery. American Journal of Gastroenterology 83:510–512.

Sbarbati A., Deganello A., Bertini M., Gaburro D. and Osculati A. (1993) Reflux oesophagitis in children: a scanning and transmission electron microscope study. Journal of Submicroscopic Cytology and Pathology 25:603–611.

Schneider H. A., Yonker R. A., Longley S., Katz P., Mathias J. and Panush R. S. (1984) Scleroderma esophagus: a nonspecific entity. Annals of Internal Medicine 100:848–850.

Schroeder W. W., Myer C. M. and Schechter G. L. (1987) Ectopic gastric mucosa in the cervical esophagus. Laryngoscope 97:131–135.

Schuffler M. D. and Pope C. E. II. (1976) Esophageal motor dysfunction in idiopathic intestinal pseudo-obstruction. Gastroenterology 70:677–682.

Scott B. B. and Jenkins D. (1982) Gastro-oesophageal candidiosis. Gut 23:137–139.

Seefeld U., Krejs G. J., Siebenmann R. E. and Blum A. L. (1977) Esophageal histology in gastroesophageal reflux. American Journal of Digestive Diseases 22:956–964.

Seifert E., Borst H. H., Ostertag H., Stender H. St., Braschke M., Misaki F. and Atay Z. (1973) Carcinoma in situ of the esophagus (early esophageal cancer). Endoscopy 5:147–153.

Seivewright N., Feehally J. and Wicks A. C. B. (1984) Primary tuberculosis of the esophagus. American Journal of Gastroenterology 79:842–843.

Shah K. K., DeRidder P. H. and Shah K. K. (1986) Ectopic gastric mucosa in proximal esophagus. Journal of Clinical Gastroenterology 8:509–513.

Sheahan D. G. and West A. B. (1985) Focal lymphoid hyperplasia (pseudolymphoma) of the esophagus. American Journal of Surgical Pathology 9:141–147.

Sherrill D. J., Grishkin B. A., Galal F. S., Zajtchuk R. and Graeber G. M. (1984) Radiation-associated malignancies of the esophagus. Cancer 54:726–728.

Siegel C. I. and Hendrix T. R. (1963) Oesophageal motor abnormalities induced by acid perfusion in patients with heartburn. Journal of Clinical Investigation 42:686–695.

Stadelmann O., Elster K. and Kuhn H. A. (1981) Columnar-lined oesophagus (Barrett's syndrome): congenital or acquired? Endoscopy 13:140–147.

Steadman C., Kerlin P., Teague C. and Stephenson P. (1988) High esophageal stricture: a complication of "inlet patch" mucosa. Gastroenterology 94:521–524.

Stephens W. P., Mossman A., Ratcliffe J. F., Gould D. A. and Oleesky S. (1986) Intramural pseudodiverticulosis: an unusual cause of benign oesophageal stricture. Postgraduate Medical Journal 62:201–204.

Stern Z., Sharon P., Ligumsky M., Levij I. S. and Rachmilewitz D. (1980) Glycogenic acanthosis of the esophagus. American Journal of Gastroenterology 74:261–263.

Stoschus B. and Allescher H. D. (1993) Drug-induced dysphagia. Dysphagia 8:154–159.

Streitz J. M. Jr (1994) Barrett's esophagus and esophageal cancer. Chest Surgery Clinic of North America 4:227–240.

Streitz J. M. Jr, Andrews C. W. Jr and Ellis F. H. Jr (1993) Endoscopic surveillance of Barrett's esophagus: does it help? Journal of Thoracic Cardiovascular Surgery 105:383–387.

Tateishi R., Taniguchi H., Wada A., Horai T. and Taniguchi K. (1974) Argyrophil cells and melanocytes in esophageal mucosa. Archives of Pathology 98:87–89.

Thompson J. J., Zinsser K. R. and Enterline H. T. (1983) Barrett's metaplasia and adenocarcinoma of the esophagus and gastroesophageal junction. Human Pathology 14:42–61.

Tishler J. M. A. and Helman C. A. (1984). Crohn's disease of the esophagus. Journal of Canadian Association of Radiologists 35:28–30.

Toet A. E., Dekker W., Op den Orth J. O. and Blok P. (1985) Squamous cell papilloma of the esophagus: report of 4 cases. Gastrointestinal Endoscopy 31:77–79.

Trier J. S. (1970) Morphology of the epithelium of the distal esophagus in patients with midesophageal peptic strictures. Gastroenterology 58:444–461.

Truong L. D., Stroehlein J. R. and McKechnie J. C. (1986) Gastric heterotopia of the proximal esophagus: a report of 4 cases detected by endoscopy and review of the literature. American Journal of Gastroenterology 81:1162–1166.

Tummala V., Barwick K. W., Sontag S. J., Vlahcevic R. Z. and McCallum R. W. (1987) The significance of intraepithelial eosinophils in the histologic diagnosis of gastroesophageal reflux. American Journal of Clinical Pathology 87:43–48.

Vadva M. D. and Triadafilopoulos G. (1993) Glycogenic acanthosis of the esophagus and gastroesophageal reflux. Journal of Clinical Gastroenterology 17:79–83.

Van Maercke Ph., Gunther M., Groth W., Gheorghiu Th. and Habermann U. (1988) Lichen ruber mucosae with esophageal involvement. Endoscopy 20:158–160.

Van Rensburg E. J., Venter E. H. and Simson I. W. (1993) Human papillomavirus DNA in aerodigestive squamous carcinomas demonstrated by means of in situ hybridisation. South African Medical Journal 83:516–518.

Villar L. A., Massanari R. M. and Mitros F. A. (1984) Cytomegalovirus infection with acute erosive esophagitis. The American Journal of Medicine 76:924–928.

Volpicelli N. A., Yardley J. H. and Hendrix T. R. (1975) A histopathologic demonstration of the association between gastritis and reflux esophagitis. Gastroenterology 68:1007.

Walker J. H. (1978) Giant papilloma of the thoracic esophagus. American Journal of Roentgenology 131:519–520.

Walsh T. J., Belitsos N. J. and Hamilton S. R. (1986) Bacterial esophagitis in immunocompromised patients. Archives of Internal Medicine 146:1345–1348.

Wang G-Q. (1981) Endoscopic diagnosis of early oesophageal carcinoma. Journal of the Royal Society of Medicine 74:502–503.

Wang M. M. J., Spear M. and McGrew W. (1986) Heterotopic gastric mucosa of the esophagus. Southern Medical Journal 79:633–635.

Waterfall W. E., Somers S. and Desa D. J. (1978) Benign oesophageal papillomatosis. Journal of Clinical Pathology 31:111–115.

Weinstein W. M., Bogoch E. R. and Bowes K. L. (1975) The normal human esophageal mucosa: a histological reappraisal. Gastroenterology 68:40–44.

Weller I. V. D. (1985) AIDS and the gut. Scandinavian Journal of Gastroenterology 20(suppl 114):77–89.

Wilkins W. E., Ridley M. G. and Pozniak A. L. (1984) Benign stricture of the oesophagus: role of non-steroidal anti-inflammatory drugs. Gut 25:478–480.

Winkler B., Capo V., Reumann W., Ma A., la Porta R., Reilly S., Green P. M. R., Richart R. M. and Crum C. P. (1985) Human papillomavirus infection of the esophagus. Cancer 55:149–155.

Winter H. S., Madara J. L., Stafford R. J., Grand R. J., Quinlan J-E., and Goldman H. (1982) Intraepithelial eosinophils: a new diagnostic criterion for reflux esophagitis. Gastroenterology 83:818–823.

Wood D. R., Patterson J. B. and Orlando R. C. (1982) Pemphigus vulgaris of the esophagus. Annals of Internal Medicine 96:189–191.

Yamamoto H., Kozawa Y., Otake S. and Shimokawa R. (1983) Pemphigus vulgaris involving the mouth and esophagus. International Journal of Oral Surgery 12:194–200.

Yamazaki K., Ohmori T., Kumagai Y., Makuuchi H. and Eyden B. (1991) Ultrastructure of oesophageal melanocytosis. Virchows Archiv (A) 418:515–522.

Zamost B. J., Hirschberg J., Ippoliti A. F., Furst D. E., Clements P. J. and Weinstein W. M. (1987) Esophagitis in scleroderma: prevalence and risk factors. Gastroenterology 92:421–428.

Zhang L., Yie G., Huang X. and Xie Y. (1994) Esophageal Crohn's disease: a case report. Chinese Medical Science Journal 9:59–60.

Zweiban B., Cohen H. and Chandrasoma P. (1986) Gastrointestinal involvement complicating Stevens-Johnson syndrome. Gastroenterology 91:469–474.

II

Gastric Biopsy

5

NORMAL APPEARANCES IN GASTRIC BIOPSY SPECIMENS

The pyloric glands occupy a roughly triangular area in the lower third of the stomach. On the greater curve they occupy the immediate pyloric region, but on the lesser curve the upper limit, although commonly held to be in the region of the incisura angularis, is quite variable and rarely extends to the oesophagus. The cardiac glands are found distal to the cardio-oesophageal junction for a distance of about 1 cm, and the remaining mucosa is of body type. The junction among the three areas may be abrupt but is often occupied by a narrow transitional zone. At the pylorus-body junction in the lesser curve region the width of the transitional zone is variable, and rarely does the whole lesser curve show a transitional appearance.

Transitional zones also occur where the cardiac mucosa abuts the oesophagus and where the antral mucosa abuts the duodenum. At the former site the transition is usually abrupt, although in the gross it takes the form of the irregular or serrated so-called Z line. The transition zone between gastric and duodenal mucosae also tends to be serrated and up to 3 mm wide, but beyond this for another 3 mm a mucosa with mixed histological features may also be seen. In this zone, adjacent villi may be covered by antral-type superficial epithelium or small bowel–type epithelium in a varying mix (Lawson 1988).

The basic structure of the gastric mucosa is similar in the three main areas. The superficial epithelium dips down to be continuous with the gastric pits, which in turn are continuous with the gastric glands. Autoradiographic studies have shown that the component cells of the gastric mucosa are produced in the area of cell division that is localised to the region of the neck of the gastric glands at the junction with the lower crypts (Toner and Cameron, 1995).

BODY MUCOSA

Throughout the stomach the superficial epithelium is composed of a single layer of cells with a basal rounded nucleus usually without nucleoli, below a typical cup-shaped column of clear or faintly granular mucin. Occasionally an intraepithelial lymphocyte that has insinuated itself between adjacent epithelial cells can be observed. The surface epithelium dips to form shallow gastric pits, into which open approximately four gastric glands. These are simple straight tubules, tightly packed together, roughly the same length, that occupy three quarters of the thickness of the mucosa. Most cells lining the upper part of the glands are parietal cells. These are eosinophilic and triangular with a central nucleus. Their longest side is applied to the basement membrane, and sometimes intracellular canaliculi are visible. At the junction of the glands with the pits, scattered among the parietal cells and sometimes deeper, there are mucin-secreting neck cells that, like the superficial epithelium,

Figure 5–1. Normal body mucosa. Note the regular superficial epithelium, short gastric pits, predominance of parietal cells in the upper half, and chief cells in the lower half of the tubules (H&E ×75).

contain periodic acid–Schiff (PAS)-positive and diastase-resistant mucin. The lower half of the glands contain the chief cells, which mingle with the parietal cells in the region of the middle third (Fig. 5–1). Chief cells have a basal nucleus and a cytoplasm filled with basophilic pepsinogen granules. The extent of basophilia of the granules varies from biopsy to biopsy. Sometimes in old age, gastric body gland cells show a focal cytoplasmic eosinophilic appearance similar to that which occurs in other glandular tissues and is usually referred to as oncocytic change (Fig. 5–2). Occasionally, toward the base there is an argentaffin (enterochromaffin) cell. Rarely

Figure 5–2. Oncocytic change in the gastric body gland epithelial cells (an incidental finding that is more common in old age) (H&E ×350).

are the basal parts of the tubules cystic (Fig. 5–3), but the flattened cells always retain their special staining characteristics. An extreme form of this change, which produces elevations of the mucosa, is referred to in Chapter 8. However, this is in contrast to the cystic change that occurs in Menetrier's disease, in which the cysts are invariably larger and associated with abnormalities of the muscularis mucosae (see Chapter 8).

The lamina propria is most obvious between the gastric pits, where it contains a small number of plasma cells, lymphocytes, eosinophils, and histiocytes, together with a fine capillary plexus and nonmyelinated nerves. Owen (1986) claimed that in a normal gastric mucosa lymphatic capillaries are present in the superficial lamina propria and extend down between the gland tubules to form a plexus just superficial to the muscularis mucosae, which then drains into large lymphatics in the submucosa. However, in a combined light microscopic, electron microscopic, and immunohistochemical study Listrom and Fenoglio-Preiser (1987) showed that in a normal mucosa the upper two thirds and the lamina propria are normally devoid of lymphatics. In such circumstances the ability of intramucosal gastric carcinoma to metastasize (Bogomoletz 1984a) becomes difficult to understand. However, in a mucosa that exhibits atrophic gastritis and is thin, lymphatic channels do in fact reach the surface. Because gastric cancer often arises in a background of atrophic gastritis, the access of malignant cells to lymphatics is thus understandable.

There are no objective guidelines as to what constitutes a normal number of cells in the lamina propria. This, of course, is only a reflection of the difficulty, first, in defining a normal population and, second, in acquiring biopsy specimens from such a group. An example of this is seen in the study of Myren and Serck-Hanssen (1975), who found what they subjectively considered to be an increase in inflammatory infiltration in the interfoveolar lamina propria of four antral, three lesser curve, and two greater curve biopsies from 10 healthy medical student volunteers. In another study on nine healthy volunteers (Toner and Cameron 1995), it was shown that mononuclear cells are more common than polymorphs, but there is a wide variation in numbers and at present it appears that there is no acceptable definition of normality. Nevertheless, biopsies, in which neither acute nor chronic inflammatory cells form an obvious infiltrate at relatively low magnification and in which there is good preservation of the epithelial and glandular cells, can be regarded as within the "normal" range. At intervals along the mucosa the muscularis mucosae sends

Figure 5–3. Body mucosa shows cystic change at the base of the gland tubules (H&E ×188).

infrequent groups of smooth muscle fibres upward between the glands. In reticulin preparations (Fig. 5–4) the basement membrane of the surface epithelium, pits, and glands appears as a single layer of fibres, between which a delicate mesh of strands represents the supporting connective tissues between and in relation to the capillaries. The sharp division between the reticulin pattern of the lamina propria and the denser network around the fibres and vessels of the muscularis mucosae is broken only by occasional tent-shaped skeins of fibres that surround the upward muscularis prolongations.

PYLORIC MUCOSA

In the pyloric mucosa (Fig. 5–5) the gastric pits are deeper and sometimes branched, and the glands are shorter and less tightly packed than in the body, ending at different levels and occupying one half or less of the mucosal thickness. They are simple or branched coiled tubules, composed of mucin-secreting cells and occasional parietal cells (Fig. 5–6), especially near transitional zones. The incidence and distribution of parietal cells in antral mucosa were studied in an autopsy series by Tominaga (1975). They were found in 98.3% of cases throughout the range from newborn to old age and were considered to be a normal constituent of antral mucosa and not due to either metaplasia or dystopia. Very infrequently an isolated zone of chief cells may be seen (Fig. 5–7). Argentaffin cells are more frequent in this area of the gastric mucosa. They have a nucleus near the lumen of the gland and a strongly eosinophilic cytoplasm due to granules too small to be resolved by the light microscope (Fig. 5–8). The interdigitation of fibres from the muscularis mucosae is

Figure 5–4. Normal body mucosa with typical reticulin distribution (reticulin stain ×102).

Figure 5–5. Pyloric mucosa. The pits are relatively long and some branch; they occupy one half the thickness of the mucosa. The glands are a simple mucin-producing type (H&E ×75).

more marked, and there is more intertubular reticulin, so that the pattern is quite distinctive (Fig. 5–9).

In the absence of any other discernible abnormality the lamina propria frequently shows a light scattering of lymphocytes and plasma cells. This is in contrast to the body mucosa in the normal state. The exact relationship of this infiltrate to other forms of gastritis has not been established nor is it known if it is abnormal (see the next section).

CARDIAC MUCOSA

The cardiac mucosa (Fig. 5–10) is essentially similar to the pyloric mucosa, except that the glands are even less tightly packed together. As a rule, parietal cells

Figure 5–6. Pyloric mucosa. Occasional parietal cells *(arrows)* in otherwise typical mucin-producing pyloric glands (H&E ×400).

Figure 5–7. Pyloric mucosa. In addition to the scattered parietal cells in other tubules, one tubule is filled predominantly with chief cells (H&E ×375).

Figure 5–8. Pyloric gland, argentaffin cell *(arrow)*. Note that the nucleus is nearer to the lumen of the tubule than to the basement membrane (H&E ×500).

Figure 5–9. Pyloric mucosa. Distinctive reticulin pattern with more intertubular reticulin than in the body mucosa (reticulin stain ×42).

and argentaffin cells are absent. A characteristic feature is the presence of one or more dilated or cystic glands with a thin epithelial wall.

It is not unusual for the cardiac mucosa to show a slight lymphocyte and plasma cell infiltration of the lamina propria when the body mucosa areas are normal. In this respect the cardiac mucosa is similar to the antral mucosa, with which it shares other features as already noted. It is a matter of conjecture whether this is an indication that both sites are "watershed" areas and more obviously exposed to

Figure 5–10. Cardiac mucosa. As in the pyloric mucosa the pits occupy one half of its thickness. The cystic gland is typical (H&E ×85).

Figure 5–11. Transitional mucosa, from region of junction of body with pyloric area (H&E ×75).

changes in "milieu" due to first exposure to food intake or refluxate than the body mucosal areas. It is of some interest that Genta, Huberman and Graham (1994) have also shown that when significant antral gastritis is present, although there may be relative sparing of the body and fundus mucosa, the cardiac mucosa shows similar changes, although not with respect to lymphoid follicle formation.

TRANSITIONAL MUCOSA

The transitional mucosa (Figs. 5–11 and 5–12) is composed of body and pyloric or cardiac-type glands. As in the pyloric and cardiac mucosa, the pits occupy about half of the mucosal thickness.

Electron microscope, histochemical, and immunological studies have shown that

Figure 5–12. Detail of Figure 5–11 shows pyloric *(left)* and body *(right)* glands (H&E ×150).

Figure 5–13. Pyloric mucosa. Note the numerous clear cells *(arrowheads)* (H&E ×300).

in addition to argentaffin cells several other endocrine polypeptide cells are present in the gastric mucosa (Dawson 1970, Pearse et al 1970), but the characterisation of this complex system of cell types is still the subject of investigation.

In ordinary hematoxylin and eosin (H & E) preparations many of the nonargentaffin endocrine cells appear as clear cells or halo cells (Fig. 5–13). The gastrin-producing cells of the antrum belong to this group and constitute some 50% of the endocrine cells in this site.

Approximately 30% produce serotonin, and 15% produce somatostatin. In the body mucosa the major portion of endocrine cells belongs to the so-called enterochromaffin-like group and secretes histamine, bombesin, and vasoactive intestinal peptide. Other endocrine cells secrete serotonin, and in some identified by a variety of histochemical techniques the secretions produced remain to be identified. Thus the list of hormones secreted by these cells in the gastric mucosa as elsewhere in the gut is growing rapidly. Comprehensive accounts of the gut hormone system are in a multiauthor book edited by Bloom and Polak (1981) and, more recently, in a chapter by Falkmer and Wilander (1995). Also being increasingly appreciated is that with intestinalisation of the gastric mucosa due to metaplasia new endocrine cell types also appear (Mingazzini et al 1984). Another cell type occasionally described in the gastric mucosa is the fibrillovesicular cell, or tuft cell, but it has only been identified in electron microscope studies (Wattel and Geuze 1978, Blom 1984).

6

GASTRITIS

Gastritis has usually been divided into acute and chronic forms. However, accurate information concerning the mucosal histology of the putative "acute gastritis" used in reference to the symptom complex associated with alcohol and food overindulgence, drug ingestion, and viral infections is meagre. It is only since the use of fibreoptic biopsy instruments that the spectrum of these changes has been better delineated. As a result many of the lesions produced by ingestion of certain drugs are more accurately described as acute haemorrhagic erosions than as acute gastritis.

The capacity of the gastric mucosa to withstand the deleterious effects of its own secretions is probably the result of several interacting phenomena that effectively constitute a mucosal barrier (Rees and Turnberg 1982, Rees 1987). All has yet to be revealed, but some of the mechanisms involved are its capacity for regeneration, factors that control its blood flow, its ability to maintain a lumenal mucous layer and to secrete bicarbonate, the protective effect of prostaglandins, and epidermal growth factors. Presumably any one or a combination of several circumstances that tend to interfere with this complex barrier may precipitate mucosal self-injury, which is manifested by superficial necrosis and haemorrhage. Cell death may be followed by an inflammatory reaction so that, by a common pathway, an acute gastric inflammation is a predictable course of events following tissue damage initiated by several different means. In experimental animals there is ample evidence for the induction of mucosal injury by alcohol, aspirin and other nonsteroidal anti-inflammatory drugs (NSAIDs), bile, pancreatic juice, and a variety of stresses that induce a decreased mucosal blood flow.

Since the widespread use of fibreoptic biopsy instruments, clear pathophysiological subgroups of chronic gastritis have been delineated. The importance of the classification is in the identification of patients at greatest risk of developing pernicious anaemia, peptic ulcer, gastric adenocarcinoma, and malignant lymphoma. It is the morphology and topographical distribution in the stomach of the mucosal changes that is the basis for the current recognition of the subgroups of chronic gastritis, and the aetiology involves immune phenomena, bacterial infection, diet, bile reflux, and the effects of ingesting NSAIDs.

ACUTE (GASTRITIS) MUCOSAL INJURY

Clearly, the gastric mucosa is injured by a variety of chemicals and strong acids and alkalis. There is a report of extensive damage due to a saline emetic (Calam, Krasner and Haqqani 1982). In circumstances when damaging agents are inadvertently ingested a varied histological lesion results, ranging from hyperaemia and surface erosion to more massive mucosal necrosis and sloughing with or without secondary haemorrhage. These changes are rarely seen in biopsy specimens; available information is based on findings in surgical and autopsy material. In milder forms of injury the initial lesion stimulates an acute inflammatory reaction so that at some stage if resolution occurs, acute gastritis occurs. Furthermore acute injuries may be superimposed on a mucosa showing chronic inflammatory changes.

Acute mucosal damage is induced by external x-ray therapy for peptic ulceration. Two weeks after treatment there is a patchy but severe coagulative necrosis with subsequent secondary inflammatory infiltration (Goldgraber et al 1954) and a tendency to revert to normal after about 4 months. After intragastric irradiation, however, permanent and histologically characteristic tissue damage occurs with ulceration, fibrosis, and obliterative vascular hyalinisation (Fruin, Littman and Littman 1963, Berthrong and Fajardo 1981).

The majority of instances of acute mucosal injury in the form of haemorrhages or haemorrhagic erosions are due to the ingestion of aspirin or other NSAIDs (Pemberton and Strand 1979, Laine and Weinstein 1988a). In a group of healthy volunteers Hoftiezer, O'Laughlin and Ivey (1982) showed that this is true of aspirin even if buffered and when used in recommended daily doses. Aspirin and related drugs probably act by damaging the mucosal barrier; this was reviewed by Silen (1985), who highlighted that this barrier is a complex physiological mechanism involving mucosal blood flow and events involving local acid and alkaline metabolites. Salicylates accelerate epithelial cell turnover (Croft 1963), cause back diffusion of acid (Davenport 1967), and in common with many NSAIDs inhibit prostaglandin synthesis. Prostaglandins and epidermal growth factor are known to be cytoprotective for the gastric mucosa in a variety of experimental situations (Konturek et al 1981, Lacy and Ito 1982, Rainsford and Willis 1982). The overall result is to produce haemorrhagic erosions (Lanza 1984). These are frequently the cause of acute intragastric bleeding and are commonly viewed endoscopically though rarely subjected to biopsy (Figs. 6–1 and 6–2). Sometimes aspirin-induced erosion and haemorrhage is diffuse, and urgent radical surgery is indicated. In the excised specimen histological examination reveals loss of the superficial epithelium and upper gastric pits with

Figure 6–1. Acute gastric erosion in body mucosa following aspirin. The region of mucosa normally composed of pits is absent centrally, and there is haemorrhage into the upper lamina propria (trichrome ×80).

Figure 6–2. Biopsy of a healing acute erosion in its early stage. Note the mainly acute inflammatory reaction (H&E ×150).

a diffuse haemorrhage into the upper layers of the mucosa (Fig. 6–3). This so-called acute haemorrhagic gastritis is sometimes the result of stress when ulceration either in the form of multiple erosions or as a diffuse lesion occurs mainly in the body of the stomach. It may be seen after major surgery or trauma (Flowers, Kyle and Hoerr 1970), sepsis, burns, or head injury and is probably related to a reduced mucosal blood flow (Skillman and Silen 1972, Miller 1987) and tissue acidosis (Silen 1987).

Apart from diffuse lesions that necessitate surgery, evidence suggests that most acute mucosal erosions heal completely, leaving a normal mucosa, but may be subjected to biopsy when the lesions are only partially resolved (Fig. 6–4). Chronic use of aspirin and NSAIDs, however, has been implicated in chronic peptic ulceration, although this is still controversial (Duggan et al 1986, Graham and Smith 1986). It seems possible that, in some patients at least, chronic use is associated with a mucosal adaptation response and does not necessarily lead to chronic ulceration. Metzger et al (1976) described the gastric mucosa in biopsy specimens from patients with rheumatoid arthritis during continuous or interrupted ingestion of aspirin. Although there was focal mucosal injury with haemorrhage and erosion, there was no significant increase in gastritis in the mucosa away from the focal lesions. MacDonald (1973) and Hamilton and Yardley (1980) showed that in gastric resections for gastric ulcer in patients who used aspirin regularly, about 50% showed a normal mucosa around the ulcer. This has practical applications in reporting biopsy tissues taken from gastric ulcer margins. The lack of a significant gastritis and an absence of pyloric or intestinal metaplasia raise the likelihood that an ulcer is drug-induced; this clearly has important implications for management and prognosis. With the recognition of so-called type C or reactive gastritis (Quinn et al 1993), it has been more recently shown that the use of NSAIDs is a potent cause of this type of gastric lesion. This is discussed in Chapter 7.

Figure 6–3. Body mucosa shows acute haemorrhagic gastritis. The superficial epithelium and gastric pits are eroded, and a diffuse haemorrhagic zone occupies the surface layer (H&E ×70).

Figure 6–4. Acute erosion in the stage of partial healing. Note histiocytes in the often-dilated atrophic tubules and a mild, mainly chronic inflammatory infiltrate of the lamina propria. The repair of the superficial epithelium is relatively more advanced (H&E ×300).

It has long been held that alcohol ingestion is a cause of acute mucosal damage; whereas changes due to alcohol can be induced in experimental animals, the doses used are not always comparable to the amounts consumed by humans. Palmer (1954) reported without illustration an acute superficial gastritis in all of 34 men subjected to biopsy within 6 hours of a bout of acute alcohol intoxication. In 9 of 11 on whom biopsies were performed 3 weeks later, the mucosa was said to have returned to normal. Gottfried, Korsten and Lieber (1978) observed the gastric mucosa in seven male alcoholic volunteers after the ingestion of the equivalent of 6–7 oz of an 86 proof beverage. The changes described at 3 hours after ingestion consisted of an extravasation of red cells into the upper lamina propria in four of seven subjects. The superficial epithelium remained ostensibly normal, however, and appears so in their illustration. Similar changes were reported by Laine and Weinstein (1988b) about a group of actively drinking alcoholics, but it is interesting that the extent of haemorrhage observed was only statistically more severe in the alcoholics than in a nonalcoholic control group. Certainly these changes are not regarded by this author as specific for alcohol damage as similar haemorrhages are seen in gastric biopsies in nonalcoholic patients who otherwise have a normal mucosa; they could easily be a traumatic biopsy artefact. It is possible that alcohol affects the gastric mucosa in such a way that a biopsy procedure is more likely to result in subepithelial haemorrhage.

Virtually nothing is known of the morphological changes that may be induced by the many oral drugs associated with gastric upsets or by the vast variety of exotic foodstuffs and condiments consumed. Certainly the ingestion of pickles can produce epithelial degeneration (Fig. 6–5), and it is tempting to postulate that repeated minor damage of this type determined by dietary habits is responsible for the high incidence of chronic gastritis that occurs in countries such as Finland and Japan. Indeed, Fontham et al (1986) and Burr et al (1987) produced evidence that in populations whose diet is rich in salt and deficient in fresh fruit and vegetables there is a high incidence of gastritis.

ACUTE GASTRIC INFECTIONS

In humans, unlike some animals, the stomach does not harbour a permanent microbial flora. Bacteria entering with food are quickly killed by the action of free hydrochloric acid, but some, such as lactobacilli, are more resistant than usual and may persist for short periods. The achlorhydric stomach therefore, as expected, is usually heavily colonised. Gastric acidity is thus important in protecting the small bowel from potential pathogens. It is not surprising that in a normal stomach bacterial infection is unusual.

Pastore et al (1976) have described reversible gastric mucosal alterations due to infestation by *Vibrio cholerae*. These included degenerative changes of the superficial epithelium, oedema, vascular congestion, and mononuclear cell infiltration of the lamina propria. The changes that Palmer (1951) described in acute staphylococcal food poisoning were principally those of epithelial necrosis and intralumenal sloughing in the region of the gastric pits. However, a critical appraisal of the illustrations published shows only a series of traumatic artefacts. Rarely is the gastric mucosa invaded by the haemolytic streptococcus (Gonzalez-Crussi and Hackett 1966, Nevin et al 1969). The invasion is usually the consequence of a severe generalised infection presenting elsewhere as an acute abdominal crisis; a diagnosis based on biopsy is unlikely. This is largely because the disease is an acute purulent necrotising lesion due to a diffuse spread of organisms throughout the mucosal, submucosal, and muscular layers of the bowel. The mucosa sloughs and the stomach wall is grossly thickened, hyperaemic, or infarcted and shows extensive vascular thrombosis. It is possible that the condition of emphysematous gastritis is a related lesion due to the involvement of gas-forming organisms. Ross and Vincenti (1994), in a study of

Figure 6–5. Normal human volunteer *(A)* before and *(B)* 1 hour after consuming 8 ounces of pickled gherkins. There are appreciable changes of possible damage to the surface epithelium (H&E ×420).

acute phlegmonous gastritis, reviewed this rare phenomenon and stressed an association with an immunosuppressed state.

With the exception of herpes simplex virus and cytomegalovirus infection in immunosuppressed patients (Gazzard 1988, Malfertheiner 1988), the putative gastritis that occurs as part of systemic viral illness has not been studied by biopsy. In cytomegalovirus infection, however, typical inclusions are often seen in the epithelial cells in the base of superficial erosions or the neighbouring mucosa (Fig. 6–6). An uncommon presentation in cytomegalovirus gastritis is an appearance at endoscopy of multiple hyperaemic nonulcerated nodules (Shuster et al 1989).

Gastric involvement in syphilis is rarely recognised, but in four cases the diagnosis was made in endoscopic biopsies by demonstrating the organisms in the edges of erosions or ulcers. The latter tended to have raised edges, and the patients presented with gastric bleeding (Fyfe et al 1993). Gastric syphilis rarely presents as linitis plastica (Abdu, Carter and Pomidor 1993).

Figure 6–6. Biopsy of the edge of a gastric ulcer. There is marked gastritis and typical cytomegalovirus inclusions in the epithelial cells *(arrows)* (H&E ×500).

Candida can also invade the gastric mucosa in the immunocompromised person and is fairly common complicating systemic candidiasis in prolonged antibiotic use, steroid and cytotoxic therapy (Eras, Goldstein and Sherlock 1972), and in AIDS patients (Gazzard 1988), but it is more common as an invader of the base of chronic peptic or malignant ulcers (Katzenstein and Maksem 1979, Scott and Jenkins 1982). This was studied in detail by Kalogeropoulos and Whitehead (1988), who found the organism in 26% of gastric ulcers, 20% of duodenal ulcers, and 24% of the ulcers associated with Barrett's oesophagus. In these circumstances it is regarded as a commensal, but it is natural to wonder if its presence in a peptic ulcer has an influence on the chronicity of the lesion and its response to antiulcer therapy.

GASTRITIS AND *HELICOBACTER PYLORI, GASTROSPIRILLUM HOMINIS,* AND *GIARDIA LAMBLIA*

Helicobacter pylori

Ramsey et al (1979) described an epidemic of transient gastritis characterised by abdominal pain, nausea, and vomiting that occurred in a group of volunteers being used for gastric secretory studies. Acute inflammatory changes mainly in the superficial parts of the gastric mucosa were coincident with decreased acid secretion, although the parietal cells were largely uninvolved in the inflammatory process. The agent responsible for the epidemic was not discovered at that time, but has been ascribed to *Campylobacter pyloris* (Gledhill et al 1985). This organism is now known as *Helicobacter pylori*. There are other, isolated reports supporting the claim that *H. pylori* can cause acute gastritis (Frommer et al 1988). This organism and its relationship to gastritis, intestinal metaplasia, duodenitis and peptic ulcer, and gastric lymphoma and adenocarcinoma are now the subject of a vast supporting literature. It is said that *H. pylori* causes an acute gastritis because it is usually seen in association with polymorph infiltration of the gastric epithelium (Fig. 6–7); it can affect children and adults; it is associated with the type B gastritis seen in prepyloric and duodenal ulcers; it affects the metaplastic gastric epithelium in the duodenum, which is often

Figure 6–7. Gastric pits show epithelial degenerative changes, polymorph infiltration, and *Campylobacter* organisms applied to the mucous layer and in the lumen (H&E ×1,000).

present in association with duodenal ulcers; and it is always associated with a neutrophil polymorph inflammatory cell infiltration of the epithelium in whose mucinous layer it resides. *H. pylori* is also said to result in gastric adenocarcinoma; in the acquisition of mucosal lymphoid aggregates, thus predisposing to lymphoma; and may even be involved in the evolution of the mucosal lesion in pernicious anaemia (Barthel et al 1988, Bartlett 1988, Price 1988, Rauws et al 1988, Graham 1989, Eidt and Stolte 1993, Sipponen and Hyvarinen 1993, Varis, Valle and Siurala 1993, Craanen et al 1994, De Boni, De Bona and Cielo 1994, De Koster et al 1994, Dixon 1994, Eidt and Stolte 1994; Eidt, Stolte and Fischer 1994, Genta and Hamner 1994, Genta, Huberman and Graham 1994, Sipponen 1994, Yamashiro et al 1994, Correa 1995, Sipponen 1995, Wyatt 1995). Some advocate the use of therapy aimed at eradicating the organism when it is demonstrated in biopsy specimens of patients investigated for any upper gastrointestinal symptoms (Marshall 1988). Of interest however, in this respect, is the report by Berstad et al (1988) that antacids reduce *H. pylori* colonization without affecting the gastritis in patients with nonulcer dyspepsia and erosive prepyloric changes. There is an equally impressive literature that casts some doubt over some of these enthusiastic claims. The organism is uncommon in association with gastric metaplasia of the duodenum in some circumstances, e.g., chronic renal failure (Shousha, Keen and Parkins 1989). It is not associated with some 30% of gastric ulcers. It is not always associated with a neutrophil polymorph tissue reaction (Fig. 6–8), and the latter may be extreme in its absence (Fig. 6–9). It is seen in association with the gastritis and duodenitis found in asymptomatic people (Fitzgibbons et al 1988) and in as many as 25% of humans with a normal gastric body mucosa. It is found fairly commonly in association with the gastric metaplastic epithelium in Barrett's oesophagus and in association with ectopic gastric mucosa (the inlet patch), but it has no consistent relationship to either inflammation or peptic ulceration in these circumstances (Kalogeropoulos and Whitehead 1988, Talley et al 1988, Borhan-Manesh and Farnum 1993). Indeed, in Barrett's oesophagus the role of gastric reflux in the pathogenesis of ulceration seems to be confirmed in view of the report that it is known to regress under the influence of omeprazole therapy (Deviere et al 1989). That the relationship of *H. pylori* to gastric mucosal disease is not a simple one is also highlighted by epidemiological evidence. Much of

Figure 6–8. Gastric surface epithelium with numerous *Campylobacter* organisms but a conspicuous absence of neutrophil polymorph leukocytes (Dieterle's ×750).

the data upon which claims have been made come from the developed countries; yet in parts of Africa and India, for example, despite a nearly 100% incidence of *H. pylori* in the adult population, peptic ulcer and gastric adenocarcinoma are rare (Holcombe 1992, Gill and Desai 1993, Holcombe et al 1994). In Colombia, South America (Correa et al 1990) *H. pylori* is associated not with diffuse antral gastritis (type B) but with multifocal atrophic gastritis; whereas gastric ulcer and adenocarcinoma are common, duodenal ulcer is rarely seen. Doubt has been cast by others, however, on the extent of the role played by *H. pylori* in the aetiology of adenocarcinoma (Wee, Kang and Teh 1992, Clarkson and West 1993, Farinati et al 1993,

Figure 6–9. Gastric pit with marked epithelial polymorph infiltration but no *Campylobacter* organisms (H&E ×1,000).

Shousha et al 1993, Takahashi et al 1993). In children infected with *H. pylori* there is also an apparent serious difficulty in the lack of correlation between duodenitis and gastric metaplasia and the presence of duodenal ulceration (Shabib et al 1994). A notable lack of correlation also exists between blood group secretor status and *H. pylori* infection in patients with duodenal ulcer (Dickey et al 1993). There is some concern over the claims for an aetiological role of *H. pylori* infection in gastric lymphoma. Gastric lymphoma is relatively uncommon in the region of the cardia, which nevertheless often exhibits gastritis when the antrum is involved, although the phenomenon of lymphoid follicle development is not seen as often as in the antrum when *H. pylori* are harboured in the stomach (Genta, Huberman and Graham 1994). However, this is possibly outweighed by the fact that lymphoid follicles in *H. pylori*–positive stomachs tend to persist when the organisms have been eradicated by appropriate therapy (Genta, Hamner and Graham 1993, Genta, Lew and Graham 1993, Genta and Hamner 1994). Others have expressed surprise that despite the prevalence of histologically active gastritis in AIDS patients, *H. pylori* colonisation of the stomach is very low (Marano, Smith and Bonanno 1993). *H. pylori* and the other putative mucosal damaging agents, the NSAIDs, do not appear to be synergistic in causing gastric mucosal damage, which is somewhat idiosyncratic (Laine 1993); in the elderly at least, NSAIDs play a much greater role in ulcer disease than does the presence of *H. pylori* (Wyatt et al 1992). Similarly it is bile reflux in the elderly, rather than the presence of *H. pylori,* that seems most strongly related to intestinal metaplasia and adenocarcinoma (Sobala et al 1993).

Gastrospirillum Hominis and *Giardia*

Not all spiral or curved organisms in gastric mucosa are the *H. pylori* species (McNulty et al 1989). In some ways the presence of *H. pylori* in the stomach and duodenum in association with peptic ulceration has been compared with the presence of other commensal organisms such as *Candida albicans;* it has been suggested that much more research is needed before a direct as opposed to an accessory causal role for *H. pylori* in gastric peptic ulceration and gastric cancer is accepted (Marcheggiano et al 1987, Sethi et al 1987, Graham and Michaletz 1988, Kalogeropoulos and Whitehead 1988, Nedenskov-Sorensen et al 1988, Price 1988, Queiroz et al 1988).

It is being increasingly recognised, for example, that on occasion in the gastritic stomach another organism, *Gastrospirillum hominis,* may be demonstrated (Fig. 6–10). This has been described in adults and children (Lopez et al 1993, Oliva, Lazenby and Perman 1993, Tanaka et al 1994). Even *Giardia lamblia* has been cited as a possible cause of gastritis (Berney, Rampton and van der Walt 1994).

CHRONIC GASTRITIS: AN HISTORICAL PERSPECTIVE

It is usual to use the pathological term chronic gastritis in reference to an inflammatory lesion of the stomach that affects more or less of the mucosa, that may or may not be associated with peptic ulcer or pernicious anaemia, and that increases in frequency with age. Histologically it is characterised by mucosal inflammation, with or without destruction, and architectural modification of the epithelial components. It emerged as an entity as a result of the work concerned with the lesion of pernicious anaemia (Faber 1935, Magnus and Ungley 1938). Further studies were made by examination of laparotomy biopsies (Schindler 1947) and excised stomach specimens (Magnus 1946, 1952). It was, however, the advent of the flexible tube biopsy instruments (Wood et al 1949, Tomenius 1950) that marked the beginning of a new era of interest and investigation into mucosal lesions of the stomach. A mass of literature soon ensued concerning the association of chronic gastritis with the anaemias, peptic ulceration, malignancy, and autoimmune phenomena. A good

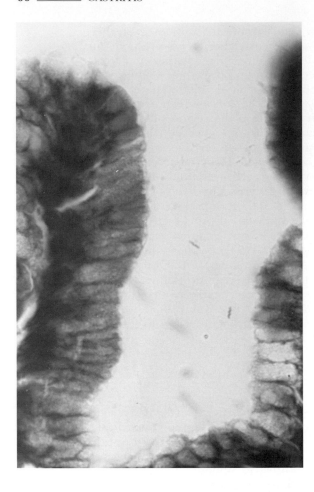

Figure 6–10. *Gastrospirillum hominis.* Two examples located centrally in the gastric pit (Giemsa ×600).

deal of discrepancy arose, and this was in part due to the lack of good control studies in normal populations, but mainly to the inherent shortcomings of the biopsy instruments. They could provide biopsies only from a limited area of the stomach, never from high in the fundus and hardly ever from the antrum. The site of the biopsy usually taken from the greater curve on the anterior wall was never accurately known. It was with justification that MacDonald and Rubin (1967) wrote "the definition and classification of chronic gastritis remains unsatisfactory."

With the advent of fibreoptic gastroscopes equipped with biopsy facilities, specimens could be obtained from all parts of the gastric mucosa and clearly viewed and photographed at the same gastroscopic examination. The biopsy specimens, although small, usually include the muscularis mucosa.

Multiple biopsies can be taken from different anatomical sites. Their accurate evaluation and the facility of sequential studies have resulted in considerable advances in the knowledge of chronic gastritis, particularly in the recognition of subtypes. Most recent has been the recognition of the aetiological roles of *H. pylori,* bile reflux, and the NSAIDs.

Evaluation of Chronic Gastritis in Biopsies

In order to categorise chronic gastritis the importance of the histological character of the mucosa, the geographical distribution of the changes within the stomach, and the presence of antibodies to gastric cell components has become increasingly clear; to a far lesser extent is the importance of the macroscopic appearances at endoscopy. The subtypes of chronic gastritis that are recognised have certain histological features in common. Thus in each biopsy the different components of the mucosa should be assessed separately and variations from normal noted carefully. The different combinations of features taken in conjunction with the other factors mentioned previously will then allow the gastritis to be typed. The importance of the topographical distribution in classifying gastric changes cannot be stressed too heavily. It is for this reason that the so-called Sydney system (Price 1991) of classifying chronic gastritis has been so severely criticised (Correa and Yardley 1992). Particularly so has been the advocacy of only two antral and two body biopsies for assessing and classifying any particular case of chronic gastritis, especially when multifocal chronic gastritis (type AB) characteristically begins at the angulus before spreading to other mucosal areas and thus can easily be miscategorised.

Superficial Epithelium. This epithelium may show features suggesting degenerative or regenerative processes. The cells may appear flattened or cuboidal with hyperchromatic nuclei, show partial or complete loss of the mucin column, and have increased basophilia of the diminished cytoplasm (Fig. 6–11). The cells may form a layer several cells thick, their limiting membranes becoming blurred and indistinct so that bud-like syncytial masses are formed (Fig. 6–12), and may seem to be in the process of exfoliation. On occasion mitotic figures occur in the superficial epithelium (Fig. 6–13). Normally they are rare and are seen only in the regenerative zone of the mucosa at the base of the gastric pits, and thus it seems that very immature cells still capable of cell division are reaching the surface. When degenerative changes are most marked the epithelium may show invasion by polymorphonuclear leukocytes; this constitutes a striking picture (Fig. 6–14) suggestive of an active inflamma-

Figure 6–11. Gastric body mucosa in chronic gastritis shows degenerative changes of the superficial epithelium (H&E ×188).

Figure 6–12. Gastric superficial epithelium shows regenerative syncytial masses of hyperchromatic cells, some of which appear to be in the process of exfoliation (H&E ×450).

Figure 6–13. Gastric pit contains pus cells. Note the mitotic figure in the superficial epithelium *(arrow)* (H&E ×450).

Figure 6–14. Gastric superficial epithelium and pits show degenerative and regenerative features with an active inflammatory infiltration and distortion. Note intraepithelial polymorphs and lymphocytes seemingly in a vacuole (H&E ×425).

tory destruction of the epithelium and may be associated with epithelial erosions. Sometimes intraepithelial lymphocytes are the predominant feature; when these are numerous in the absence of a polymorph component they frequently appear with a surrounding clear space or vacuole. The surface epithelium in this circumstance may show little change and appear relatively normal. This may also occur in the absence of intraepithelial lymphocytes, especially when the inflammatory infiltrate of the lamina propria is also minimal despite marked glandular atrophy. The superficial epithelium may also be the site of small intestinal metaplasia (see the subsequent section on metaplasia).

Pits. These epithelial changes also may be seen in the gastric pits. Polymorph invasion of the crypt epithelium, with collections of polymorphs in the dilated lumen (Fig. 6–13), mimics the appearance of a crypt abscess in ulcerative colitis. The increased activity of the regenerative zone is reflected not only in an increased basophilia and mitotic activity but also by a tortuosity and elongation of the pits. This may be a striking feature in some circumstances. The pits may also be separated by inflammatory oedema of the lamina propria and congestion of capillary vessels. The pits may thus appear reduced in number. But a reduction in number and distortion of the normal pattern is usually the result of degenerative atrophy and incomplete restoration due to previous episodes of inflammation. An intraepithelial lymphocyte population similar to that in the superficial epithelium may also be a striking feature (Fig. 6–14).

Helicobacter pylori. *H. pylori* organisms are commonly recognisable in ordinary hematoxylin and eosin (H & E)-stained sections, but they can readily be demonstrated by Dieterle's silver stain method (see Fig. 6–8). Many rely on the much less tedious Giemsa's method, which stains them blue. Genta, Robason and Graham

Figure 6–15. Gastric body gland tubules show inflammatory destruction. Note the generalised cellular infiltrate and prominence of polymorphs in the lamina propria (H&E ×200).

(1994) described a new stain that allows simultaneous viewing of _H. pylori_ and the mucosal morphology.

Gland Tubules. These may remain normal despite severe changes in the superficial epithelium and gastric pits. Frequently, however, a shrinkage or complete disappearance of groups of tubules occurs. The number that disappears varies, and no normal tubules may remain. Sometimes an acute inflammatory destruction is observed similar to that in the superficial epithelium and gastric pits (Fig. 6–15).

Metaplasia. Pseudopyloric metaplasia (Figs. 6–16 and 6–17) is recognised only

Figure 6–16. Body mucosa shows diffuse inflammatory infiltration and, centrally, loss of gland tubules with the earliest stage of pseudopyloric metaplasia in others (H&E ×70).

Figure 6–17. Body mucosa shows marked pseudopyloric metaplasia of glands. Note intestinal metaplasia of the pits and superficial epithelium (H&E ×70).

in body glands, whereas intestinal metaplasia affects all types of glands, the superficial epithelium, and pits. The earliest stage of pseudopyloric metaplasia consists of an increase in mucous neck cells, which later replace the remaining specialised cells in the rest of the tubule so that the appearance mimics normal pyloric glands. This may reflect deficient differentiation, whereas in the normal course of events mucous neck cells descend into the gastric glands and become chief and parietal cells. When there is intestinal metaplasia (Figs. 6–18 and 6–19), epithelial cells of small intestinal type, including absorptive cells in various stages of maturation, goblet cells, and Paneth's cells, can be recognised. Argentaffin cells are also present in increased numbers. Sometimes structures covered by intestinal epithelium project from the surface, thus simulating intestinal villi closely; rarely does the transformation closely mimic a small intestinal mucosa with villi and a gland layer (Fig. 6–20). However, the transformation of gastric cells into intestinal cells results in intermediate forms. When the transformation is complete, with enterocytes, intestinal goblet cells, and Paneth's cells, the cells have all the characteristics of small intestine cells, both ultrastructurally and histochemically (Lev 1966, Goldman and Ming 1968). An intermediate or incomplete form is also recognised (Iida, Murata and Nagata 1978), which has the combination of goblet cells and columnar cells with features resembling gastric foveolar cells. This type of intestinal metaplasia has been further subdivided on the basis of the histochemistry of the mucus it contains. In type IIA, neutral mucins are said to predominate whereas in type B they are sulphomucins. Using immunohistological methods Nardelli et al (1983) showed that incomplete intestinal metaplasia has antigens common to foetal duodenum. Complete and incomplete intestinal metaplasia types A and B are now referred to as types I, II, and III, respectively. It is claimed that any person with extensive metaplasia is at high risk for gastric adenocarcinoma and should be subject to periodic screening. The extent of the metaplastic process is probably more important than the subtype (Stemmer-

Figure 6–18. Metaplastic intestinal absorptive cells and goblet cells *(right and above)*; note the brush border *(arrowhead)*. Typical gastric superficial epithelium *(left)* (H&E ×420).

mann 1994). The association of intestinal metaplasia with other cell types normally not present in the gastric mucosa is also worthy of note.

In Japanese subjects with peptic ulcer, epithelial dysplasia, or early cancer seen in association with areas of intestinal metaplasia, it is not that unusual to find cystically dilated glands containing ciliated cells (Rubio and Kato 1986). Sometimes such cells also contain argyrophilic basal granules. Ultrastructural studies show that the cilia have a shaft, neck, and basal body comparable to those seen in the respiratory epithelium (Torikata et al 1986, Torikata, Mukai and Kawakita 1989). Similar cells are apparently less common in Europeans (Rubio and Serck-Hanssen 1986). Another cytological phenomenon sometimes related to ciliated cells is the presence of cytoplasmic vacuolisation. The vacuoles may be mucin-positive and may also contain neuroendocrine granules, but also they may be mucin-negative and

Figure 6–19. Metaplastic Paneth's cells with typical refractile granules *(arrowhead)* (H&E ×420).

Figure 6–20. Gastric body mucosa shows a virtually complete small intestinalisation with villous processes and a gland layer. Note there is still a prominent inflammatory infiltrate of the lamina propria (H&E ×45).

devoid of cilia, and the vacuole appears infranuclear in position. A further type is the vacuole that seemingly surrounds intraepithelial lymphocytes (Rubio and Kato, 1987 and 1988). In association with type IIB or III intestinal metaplasia Newbold, MacDonald and Allum (1988) have also described probable precursor cells that occur in the surface epithelium between gastric pits. They occur as groups of up to 25 cells, exhibit no mitotic activity, are mucin-negative, and have no brush border. Doglioni et al (1993) described pancreatic-acinar cells in gastric mucosa that are morphologically, immunocytochemically, and electron-microscopically identical to the same cells in the pancreas. They tend to be arranged in nests or small lobules among the gastric glands, have abundant cytoplasm, and are acidophilic and finely granular in the apical and middle regions and basophilic in the basal compartment. Their presence is unrelated to pancreatic heterotopia of the stomach.

Lamina Propria. This may show an inflammatory infiltrate that includes plasma cells, lymphocytes, and eosinophil and neutrophil polymorphs. Neutrophil polymorphs or a mixture of lymphocytes and plasma cells may predominate. The infiltrate may be restricted to a part or the whole of the area between the gastric pits and, in addition, may involve part or the whole of the deeper parts when it is usually associated with glandular atrophy. A polymorph-rich infiltrate is commonly associated with vascular dilation and a serofibrinous oedema with destructive inflammation of the related epithelium. When chronic inflammatory cells predominate, plasma cells are seen in the upper layers and lymphocytes in the lower layers, where follicular aggregates with or without germinal centres may form (Fig. 6–21). In the past this was called follicular gastritis; more recently it is considered a reaction to *H. pylori* (Genta, Hamner and Graham 1993) and a possible precursor of gastric lymphoma (Isaacson and Spencer 1993). In a mucosa with only minimal epithelial degenerative changes or widespread atrophy and metaplasia, the inflammatory infiltrate is often very scanty and always the plasma cell and lymphocyte preponderance type. Foci of fatty infiltration may appear in the lamina propria (Fig. 6–22) and in any lymphoid follicles present, which also will appear atrophic, being without germinal centres.

Sometimes the lamina propria shows only oedema, vascular hyperaemia, and particularly in the antrum a tendency for new strands of smooth muscle to grow up into the upper layers.

The reticulin fibres may appear more widely spaced than normal when there is inflammatory oedema. A more frequent change is seen in association with atrophy.

Figure 6–21. Gastric body mucosa shows pseudopyloric metaplasia and lymphoid hyperplasia (H&E ×14).

Under the superficial epithelium and in the interpit and intergland areas a felt-like mesh results when the reticulin fibres collapse together, as the tubules disappear and new fibres are formed as part of the inflammatory reaction. In severe atrophy the junction between the muscularis mucosa and lamina propria is less well defined than normal, and the whole of the normal reticulin pattern is obscured (Figs. 6–23 and 6–24).

Sometimes in biopsy interpretation there are difficulties in recognising mucosal type if severe gastritis is present and there is atrophy or metaplasia. When only metaplastic pseudopyloric or intestinal tubules remain, the mucosa cannot be classified, but if residual body glands remain and their recognition is facilitated by Maxwell's preparations, the mucosa must be of body or junctional type. If all the tubules that remain are of pyloric type, the mucosa could have originated in any part of the stomach, because gastritis in pyloric or cardiac mucosa is similar to

Figure 6–22. Gastric body mucosa shows intestinal metaplasia and fatty infiltration of the lamina propria (H&E ×150).

Figure 6–23. Gastric body mucosa in atrophic gastritis. There are subepithelial and intertubular condensation and deposition of new reticulin. Compare with Figure 5–4 (reticulin stain ×75).

gastritis with complete pseudopyloric metaplasia in body or junctional mucosa. When fibreoptic instruments are used, the site of the biopsy specimen is fairly accurately located, except in stomachs altered by previous operations. Thus in usual practice difficulty arises only in biopsy specimens from the lesser curve area, where even in the normal stomach the demarcation of one region from its neighbour is often poorly defined. A helpful point in the differentiation of normal pyloric glands from pseudopyloric glands is that whereas the former may contain occasional parietal cells, the latter do not.

If the inflammatory and reactive changes already outlined affect only the superficial epithelium, gastric pit region, and related lamina propria, it is convention to refer to this as superficial gastritis. Atrophic gastritis, on the other hand, occurs if the changes affect the gland layer, and the difficult line of demarcation is between superficial gastritis and early atrophic gastritis, the later and more severe grades of atrophic gastritis being obvious. Deep extension of the inflammatory infiltrate around the tubules may be helpful in the recognition of atrophic gastritis, but the only satisfactory criterion is recognition of atrophy of the tubules. In this respect the

Figure 6–24. Gastric pyloric mucosa in atrophic gastritis (features similar to those of Figure 6–23). Compare with Figure 5–9 (reticulin stain ×75).

preparations stained for reticulin are most valuable as loss of tubules, even in small numbers, is reflected by the changes in reticulin pattern already outlined.

Atrophic gastritis could be quantitated by accurately measuring the number of glands that remain, but a convenient subdivision is into mild, moderate, and severe. If only one or two groups of tubules have disappeared, the mucosa is classified as showing mild atrophy. It is this severity of involvement that is sometimes called focal atrophic gastritis. If all normal tubules are lost or only one or two groups remain, the diagnosis is severe; all appearances between these two extremes are classed as moderate. It is important for this scheme that only normal glands be considered and those showing metaplasia be discounted.

In severe atrophic gastritis with widespread metaplasia, a negligible inflammatory cell infiltrate, atrophic lymphoid aggregates, and fatty infiltration of the lamina propria, the appearances are often classified as gastric mucosal atrophy (Figs. 6–25 and 6–26). A further feature in severe atrophic gastritis is an increase in the number of endocrine cells induced by hypergastrinaemia (Rubin 1969, Bordi, Ravazzola and De Vita 1983, Belaiche et al 1993). In addition to cell types normally present in the stomach, new forms are acquired. By immunofluorescence cells positive for somatostatin, motilin, glicentin, and cholecystokinin have been demonstrated (Bordi and Ravazzola 1979). In some instances endocrine cells are so numerous that they can be recognised in ordinary H & E-stained sections (Figs. 6–27 and 6–28) and confirmed in a Grimelius's preparation. It is now well recognised that pernicious anaemia or achylia are conditions most closely associated with carcinoids (Wilander 1981), and cases have been recorded (Black and Haffner 1968, Hodges, Isaacson and Wright 1981) of multiple gastric carcinoid tumours and endocrine cell hyperplasia that is grossly nodular (Sjoblom et al 1989).

Some biopsy specimens exhibit an invasion of polymorphs into, and degenerative changes of the epithelial elements of, the gastric mucosa. Crypt abscess formation may be present, and if these features reflect an acute inflammatory epithelial destruction, as seems likely, then clearly its presence should be recorded. It is surprising that this phenomenon received scant mention in the literature until reported by Whitehead, Truelove and Gear (1972). If epithelial degenerative changes are associated with an infiltrate of chronic type, this could be regarded as chronic activity, and in both types the activity could be graded simply on the basis of whether it was

Figure 6–25. Gastric body mucosa shows gastric atrophy. There is partial intestinal metaplasia but no evidence of epithelial degeneration. The density of the cellular infiltrate is comparable to that in the normal mucosa, considering that there is severe tubular atrophy and a secondary condensation of the lamina propria (H&E ×75).

Figure 6–26. Gastric body mucosa shows gastric atrophy and complete intestinal metaplasia (H&E ×75).

diffuse throughout the mucosa or patchy in distribution. In some cases the mucosa shows little or no epithelial degenerative change and either a very slight or imperceptible chronic inflammatory infiltrate, in spite of the fact that there may be evidence of distortion and atrophy of the normal mucosal architecture. These appearances are clearly suggestive of a quiescent or burnt-out stage of a previous inflammatory process. This quiescent phase is seen in mucosae with severe atrophy and metaplasia, those showing so-called gastric atrophy.

Intestinal metaplasia nearly always occurs in a mucosa that is the site of atrophic gastritis. Sometimes it is present in the superficial epithelium and pits in superficial

Figure 6–27. Severe atrophic gastritis with islands of endocrine cell hyperplasia in association with the basal glands and in the neighbouring lamina propria (H&E ×500).

Figure 6–28. Field comparable to that of Figure 6–27 and stained specifically for endocrine cells (Grimelius's ×600).

gastritis, and very occasionally isolated islands are seen in biopsy specimens consisting of otherwise normal mucosa (Fig. 6–29). For practical purposes the presence of epithelium with intestinal morphology should always be regarded as abnormal. Pseudopyloric metaplasia also occurs invariably only in atrophic gastritis, but occasional gland tubules of simple mucus-secreting type are rarely seen among specialised gland tubules in an otherwise normal body mucosa. There is some evidence, based on surgically induced trauma of body mucosa, that initially causes a reversion to the more simple pyloric structure followed by recovery, that at least in some circum-

Figure 6–29. Normal pyloric mucosa with isolated island of intestinal metaplasia (H&E ×75).

stances this type of metaplasia may be reversible (Harvey 1907). Similar findings have been recorded in the repair of aspirin-induced erosions (Yeomans 1976). Both types of metaplasia should be recorded separately because they may have different significance, and the extent to which they are present can be conveniently graded. Reference has already been made to the possibility of subdividing intestinal metaplasia according to the mucins that predominate. Although there are claims as to the greater malignant potential of the incomplete type of metaplasia (Filipe 1983, Silva and Filipe 1986), which resembles colon rather than small intestine, there is a clear need for further elucidation of this; it may be that the metaplasia is a paraneoplastic rather than a preneoplastic phenomenon (Bedossa, Lemaigre and Martin 1987, Ramesar, Sanders and Hopwood 1987, Rubio et al 1987).

Thus in evaluating chronic gastritis according to the preceding principles, the following features should be considered.

Mucosal Type

Aided by knowledge of the site of biopsy it is usually possible to type the mucosa as of pyloric, body, cardiac, or junctional zone origin. Junctional mucosa occurs not only at the sites of change between the main mucosal areas in the stomach, namely antral, body, and cardiac, but also between the pylorus and duodenum and between the cardiac region and the oesophagus.

Site of Gastric Process

It is of considerable value to register the predominant site of the inflammatory process in gastritis. A superficial inflammation is arguably an earlier or less severe form of tissue damage than a deeper form, which is invariably associated with glandular destruction and atrophy.

Type of Inflammation

The inflammatory infiltrate that characterises gastritis may be mainly acute, mainly chronic, or mixed acute and chronic. This is a reflection of the activity of the pathogenetic process related to the factors causing the gastritis. It is also possible that differences in aetiology may be concerned in determining whether the inflammation also seems to centre on the epithelium as well as the lamina propria or even in preference to it.

Metaplasia

Pseudopyloric and intestinal metaplasia are important histological features because they represent a reaction by the mucosa to a significantly severe pathological process tending to destroy the native cellular elements. There is some evidence that intestinal metaplasia represents a more severe expression of mucosal injury. It is largely a nonreversible change and has an association with an increased malignant potential, the precise nature of which needs elucidation.

Lamina Propria Changes

Apart from inflammatory cell infiltration, important lamina propria changes include collapse of the reticulin framework and approximation of the surface and crypt epithelium to the deeper-lying lymphoid plexus, which is important in the metastatic process involved in early gastric cancer. In addition, the oedema, neomuscularisation, and vascular ectasia appear to be a reaction to some forms of tissue injury, notably bile reflux and following prolonged use of NSAIDs.

The different combinations of these features in conjunction with other known circumstances, such as the presence of autoantibodies, family history, and the geographical distribution of the lesions in the stomach, usually allows allocation of the gastritis to one or another category, which may have pathogenetic and clinical significance in terms not only of possible therapy but also of likely complications, such as anaemia, peptic ulcer disease, or malignancy. Thus it has become possible to classify several subtypes of chronic gastritis.

7

THE CLASSIFICATION OF CHRONIC GASTRITIS: CURRENT STATUS

The human organism has a restricted number of patterns of responses to noxious stimuli. Nevertheless, even at a morphological level it is often possible to define specific disease processes and ascribe patterns of tissue reaction to a narrow range of aetiological agents. Combine histological variables with epidemiological and functional disturbances and it is often possible to divide what was once regarded as a single entity into a number of separately identifiable groups so that the pathophysiological significance of each can be further characterised. Such is the case with chronic gastritis, which excludes the relatively well-defined entities like granulomatous gastritis, sarcoidosis, eosinophilic gastritis, and the gastritis associated with specific infectious agents. By identifying combinations of microscopic features, topographical distribution of the abnormalities, and the association with other variables, it is possible to identify different types. One of the primary histological features of all of them is inflammation that is mainly chronic, i.e., composed of lymphocytes and plasma cells, and may have a variable acute component characterised by neutrophils. Inflammation of the gastric mucosa is relatively easily recognised and categorised because in the normal state the mucosa has little, if any, of the cellularity that characterises the lamina propria of the small and large intestines. Another feature is the tendency towards inflammatory destruction of the glandular elements, which results with time in atrophy. This is frequently associated, during the atrophic process, with a metaplasia of the epithelial components of the mucosa. The specialised glands and the simple mucous glands may not just undergo inflammatory destruction, a process similar to that which occurs in the colon in, for example, ulcerative colitis, but the body glands may be replaced by pseudopyloric mucous glands, and any surface, pit, and glandular epithelium may be replaced by elements more usual to the intestine. Intestinalisation is important because it is believed to be an inaugural step in a chain of events that can lead to malignancy.

Because the tendency for development of malignancy is much greater in the large intestine than in the small intestine, evaluation of intestinal metaplasia of the colonic rather than the small bowel type is important. There is a good deal of evidence that gastric adenocarcinoma develops through stages of increasing dysplasia, especially when the malignancy concerned is of the so-called intestinal type deriving from large bowel metaplasia. There is also increasing evidence that the acquisition of significant lymphoid tissue by the mucosa in the process of development of chronic gastritis has implications for subsequent so-called mucosa-associated lymphoid tissue (MALT) malignant lymphoma. The stomach, which is affected by chronic inflammation of certain subtypes, also appears susceptible to peptic ulceration, another serious disease.

Thus, it seems that chronic gastritis, which is arguably an entity not easily or possibly not definable at all, in strictly clinical terms and symptomatology, is nevertheless of considerable significance because of its intimate relationship with more serious conditions, namely gastric cancer, malignant lymphoma, and peptic ulcer. Perhaps this is one of the reasons why attempts have been made to categorise the types of chronic gastritis. Certainly, unless such attempts are made and the types are subject to more intensive individual study, advances in the management and prevention of these serious consequences may not be made. It should be realised, however, that in individual cases the cause may be multifactorial, and clearly this may well result in difficulties in assigning such cases to a specific category.

TYPES OF CHRONIC GASTRITIS

Type A

Strickland and Mackay (1973) designated this as type A, but it is also known as autoimmune gastritis and as diffuse atrophic corporal gastritis. It is characterised by progressive atrophy of body glands, loss of the parietal and chief cell components, and replacement by simple pseudopyloric mucus cells or by intestinal epithelial components. There is a mainly chronic inflammatory cell infiltration of the lamina propria, and it is assumed that the epithelial damage is immune mediated; certainly even in its early stages neutrophil infiltration, such as characterises some other forms of gastritis, is not a significant feature. Eventually the whole body portion of the gastric mucosa is replaced by intestinalised or pseudopyloric epithelium, and with time the density of the inflammation of the lamina propria gradually diminishes. This type of chronic gastritis is not generally characterised by the presence of *Helicobacter pylori*, particularly in the later stages. Type A chronic gastritis, which some prefer to call gastric atrophy, especially as the name is arguably more apt in the disease's fully developed state, is associated with other autoimmune diseases, is characterised by antibodies to gastric mucosal constituents, and causes vitamin B_{12} deficiency due to lack of intrinsic factor. It is rare for peptic ulcers, either duodenal or gastric, to coexist. The antrum of the stomach, in addition to showing G cell hyperplasia, which appears as an increase in clear cells in the antral mucosa in ordinary haematoxylin and eosin (H&E) histological preparations, may also show in the early stages of the pathological process a variable inflammation that tends to disappear with time. Mucosal polyps of regenerative or hyperplastic type, which are sometimes transitory, have also been described (Lewin et al 1976, Elsborg et al 1977). In addition, Kekki et al (1983) have shown that the antral mucosa may also show gastritis of variable degree that tends to revert to normal in the later stages, especially if the initial gastritis was superficial.

In the remainder of the stomach the body and fundal areas show a severe atrophic gastritis that, in the later stages, when the lamina propria inflammatory cell component tends to disappear, is better described as gastric mucosal atrophy. There is a progressive loss of the specialised body glands, which are replaced by pseudopyloric or intestinal metaplastic elements. There is also an epithelial endocrine cell proliferation and a predisposition to carcinoid tumours (Borch et al 1986, Bordi et al 1986, Mueller, Kirchner and Mueller-Hermelink 1987, Itsuno et al 1989) that is driven probably by the hypergastrinaemia. A biopsy showing all these features is not diagnostic, however, because similar changes are seen in other forms of chronic atrophic gastritis. Apart from minor changes, from megaloblastosis back to normal, the lesion is not reversed by vitamin B_{12} therapy, although it has been claimed that vitamin B_{12} absorption and histology may improve following cortisone administration (Jeffries 1965). This was not confirmed, however, in a similar study by Strickland et al (1973).

In latent pernicious anaemia, achlorhydria, low intrinsic factor secretion, and atrophic gastritis are present, but although serum levels of vitamin B_{12} may be low there are no manifestations of vitamin B_{12} deficiency. A proportion go on to develop pernicious anaemia, but the factors that determine this progression are not fully understood. Pernicious anaemia may occur rarely in juveniles, and it appears to have several causes. There may be inadequate synthesis of intrinsic factor, a block to its secretion, or the secretion of abnormal intrinsic factor (Levine and Allen 1985). Acid secretion and gastric mucosal histological conditions are normal. In Imerslund's syndrome (Imerslund 1960) the same features are associated with the production of normal intrinsic factor, but the syndrome is not effective in promoting vitamin B_{12} absorption, and there is a coexistent proteinuria.

The literature concerning immunological studies in chronic gastritis is enormous and often contradictory (Glass 1977). Limited sampling of the gastritic mucosa and the technical difficulties inherent in the immunological methods used have probably contributed to this. Antibodies against a microsomal fraction of parietal cells can be demonstrated by fluorescence and by complement fixation methods. Two antibodies active against intrinsic factor have been demonstrated. One blocks the interaction of vitamin B_{12} with intrinsic factor, and the other combines with the vitamin B_{12} intrinsic factor complex.

Parietal cell antibodies are rarely found if the body mucosa is normal, and the incidence of antibodies rises with increasing severity of the histological lesion. The production of parietal cell antibodies in a case of chronic gastritis seems to depend on the type of patient in which the gastritis occurs rather than on the gastritis itself. For example, these antibodies are commonly associated with gastritis in patients with pernicious anaemia, iron deficiency anaemia, diabetes, or thyroid autoimmune disorders (Wright et al 1966).

Antibodies to intrinsic factor are less common than parietal cell antibodies and are associated with the more severe grades of gastritis. They are usually found in patients with pernicious anaemia or latent pernicious anaemia. When present in other conditions, e.g., thyroid diseases, they appear in the serum and not in the gastric juice. It seems that it is the gastric juice antibodies that are important in interfering with vitamin B_{12} absorption. There is no relationship between serial serum intrinsic factor antibody titres and the liability to develop the disease (Irvine, Cullen and Mawhinney, 1974).

The antibodies probably do not initiate the gastritis, although a lesion in monkeys equivalent to gastritis has been produced by Freund's adjuvant and gastric mucosal injections (Andrada and Rose 1969) Cell-mediated immunity against intrinsic factor has also been shown (Chanarin and James 1974). Cytotoxicity of the antibodies has not been demonstrated, but this may reflect only the present difficulties in growing gastric mucosal constituents in tissue culture. Cell-mediated immunity against other mucosal antigens has, however, been demonstrated by Uibo and Salupere (1981) in patients who have no parietal cell antibodies. Clearly, the question of the role of immune phenomena in the production of gastritis is still to be resolved, but the role of cytotoxic antibodies seems to be gaining acceptance (De Aizpurua et al 1983, Kaye, Whorwell and Wright 1983). It is possible that gastritis may well be initiated by environmental factors and subsequently perpetuated by autoimmune phenomena, especially in a prone and genetically determined group. It is pertinent in this respect that there is a considerable immunological overlap among pernicious anaemia, thyroid autoimmune disease, and diabetes and that patients with severe atrophic gastritis following gastrectomy operations rarely develop antibodies.

Type B

Type B (Strickland and Mackay 1973, Correa 1980, Varis 1981, Correa 1988), or diffuse antral, gastritis in its pure form is not primarily atrophic, but characterised by a mixed acute and chronic mucosal inflammation, often with prominent lymphoid follicles tending to occupy the deeper lamina propria and to display reaction centres.

This type tends not to extend beyond the antrum and is strongly associated with the presence of *H. pylori* (Wyatt and Dixon 1988). With time there is a tendency for intestinal metaplasia to occur, but this is never a striking feature in the usual case. Type B gastritis is frequently accompanied by peptic duodenitis; patients with this type are prone to both prepyloric and duodenal ulceration (Correa 1980, Kekki and Villako 1981). Varis (1981) and Correa (1988) have stressed the density of the lymphoid infiltrates with reactive germinal centres. Wyatt and Dixon (1988), on the other hand, proposed that type B gastritis is closely related to colonisation with *H. pylori* predisposing both gastric mucosa and gastric metaplasia of duodenal mucosa to ulceration. The relationship between gastritis and peptic ulcer is nevertheless far from clear. From the very earliest of observations (Cruveilhier 1862) it became evident that ulcer and gastritis were invariably present in the same stomach.

The gastritis has a type B distribution in prepyloric and duodenal ulcers, but in ulcers higher in the stomach it extends proximally to involve a larger area, although in a patchy fashion (Gear, Truelove and Whitehead 1971). This is referred to again in consideration of the entity that has been called type AB gastritis. All chronic peptic ulcers are situated in a pyloric type of mucosa and thus occur either just distal to the junction of body with the pyloric mucosa or in the pyloric mucosa beyond (Oi, Oshida and Sugimura 1959). Consequently, when the ulcer occurs high in the stomach the antrum appears to be enlarged. This could be the clear result of atrophic gastritis and pseudopyloric metaplasia involving the more proximal as well as the distal part of the stomach in a way that suggests that there is backwards extension of the process, but it could also be interpreted to mean that those individuals who possess an abnormally large antrum are prone to ulcer. There is some evidence that the former is the case and that high gastric ulcers are always associated with gastritis in the area of the stomach distal to the ulcer (Tatsuta and Okuda 1975). However, the possibility of mixed forms of gastritis indicates the need for further research. There does not seem to be a significant risk in type B gastritis patients for the development of gastric adenocarcinoma.

Type AB

Type AB (Correa 1980, Varis 1981, Correa 1988), or multifocal atrophic, gastritis is in numerical terms possibly the most important type, especially because of its relationship with and susceptibility to lead to adenocarcinoma. It is a chronic gastritis, which begins at the incisura and spreads out radially from there with time as it involves more and more of the gastric mucosa. Inevitably it causes progressive atrophy of the body and antral glands. Intestinal metaplasia is a usual accompaniment of the process, and the inflammation frequently has a mixed acute and chronic component. There is a controversial and less consistent association with the presence of *H. pylori* than is the case with type B gastritis. Type AB gastritis is associated with gastric ulcer rather than duodenal ulcer; arguably, of most importance in association with it is an increased incidence of gastric adenocarcinoma.

The AB gastritis of Kekki and Villako (1981) and Varis (1981) corresponds to the multifocal atrophic gastritis of Correa (1980 and 1988). It tends to occur with a geographical distribution in populations with a high risk of gastric cancer and also appears to be associated with gastric peptic ulcers, which are situated high in the stomach. It is initially a patchy proximal atrophic gastritis that affects the antrum and lesser curve and develops as a more widespread lesion associated with increasing intestinal metaplasia involving the higher lesser curve region and the anterior and posterior walls of the body. The foci increase in size with duration and tend to coalesce, thus affecting most of the gastric mucosa, but the high fundus is usually spared. The associated gastric ulcer may heal as the disease progresses, which is possibly related to the tendency to develop hypochlorhydria. However, coexistent intrinsic factor and parietal cell antibodies are unusual, and vitamin B_{12} deficiency does not occur. The progressive nature of this disease has been monitored in biopsy studies (Gear, Truelove and Whitehead 1971, Aukee and Krohn 1972, Kekki, Hakkiluoto and Siurala 1976, Pulimood, Knudsen and Coghill 1976, Ormiston, Gear and Codling 1982) and shown to be uninfluenced by ulcer treatment using histamine H2-receptor-antagonists (Pounder et al 1976).

Although there may well be a genetic susceptibility to acquire this type of gastritis in that it appears to run in families (Bonney et al 1986), the high incidence in populations consuming diets high in salt and deficient in fresh vegetables and fruit makes it highly likely that environmental influences are also important (Fontham et al 1986). In low incidence areas, however, genetic influences seem to be of prime importance and may account for the familial occurrence of gastric carcinoma.

Type C

Type C, or chemical reactive, gastritis is seen in sites of bile reflux following gastrojejunostomy, Billroth's I and II operations, and vagotomy and pyloroplasty. In these circumstances other forms of chronic gastritis may already be present. When due to bile reflux it affects the areas where significant bile containing refluxate bathes the gastric mucosa, and there is increasing evidence that bile reflux can also occur in the ostensibly normal stomach, i.e., without the altered physiology secondary to the gastric operations (Dixon et al 1986, Bechi et al 1987, Sobala et al 1990 and 1993). The subject has, however, been controversial. There is good experimental evidence for a damaging effect of bile and pancreatic juice on the gastric mucosa (Davenport 1968, Cheng, Ritchie and Delaney 1969, Brooks, Wenger and Hersh 1975, Eastwood 1975, Mann 1976, Orchard et al 1977), and thus there has been increasing acceptance that alkaline or enterogastric reflux may be of clinical importance in humans (Ritchie 1984 and 1986). Others claim that reflux is rare in normal people (Cocking and Grech 1973). Still others have claimed that it is commonplace in patients attending gastroenterology clinics who do not have a gastric ulcer or a history of previous gastric operations (Niemela et al 1987), and when present at endoscopy it has no clinical relevance and is not associated with histological injury (Nasrallah et al 1987). In patients who have had gastric operations for peptic ulcer, either duodenal or gastric, it is the accepted view that enterogastric bile alkaline reflux is usual (Hoare et al 1977), and concern has been expressed over a relationship between this and the subsequent development of gastritis, gastric mucosal dysplasia, and carcinoma (Aukee and Krohn 1972, Watt, Sloan and Kennedy 1983, Watt et al 1983, Langhans, Bues and Bunte 1984, Houghton et al 1986), although the results of other researchers indicate that the case has been overstated (Ovaska et al 1986). The matter is further complicated by reports that in patients with gastric ulcer treated by certain types of operations, e.g., highly selective vagotomy, there may be a decrease in the extent of bile reflux, but that this has no effect on the gastritis present (Dewar, Dixon and Johnston 1984).

Clearly there are problems with many of these previous studies in definitions of what constitutes "bile reflux," in the parameters chosen for assessing gastric mucosal damage and the fact that in patients with peptic ulcers there is an associated chronic gastritis that may or may not be related to bile reflux. It has long been known that the gastritis associated with peptic ulcer persists and progresses in severity even when the ulcer has healed (Gear, Truelove and Whitehead 1971, Pulimood, Knudsen and Coghill 1976), and this may be independent of reflux. Of the different morphological aspects of chronic gastritis it seems theoretically possible that one or more parameters are aetiologically more closely related to reflux than the others. Thus, Mosimann et al (1981) drew attention to elongation and tortuosity of the gastric pits as a specific association of bile in the stomach. Some further confirmation of this was supplied by Mosimann et al (1984) when this lesion was seen to regress in postoperative duodenal ulcer patients if bile diversion was achieved by a Roux-en-Y gastrojejunostomy procedure. A study by Dixon et al (1986) led to the claim that reflux-associated features in gastric biopsies are foveolar hyperplasia, oedema and smooth muscle fibres in the lamina propria, vasodilatation and congestion of superficial mucosal capillaries, and a paucity of acute and chronic inflammatory cells. It is not clear from this study, however, what was the extent of changes in the stomach that would normally be regarded as part of the forms of chronic gastritis that are typically present in at least part of the stomach in association with peptic ulcer. Bechi et al (1987) addressed this issue and showed that, whereas foveolar hyperplasia is reflux-related, chronic atrophic gastritis is not. These histological features can certainly occur in the stomach when obvious bile reflux is seen endoscopically (Figs. 7–1 to 7–4). However, such changes are not entirely specific for reflux; they can in fact be seen in other states of the gastric mucosa, such as the edge of erosions or ulcers, in Ménétrier's disease, gastritis cystica profunda, hyperplastic polyps, and the Canada-Cronkhite lesion, and they are probably part of the spectrum of the mucosa's response to injury. The claim that subnuclear vacuolisation of foveolar cells of fundic or body mucosa is a histological marker for protracted duodenogastric reflux (Rubio and Slezak 1988) requires confirmation, particularly as the vacuoles are usually empty and do not stain with mucin and mucopolysaccharide.

An identical histological type of mucosal reaction affects the antral area in patients taking nonsteroidal anti-inflammatory drugs (NSAIDs) (Sobala et al 1990). The mucosa shows elongation and tortuosity of the gastric crypts, with hyperplasia of the crypt and surface epithelium, characterised by an increase in the size of the mucus compartment of the component cells (Figs. 7–5 and 7–6). There are oedema and increased vascularity of the lamina propria, which also with time shows fibromuscularisation. Inflammation is variable and probably depends in part on the mucosal appearance prior to the use of the NSAIDs or the surgical procedure with which the inflammation may be associated. Certainly in some instances the inflammation is relatively slight and of chronic type. In type C gastritis due to bile reflux in particular, intestinal metaplasia may be present (Haot et al 1989). There is an increased risk of adenocarcinoma in the type C gastritis associated with bile

Figure 7–1. Antral mucosa showing elongation and tortuosity of gastric pits in the presence of severe endoscopic bile reflux (H&E ×50).

Figure 7–2. Body mucosa in the same stomach as in Figure 7–1. There is marked tortuosity and elongation of pits in addition to increased vascularity and muscularisation of the lamina propria. Note the relative absence of inflammation (H&E ×200).

Figure 7–3. Detail of the upper lamina propria in bile reflux. Note the oedema and increased vascularity and relatively scant inflammation (H&E ×350).

Figure 7–4. Detail of the upper lamina propria in bile reflux. Note the epithelial changes and the muscularisation of the lamina propria (H&E ×350).

Figure 7–5. Antral mucosa in chemical (type C) gastritis. The gastric pits are elongated and tortuous, and there is oedema of the lamina propria with vascular dilatation (H&E ×300).

Figure 7–6. Chemical (type C) gastritis with pronounced muscularisation. Note also the vascular dilatation and hyperplasia of surface and crypt epithelial cells (H&E ×400).

reflux, particularly in association with previous gastric surgery. Both duodenal and gastric ulceration are prone to occur in the type associated with the use of NSAIDs.

CHRONIC EROSIVE VERRUCOUS GASTRITIS, VARIOLIFORM GASTRITIS, AND LYMPHOCYTIC GASTRITIS

In the late 1970s endoscopists began to refer to certain gastric mucosal appearances as aphthous ulceration (Morgan et al 1976), chronic erosive verrucous gastritis (Green et al 1977), and varioliform gastritis (Lambert et al 1978). These had no relationship to acute haemorrhagic erosions, which are also known as erosive gastritis. One of the problems associated with the definition of this disease is the use of erosion by endoscopists for lesions that histologically have an intact surface epithelium (Karvonen et al 1983, Nesland and Berstad 1985, Nesland, Berstad and Serck-Hanssen 1986, Berstad and Nesland 1987). This was addressed in a multicentre European study in which both endoscopic and histological features were correlated (Gad 1986). It was shown that as little as 42% of lesions diagnosed endoscopically as erosions had histological evidence of surface loss of epithelium. Thus, most of the lesions diagnosed macroscopically as erosions were revealed to be foci of acute inflammation with or without surface exudate, islands of intestinal metaplasia, areas of subepithelial capillary hyperaemia, and a variety of other lesions. A further problem is the fact that as a basic principle it seems likely that an inflamed gastric mucosa is prone to erosion of its surface epithelium, so "chronic erosive gastritis" may be only a stage in the evolution of several different forms of chronic gastritis. Indeed there is evidence that chronic erosions occur frequently in patients with type B, or diffuse antral, gastritis and that there is thus an association with prepyloric and duodenal ulceration (Karvonen et al 1987). Evidence emerged gradually that a separate form of chronic erosive gastritis also existed and that this was unrelated to type B gastritis or peptic ulceration. It corresponded to the varioliform gastritis of earlier authors (Lambert et al 1978) and was sometimes characterised by raised nodular lesions with an ulcerated or an intact surface epithelium that tended to occur in rows in the body of the stomach situated on the rugae and only sometimes extended into the antrum (Elta et al 1983, Franzin et al 1984). Unfortunately some reports included inadequate histological examination of the lesions (Gallagher, Lennon and Crowe 1987).

As a follow-up study to previous work Haot et al (1988) reviewed their cases characterised previously at endoscopy as erosive, varioliform, or aphthoid gastritis. When large folds predominated in the gastric body and were accompanied by nodules and erosions, the histological appearance of the neighbouring mucosa was said to show a characteristic picture, namely lymphocytic gastritis. In this lymphocytes appear in the surface and foveolar epithelium and are surrounded by a typical clear halo (Fig. 7–7). Gastric pits are elongated and tortuous but otherwise normal. Lymphocytes and plasma cells, although present in the lamina propria, may be few in number, but the density is variable and there is no correlation with the density of the intraepithelial lymphocyte population. In the vicinity of erosions the picture is obscured by the presence of more acute inflammation and the accumulation of polymorphs within the crypts. In the remaining cases of chronic erosive gastritis examined by Haot et al, the histological findings in the surrounding mucosa was said to be "nonspecific" and would usually be described as chronic atrophic gastritis. This is also the author's experience. It is essentially a lesion representing early peptic ulcer. Seemingly, therefore, Haot claimed that lymphocytic gastritis has a typical endoscopic appearance with nodules, erosions, and large folds predominating in the body. This has been reaffirmed (Haot et al 1989) after a review of the original cases of diffuse varioliform gastritis originally published by Lambert et al (1978). Some intraepithelial lymphocytes are seen in other forms of chronic gastritis, and some

Figure 7–7. Chronic gastritis with no significant polymorph infiltration but a prominent intraepithelial lymphocyte population (H&E ×350).

objective determination of what numbers constitute a diagnosis is needed. In children in whom quantitative studies have been carried out (De Giacomo et al 1994) it is claimed that in lymphocytic gastritis there is a mean of 40.64 lymphocytes per 100 epithelial cells, which is more than 10 times the number found in normal subjects and in the mucosa in gastritis associated with *H. pylori* colonisation. These same authors showed that the lymphocytes were T cells, confirming previous work by Mosnier et al (1991), who, like Haot et al (1991), also suggested a possible relationship between lymphocytic gastritis and Ménétrier's disease. Wolfsen, Carpenter and Talley (1993) in their study concluded that the two conditions were separate and distinct. Dixon et al (1988), however, also recognise lymphocytic gastritis as a distinct entity and believe that it is possibly the result of an abnormal response to antigens produced by *Campylobacter pylori* and that the condition is comparable to coeliac disease. A more direct relationship to coeliac disease was postulated by De Giacomo et al (1994), who, in contrast to the claims by Dixon et al, found no association between the presence of lymphocytic gastritis and evidence for *H. pylori* infection, although Groisman, Rosh and Harpaz (1994) describe resolution of lymphocytic gastritis with hypoproteinaemia when *H. pylori* was eradicated by appropriate therapy. The small bowel appearances in coeliac disease are not entirely specific. Nevertheless, Kawai et al (1970) postulated an immunological pathogenesis in the aetiology of chronic erosive gastritis, and Roesch and Warnatz (1974) demonstrated a decrease in immunoglobulin (Ig)M and an increase in IgG cells in the nodular lesions. Lambert et al (1977), however, described an increase in IgE cells, but all these phenomena may be secondary. In follow-up studies spanning 6 years, Freise et al (1979) found that the lesions remained static in 50% of cases and either disappeared or decreased in size in the other half. Farthing et al (1981) reported healing in patients receiving prednisolone therapy, and Elta et al (1983) reported healing following antacid treatment. Clarke, Lee and Nicholson (1977), no doubt also describing lymphocytic gastritis, and Farahat et al (1993) have drawn attention to it as a cause of protein-losing enteropathy. Varioliform or lymphocytic gastritis has also been described as a cause of massive gastric bleeding leading to gastrectomy (Vinograd et al 1993) and in association with lymphocytic colitis (Christ et al 1993). When erosions are present in varioliform gastritis the central epithelial deficit is seen to have a necrotic base but is bordered by hyperplastic, elongated, tortuous, and branched crypts composed of relatively undifferentiated cells.

The inflammatory changes in the surrounding mucosa appear to vary in severity (Fig. 7–8). In the lamina propria it can be minimal or marked and is characterised by an intraepithelial lymphocyte population that is abnormally conspicuous. The muscularis mucosa is always intact but may show hyperplasia. Cystic dilatation of deeper glands may occur, they may also exhibit pseudopyloric metaplasia when the lesion involves the body mucosa. A combination of foveolar and pseudopyloric glandular hyperplasia adds bulk to the lesion. The overall structure of this lesion accounts for its gross polypoidal character, and the central erosion gives the lesion a classic volcano-like form easily identified radiologically and endoscopically (Figs. 7–9 and 7–10). Thus, the Japanese have classified the lesion as a form of gastric polyp. Questions still remain as to when the diagnosis of lymphocytic gastritis can be made. Is it possible at a time when the mucosa is still nonverrucous and noneroded but shows an intraepithelial lymphocyte population that exceeds that seen in any other type of chronic gastritis? (Fig. 7–11) Or is it only possible when one assumes the later stages of verrucosity and ulceration occur? Much has yet to be done in defining this form of chronic gastritis with more accuracy.

Chronic Erosive Gastritis

Pathologists know that, despite the limited number of ways that tissues can react to noxious stimuli, different diseases can be recognised by the combination of ways these reactions appear grouped together. Such examples are plentiful in the

Figure 7–8. Lymphocytic gastritis with more marked cellularity of lamina propria than in Figure 7–7 (H&E ×400).

Figure 7–9. Healed chronic erosion with persistent tortuous and irregularly branched crypts and hyperplastic pyloric-type glands. Note the occasional cystic crypts and the mainly superficial inflammation (H&E ×75).

Figure 7–10. Detail of healed chronic erosion to show xanthelasmatous foamy macrophages in the lamina propria (H&E ×300).

Figure 7–11. Detail of the margin of a chronic erosion. Note the hyperplastic appearance and the inflammation characterised by numerous intraepithelial lymphocytes (H&E ×300).

recognition of the different forms of colitis, for example, and it is being increasingly recognised that similar attention needs to be given to chronic erosive gastritis. There are two central problems. First, there is the specificity or otherwise of the erosive aspect of the condition; second, there is the specificity or otherwise of the gastritis. In the stomach or duodenum pathologists accept the definition of erosion as a focus of loss of part of or the full thickness of the mucosa, not including the muscularis mucosa. Erosion implies the probability of healing without scarring and is a convenient way of differentiating erosion from the more advanced lesion of peptic ulcer. In reality this is somewhat artificial as presumably every ulcer starts life as an erosion, no matter how brief a life this may be. However, this does not deny the possibility that erosions may have different causes and a different natural life span related to the cause. It is also likely that this cause will be reflected in the histological appearance of the mucosa immediately related to the site of the erosion. Application of this reasoning gives grounds for the view that at least one form of chronic erosive gastritis is related to type B gastritis and is associated with peptic ulceration, probably as a precursor lesion being more frequently antral (Fig. 7–12). Other forms of erosion may well be related to the use of NSAIDs in patients who already have one or another form of chronic gastritis such as described by Publig, Wustinger and Zandl (1994).

Histologically therefore, this type of erosion would simply show superficial necrosis surrounded by mucosa showing features of chronic gastritis such as is seen, for example, in that with a type B or AB distribution. This may have acute or chronic inflammatory elements and a varying amount of metaplastic features and may or may not be associated with *H. pylori*. Erosions occurring in association with pure type C gastritis when an NSAID or a bile reflux effect is not complicating a preexisting chronic gastritis of another type should probably be regarded as acute (Fig. 7–13).

AETIOLOGY AND SIGNIFICANCE OF THE TYPES OF CHRONIC GASTRITIS

Aetiology

Although there is no direct evidence that repeated gastric mucosal injury or recurrent acute gastritis leads to chronic gastritis, this is commonly assumed. Much

Figure 7–12. Chronic erosions. Early lesion with regenerative tortuosity of the marginal crypts and associated inflammatory changes (H&E ×100).

Figure 7–13. Erosion complicating chemical (type C) gastritis. Note lack of inflammatory reaction (H&E ×100).

of the work in this area predated the recognition of the various types of chronic gastritis already discussed. Nevertheless many of the observations are worthy of consideration because even in retrospect they can be related to the forms of chronic gastritis that are recognised in modern times. Chronic gastritis of the body mucosa has been linked with chronic alcoholism, although the reported incidence varies from 10% to 70% (Joske, Finckh and Wood 1955, Williams 1956, Debray et al 1957, Parl et al 1979). Indirect evidence for a link comes from Dinoso et al (1972), who demonstrated an improvement in histological appearance in 12 alcoholics following abstinence of up to 9 months. The gastritis was described as either superficial or atrophic, but as these lesions are commonplace in subjects with type AB gastritis who are not alcoholics and increase in incidence with age (Kekki et al 1977), the significance of this observation loses some of its impact. Indeed, there is other evidence that tends to refute an association. Brown et al (1981), for example, reported that in patients with alcoholic cirrhosis the incidence of chronic gastritis is no higher than in control series. In the past blind biopsy studies have also shown that the drinking of hot liquids is associated with an increased incidence of chronic gastritis of the body of the stomach (Edwards and Edwards 1956); this suggests repeated trauma as a causative factor. Indeed, Correa (1982) makes a claim for dietary trauma due to highly salted food and hard grains in the food of those living in high incidence areas of type AB chronic gastritis. This finds support in the fact that the incidence of body gastritis increases in frequency with age (Andrews et al 1967). Cigarette smoking also seems to be important in some way (Edwards and Coghill 1966), and it is perhaps significant that both age and cigarette smoking are also related to atherosclerosis. Chronic peptic ulceration, which is always associated with either type B or type AB chronic gastritis, is much more common in patients with severe atherosclerosis, especially if there is aortic calcification and particularly if atheromatous aneurysms are present (Elkeles 1964, Jones, Kirk and Bloor 1970). The effect of smoking on vessels and on the stomach may be quite separate. Jarvis and Whitehead (1980), for example, showed that administration of nicotine to rats in their drinking water resulted in a decrease in the mucus-producing component of the gastric mucosa. Theoretically this would tend to decrease its ability to withstand the effect of any other ingested agents, with a resulting propensity for gastric mucosal injury.

The association between types B and AB gastritis and chronic peptic ulcer provides presumptive evidence for an association between gastritis and chronic renal failure, hyperparathyroidism, cardiovascular disease other than hypertension, cirrhosis of the liver, and chronic respiratory disease, in all of which peptic ulcer incidence is elevated (Langman and Cooke, 1976).

Edwards and Coghill (1966) also showed an increased incidence of presumptive AB chronic gastritis in the lower social classes and in those subjects who have blue eyes, which suggests a possible genetic predisposition. Further evidence for this came from the family studies of Varis (1981) and Kekki and Villako (1981) in Finnish and Estonian populations. In a blind biopsy follow-up study Siurala and Salmi (1971) showed that superficial gastritis develops with time into atrophic gastritis.

However, this seems not to be so in all types of gastritis. Siurala, Sipponen and Kekki (1985), for example, showed that whereas type A body gastritis progresses rapidly, changes in the antrum tend to resolve. In type B associated with prepyloric or duodenal ulcer gastritis persists and gets worse in the antrum but does not seem to progress to affect the body unless antrectomy is performed. In high gastric ulcers the body gastritis associated with it tends to progress rapidly, whereas that in the antrum does not. Thus, it is becoming increasingly clear that there are different forms of simple gastritis and that the aetiology is complex. Combinations of environmental and genetic factors coupled with pathophysiological disturbances causing autoimmune phenomena, hypersecretion, or reflux of duodenal contents all seem to interplay in the production of a chronic mucosal damage. At least in some forms this chronic damage seems to be punctuated by acute episodes characterised by more obvious epithelial injury and polymorphonuclear leukocyte infiltration. There is some biopsy evidence (McIntyre, Irani and Piris 1981) that this mechanism operates in the gastritis associated with prolonged NSAID therapy, but at least in the early stages acute or chronic inflammation usually does not appear as part of the mucosal damage associated with these agents (personal observation). However, that prolonged use does cause gastric ulceration, which is most often prepyloric, seems proven (Roth and Bennett 1987), but the position is complicated by the fact that NSAIDs may be used by a large number of patients who already have a chronic gastritis related to other factors. The case for their ulcerogenicity seems proven in the face of the evidence and the fact that prevention of NSAIDs-associated peptic ulceration can be achieved therapeutically by a synthetic prostaglandin E analogue (Graham, Agrawal and Roth 1988).

It therefore seems likely both that superficial gastritis can progress to atrophic gastritis and that so-called gastric atrophy is an end stage of atrophic gastritis. This appears to be true of gastritis occurring both with and without peptic ulceration. There are claims (Roesch, Demling and Elster 1975) that although progression is usual, regression from atrophic gastritis to normal may occur in gastritis that would now probably be regarded as type AB if it is not associated with ulcers. The implication is considerable, i.e., the possible reversibility of a highly cancer-prone situation. More evidence related to this is clearly desirable.

The controversy related to the role of *H. pylori* in the aetiology of acute gastric inflammation, chronic gastritis, and peptic ulceration has already been referred to in detail. Credibility for an association stems in large measure from the claim by Marshall et al (1985) to have fulfilled Koch's postulates for the organism in that an acute transient gastritis followed ingestion of a laboratory culture by a human volunteer. The experience was repeated by another group (Morris and Nicholson 1987) with apparently similar results, but in both the organism flourished in the stomach only if drug-induced hypochlorhydria was artificially induced prior to challenge with the organism. Moreover, there is a considerable body of evidence that is counter to a simple one-to-one aetiological role for this organism in causing either acute or chronic gastritis; hence its precise relationship to peptic ulcer. It is obviously a ubiquitous bacterium and in the right circumstances can flourish in the stomach, but further investigation is required as to its precise role. Until then there will continue to be reports with conflicting accounts of its role in the cause of peptic ulceration in the duodenum and stomach (Amarapurkar et al 1993, Appelman 1994).

Significance

The ability to secrete acid, pepsinogen, and intrinsic factor is reduced as the body mucosa atrophies (Glass et al 1960), but normally the ability to produce some intrinsic factor persists longer than that to secrete appreciable acid. This is interesting because in humans both are produced by the parietal cell (Hoedemaeker et al 1964). It may be simply a reflection of the volumes of the two products secreted normally and their relative biological activity.

As atrophic gastritis progresses the pattern of mucoprotein secretion alters, and albumin and globulin in high concentrations may be found in the gastric juice (Glass and Ishimori 1961, Glass 1965). Diffuse atrophic gastritis with a persistent loss of albumin from the gastric mucosa has been postulated as a cause of otherwise obscure hypoalbuminaemia that occurs in elderly patients (Coghill 1969).

Despite these disturbances of function the evidence that chronic gastritis of the body mucosa is associated with dyspepsia is far from convincing (Joske, Finckh and Wood 1955, Shiner and Doniach 1957, Coghill 1960, Hojgaard, Matzen and Christoffersen 1987, Talley and Phillips 1988). There can be no doubt that chronic gastritis of the body mucosa can be present in patients who have no symptoms referable to the stomach, whereas many who complain of persistent dyspepsia have neither peptic ulcer nor body gastritis. In a study of dyspepsia patients in whom gross gastric, duodenal, pancreatic, and hepatic conditions were excluded as far as possible, Cheli, Perasso and Giacosa (1983) showed that the incidence of antral and body gastritis was the same as in a control group. They concluded that gastritis was not a cause of dyspepsia "sine materia."

It has been shown repeatedly that the incidence of body gastritis in patients with iron deficiency anaemia is 30%–60% (Badenoch, Evans and Richards 1957, Coghill and Williams (1958), and gastritis of the body mucosa is more common in those who have no other known cause for iron deficiency. The view that iron deficiency causes gastritis is unfounded; follow-up studies (Ikkala and Siurala 1964, Ikkala, Salmi and Siurala 1970) show that gastritis persists after the anaemia has been treated and that recurrent anaemia is seen more frequently in those patients in whom the gastritis progresses in severity. This indicates that the gastritis might be the cause of the anaemia. In postgastrectomy patients, for example, there is a significant blood loss from the atrophic gastric mucosa of the gastric remnant (Holt, Gear and Warner 1970). In addition, patients with atrophic gastritis show an increase in free iron loss (Sutton et al 1970) that undoubtedly is related to the markedly raised rate of cell turnover that occurs in this condition.

The levels of serum gastrin in relation to chronic gastritis have been studied intensively in peptic ulcer patients (Byrnes et al 1970, Korman, Soveney and Hansky 1971, 1972). The most usual findings are raised levels in patients with gastric ulcer or with Zollinger-Ellison syndrome and low levels in patients with duodenal ulcer. There is usually, however, a greater response in patients with duodenal ulcer than in normal patients or in patients with gastric ulcer after given protein foods, but the highest stimulated levels are seen in patients with Zollinger-Ellison syndrome. It has also been shown that patients with pernicious anaemia have high levels (McGuigan and Trudeau 1970). Another study has directly related gastrin levels specifically to antral gastritis. Fasting serum levels are decreased in patients with atrophic gastritis only if the antrum is relatively unaffected (Strickland et al 1971).

Morson (1955) has shown that atrophic gastritis with intestinal metaplasia is seen in more than 90% of cases of cancer of the stomach. After 25 years the incidence of cancer in patients who have had a gastrectomy or gastroenterostomy for either duodenal or gastric ulcer is six times the expected rate (Stalsberg and Taksdal 1971), and gastritis in these patients is the rule (Schrumpf et al 1977). Deaths from gastric cancer occur with three and four times the expected frequency in patients with pernicious anaemia (Mosbech and Videbaek 1950, Blackburn et al 1968). In a follow-up study of atrophic gastritis of type AB unassociated with pernicious anaemia, Siurala and Seppala (1960) showed that approximately 10% develop cancer and that as this form of gastritis occurs numerically so much more often, it constitutes a much larger risk and a more important precancerous condition than pernicious anaemia. There is evidence even for significantly greater cancer risk than normal in a stomach that is merely the site of chronic superficial gastric mucosal inflammation (Sipponen et al 1994). Indeed, in a population-based study Schafer et al (1985) could find no strong indication for endoscopic surveillance of asymptomatic patients with pernicious anaemia with a view to detecting treatable carcinoma.

There is evidence that carcinoma arising in chronic gastritis does so through progressive dysplasia involving the areas of intestinalisation (Morson et al 1980, Antonioli 1994). Furthermore, the tumour arising in such circumstances is of the so-called intestinal type (Lauren 1965); studies suggest that the intestinal mucosa from which it arises is of colonic (type 3) rather than small intestinal type. This has been based on the histochemical characterisation of epithelial mucins (Jass and Filipe 1979, 1981, Filipe et al 1985, Silva and Filipe 1986, Filipe et al 1994). This is disputed by Stemmermann (1994), who believes that it is the extent of metaplastic process that is important and not its subtype as based on the identification of enzymes and mucosubstances. It is this type of carcinoma that forms the excess of tumours in those countries with a high incidence of gastric cancer, and it would be in keeping with the relative incidence of carcinoma arising in the small and large intestine. However, Ramesar, Sanders and Hopwood (1987) found that typing intestinal metaplasia in biopsies is of little value in identifying patients at risk of gastric adenocarcinoma. Furthermore, type 3, or large intestinal–type metaplasia, is uncommon in the gastric remnant harbouring a carcinoma (Bedossa, Lemaigre and Martin 1987a). Indeed, Rubio et al (1987) believe that incomplete or type 3 intestinal metaplasia may be a paraneoplastic rather than a preneoplastic phenomenon. It would certainly seem that dysplasia and preneoplastic changes can be seen in nonintestinalised epithelium (Ghandur-Mnaymneh et al 1988), and it is postulated that this phenomenon is important in the genesis of the diffuse type of gastric carcinoma. At the same time dysplasia can also be seen in association with intestinalised epithelium in stomachs that are also the site of intestinal-type carcinomas (Saraga, Gardiol and Costa 1987). More recently the cancer risk has been equated to the presence in the intestinalised mucosa of the number of atypical mitoses (Rubio, Kato and Kitagawa 1994). There thus appears to be a strong association between chronic gastritis of type A, type B, and type AB and the development of carcinoma of the stomach. The nature of this association is still in doubt. However, electron microscope (Tarpila, Telkka and Siurala 1969), immunological (De Boer, Forsyth and Nairn 1969), and histochemical (Stemmermann 1967, Sasano et al 1969) studies have shown that almost all gastric cancers have a proportion of cells with characteristics of intestinal epithelium. Cells with intestinal characteristics are also found in normal gastric mucosa towards the bottom of the gastric pits, and this is known to be the area associated with proliferation and cell renewal. In gastritis there is a tendency for the intestinal type of cell to be produced, and in atrophic gastritis with a markedly increased cell turnover cancer might well be expected to supervene in a proportion of cases. These circumstances may explain why cancer and intestinal metaplasia are so commonly associated. What is less easily understood is why, although gastric carcinoma and pernicious anaemia occur most frequently in association with blood group A, there is no increased incidence of blood group A in those patients with atrophic gastritis who have obvious intestinal metaplasia in their gastric mucosa (Glober et al 1972).

The association of widespread atrophic gastritis and intestinal metaplasia with the development of cancer has important clinical connotations. Skinner, Heenan and Whitehead (1975) showed that the gastritis and intestinal metaplasia associated with peptic ulcer of the body of the stomach has a similar distribution and severity to that seen with gastric cancer but that it is more localised with pyloric ulcer. In cases of recurrent stomal or pyloric ulcer after gastrojejunostomy for duodenal ulcer, however, the gastrectomy specimen shows a distribution and severity of gastritis that is also like that seen in cancer. This similarity points to a higher cancer risk in the stomach with body ulcer and after gastrojejunostomy; Lundegardh et al (1988) showed that stomach cancer is indeed more common in patients operated on for gastric ulcer than those operated on for duodenal ulcer. For duodenal ulcer Polya's gastrectomy operation as opposed to varieties of vagotomy and antrectomy or drainage appears to be associated with a higher cancer risk (Lygidakis 1986). Nevertheless it is plain that the choice of surgical treatment of peptic ulcer that ensures cure must be influenced by the relative postoperative tendencies to accelerate the premalignant condition of chronic gastritis of both type B and AB and possibly that due to or accentuated by bile reflux (Kliems et al 1979, Assad and Eastwood 1980, Kekki et al 1980, Saukkonen et al 1980, Graem et al 1981, Dougherty, Foster and Eisenberg 1982). It has been argued whether the risk of cancer is wholly related to the surgical intervention for ulcer disease or whether the disease process itself is responsible and the surgery is incidental (Hermanek and Riemann 1982). It seems much more likely that it is the addition of a further dimension of disturbance of gastric function that increases the rate of the progress of the basic disease process, that is, the chronic gastritis. Thus, if some form of gastric operation is found necessary for the treatment of peptic ulcers, the chances of subsequent development of cancer is so high that a case can be made for interval gastroscopy and multiple biopsy, as early asymptomatic cancer can be present in such stomachs (Schrumpf et al 1977). At this stage the cancer is more amenable to complete cure; this was highlighted by Pointner et al (1988) in their report of early gastric cancer in the gastric remnant.

There is no convincing information beyond the anecdotal (Mosnier et al 1991) on a relationship between varioliform or lymphocytic gastritis and susceptibility to gastric cancer. The association of lymph follicle formation with *H. pylori* associated gastritis has already been cited. It has been regarded as a precursor of gastric lymphoma (Isaacson and Spencer 1987, Wotherspoon et al 1991, 1993, Harris 1993, Diss et al 1993) that opens the door to a possible cure in its developing stage by antibiotic therapy. Evidence is accumulating that this may be the case (Stolte and Eidt 1993, Chan 1994). It would be of interest to know whether gastric lymphoma incidence is high in those underdeveloped countries where *H. pylori* colonisation reaches almost 100%.

SUMMARY

Although there is some general agreement for the validity of this classification, it is still controversial and the reasons for this are manifold. The proper and careful categorisation of any individual case of chronic gastritis requires a detailed clinicopathological evaluation and demands a close working relationship between the clinician obtaining biopsy samples of the stomach and the histopathologist who examines them. The sites of biopsy must be carefully recorded. This is because of the overriding importance of the topography of the histological changes of gastritis as opposed to the changes themselves, which can be so similar even in the different types of gastritis. It is for this reason that the so-called Sydney system (Price 1991) of classifying chronic gastritis has been severely criticised (Correa and Yardley 1992, Kimura et al 1994). Advocating only two antral and two body biopsies in order to assess and classify any particular case of gastritis, especially when multifocal atrophic gastritis characteristically begins at the angulus and could thus easily be miscategorised has been emphasized.

The role of *H. pylori* in the aetiology of the various forms of gastritis is also not as clearly defined as some believe. Even in relation to diffuse antral gastritis and duodenal ulcer in particular, let alone peptic ulcer generally, intestinal metaplasia and through this to gastric adenocarcinoma, there are conflicting pieces of evidence. Much of the data has been derived from the developed countries, yet in parts of Africa, for example, despite a nearly 100% incidence of *H. pylori* in the adult population, peptic ulcer and gastric adenocarcinoma are rare (Holcombe 1992). In Colombia, South America (Correa et al 1990) *H. pylori* is associated not with diffuse antral gastritis but with multifocal atrophic gastritis; whereas gastric ulcer and adenocarcinoma are common, duodenal ulcer is rarely seen. The distinction between diffuse corporal and multifocal atrophic gastritis in those parts of the Northern Hemisphere where pernicious anaemia is common is also an obvious area of difficulty. It is claimed that views on the nature of chronic gastritis based on studies in the Scandinavian countries in particular may have confused the situation in relation to its classification (Correa and Yardley 1992). There is also an apparent discrepancy in the relative incidence of the intestinal as opposed to diffuse type of gastric cancer in areas of high incidence of *H. pylori* infestation (Wee, Kang and Teh 1992) that throws some doubt on the claimed role of *H. pylori* in inducing intestinal metaplasia and thus of having an aetiological role in adenocarcinoma. It is also claimed that in the elderly it is bile reflux, rather than the presence of *H. pylori* that seems to be most strongly related to intestinal metaplasia and adenocarcinoma (Sobala et al 1993). Also in the elderly it seems to be the use of NSAIDs rather than *H. pylori* that is aetiological for peptic ulcer disease (Wyatt et al 1992). Furthermore, the claims that lymphocytic gastritis is related to Ménétrier's disease and that lymphocytic gastritis is part of the spectrum of coeliac disease are speculative at this stage.

Clearly one is thus prompted to draw the conclusion that in many cases of chronic gastritis the causes are multifactorial. There is certainly strong evidence that genetic influences may play a part. Undoubtedly inherited tendencies acting through autoimmune mechanisms play a role in the cause of diffuse atrophic corporal gastritis and possibly lymphocytic gastritis. Hereditary factors have a role in determining the occurrence of familial gastric cancer, which is preceded by multifocal chronic atrophic gastritis in many instances; at least it frequently occurs in that background. The tendency to a high incidence of gastric cancer in certain racial groups may also be in part genetically determined. There is an increased incidence of blood group O nonsecretors in patients with duodenal ulcer and diffuse antral gastritis. Thus, for several types of chronic gastritis there is evidence that genetic or hereditary factors have a role in aetiology. As for environmental factors there is also clear evidence that several are involved. Diet probably plays a significant role; salty foods and those rich in nitrosamine compounds appear to be related to multifocal atrophic gastritis. Infection with *H. pylori* and possibly other pathogens appears to be involved with diffuse antral gastritis and possibly multifocal atrophic gastritis also. Drugs, and NSAIDs in particular, are related to chemical gastritis. Bile reflux is also a cause of chemical gastritis and particularly of the acquisition of intestinal metaplasia and hence a predisposition to adenocarcinoma.

Although more or less identifiable groups of chronic gastritis undeniably occur in any individual case, there is a good chance that more than one aetiological factor comes into play either conjointly or temporally; this tends to blur the edges of the classification groups. For example, patients with chronic gastritis primarily of one type might have this altered by gastric surgery or develop bile reflux or autoimmune mucosal damage and need to take NSAIDs. In reality, this happens and thus it needs to be realised that the classification of chronic gastritis is still evolving. Its continued study and the relationship with serious disease processes such as peptic ulcer, gastric adenocarcinoma, and malignant lymphoma provide a very important ongoing challenge.

8

GASTRIC EPITHELIAL DYSPLASIA AND EARLY GASTRIC CANCER, MUCOSAL HYPERPLASIA, EPITHELIAL POLYPS AND POLYPOSIS, LYMPHOID HYPERPLASIA AND MALIGNANT LYMPHOMA

GASTRIC EPITHELIAL DYSPLASIA AND EARLY GASTRIC CANCER

In parallel with experience in other organs and epithelial surfaces, the identification of early cancer of the stomach has resulted in the delineation of even earlier stages of the disease, namely malignant dysplasia (Schade 1974, Oehlert et al 1975, 1979, Borchard, Mittelstaedt and Kieker 1979, Cuello et al 1979, Meister et al 1979, Morson et al 1980, Farini et al 1981, Ming et al 1984). Dysplasia is commonly, but not always, associated with areas of intestinal metaplasia of incomplete type, and it occurs in flat as well as polypoidal lesions (Jass 1983). It is perhaps significant that this type of metaplasia is similar to that which occurs in Barrett's oesophagus, another site of the dysplasia-cancer sequence. However, dysplastic features occur independently of intestinalisation, and there are claims (Ghandur-Mnaymneh et al 1988) that this type of metaplasia is related more closely to the development of the diffuse as opposed to the intestinal type of carcinoma. However, the distinction between intestinal and diffuse is somewhat artificial in terms of the pathobiology of gastric cancer, although it has some value in providing insight into possible aetiology and its precursor or associated lesions. It is thus not surprising that descriptions of dysplasia have involved the use of different terminology to describe a subjective impression of increasing architectural and cytological atypia, i.e., dysplasia that at its end point qualifies as carcinoma in situ. The difficulties that such exercises created in the past have resulted in such categories as "borderline" and "probably carcinoma" (Nagayo 1972) and the suggestion that "carcinoma in situ" as a term should be abandoned. Morson et al (1980), for example, suggested that any lesion still confined by epithelial basement membrane should be designated as severe dysplasia and that when invasion of the lamina propria is demonstrated the lesion be called intramucosal carcinoma. This, however, is clearly not satisfactory for small endoscopic biopsy

Figure 8–1. Mildly dysplastic appearances largely due to nuclear size changes and staining intensity. There is also an inflammatory component (H&E ×150).

interpretation and reporting. It is not possible to make such a diagnosis unless the gastrectomy specimen is available, because the malignant tissue may not be entirely intramucosal. Consequently it is now advocated that the problem of differentiating between true dysplasia and regenerative dysplasia be recognised and that atypical features, such as nuclear enlargement, hyperchromasia, loss of differentiation, a high mitotic rate, glands sharing a common "party wall," and abnormal patterns of cell orientation and mucin secretion, produce a range of true dysplastic appearances that culminate in an appearance that is histologically similar to some carcinomas but is still confined by a basement membrane, i.e., carcinoma in situ (Figs. 8–1 to 8–6). For the time being these abnormalities are best conveyed to the clinician in terms of mild, moderate, or severe dysplasia; the use of the term "carcinoma in situ" may

Figure 8–2. Detached epithelium that appears abnormal because of nuclear abnormalities and an abnormal disposition of cells (H&E ×300).

Figure 8–3. Abnormality of nuclei and cytoplasm, with ''party-walling'' giving an appearance of in situ signet ring cells (H&E ×600).

result in overexuberant treatment, which, at our present state of knowledge, is not justified. This is reinforced by the findings in an 11-year histological follow-up study by Saraga, Gardiol and Costa (1987), who showed that in 85 patients in whom dysplasia was diagnosed, 17 out of 18 diagnosed as severe dysplasia developed a carcinoma, whereas 1 from 41 with moderate and 0 from 23 with mild dysplasia did so. More recent studies have confirmed that the chances of dysplasia evolving into invasive carcinoma increase proportionally with increasing degrees of dysplasia (Di Gregorio et al 1993, Farinati et al 1993, Fertitta et al 1993, Antonioli 1994, Rugge et al 1994). There is evidence that in patients at high risk for the development of gastric adenocarcinoma, such as those who have undergone previous gastric surgery, endoscopic surveillance and biopsy for the detection of dysplasia and early cancer

Figure 8–4. Features are sufficiently abnormal to be regarded as in situ carcinoma (H&E ×300).

Figure 8–5. Features are sufficiently abnormal to be regarded as in situ carcinoma (H&E ×300).

may be justified (Sowa et al 1993, Stael von Holstein et al 1993). In other at-risk groups, such as pernicious anaemia patients (Hsing et al 1993), evidence is accumulating that regular endoscopic surveillance may be justified, especially for young patients (Sjoblom, Sipponen and Jarvinen 1993). It was suggested in a Japanese study that atypical mitoses in gastric intestinal metaplasia may be an even earlier marker than frank dysplasia for the development of gastric adenocarcinoma (Rubio, Kato and Kitagawa 1993).

Hyperplasia and regeneration of ulcerated gastric mucosa may mimic dysplastic changes, but there is usually but not always a prominent inflammatory infiltration with polymorph invasion between the epithelial cells, which consequently may also show degenerative appearances in some areas (Figs. 8–7 and 8–8). With experience, differentiation between true dysplasia and regenerative dysplasia is usually easy, but

Figure 8–6. Features are sufficiently abnormal to be regarded as in situ carcinoma (H&E ×300).

Figure 8–7. Gastric biopsy of a benign ulcer edge. There are mild epithelial cell abnormalities due to regeneration. Note scarring of lamina propria (H&E ×300).

Figure 8–8. Gastric biopsy of a benign ulcer edge. The abnormalities are more severe than in Figure 8–7, and there is more palisading of nuclei, although the cells mature towards the surface *(arrowhead)* (H&E ×300).

from the practical standpoint, if there is doubt it is advisable to repeat the endoscopy and obtain further biopsy specimens. A useful pointer in regenerative atypia is for the cells to show a tendency to mature towards the surface, but even this may not be seen in earlier regenerative change; hence the need sometimes to perform another biopsy. There will inevitably be an unclassifiable group, but this should be progressively smaller as experience increases. It is the persistence of abnormal features in sequential biopsies that justifiably supports a diagnosis of true dysplasia. There is some evidence that dysplasia in situ may be recognisable even cytologically (Seppala, Lehtola and Siurala 1976). Efforts to diagnose these possibly earlier stages of carcinoma also include the use of dyes. Just before endoscopy the dyes are introduced into the stomach for the purpose of directing the biopsy to areas of intestinal metaplasia, dysplasia, or small foci of cancer. Methylene blue (Suzuki et al 1973), toluidine blue (Giler, Kadish and Urca 1976), indigo carmine (Ida et al 1975), and the combined Congo red–methylene blue (Tatsuta et al 1982) are just some of the dye methods that have been used. Dysplasia apparently may exist for many years before becoming invasive carcinoma (Loux and Zamcheck 1969). Obviously with the more precise delineation of dysplasia or precancer, great strides forward in the area of cancer prevention are to be made. There is evidence that morphometric methods similar to those already applied in the cytological diagnosis of malignancy (Boon et al 1981) may also be developed for use in biopsy tissues. Already the shortcomings of the subjective classification of dysplasia have been the stimulus to use a computerised measuring system in the analysis of its various features (Jarvis and Whitehead 1985), and there is also increasing evidence that such methods may have a real place in the assessment of these early stages of gastric malignancy (Tosi et al 1987). In the meantime pathologists need to begin to recognise true dysplasia so that patients can be sequentially subjected to endoscopy and further biopsies. Much more of the natural history of carcinoma of the stomach will then unfold.

The diagnosis of the earlier stages of carcinoma of the stomach is now commonplace. These show certain distinctive macroscopic appearances and have been classified by the Japanese Gastroenterological Endoscopical Society according to whether the lesion is raised above the surface and whether there is ulceration. Raised carcinomas account for only one quarter of the cases and tend to occur more often either in the distal or the proximal stomach (Mori et al 1987, Ohta et al 1987) rather than the body. The principal application of the classification appears to be in the accurate communication of endoscopy appearances between endoscopists. However, it has a greater value if it serves to draw the attention of the endoscopist to a different macroscopic form of stomach cancer that is potentially curable, as seems to be the case even in those countries that lagged behind Japan in the recognition of this form of gastric adenocarcinoma (Guadagni et al 1993, Sue-Ling et al 1992, 1993), especially if the treatment includes lymph node dissection (Baba et al 1995) as opposed to local endoscopic resection (Sano, Kobori and Muto 1992, Takechi et al 1992). Although first described in Japan, early gastric cancer has since been recognised worldwide (Evans et al 1978, Elster et al 1979, Ostertag and Georgii 1979, Seifert et al 1979, Green et al 1981, Goldstein et al 1983, Bogomoletz 1984, Grigioni et al 1984, O'Brien et al 1985, White et al 1985, Lehnert et al 1989, Olivera, Nobre-Leitao and Chaves 1992, Lin et al 1994). It is generally regarded not as a lesion fundamentally different from advanced gastric cancer, but only at an early stage of development (Leocata et al 1993). Early and late gastric cancer have been shown, for example, to have similar DNA distribution patterns (Macartney, Camplejohn and Powell 1986, Czerniak, Herz and Koss 1987). Its recognition and study have made it clear that the evolution of the advanced stage of the disease occurs during a long period of up to 15 years or more (Fujita 1978). It has even been argued on the basis of follow-up endoscopic studies in high-risk patients that delaying surgery for early gastric cancer can be justified (Bodner, Pointner and Glaser 1988). Certainly, cases are on record of early gastric cancer remaining unchanged for 7 years (Eckardt et al 1984), although very rarely early gastric cancer is associated with liver metastasis (Ohta et al 1993). Early gastric cancer is thus a useful term, for its diagnosis has meaning in a much better prognosis for the patient following appropriate therapy. There is some evidence, however, that early gastric cancers in young adults have a more aggressive behaviour than tumours arising in older age groups (Fujimoto et al 1994).

Early cancer is defined as a tumour that does not extend beyond the mucosa or submucosa, even though there may be lymph node metastases. Clearly, early gastric cancer can (1) be in situ, i.e., confined by the epithelial basement membrane; (2) be intramucosal, i.e., confined by the muscularis mucosa, but invading the lamina propria; or (3) invade the muscularis mucosa and submucosa. Histological examination reveals the same tumour types as in the usual carcinoma of stomach, and it is likely that early gastric cancer is the early stage of development of ordinary gastric cancer. Fukuda et al (1988) describe a rare small-cell early gastric carcinoma that, like its advanced counterpart, also exhibited argyrophilia and evidence of squamous differentiation. Likewise, early Epstein-Barr virus–associated early gastric cancer of typical morphology with lace-like or branching formations of carcinoma cells is surrounded by a lymphocytic infiltrate (Takano, Kato and Sugano 1994, Uemura et al 1994).

One macroscopic variety deserves special mention in that it mimics peptic ulceration (Gear et al 1969, Mountford et al 1980, Chan et al 1992), and intramucosal cancer has been observed to ulcerate and heal repeatedly (Sakita et al 1971). It cannot be stressed too forcibly that all stomach ulcers should be examined histologically. Biopsies should be taken from the base as well as the edge (Hatfield et al 1975), and six from each site appears to be the smallest number that ensures the maximum "pick-up" rate, those from the base giving only a slightly smaller yield than those from the edge (Lin et al 1989). It has been shown that early carcinoma may be revealed only after repeated endoscopy and biopsy of apparently benign ulcers (Farinati et al 1987). When biopsy examination is combined with brush cytology the success rate is highest (Witzel et al 1976, Halter et al 1977, Chambers and Clark 1986), 95%–100%.

To the pathologist the diagnosis of early cancer does not differ from that of established cancer. The difficulties are the same, the problem of arriving at a definite diagnosis on relatively minute tissue samples. The histological diagnosis of carcinoma may be obvious where there is invasion beyond the muscularis mucosa (Fig. 8–9). However, the biopsy specimens frequently do not contain tissue deep to the muscularis mucosa, and some other guidelines are then necessary. A common situation is the presence of abnormal but gland-forming epithelium in which the component cells are so bizarre that the diagnosis of carcinoma can be made with confidence. The question arises whether this epithelium is still confined by the epithelial basement membrane, i.e., is it an in situ growth or is it invasive? The only guide to invasiveness when the biopsy is small and does not include deeper structures is the nature of the tissue that surrounds the abnormal glandular epithelium. Invasive carcinoma invariably excites around itself a more or less dense desmoplastic stromal reaction (Fig. 8–10). If abnormal glandular epithelium is surrounded by normal lamina propria, therefore, it should be regarded as carcinoma in situ (Fig. 8–11). Biopsies from benign gastric ulcers can mimic this appearance when the healing process traps glandular elements. Generally the glands are not atypical, and the fibrous tissue is not usually as homogeneous or dense but possesses more of the characteristics of granulation tissue (Fig. 8–12). Invasive carcinoma can also be diagnosed with confidence when individual or small abnormal groups of malignant cells can be identified in the lamina propria (Fig. 8–13). This may occur on occasion without an obvious stromal reaction, especially with signet ring cell carcinoma. Slides stained by a method for mucin are particularly useful in the diagnosis of this type of carcinoma. Sometimes only a few malignant cells are present that may be inconspicuous in ordinary haematoxylin and eosin (H&E) preparations but that become obvious with a mucin stain (Fig. 8–14). Microscopically, therefore, early gastric cancer may have an adenocarcinomatous or tubopapillary pattern or it may be anaplastic. The latter

Figure 8–9. Carcinomatous tissue mingling with and deep to elements of the muscularis mucosa *(left)*. Compare with the uninvolved but traumatised mucosa *(right)* (H&E ×60).

Figure 8–10. Malignant acini surrounded by a dense fibrous tumour stroma (H&E ×90).

Figure 8–11. In situ malignant acini surrounded by a normal lamina propria (H&E ×90).

Figure 8–12. Normal acini surrounded by granulation tissue in a benign ulcer margin (H&E ×150).

Figure 8–13. Individual signet ring carcinoma cells in the lamina propria (H&E ×350).

Figure 8–14. Individual malignant cells *(dark dots)* stained by the PAS method (PAS ×40).

is usually of classic signet cell ring cell type or mucocellular, but mixtures of the two are also seen. The appearances do not differ from that of late gastric carcinoma (Elster et al 1979). It is of some interest that it is the tumours of adenocarcinomatous pattern that are more likely to metastasise and, in contrast to advanced carcinoma of this type, have a worse prognosis than the diffuse form.

There seems to be no reason why superficial spreading carcinoma (Figs. 8–15 and 8–16) should be regarded as a separate entity. Unless it can be shown that it always remains intramucosal despite involving large areas of the stomach, it is sensible to regard it as another macroscopic form of early cancer because, histologically, it is usually anaplastic or the signet ring type.

Since Balfour (1922) first described carcinoma in patients treated for ulcer by partial gastrectomy, the subject has generated a considerable literature (Farrands et al 1983, Totten, Burns and Kay 1983, Offerhaus et al 1984a, 1984b, Pickford et al 1984, Clark, Fresini and Gledhill 1985, Lundegardh et al 1988, Pointner et al 1988). Although there are opinions to the contrary, most authors advocate follow-up endoscopy and biopsy of patients who have had previous gastric surgery. There is controversy, however, as to when this surveillance should begin and how often it should be carried out. Certainly 20 to 25 years after the operation the chance of finding cancer is very real. In view of the probable time span associated with the development of advanced carcinoma in a nonoperated stomach, a case for beginning surveillance soon after surgery could and has been made (Sowa et al 1993, Stael von Holstein et al 1993).

MUCOSAL HYPERPLASIAS, MÉNÉTRIER'S DISEASE, CRONKHITE-CANADA SYNDROME, EPITHELIAL POLYPS AND POLYPOSIS

Fibreoptic gastroscopy has revealed that gastric polyps are not as rare as was once believed. In particular it is now commonplace for polyps of 1 cm or less in size to be removed at endoscopic examination. Because of the diverse pathological nature of polypoidal lesions, polypectomy by snare may be neither possible nor the best form of treatment. Each case should be considered on its merits, but there

Figure 8–15. Excised stomach specimen, normal pyloric mucosa on the left and intramucosal carcinoma on the right (H&E ×315).

Figure 8–16. Detail of intramucosal carcinoma in Figure 8–15 (H&E ×375).

would seem to be a place for biopsy of a majority of large polypoidal lesions so that something of their nature can be ascertained before deciding appropriate therapy.

However, polypoidal lesions caused by abnormalities of the deeper gastric tissues may not be revealed in the relatively superficial fibreoptic biopsy unless the lesion is ulcerated. Although the term "polyp" embraces all lesions of the mucosa, submucosa, and muscularis that cause a protrusion into the gastric lumen, from the clinical standpoint the term is most commonly used in reference to lesions composed of the mucosal elements. The particular importance of epithelial polyps lies in their relationship to carcinoma, for more than half of all polyps are asymptomatic. Symptoms are usually the result of erosion and bleeding or are secondary to the polyp's bulk or its obstruction of cardia or pylorus. There are several classifications of gastric polyps and polyposis syndromes (Nakamura 1970, Elster 1976, Ming 1977, Nakamura and Nakano 1985); whereas it is possible to match one type in one classification with a similar one in another, the lack of uniformity of nomenclature and omission of certain polyp types is unsatisfactory. Furthermore, not all classifications address themselves to the problem of the definition of "polyposis" and its relationship, if any, to the stomach with more than one polyp, on the one hand, and a diffuse, polypoidal, hyperplastic mucosal lesion on the other. Biopsy and the facility for excision of epithelial polyps demand a clear and comprehensive classification. Epithelial polyps presumably arise either by an abnormal stimulation of cell growth, i.e., hyperplasia, in excess of that required for normal mucosal integrity or by a more complete loss of control over mucosal kinetics, i.e., neoplasia. Thus, whereas a hyperplastic group and a neoplastic group of polyps might be recogised, there is reason to believe that a hyperplastic process may at any time revert to normal or, alternatively, become truly neoplastic. By this reasoning it is possible to predict that hyperplastic polypoidal reactions will have histological similarities not only if focal in form but also if they involve more or less the whole of the gastric mucosa, thus constituting a diffuse mucosal hyperplasia or a polyposis. Furthermore, the occasional development of neoplasia in a longstanding hyperplastic condition is also, as in other organs, predictable. The turnover of gastric surface epithelial mucous cells is rapid, with a cell cycle time of 2–3 days and replacement in 4–6 days. Parietal and chief cells are replaced much more slowly, probably in excess of 3 months (Lipkin 1981). It seems that all these cell types are derived from a common precursor in the region of the base of the gastric pit, only this population being capable of cell division in normal mucosa. The controlling mechanisms for gastric cell turnover are largely unknown. Clearly there must be local ones that promote orderly healing of focal lesions, but there are others, such as the hormone gastrin, that exert a generalised trophic action. Disorder of these mechanisms, which may be the result of exogenous or endogenous factors, could clearly result in local as well as generalised mucosal hyperplasia and both focal and more widespread dysplastic or neoplastic lesions. In a consideration of gastric polyps, therefore, these facts need to be taken into account. If in prospective observations a lesion proves to be reversible, it would be logical to argue that it was hyperplastic rather than neoplastic in nature, even though the original stimulus was not known.

The basic pathological process in all forms of hyperplasia is essentially the same and differs only in extent of severity of variation or combination of the individual histological features in each instance. Similar changes are seen in the margins of a healing gastric ulcer, and the mechanism of polyp formation seems to be an exaggeration of the normal response of proliferation in the process of healing. However, an erosion or ulcer is not always present, and the stimulus for hyperplasia is often obscure.

There is a proliferation of the foveolar cells and a tendency towards so-called pseudopyloric metaplasia of glands if body mucosa is involved. The foveolae, or pits, elongate and become tortuous, and individual cells appear hypertrophied and sometimes have a metaplastic appearance with an eosinophilic cytoplasm. The simple mucinous glands have a tendency to form cysts. The lamina propria usually contains a mixture of lymphocytes, plasma cells, and a few eosinophils and, especially if there is associated surface erosion, a population of polymorphs. Sometimes any increase in cellularity is minimal, but usually the intervening lamina propria is oedematous in places; near the surface, particularly, it shows a profusion of thin-walled dilated vascular spaces. Another variable feature is a proliferation of muscular elements that spring from the muscularis mucosa and extend for varying distances into the lamina, sometimes almost reaching the surface. Sometimes intestinal metaplasia is present, but rarely is this extensive and is probably accounted for by the development of the polypoidal process on a background mucosa involved by chronic gastritis. Uncommonly, and usually in association with ulceration or other specific clinical situations, the cyst formation of the simple mucinous glands and the muscular hyperplasia is an extremely prominent feature. The resulting appearances have prompted the use of somewhat elaborate terminology. This is true for all of the hyperplastic polypoidal states of the gastric mucosa; whereas the basic tissue reactions are similar, clinical and other features seen in association with the various combinations of these reactions vary widely. Hence several types of hyperplastic lesions can be recognised.

Hyperplastic Polyps

These polyps (Fig. 8–17) often constitute up to 90% of gastric polyps in different reported series (Ming 1977, Nakamura and Nakano 1985, Rattan et al 1993), but more recent work (Stolte et al 1994) places them second in frequency to gastric body gland polyps. They rarely exceed 2 cm in largest diameter and are then commonly pedunculated. Usually they are much smaller and sessile with a smooth surface. Although they are usually single and most common in the antrum, multiple polyps can be seen in the same stomach and may involve all mucosal areas. Extensive

Figure 8–17. Sessile hyperplastic polyp removed endoscopically. Note the epithelial cysts and tortuous branched foveolae (H&E ×25).

multiple polyposis is uncommon. The background mucosa on which they occur may be essentially normal or it can show chronic gastritis.

Histologically the polyp consists of hyperplastic foveolae lined by tall epithelial cells with copious cytoplasm but basal nuclei (Fig. 8–18). This epithelium extends onto the surface, which is generally nonulcerated. The foveolae usually have complex branched outlines or are cystically dilated. The lamina propria contains a variable number of inflammatory cells; especially in polyps that are not ulcerated, they may be scant. Heavy infiltration is unusual, and it may have a neutrophil component. The lamina is also frequently oedematous and exhibits a profusion of thin-walled vessels. Another usual but variable feature in terms of its extent is proliferation of strands of smooth muscle that run between the glandular elements (Fig. 8–19). The deeper parts of the polyp frequently show a few pyloric-type glands even when the polyp is located in the body region and residual chief and parietal cells are unusual (Fig. 8–20). Intestinal metaplasia is never a prominent feature but occurs as small foci in approximately 15% of polyps (Fig. 8–21). There is usually no evidence of significant dysplasia of the epithelial elements, although when surface ulceration is seen the neighbouring epithelium often reverts to a lower, more basophilic, proliferative type. A characteristic feature of the hyperplastic polyp, especially the sessile type, is the gradual transition of the appearances at the junction of the polyp and neighbouring mucosa (Fig. 8–22). As asserted by Ming (1977) there seems to be little point in recognising a subgroup, the so-called foveolar hyperplastic polyp (Elster 1974), because this lesion is nothing more than an early hyperplastic polyp (Fig. 8–23). There is increasing evidence that a proportion of hyperplastic polyps develops as an overexuberant reaction in the process of erosion (Mitsufuji, Tsuchi-hashi and Kodama 1994).

There is also evidence that the hyperplastic polyp is not a significant precancer-ous lesion, although in the same stomach it may coexist with carcinoma. This evidence was provided by Kamiya et al (1981) in a prolonged follow-up study of 5–12 years that even showed the disappearance of a few lesions. However, the same authors also describe the development of increasing atypia and eventual carcinoma in 2 of more than 2,000 lesions. Polyps with mixed hyperplastic and adenomatous features are also encountered; this subject is considered in the section on adenoma-

Figure 8–18. Hyperplastic branched foveolae composed of mucus-secreting cells with copious cytoplasm. Note the vascularity of the oedematous lamina propria and the inflammatory infiltrate (H&E ×300).

tous polyps later in this chapter. Carneiro et al (1993) have reported a form of hyperplastic polyposis with an autosomal dominant form of inheritance that is associated with a high incidence of diffuse type carcinoma of the stomach. Hyperplastic gastric polyps also occur in Cowden's disease (Hizawa et al 1994).

Gastritis Cystica Polyposa (et profunda)

This is a lesion characterised by all the histological features described in the section on hyperplastic polyps. In addition, however, there is a marked proliferation of muscular elements and entrapment of numerous epithelial cysts. Sometimes, but not always, the lesion appears below the split and hypertrophied muscularis mucosa, hence the use of "profunda" in the terminology (Figs. 8–24 and 8–25). The lesion has been described at gastroenterology stomas, at peptic ulcer edges, and in association with carcinoma (Ignatius, Armstrong and Eversole 1970, Mori, Shinya and Wolff 1971, Littler and Gleibermann 1972, Honore, Lewis and Ohara 1979, Stemmermann and Hayashi 1979, Franzin and Novelli 1981, Jablokow, Aranha and Reyes 1982, Fonde and Rodning 1986, Ozenc, Ruacan and Aran 1988). Occasionally it presents as a polypoidal mass in an otherwise normal stomach (Wu et al 1994). Because of the frequent association with chronic gastritis the lesion is also fairly frequently associated with areas of intestinal metaplasia. The condition has commanded attention because of its florid gross appearance. A typical lesion at a gastroenterostomy stoma is often several centimetres in diameter and consists of a local massive

Figure 8–19. Muscle hyperplasia is sometimes seen extending almost to the surface (H&E ×300).

Figure 8–20. The deeper glands in this hyperplastic polyp are the pyloric type, and there is obvious muscle hyperplasia (H&E ×300).

Figure 8–21. Hyperplastic polyp with intestinal metaplasia (right) (H&E ×300).

Figure 8–22. Pyloric mucosa near a hyperplastic polyp. There is noticeable foveolar tortuosity due to hyperplasia and occasional glandular cysts (H&E ×125).

Figure 8–23. So-called foveolar hyperplastic polyp, which is only an early hyperplastic polyp without the features seen in large lesions (H&E ×175).

Figure 8–24. Gastritis cystica profunda. Note the inflammatory infiltration, intestinal metaplasia *(arrow)*, and the deep cysts (H&E ×25).

Figure 8–25. Detail of Figure 8–24. Cystic simple mucinous glands lie below the splayed and hyperplastic muscularis mucosa running across the centre (H&F. ×175).

exaggeration of the normal mucosal rugal pattern. Presumably the lesion is due to a prolonged stimulated hyperplastic response to mucosal injury or erosion. Erosions are common in the region of gastroenterostomy stomas, and the regurgitation of bile and pancreatic juice, which is a regular event in this postoperative state, could well account for a prolonged mucosal injury. Indeed, in exaggerated form, most of the histological features seen in this condition are similar to those present in bile-reflux gastritis. Given the increased incidence of cancer in the postoperative stomach it is not surprising that dysplastic changes have been described in this condition (Franzin et al 1985), which may also account for its coexistence with frank adenocarcinoma (Bogomoletz et al 1985).

Other Forms of Mucosal Hyperplasia

The unusual prominence of normal gastric rugae was called état mammelonné by early French pathologists (Magnus 1952). An abnormal rugal hyperplasia, however, occurs in some patients with duodenal ulcer and the Zollinger-Ellison syndrome (Krag 1966, Zollinger and Moore 1968). Mucosal biopsies afford the means of estimating parietal cell mass by quantitative methods. Schmidt-Wilcke, Haake and Riecken (1974), for example, showed a close relationship between parietal cell density and maximal acid output in duodenal ulcer patients.

Epithelial hyperplasia involving the gastric pits, glands, or both (Fig. 8–26) has been described in association with carcinoma of the stomach and with peptic ulcer, both gastric and duodenal (Monroe, Boughton and Sommers 1964, Stamm and

Figure 8–26. Antral-type mucosa near a prepyloric peptic ulcer. There is pit, neck, and glandular hyperplasia. Compare with Figure 5–5 (H&E ×100).

Saremaslani 1989). Usually, but not always, it occurs close to the primary lesion, and similar changes occur in the mucosa adjacent to colonic carcinoma (Saffos and Rhatigan 1977). It is important that this entity is recognised as being different from the lesion that results from gastritis with pseudopyloric metaplasia of body glands, which is seen in the distal stomach in relation to peptic ulcer. It is universally accepted that carcinoma of the stomach and peptic ulcer are associated with a degree of type AB or B chronic gastritis involving the pyloric antrum, and to a variable degree more proximal parts of the stomach. The gastritis is commonly severe, especially in conjunction with high gastric ulcer and carcinoma, and is frequently associated with both pseudopyloric and intestinal metaplasia. Distortion of the gastric pits by inflammatory oedema, and inflammatory infiltration with lymphoid aggregates when there is also pseudopyloric metaplasia of body glands, is easily interpreted as a hyperplastic state of the pyloric mucosa. For this reason, some authors, misinterpreting these changes, claim that high gastric ulcers occur in stomachs with an unusually large antrum. It has already been pointed out, however, that pyloric mucosa can often be differentiated from pseudopyloric metaplasia by the presence of parietal cells in the former.

Ménétrier's Disease

Ménétrier's disease (Ménétrier 1888) is frequently referred to as hypertrophic gastritis. In hypertrophy of a tissue or an organ there is an increase in size and not in number of its constituent parts, the latter being hyperplasia. Both may exist concomitantly, but in the case of Ménétrier's disease the lesion is a hyperplasia and not hypertrophy.

Figure 8–27. Gastric body mucosa in Ménétrier's disease. There is overall thickening of the mucosa, and simple surface-type mucin-secreting epithelium extends into and lines deep cystic spaces (H&E ×56).

The thickened mucosa (Fig. 8–27) is thrown into folds into which a spur of muscularis mucosa often projects. The pits are elongated, as are the glands, which nevertheless may retain a normal cellular component. There are areas, however, where simple mucin-secreting epithelium similar to gastric surface epithelium extends into the basal parts of the glands, which frequently show cystic change. This mucin-secreting epithelium may be flattened but usually shows histochemical evidence of a transition from gastric to intestinal type (Whitehead, unpublished observation). Sometimes frank intestinal metaplasia is seen (Fig. 8–28), but this seems to occur more commonly in areas where there is also inflammatory infiltration.

Figure 8–28. Cystic basal glands in Ménétrier's disease tending to split the muscularis mucosa. Note the small-intestinal type of goblet cells *(arrowheads)* as compared with the gastric type of mucin-secreting epithelium lining other cysts (PAS ×150).

Smooth-muscle bundles can be traced from the muscularis mucosa between the glands and often right up to the surface (Fig. 8–29). There is hyperplasia; splitting and irregularity of the muscularis mucosa, which is exaggerated where cystic glandular changes are most marked; and cystic glands may appear in the submucosa.

In some cases there is an overall depletion of specialised oxyntic and peptic cells, and it is not unusual for low acid secretion to accompany the disease. Parietal and peptic cells may be very obvious, however, and some cases are also associated with a normal (Gabreau et al 1982) or a high acid output (Brooks, Isenberg and Goldstein 1970, Overholt and Jeffries 1970, Kristensen and Nilsson 1985). Lam et al (1983) describe two brothers with pachydermoperiostosis, Ménétrier's disease, and peptic ulcer, and in large series of cases peptic ulcer disease appears to be common (Searcy and Malagelada 1984, Leardi et al 1993). Although other familial cases are on record (Larsen, Tarp and Kristensen 1987), heredity seems to be of minor significance in pathogenesis. Celik, Ettinger and Satchidanand (1984) describe a case associated with massive bleeding from a coexistent arteriovenous malformation, which in all probability is a fortuitous relationship.

The degree and distribution of an inflammatory infiltration or true gastritis vary in different cases, and at least some are related to rupture of cystic lesions (Fig. 8–30). The mucus released seems to evoke an inflammatory reaction characterised by an occasional giant cell.

There is ample evidence that Ménétrier's disease is sometimes reversible (Berry, Ben-Dov and Freund 1980, Walker 1981), and occasionally this has followed treatment with cimetidine (Vendelboe and Jespersen 1981, Gabreau et al 1982). An interesting case of Ménétrier's lesion ascribed to increased local synthesis of prostaglandin E_2 was described (Boyd et al 1988) in which the lesion regressed after successful treatment of a carcinoid syndrome.

Transient Ménétrier's disease seems to occur particularly in childhood

Figure 8–29. Gastric mucosa in Ménétrier's disease shows smooth-muscle bundles extending almost to the surface epithelium (H&E ×255).

Figure 8–30. Ruptured cystic lesion in Ménétrier's disease with secondary inflammatory reaction and mucin granuloma (H&E ×375).

(Scharschmidt 1977, Bloom 1981, Kraut et al 1981, Stillman et al 1981). In childhood it also appears that the mucosa can revert to normal (Baker et al 1986), whereas in adults resolution may result in residual atrophic gastritis (Berenson, Sannella and Freston 1976).

It is interesting that certain cases with typical histological features of Ménétrier's disease are associated with multiple endocrine adenomas (Kenny, Dockerty and Waugh 1954) and sometimes with Zollinger-Ellison syndrome, a pancreatic islet cell tumour, marked gastric hypersecretion, and peptic ulceration (Whitehead, unpublished observation). Ménétrier's disease has also been described in association with vitiligo, and Cieslak et al (1993) reported two cases in children associated with cytomegalovirus infection. Sometimes it occurs in the newborn (Beneck 1994) and rarely in conjunction with retinopathy, a nephrotic syndrome, and diabetes (Masugi et al 1994). It has also been cited as a cause of gastroduodenal intussusception (Deutsch et al 1994). Berkowitz, Passaro and Isenberg (1977) and Ming (1977) identified three types of hyperplasia of the gastric mucosa, one primarily involving mucous cells of foveolar origin, one involving chief and parietal cells only, and a third affecting all cell types. However, cases reported in the literature make it plain that the gastric mucosal hyperplasia, which characteristically spares the antrum, presents a spectrum of clinical and histological features. The more severe and prolonged disturbances of mucosal dynamics, whatever the precipitating stimulus, are associated with the most severe histological disturbances whereas relatively milder and shorter-lived stimuli give rise to milder and potentially reversible lesions. This does not require the elimination of terms such as Ménétrier's disease or Zollinger-Ellison syndrome because they also have other clinical implications. There has been some confusion in the literature between lymphocytic gastritis, when associated with a thickening of the mucosa, and Ménétrier's disease (Groisman et al 1994); there have also been claims that lymphocytic gastritis is a treatable form of Ménétrier's disease, achievable by eradicating *Helicobacter pylori* from the mucosa (Bayerdorffer et al 1994). Wolfsen, Carpenter and Talley (1993), however, make a strong case for lymphocytic gastritis and Ménétrier's disease as being distinctly different entities.

Diffuse gastrointestinal mucosal thickening and irregularity, often referred to as polyposis, together with abnormal skin pigmentation, dystrophy of the nails, baldness, and various biochemical abnormalities secondary to the gastrointestinal loss of protein and tissue fluid was first described by Cronkhite and Canada in 1955. The syndrome often has a prolonged course and only a minority of patients have been observed to recover spontaneously (Aanestad et al 1987).

The intestinal mucosal lesion is not a true neoplastic polyposis, and in the stomach it shares many features with Ménétrier's disease. Not only in the stomach but also in the rest of the intestine (see Fig. 18–35) the lesions appear to be the result of a functional disorder of the mucin glands. Early lesions in the stomach show a progressive loss of specialised body glands by a process of mucin cell transformation. These become increasingly numerous, enlarged, and often bizarre in morphology, and because of excessive and perhaps abnormal secretion the glands become cystic. Consequently there is deformity and thickening of the mucosa (Fig. 8–31). Some cysts are invaded by inflammatory cells, and others rupture into the lamina propria causing a further secondary inflammatory response that has a conspicuous histiocytic element (Fig. 8–32). It is this excessive secretion, cystic dilatation of glands and their rupture, and increased bulk of the lamina propria (Fig. 8–33) that account for the grossly polypoidal appearance of the mucosa. It is also because of these features that Johnson et al (1972) regarded the lesions as a diffuse gastroenterocolitis with inflammatory pseudopolyposis. There is evidence that the nonpolypoidal mucosa is also abnormal with a tendency for specialised cell type to be replaced by mucous cells (Freeman et al 1985). It has been postulated, based on an electron microscope study, that the primary process or defect affects the regenerative zones of the involved mucosa (Jenkins, Stephenson and Scott 1985).

Cronkhite-Canada Syndrome

The Cronkhite-Canada syndrome has been reported in association with multiple myeloma (Rubin et al 1980) and cytomegalovirus infection (Lipper and Kahn 1977), but both are probably fortuitous. Nonomura et al (1980) described a case associated with sigmoid carcinoma and, in a review of the literature, noted a 15% prevalence of complicating carcinoma in this rare condition. In cases described by Katayama, Kimura and Konn (1985) and Malhotra and Sheffield (1988), not only was colon carcinoma present but there were also adenomatous changes in the epithelium of the polypoidal lesions. Murai et al (1993) have even suggested that the syndrome

Figure 8–31. Gastric biopsy in Cronkhite-Canada syndrome. The mucosa is thickened, and some glands are cystic. Note the apparent excess of lamina propria (H&E ×14).

Figure 8–32. Gastric mucosa in Cronkhite-Canada syndrome. The ruptured cyst has produced secondary inflammation and a marked histiocytic reaction (H&E ×105).

Figure 8–33. Gastric mucosa in Cronkhite-Canada syndrome. The lamina propria is bulky and distinctly oedematous. Note the enlargement and irregularity of form of the mucinous epithelium (H&E ×105).

may be a premalignant disorder; this has been echoed by Harned, Buck and Sobin (1995). Colonic tumours are not that rare, but in their review of 55 cases in the literature Daniel et al (1982) found only one complicated by gastric cancer. In contrast, an association between Ménétrier's disease and gastric carcinoma appears real (Scharschmidt 1977). This does not mean that Ménétrier's disease and Cronk-hite-Canada syndrome are entirely unrelated. They share histological similarities in the gastric mucosa and, as in cases of Ménétrier's disease, the features of Cronkhite-Canada syndrome are known to be completely reversible (Russell, Bhathal and St. John 1983, Peart et al 1984). The interrelationships of all the hyperplastic lesions of the stomach, although often distinct clinicopathological entities, can be illustrated by the reports of Krentz and Gohrband (1976), who followed up 45 patients with gastric erosions for 5 years and witnessed the evolution in 26 of hyperplastic folds. Similarly, as Roesch (1978) reports, chronic erosions are frequently seen at the apices of the giant hyperplastic folds in Ménétrier's disease. It seems that hyperplastic lesions of the stomach are in some instances a reaction to mucosal damage or ulceration, in others the result of the trophic action of gastrin, but in the majority of cases the stimulus to hyperplasia is as yet not determined.

Hamartomatous and Heterotopic Polyps

Primarily epithelial polyps may also be due to errors of development, i.e., they are hamartomas or heterotopias. In Peutz-Jeghers syndrome gastric involvement occurs in approximately one quarter of cases. The lesions, as elsewhere, are composed of a somewhat disorganised arrangement of the glandular elements normally present in that part, i.e., antral, body, or cardiac, together with muscle bundles extending from the muscularis mucosa (Figs. 8–34 and 8–35). In Peutz-Jeghers syndrome as a whole there is now a well-recognised increased incidence of cancer not only of the intestine and stomach but also in a variety of other organs (Utsunomiya et al 1974, Halbert 1982, Hizawa et al 1993b, Rodriguez et al 1993). The exact relation-

Figure 8–34. Peutz-Jeghers gastric polyp with branching muscular core and cystic deep mucous glands (H&E ×125).

Figure 8–35. Peutz-Jeghers gastric polyp in its upper part with irregularly branching abnormal crypts and strands of interfoveolar muscle tissue (H&E ×250).

ship between gastric polyps and the evolution of carcinoma of the stomach still requires elucidation. In colonic juvenile polyposis, gastric involvement may also occur. Like juvenile polyps elsewhere the sparse, often cystic, glandular elements are set in abundant lamina propria devoid of muscle. They are commonly infiltrated by inflammatory cells and have a rounded appearance and a smooth surface. Malignant potential is only rarely recorded (Sassatelli et al 1993). In the case of familial juvenile polyposis of the stomach described by Watanabe, Nagashima and Motoi (1979), who also review the previous literature, there is a remarkable similarity of the illustrated pathology to the lesions of Cronkhite-Canada syndrome. Another form of gastric polyposis, which occurs in the region of the gastric body mucosa, is also included in the hamartomatous group (Parks, Bussey and Lockhart-Mummery 1970, Tatsuta et al 1982). It occurs in patients with familial polyposis coli, or Gardner's syndrome (Church et al 1992, Seow-Choen et al 1992), and in the hereditary flat colonic adenoma syndrome (Lynch et al 1993) but much more frequently is unassociated (Elster 1976, Lee and Burt 1986, Bedossa, Lemaigre and Martin 1987a, Justrabo et al 1987, Hizawa et al 1993a, Kinoshita et al 1993), although fundic gland polyposis itself may be familial on occasion (Tsuchikame et al 1993). The lesions are usually just a few millimetres in diameter and are rarely as large as 1 cm. They are caused by a cystic dilatation of the gastric body glands and, although flattened, the lining cells usually retain the features of parietal and chief cells, although occasional cysts are lined by mucous neck cells (Figs. 8–36 and 8–37). The gastric pit zone and surface epithelium are largely normal although stretched over the underlying cystic glands, and usually there is not a significant inflammatory change in the lamina propria unless a coincidental and probably unrelated gastritis is present. It is probably incorrect to regard these lesions as hamartomatous because the basic structure of the gastric mucosa is normal, the only abnormality being gland dilatation. Iida et al (1980) described three patients in whom multiple polyps of this type spontaneously resolved; they are thus more likely to be the result of disordered function and secretion of the gastric glands. Watanabe et al (1978), in common with other Japanese pathologists, have called these lesions fundic gland polyps. "Cystic glandu-

Figure 8–36. Cystic body gland polyp (H&E ×125).

Figure 8–37. Detail of Figure 8–36 showing the characteristic lining of chief and parietal cells (H&E ×400).

lar fundic polyposis" is a similar terminology that is favoured by Voigt et al (1983), but these polyps can occur in all areas of the gastric mucosa that is of body type, the use of "fundic," which is only part of the body mucosa, is incorrect. Elster (1976) prefers the descriptive term "cysts of the gastric glands," whereas Chakravorty and Schatzki (1975) called the lesion "gastric cystic polyposis." A more accurate descriptive terminology is, however, "cystic body gland polyp," or "cystic body gland polyposis" if multiple.

Carfagna et al (1987) reported a fundic polypoidal hamartoma in a patient with widespread gastritis. It consisted of cystic glands set in a framework of smooth muscle tissue. The glands were body and antral in type and included endocrine cells.

Heterotopic pancreatic tissue, or Brunner's glands, may also present as a polypoidal lesion, usually in the region of the antrum (Stolte et al 1994). A rare entity, "Devon polyposis syndrome," a condition in which recurrent multiple inflammatory fibroid polyps occur in the stomach or ileum, has also been described (Allibone, Nanson and Anthony 1992). Solitary inflammatory fibroid polyps (see Chapter 9) are by comparison less rare but still uncommon. For accurate diagnosis, examination of the whole lesion rather than a surface biopsy is required because of its nature. These lesions appear to be different from inflammatory pseudotumour described by Kojimahara et al (1993).

Adenomatous Polyps

These lesions arising in intestinalised gastritic mucosa exhibit a range of macroscopic appearances identical to adenomatous polyps of the colon. It appears that smaller sessile lesions are common in Japan (Nakamura 1970, Nakamura and Nakano 1985), whereas in most other countries polyps tend to be rather more pedunculated, larger, and sometimes villous. Adenomatous polyps are the more common of the two types of lesion seen in the stomach in familial adenomatosis patients, the other being cystic fundic gland polyps (Iida et al 1988). Because of the usual distribution of simple chronic gastritis, adenomatous polyps in nonadenomatosis patients are most frequent in the antrum, but they may occur in any site. In essence they constitute a focus of dysplastic epithelium whose growth characteristics determine that an accumulation of cells occurs at the site, thus raising them above the surrounding mucosa. The individual cytological features are the same whether the dysplastic focus is flat or polypoidal, and the arguments relating to the use of the term "carcinoma in situ" are the same. As in colonic polyps, tubular and villous patterns may predominate, although most are mixed. There is no doubt as to the malignant potential of adenomatous polyps, and all the arguments relating to the adenoma-cancer sequence in the colon apply to the stomach. Up to approximately half of adenomatous polyps also show invasive carcinoma, and this is more likely to be seen the larger the lesion. In addition to the cystic body gland polyps seen in patients with familial polyposis coli, adenomatous polyps of the gastric antrum also occur (Sugihara et al 1982, Jarvinen, Nyberg and Peltokallio 1983). It is also being recognised more commonly that adenomatous change may be superimposed on a hyperplastic polyp (Figs. 8–38 and 8–39). Nakamura and Nakano (1985) regard this type of lesion (type III) as being fundamentally different from the wholly adenomatous polyp (type IV), which has a greater malignant potential (Muratani et al 1989). Thus, whereas hyperplastic polyps are predominantly without a significant cancer risk, they may on occasion progress to exhibit adenomatous features, when as in an adenomatous polyp de novo a further loss of cell growth control mechanisms may result in increased malignant potential and invasion. This no doubt accounts for the examples of malignancy occurring in hyperplastic polyps (Nakamura 1970, Ming 1977, Hattori 1985, Daibo, Itabashi and Hirota 1987), but the prevalence of this change is less than 5%.

Adenomatous and carcinomatous lesions consisting predominantly of neoplastic

Figure 8–38. Gastric polyp with hyperplastic and adenomatous features (H&E ×125).

Paneth's cells are also described sometimes in association with pernicious anaemia (Lev and DeNucci 1989, Rubio 1989, Caruso and Famulari 1992).

LYMPHOID HYPERPLASIA AND MALIGNANT LYMPHOMA

The diagnosis of lesions that raise suspicions of being malignant because of their endoscopic appearance is a particularly difficult task when the lesions are of lymphoid origin. Lymphoid infiltrates may be reactive as part of the picture of chronic gastritis, or as a tissue response to ulceration (Hyjek and Kelenyi 1982), or they may be malignant. The difficulty for the pathologist in differentiating between benign and malignant infiltrates is accentuated by the fact that they may coexist in the same lesion. Furthermore, lymphoid tissue is absent from the gastric mucosa at birth (Takaki 1986) and appears during life in association with the various inflammatory states of the mucosa and ulceration, particularly in association with mucosal colonisation by *H. pylori* (Eidt and Stolte 1993, Eidt, Stolte and Fischer 1994, Genta and Hamner 1994). Thus, one would expect to find a reactive element in any malignant lymphoid process that supervened. If the malignancy derives from preexisting reactive elements a further difficulty is predictable, namely, the criteria for deciding when the malignant process has definitively established itself. With the burgeoning of immunochemistry in histopathology much new light is being cast on this problem area. Claims in the past (Katz et al 1973) that gastroscopic appearances are of greater importance than biopsy histology or brush cytology for the diagnosis of some forms of gastric lymphoma can no longer be sustained and, since the use of

Figure 8–39. Detail of the polyp in Figure 8–38. The adenomatous features are mainly of tubular pattern, and the dysplasia is moderate in degree (H&E ×300).

Kiel's classification and cell characterisation by the use of monoclonal antibodies, great progress has been made (Van den Heule, Van Kerkem and Heimann 1979, Spinelli, Lo Gullo and Pizzetti 1980, Saraga, Hurlimann and Ozzello 1981, Brousse et al 1983, Isaacson and Wright 1984, Isaacson, Spencer and Finn 1986, Myhre and Isaacson 1987). Nevertheless claims are still made for the existence of a tumour-like lesion, called gastric pseudolymphoma occurring in association with past or present peptic ulcer (Graffner and Hesselvik 1987, Tokunaga, Watanabe and Morimatsu 1987). There are claims that gastric pseudolymphoma may resolve if *H. pylori* is eradicated from the stomach by appropriate therapy (Weston et al 1994). The balance of opinion, however, is changing; with the newer methods of investigation, including gene rearrangement studies, it appears that many if not most of the so-called pseudolymphomas are low-grade lymphomas of the mucosa-associated lymphoid tissue (Myhre and Isaacson 1987, Isaacson 1992, Fend et al 1994, Uemura et al 1994). Light chain restriction has been convincingly demonstrated in lesions that would otherwise be diagnosed as pseudolymphoma (Isaacson, Spencer and Finn 1986, Burke et al 1987, Ono et al 1993). Most gastric lymphomas are thus B cell in type, of follicle centre cell origin, and contain centrocyte-like cells or have plasma cell differentiation in a minority (Myhre and Isaacson 1987). Plasmacytomas have, of course, been recognised on simple morphological grounds for some time (Nakani-shi et al 1982, Ishido and Mori 1992), some even containing crystalline cytoplasmic inclusions (Ferrer-Roca 1982); cases have also been characterised adequately using advanced immunoperoxidase and immunogold techniques (Ooi, Nakanishi and Hashiba 1987). Some have been associated with serum alpha heavy chain (Guardia et al 1980), and gastric immunoblastic lymphomas have been described in patients with a preexisting angioimmunoblastic lymphadenopathy (Bauer et al 1982). Thus, early claims that so-called pseudolymphoma was a premalignant lesion (Wolf and

Figure 8–40. Chronic atrophic gastritis. Cellular infiltrate, although deep, is not particularly dense, and although there is glandular atrophy and intestinal metaplasia, an overall preservation of mucosal architecture is present but somewhat collapsed (H&E ×100).

Spjut 1981, Brooks and Enterline 1983) seem now to be partly substantiated, although there are those who might argue that so-called pseudolymphoma is already a low-grade lymphoma (Isaacson, Spencer and Finn 1986).

Isaacson and Spencer (1987) argued that primary gastric B cell lymphoma, which often remains localised for long periods, involving regional lymph nodes in a minority of cases and responding well to therapy, even surgical removal, is a tumour arising in centrocytic-like cells that are immunologically distinct from centrocytes proper. The malignancy arises in interfollicular areas but may invade the reactive follicles secondarily. These authors draw comparison with B cell lymphomas of similar type arising in the lymphoid tissue associated with other mucosal surfaces, which are also known for their good prognosis, e.g., in the lung, salivary glands, and thyroid but not all gastric lymphomas behave in a nonaggressive fashion (Kath et al 1995). Mohri (1987), however, apparently believes that primary gastric lymphomas

Figure 8–41. Malignant lymphoma. Note the obliteration of glandular elements and the density of infiltrate, although the surface epithelium is intact. Two abnormal follicles are present, and there is a biopsy artefact above these (H&E ×100).

Figure 8–42. Lymphoepithelial lesions in biopsies of a malignant lymphoma. *A, B, C,* Note progressive destruction of the epithelial element by the infiltrating islands of malignant cells (H&E ×500).

Figure continued on following page

may arise not only in interfollicular cells but also in follicular centre cells. This is clearly a field for further study, but from the viewpoint of diagnosis of biopsy tissues several points can be made. The density of the infiltrate and the relative preservation of the native mucosal architecture, despite some glandular atrophy in the absence of ulceration, can sometimes be helpful in allaying a suspicion of lymphoma (Fig. 8–40). In lymphoma the phenomenon of epithelial tropism of the malignant cells and the formation of so-called lymphoepithelial lesions (Isaacson and Wright 1983, 1984) tend to lead to epithelial and glandular destruction (Figs. 8–41 and 8–42). These lymphoepithelial lesions tend to occur only in better differentiated tumours, and when cells resemble centroblasts or immunoblasts they are absent. The cells can usually be differentiated from nonmalignant intraepithelial lymphocytes, which tend to occur as single cells surrounded by a clear halo, whereas tumour cells occur as

Figure 8–42 *Continued*

Figure 8–43. Malignant lymphoma of a predominantly centroblastic type (H&E of resin section ×200).

Figure 8–44. Detail of Figure 8–43. The majority of nuclei are large and irregular with multiple, often peripheral, nucleoli. A few immunoblasts with central nucleoli are also seen (H&E of resin section ×500).

groups or clusters often obliterating the lumen by bulging into it. Plasma cell differentiation may be seen, but these cells do not seem to have epitheliotropism. As with lymphoma diagnosis in other sites, cytological evaluation of the suspicious cells is important and is made easier if ultrathin resin-embedded sections are available (Figs. 8–43 to 8–45). Many laboratories are now able to type suspicious cells using immunohistochemical methods even on paraffin sections, and this is beginning

Figure 8–45. Immunoblastic sarcoma with a majority of large cells having prominent central and single nucleoli (H&E of resin section ×350).

Figure 8–46. Malignant histiocytoma. Apart from some normal lymphocytes the malignant cells appear with bizarre irregular nuclei, frequent nucleoli, and a prominent copious cytoplasm (H&E of resin section ×350).

Figure 8–47. Malignant histiocytoma shows marked nuclear enlargement. The cytoplasm is less obvious than in Figure 8–46, but the tumour was typed histochemically (H&E of resin section×500).

to take on a more important aspect. Perhaps typing of lymphoma cells will be based eventually more on which markers they carry rather than on their morphological resemblance to cells that occur in normal lymphoid tissues. For the moment, however, a combination of these is proving extremely valuable. Tumours composed mainly of large bizarre cells without a tendency to form follicles behave more aggressively than those with cells exhibiting at least some tendency to differentiate towards similar cells in normal lymphoid tissue. A curious subtype of gastric lymphoma is one which by light microscopy appears as a signet ring cell lesion (Hernandez and Sheehan 1985). It is clearly important that a correct diagnosis be reached in such cases because of the much worse prognosis and the different therapeutic approach for signet ring cell adenocarcinoma.

Other forms of primary or secondary gastric lymphomas not of B cell origin seem to be uncommon. Hodgkin's disease, for example, is so rare that any such diagnosis should be seriously questioned. The problem with the remainder such as have been described in the past as histiocytic lymphomas, for example (Isaacson et al 1979, Seo et al 1982), is that they were defined before the era of more specific immunohistochemical markers. As compared with B cell tumours, other primary gastric lymphomas deriving from other lymphoid cell lines appear to be quite uncommon. A malignant histiocytic tumour confirmed by histochemistry is illustrated in Figures 8–46 and 8–47.

9

OTHER TYPES OF GASTRITIS AND MISCELLANEOUS LESIONS

OTHER TYPES OF GASTRITIS

Eosinophilic Gastroenteritis

The stomach is always involved in eosinophilic gastroenteritis, and a diagnosis can frequently be made in a gastric biopsy (Navab et al 1972, Katz, Goldman and Grand 1977). It is a disease affecting all age groups, from infancy to old age, and may also involve the oesophagus, the small intestine, and occasionally the colon (Ashby, Appleton and Dawson 1964, Tedesco et al 1981, Matzinger and Daneman 1983, Stringel et al 1984, Zora et al 1984, Naylor and Pollet 1985, Moore et al 1986, Rumans and Lieberman 1987, Snyder et al 1987, Steele et al 1987, Lee et al 1993, Olson and Fukui-Miner 1994). If mucosal involvement predominates, protein loss and malabsorption result; muscular involvement causes obstruction because of the attendant fibrosis, and serosal disease is characterised by ascites (Klein et al 1970, Trounce and Tanner 1985, Kuri and Lee 1994). Mucosal ulceration and haemorrhage are reported infrequently (Lucak et al 1982). A peripheral blood eosinophilia is often present at some stage in the disease (Kamal et al 1985, Van Rensberg, Keet and Adams 1986, Fortman et al 1993), and only about a quarter of the patients have a history of allergy. However, occasional cases of eosinophilic gastroenteritis seem to occur in the setting of the hypereosinophilic syndrome (Shah and Joglekar 1987). There are also claims based on immunohistochemical studies that in eosinophilic gastroenteritis there is an immunoglobulin E (IgE) mast cell–mediated tissue reaction characterised by eosinophil degranulation (Oyaizu et al 1985, Keshavarzian et al 1985). A previously uncategorised subgroup is that associated with connective tissue diseases such as scleroderma and its variants and dermatomyositis (DeSchryver-Kecskemeti and Clouse 1984). The gastric lesion usually takes the form of thickening of the antrum and pylorus, but less commonly the whole stomach may be involved. Histologically the diffuse form shows capillary and lymphatic dilatation of the mucosa and oedema of the lamina propria that pushes the gland tubules and crypts aside. There is always a conspicuous eosinophil polymorph leukocyte infiltration that varies in intensity from field to field and case to case. In addition it is usual to see occasional histiocytes, and these are sometimes multinucleate. Mucosal ulceration is distinctly uncommon, and in deep biopsies it becomes clear that it is the submucosa that is most heavily infiltrated (Fig. 9–1). It is also usual in this zone to find a degree of inflammatory fibrosis, and this is responsible for much of the thickening seen macroscopically. In addition to the tissue eosinophilia, IgE plasma cells are increased in number (Lucak et al 1982).

Figure 9–1. Pyloric mucosa in eosinophilic gastritis. The cellular infiltration and fibrosis is most marked in the submucosa (H&E ×60).

The disease usually responds dramatically to steroids, but this is not always so, and deaths despite steroid therapy have been recorded in the adult (Tytgat et al 1976) and in childhood (Konrad and Meister 1979). It has been assumed that the disease has an allergic basis and constitutes a reaction to ingested antigenic material. Leinbach and Rubin (1970) carried out detailed investigations in a 23-year-old man in order to determine a possible aetiological role for specific antigens, but they could conclude only that the disease was not a simple reversible allergic reaction to dietary substances. Rather, they postulated that it was a self-perpetuating process that may be symptomatically aggravated by different foods. Sherman and Cox (1982), however, described a neonatal case apparently related to transplacental sensitization of the colon by bovine milk antigens. The real situation is that the disease is incompletely understood and may be a manifestation of a variety of antigenic insults or allergic mechanisms. It has been ascribed to the drug clofazimine in patients with acquired immunodeficiency syndrome (Ravi et al 1993) and sometimes is accompanied by necrotising granulomas (Fraile et al 1994).

It is of interest that some cases have been ascribed to the ingestion of the eggs or larvae of *Eustoma rotundatum,* which is classified under the genus *Anisakis,* a parasite of the North Sea herring (Kuipers, Theil and Roskam 1960). It seems unlikely that this parasite is involved in all cases, but Watt et al (1979) described a case in Scotland due to the larvae of an *Anisakis* species and pointed out that several hundred cases of human infection by these larvae had been documented in Japan, Holland, and North America. The disease seems to be acquired by eating raw, slightly salted, or pickled sea fish and is probably that part of the broader spectrum of eosinophilic gastroenteritis in which a definite allergen has been identified.

Inflammatory Fibroid Polyp

Before the two papers by Johnstone and Morson (1978), the inflammatory fibroid polyp was widely regarded as a localised form of eosinophilic gastroenteritis, although as early as 1970 (Klein et al) doubt had been cast on their interrelationship. One of the reasons for confusion is that eosinophilic gastroenteritis can take the form of localised polypoidal disease (Bogomoletz 1984b). Inflammatory fibroid polyp, however, seems to differ in that it occurs in an older age group, a history of allergy is usually absent, and there is no blood eosinophilia. But they do have a similar distribution in the gut, and the fibroblastic tissue comprising their bulk is infiltrated by eosinophils, which, although in variable numbers, are a prominent feature in just over half of the reported cases (LiVolsi and Perzin 1975, Blackshaw and Levison 1986). They frequently cause obstructive symptoms and occasionally result in intussusception (Winkler et al 1986). Suen and Burton (1979) also describe two other shared histological features in occasional cases, namely, necrotising eosinophil granulomas and vasculitis. They considered a relationship to other hypereosinophilic syndromes, allergic granulomatosis, and the angiitis of Churg and Strauss (1951) as well as polyarteritis nodosa. Some still maintain that there are grounds for posing the question of a possible relationship between the two conditions (Battin-Bertho et al 1987).

In biopsy tissues the lesion may or may not be ulcerated, but usually it is seen to be an essentially submucosal proliferation of vascular fibrous tissue with a sprinkling of lymphocytes and plasma cells and a variable number of eosinophil leukocytes. Whereas Shimer and Helwig (1984) described the appearances as having a close resemblance to granulation tissue, Widgren and Pizzolato (1987) made a claim based on immunohistochemistry and electron microscopy that the main cellular component of this granulation tissue is the myofibroblast.

Granulomatous Lesions

It has been claimed that gastric biopsy will reveal granulomas in 10% of patients who have a confirmed diagnosis of systemic sarcoidosis but no gastrointestinal symptoms (Palmer 1958). Infrequently, however, the stomach involvement produces a granulomatous and fibrotic rigid deformity of the pylorus and, as a consequence, the appropriate clinical picture of pyloric obstruction (Sirak 1954, Croxon, Chen and Davidson 1987). A less common form of presentation is upper gastrointestinal haemorrhage (Berens and Montes 1975, Fung, Foo and Lee 1975, Ona 1981, Chlumsky, Krtek and Chlumska 1985), and it can mimic peptic ulceration (Gallagher et al

Figure 9–2. Pyloric biopsy in gastric sarcoidosis. There is a diffuse inflammatory cell infiltration with focal granulomas beneath the intact superficial epithelium (H&E ×35).

Figure 9–3. Detail of Figure 9–2 shows two granulomas (H&E ×105).

1984) and Ménétrier's disease (Chinitz et al 1985). When typical systemic sarcoidosis is present the diagnosis of gastric sarcoidosis can be based on finding typical granulomas in biopsy specimens (Figs. 9–2 to 9–4).

By themselves, however, granulomas might also denote gastric Crohn's disease, although in this circumstance it is likely that more marked diffuse cellular infiltration, lymphoid aggregates, oedema, fibrosis, and ulceration would also be present, i.e., those histological features that help to characterise Crohn's disease elsewhere in the gastrointestinal tract (Fig. 9–5).

Experience with rectal biopsy demonstrates that Crohn's disease may show minimal diffuse mucosal infiltrate with scattered granulomas; a similar pattern of involvement has been described in the stomach that is radiologically normal (Korelitz et al 1981), which makes histological distinction from sarcoidosis extremely difficult

Figure 9–4. Detail of Figure 9–2 shows a Schaumann's body in a giant cell (H&E ×210).

Figure 9–5. *A,* Crohn's disease of stomach in bottom right area of mixed inflammation (H&E ×300). *B* and *C,* Well-defined epithelioid granulomatous component (*B,* H&E ×300; *C,* H&E ×500).

if not impossible. Thus, if granulomas are found in a gastric biopsy, every effort should be made to differentiate between sarcoidosis and Crohn's disease because of the different implications of the two diseases. Consequently, full clinical and laboratory investigation is indicated and should include liver biopsy and perhaps lymph node biopsy. Differentiation even then may prove difficult, because the two diseases may share many common features, including liver granulomas and an abnormal Kveim's test result, but granulomas in lymph nodes other than those draining areas involved by Crohn's disease have not been described.

On occasions giant cell granulomas are seen in the stomach wall in relation to food debris or other foreign bodies. In the usual circumstances there is an association with peptic ulceration, perforation, trauma, or other obvious mechanical cause for the introduction of foreign material into the tissues. Sometimes, however, granulomas that show foreign material in close association with the giant cell reactions occur in mucosal biopsies without an apparent predisposing cause. Such "food granulomas" are probably the result of minor trauma to the mucosa and as such have no great significance. Rare causes of gastric granulomas are Whipple's disease and vasculitis, and there are some that occur in association with tumour (Ectors et al 1993).

A granulomatous gastritis, unassociated with a foreign body or with granulomatous involvement of other organs, has been called isolated granulomatous gastritis (Fahimi et al 1963). Although usually an adult disease, it has also been described in children (Hirsch et al 1989) and rarely in association with oesophageal and colonic granulomas (Zuckerman, al-Samman and Boman 1994). In a case studied by the author it was an incidental finding in a gastrectomy specimen from a patient with a large bleeding peptic ulcer. The granulomatous gastritis was widespread, although the lesions tended to occupy the deep aspect of the mucosa (Figs. 9–6 and 9–7). There was no evidence of systemic disease.

Other Forms of Gastritis or Infections

Tuberculous involvement and syphilitic involvement of the stomach are rare. The necessity for a diagnosis of these conditions on gastric biopsy alone hardly ever occurs but there could be difficulty in the differential diagnosis of tuberculosis and Crohn's disease in the absence of caseation necrosis. In tuberculosis, however, the more florid reaction and the confluence of granulomas and their hyalinisation are helpful features. Misra et al (1982) reviewed the literature on gastric tuberculosis and reported a case presenting as a gastric ulcer, which is the usual clinical picture (Mathis, Dirschmid and Sutterlutti 1987). Subei et al (1987) described a mass-like tuberculous lesion at the pylorus in a young man with no evidence of tuberculosis elsewhere. Occasionally tuberculosis is diagnosed at endoscopic biopsy (Al-Quorain 1992).

In syphilitic gastropathy the mucosa is described as oedematous and friable with superficial discrete erosions (Reisman et al 1975). Biopsy revealed dense infiltration of the mucosa by mononuclear cells with a prominent plasma cell component. Neutrophils were also numerous, and in a Warthin-Starry preparation several spirochetes were seen. Preparations were also positive for immunofluorescence. A similar case of ulceroinfiltrative gastropathy was also described by Besses et al (1987). Gastric syphilis is increasingly being recognised (Fyfe et al 1993); it can present as gastric ulceration (de Escalante-Yanguela et al 1993) or mimic linitis plastica (Abdu, Carter

Figure 9–6. Isolated granulomatous gastritis. The giant cell granulomas are located near the muscularis mucosa. Note the coincident chronic atrophic gastritis. This was an incidental finding in a patient with a chronic peptic ulcer (H&E ×75).

Figure 9–7. Detail of granulomas in Figure 9–6 (H&E ×120).

and Pomidor 1993). So-called emphysematous gastritis is a rare form of infectious gastritis caused by gas-forming organisms that invade the gastric wall (McKelvie and Fink 1994).

Scott and Jenkins (1982) reported a 20% incidence of secondary monilial infection in gastric cancer and a 16% incidence in gastric ulcer. The incidence reported by Gotlieb-Jensen and Andersen (1983) was higher at 36%. The subject of *Candida* infection of peptic ulcers in the oesophagus, stomach, and duodenum is discussed by Kalogeropoulos and Whitehead (1988). Primary gastric involvement, although unusual, does occur and is usually, but not always, associated with debility or immune deprivation (Minoli, Terruzzi and Rossini 1979, Minoli et al 1982, Terruzzi and Minoli 1984).

Rarer forms of fungal colonisation of gastric ulcers are due to *Aspergillus fumigatus* (Smith 1969). In histoplasmosis gastric ulceration may occur as part of a generalised infection (Pinkerton and Iverson 1952). Primary gastric mucosal infection with mucormycosis, which causes erosions and ulcers, has also been described (Kahn 1963).

Cytomegalovirus inclusion disease usually occurs as an opportunistic infection. It is being diagnosed endoscopically with increasing frequency in patients with immunodeficiency or immunosuppressed states and malignancy (Kodama et al 1985, Iwasaki 1987, Spiller, Lovell and Silk 1988). Gastric involvement may be part of a generalised infection or it may be localised, possibly due to secondary infection of a peptic ulcer (Andrade et al 1983). It is characterised by the presence of typical inclusions (see Fig. 6–6) in epithelial cells, endothelial cells, and sometimes fibroblasts (Henson 1972, Allen et al 1981, Franzin, Muolo and Griminelli 1981, Strayer et al 1981, Iwasaki 1987).

Primary gastric actinomycosis is extremely rare, but Van Olmen et al (1984) described a case presenting as a bleeding gastric tumour and reviewed the literature. Other rare inflammatory lesions in which endoscopic examination and biopsy were considered to be of value are gastric anisakiasis (Hsiu et al 1986), emphysematous gastritis that followed acute pancreatitis (Bloodworth et al 1987), and localised phlegmonous gastritis (Aviles et al 1988).

MISCELLANEOUS

Gastric Xanthelasma (Xanthoma)

Gastric xanthelasma (Kimura 1969) may occur in any part of the stomach as rounded or oval, yellow or yellow-white macules or nodules 1–5 mm in diameter. Histologically they are usually superficial and are characterised by collections of large histiocytes with a clear cytoplasm and peripheral nucleus (Fig. 9–8). The cells tend to push the glandular elements aside. They contain neutral fat and cholesterol but have no consistent relationship to blood lipid levels. Sometimes the collections of cells are multiple, and they have been noted to disappear spontaneously (Mast et al 1976). There is some evidence that at least some of these lesions are related to previous ulceration or gastric surgery (Domellof et al 1977, Terruzzi et al 1980), and similar collections of cells occur in the region of healed chronic erosions (see Fig. 7–10). There seems to be a particular relationship of xanthelasmas with forms of chronic gastritis and intestinal metaplasia (Moreto et al 1985). Coates et al (1986) reported two cases in which severe gastric involvement by xanthelasmas disappeared with resolution of cholestasis and hypercholesterolaemia but, as already stated, there is no relationship with blood cholesterol levels in the usual case. Xanthelasmas become increasingly common with age, whether associated with earlier surgery or not, and are seen in approximately 60% of all autopsies. Boger and Hort (1977) showed in an electron microscope study that the lipid-laden cells can originate as smooth muscle cells as well as histiocytes. The importance of this lesion relates to the possibility of a misdiagnosis of signet ring carcinoma in ordinary haematoxylin and eosin–stained slides (Drude et al 1982, Pieterse, Rowland and Labrooy 1985). The material within the histiocytes, however, can easily be shown to be normal in periodic

Figure 9–8. Gastric biopsy shows superficial aspect of an atrophic mucosa with pale histiocytes separating crypts and upper gland tubules (H&E ×240).

acid–Schiff and Alcian blue stains. In frozen sections the cells show abnormalities with oil red O or Sudan black stain.

Angiodysplasia

Endoscopic yellowish plaques have been described by Cocco et al (1969) in patients with pseudoxanthoma elasticum. Histologically the lesions have an appearance similar to the other vascular lesions in this disease affecting primarily the submucosal vessels, which show microaneurysms, intimal obliteration, and dystrophic calcification (Berlyne 1960, Kundrotas et al 1988) (Figs. 9–9 to 9–11). The angiomatous lesions of Rendu-Osler disease have also been diagnosed in endoscopic biopsies (Ponsot et al 1983). Acquired angiodysplastic lesions of the stomach have also been described in gastroscopic biopsies (Bank et al 1983), and they have been attributed to cholesterol embolisation of the gastric mucosa due to aortic atheroma. They have been compared with the more commonly encountered colonic angiodysplasia and basically consist of submucosal and mucosal capillary ectasia, sometimes involving draining veins. In the majority of cases, as in the colon, the aetiology appears obscure, and endoscopic descriptions of the lesions vary from hyperaemic mucosal spots to longitudinally arranged rugae converging on the pylorus, each containing dilated vessels that give an appearance resembling a watermelon (Jabbari et al 1984, Fraser et al 1992). Sometimes in biopsy material and usually only in the later stages, capillary ectasia and vascular thrombosis occur (Ruhl et al 1994). Gastric angiodysplasia of this type has been described in association with chronic haemodialysis (Cunningham 1981), portal hypertension (Papazian et al 1986), cirrhosis (Quintero et al 1987, Baxter and Dobbs 1988, Balazs 1993, Cales 1993, Payen et al 1995), and marrow transplantation (Marmaduke et al 1994), but it occurs in their absence (Arendt et al 1987, Tung and Millar 1987, Peny et al 1994). It can be a cause of gastric bleeding (Schwartz et al 1993, D'Elia et al 1994) and is described even in children (Hyams and Treem 1993).

Another increasingly recognised cause of gastric haemorrhage is so-called Dieulafoy's ulcer (Goldman 1964, Sarles et al 1984). This is basically a shallow ulcerated lesion related to an abnormal arterial or arteriovenous malformation of

Figure 9–9. Gastric mucosa in pseudoxanthoma elasticum. Note abnormal submucosal vessels (H&E ×120).

Figure 9–10. Pseudoxanthoma elasticum. Abnormal vessels are partially or totally occluded and elastica is abnormal. Overlying mucosa is necrotic (*A*, H&E ×120, *B*, elastic stain ×120).

the submucosa frequently situated in the proximal stomach. The disease has been reviewed (Mower and Whitehead 1986, Veldhuyzen van Zanten et al 1986), and there is a report (Richter 1975) of actual endoscopic resection of the lesion.

Other Abnormalities

Gastric biopsy will reveal systemic amyloidosis (Filipe and Correia 1963), but it is generally held that rectal biopsy is technically easier and more likely to be diagnostically helpful.

In one study, however, evidence was produced from an autopsy examination that in primary amyloidosis and myeloma-associated disease gastric biopsy would give a superior diagnostic yield (Yamada, Hatakeyama and Tsukagoshi 1985). This has been challenged (Ohno et al 1982), as it seems that gastric biopsy and rectal biopsy give good yields, but rectal biopsy has the highest yield (Lee, Wilson and Gottfried 1994). The deposition sometimes has a curious globular appearance (Fig. 9–12) and may cause haematemesis, nausea, and weight loss (Menke et al 1993). Localised amyloid tumour of the stomach may also be diagnosed by biopsy (Ikeda and Murayama 1978, Balazs 1981). It is a lesion of some importance in that it mimics carcinoma grossly and may or may not occur in association with systemic amyloidosis. The chief cells contain haemosiderin pigment in most patients with haemachromatosis (Joske, Finckh and Wood 1955), and gastric biopsy provides an alternative to liver biopsy if this is difficult or contraindicated. The gastric mucosa sometimes is the site of metastatic calcification (Fig. 9–13) in states of parathyroid hyperfunction.

Figure 9–11. Pseudoxanthoma elasticum. Abnormal vessels show calcification of elastica (von Kossa's ×250).

Figure 9–12. Gastric amyloidosis. The amyloid has an intertubular globular appearance (H&E ×500).

Figure 9–13. Gastric body mucosa with peritubular metastatic calcification *(arrowheads)* in hyperparathyroidism (H&E ×150).

Gastric mucosal calcinosis also occurs in organ transplant patients. The deposits range 40–250 μm in diameter and can be seen under the interfoveolar epithelium (Greenson et al 1993).

With increasing use of hepatic arterial infusion chemotherapy for the treatment of metastatic colon cancer, there has been a recognition of its association with gastric ulceration. Biopsies from such ulcers may easily be mistaken for primary gastric carcinoma (Petras, Hart and Bukowski 1985, Kwee et al 1994). Features that indicate that the lesions are produced by the chemotherapy include the bizarre nature of the cellular atypia yet a low nuclear cytoplasmic ratio, few or no mitotic figures, and relative preservation of mucosal architecture in the histologically abnormal areas (Figs. 9–14 and 9–15). The more basal aspects of the glands appear to be maximally involved, and there may be radiation-like atypia in endothelial cells and fibroblasts. Canioni et al (1995) described gastric changes attributable to busulphan, which closely mimicked cytomegalovirus gastric infection.

Changes in the gastric mucosa may also result in graft versus host disease. The changes are often minimal and consist of single cell necrosis most likely to be seen in the foveolar region of the mucosa. The foveolae may be dilated and occasionally contain polymorphonuclear leukocytes (Snover et al 1985). Langerhans's cell histiocytosis may affect the stomach (Jaffe et al 1993) and at endoscopy can appear as a polyposis. It is, however, histologically characteristic on biopsy (Groisman, Rosh and Harpaz 1994). Doglioni et al (1993) described epithelial cells in the gastric mucosa that morphologically resembled pancreatic acinar cells and contained pancreatic lipase, trypsinogen, and alpha-amylase. There was a significant correlation between their presence and chronic inflammation and with pyloric and intestinal metaplasia. This observation merits further investigation.

Figure 9–14. Gastric biopsy of base of an ulcer produced by hepatic intra-arterial infusion of mitomycin C and 5-fluorouracil. In the base of the ulcer there is marked nuclear pleomorphism, but the tubules, although deformed, have an overall general architecture and an inflamed though normal lamina propria (H&E ×500).

Figure 9–15. Ulcer edge from the same patient as in Figure 9–14. Note abnormal tubule forms and gross nuclear pleomorphism (H&E ×500).

Figure 9–16. Antral mucosa showing changes of prolapse. This rare lesion is presumably related to incoordinate action of the pyloric sphincter mechanism (H&E ×250).

Changes similar to those seen in the colon in mucosal prolapse rarely affect the mucosa of the gastric antrum. In addition to elongation and tortuosity of the gastric pits, muscularisation sometimes of quite a marked degree occurs (Fig. 9–16). The cause of mucosal prolapse is open to conjecture but may be related to gastric motility or emptying problems related to uncoordinate muscular function at the pylorus.

REFERENCES—SECTION TWO: GASTRIC BIOPSY

Aanestad O., Raknerud N., Aase S. T. and Narverud G. (1987) The Cronkhite-Canada syndrome. Acta Chirurgica Scandinavica 153:143–145.

Abdu R. A., Carter K. and Pomidor W. J. (1993) Gastric syphilis mimicking linitis plastica. Archives of Surgery 12:103–104.

Allen J. I., Silvis S. E., Sumner H. W. and McClain C. J. (1981) Cytomegalic inclusion disease diagnosed endoscopically. Digestive Diseases and Sciences 26:133–135.

Allibone R. O., Nanson J. K. and Anthony P. P. (1992) Multiple and recurrent inflammatory fibroid polyps in a Devon family ("Devon polyposis syndrome"): an update. Gut 33:1004–1005.

Al-Quorain A. (1992) Primary gastric tuberculosis: a case report. Annals of Saudi Arabia 12:578–580.

Amarapurkar D. N., Parikh S. S., Prabhu S. R., Kalro R. H. and Desai H. G. (1993) Is gastric metaplasia essential for duodenal ulcer? Journal of Clinical Gastroenterology 17:204–206.

Andrada J. A. and Rose N. R. (1969) Experimental auto-immune gastritis in the Rhesus monkey. Clinical and Experimental Immunology 4:293–310.

Andrade J. De S., Bambirra E. A., Lima G. F., Moreira E. F. and De Oliveira C. A. (1983) Gastric cytomegalic inclusion bodies diagnosed by histologic examination of endoscopic biopsies in patients with gastric ulcer. American Journal of Clinical Pathology 79:493–496.

Andrews G. R., Haneman B., Arnold B. J., Booth J. C. and Taylor K. (1967) Atrophic gastritis in the aged. Australasian Annals of Medicine 16:230–235.

Antonioli D. A. (1994) Precursors of gastric carcinoma: a critical review with a brief description of early (curable) gastric cancer. Human Pathology 25:994–1005.

Appelman H. D. (1994) Gastritis: terminology, etiology and clinicopathological correlations: another biased view. Human Pathology 25:1006–1019.

Arendt T., Barten M., Lakner V. and Arendt R. (1987) Diffuse gastric antral vascular ectasia: cause of chronic gastrointestinal blood loss. Endoscopy 19:218–220.

Ashby B. S., Appleton P. J. and Dawson I. (1964) Eosinophilic granuloma of gastrointestinal tract caused by herring parasite Eustoma rotundatum. British Medical Journal i:1141–1145.

Assad R. T. and Eastwood G. L. (1980) Epithelial proliferation in human fundic mucosa after antrectomy and vagotomy. Gastroenterology 79:807–811.

Aukee S. and Krohn K. (1972) Occurrence and progression of gastritis in patients operated on for peptic ulcer. Scandinavian Journal of Gastroenterology 7:541–546.

Aviles J. F., Fernandez-Seara J., Barcena R., Dominguez F., Fernandez C. and Ledo L. (1988) Localized phlegmonous gastritis: endoscopic view. Endoscopy 20:38–39.

Baba H., Maehara Y., Takeuchi I. et al (1995) Effect of lymph node dissection on the prognosis in patients with node-negative early gastric cancer. Surgery 117:165–169.

Badenoch J., Evans J. R. and Richards W. C. D. (1957) The stomach in hypochromic anaemia. British Journal of Haematology 3:175–185.

Baker A., Volberg F., Sumner T. and Moran R. (1986) Childhood Menetrier's disease: four new cases and discussion of the literature. Gastrointestinal Radiology 11:131–134.

Balazs M. (1981) Amyloidosis of the stomach: report of a case with ultrastructure. Virchows Archiv (A) 391:227–240.

Balazs M. (1993) Gastric vascular ectasia in cirrhosis. Zentralblatt für Pathologie 139:11–16.

Balfour D. C. (1922) Factors influencing the life expectancy of patients operated on for gastric ulcer. Annals of Surgery 76:405–408.

Bank S., Aftalion B., Anfang C., Altman H. and Wise L. (1983) Acquired angiodysplasia as a cause of gastric hemorrhage: a possible consequence of cholesterol embolization. American Journal of Gastroenterology 78:206–209.

Barthel J. S., Westblom T. U., Harvey A. D., Gonzalez F. and Everett E. D. (1988) Gastritis and Campylobacter pylori in healthy, asymptomatic volunteers. Archives of Internal Medicine 148:1149–1151.

Bartlett J. S. (1988) Campylobacter pylori: fact or fancy? Gastroenterology 94:229–238.

Battin-Bertho R., Dauge M. C., Toublanc M., Grossin M., Marche C. I. and Bocquet L. (1987) Helwig's gastric pseudo-tumour: report of three cases and review of the literature. Annals of Pathology 7:176–183.

Bauer T. W., Mendelsohn G., Humphrey R. L. and Mann R. B. (1982) Angioimmunoblastic lymphadenopathy progressing to immunoblastic lymphoma with prominent gastric involvement. Cancer 50:2089–2098.

Baxter J. N. and Dobbs B. R. (1988) Portal hypertensive gastropathy. Journal of Gastroenterology and Hepatology 3:635–644.

Bayerdorffer E., Ritter M. M., Hatz R., Brooks W., Ruckdeschel G. and Stolte M. (1994) Healing of protein-losing hypertrophic gastropathy by eradication of Helicobacter pylori: is Helicobacter pylori a pathogenic factor in Menetrier's disease? Gut 35:701–704.

Bechi P., Amorosi A., Mazzanti R., Romagnoli P. and Tonelli L. (1987) Gastric histology and fasting bile reflux after partial gastrectomy. Gastroenterology 93:335–343.

Bedossa P., Lemaigre G. and Martin E. D. (1987a) Histochemical study of mucosubstances in carcinoma of the gastric remnant. Cancer 60:2224–2227.

Bedossa P., Lemaigre G. and Martin E. (1987b) Fundic gland polyps and polyposis. Annales Pathologie 7:171–175.

Belaiche J., Delwaide J., Vivario M., Gast P., Louis E. and Boniver J. (1993) Fundic argyrophil cell hyperplasia in atrophic gastritis: a search for a sensitive diagnostic method. Acta Gastroenterologique Belgique 56:11–17.

Beneck D. (1994) Hypertrophic gastropathy in a newborn: a case report and review of the literature. Pediatric Pathology 14:213–221.

Berens D. L. and Montes M. (1975) Gastric sarcoidosis. New York State Journal of Medicine 75:1290–1293.

Berenson M. M., Sannella J. and Freston J. W. (1976) Menetrier's disease: serial morphological, secretory, and serological observations. Gastroenterology 70:257–263.

Berkowitz D. M., Passaro E. Jr and Isenberg J. I. (1977) Hypertrophic protein-losing gastropathy and vitiligo: report of a second case. Americal Journal of Digestive Diseases 22:554–558.

Berlyne M. (1960) Pseudoxanthoma elasticum. Lancet 1:77–88.

Berney D. M., Rampton D. and Van Der Walt J. D. (1994) Giardiasis of the stomach. Postgraduate Medical Journal 70:237–238.

Berry E. M., Ben-Dov Y. and Freund U. (1980) Spontaneous remission of protein-losing gastropathy associated with Menetrier's disease. Archives of Internal Medicine 140:99–100.

Berstad A., Alexander B., Weberg R., Serck-Hanssen A., Holland S. and Hirschowitz B. I. (1988) Antacids reduce *Campylobacter pylori* colonization without healing the gastritis in patients with nonulcer dyspepsia and erosive prepyloric changes. Gastroenterology 95:619–624.

Berstad A. and Nesland A. (1987) Erosive prepyloric changes (EPC): a new entity. Scandinavian Journal of Gastroenterology 128:94–100.

Berthrong M. and Fajardo L. F. (1981) Radiation injury in surgical pathology: part II—alimentary tract. American Journal of Surgical Pathology 5:153–178.

Besses C., Sans-Sabrafen J., Badia X., Rodriguez-Mendez F., Salord J. C. and Armengol J. R. (1987) Ulceroinfiltrative syphilitic gastropathy: silver stain diagnosis from biopsy specimen. American Journal of Gastroenterology 82:773–774.

Black W. C. and Haffner H. E. (1968) Diffuse hyperplasia of gastric argyrophil cells and multiple carcinoid tumours: an historical and ultrastructural study. Cancer 21:1080–1099.

Blackburn E. K., Callendar S. T., Dacie J. V., Doll R., Girdwood R. H., Mollin D. L., Saracci R., Stafford J. L., Thompson R. B., Varadi S. and Wetherly-Mein G. (1968) Possible association between pernicious anaemia and leukaemia: a prospective study of 1625 patients with a note on the very high incidence of stomach cancer. International Journal of Cancer 3:163–170.

Blackshaw A. J. and Levison D. A. (1986) Eosinophilic infiltrates of the gastrointestinal tract. Journal of Clinical Pathology 39:1–7.

Blom H. (1984) Light- and electron microscopy of normal and regenerating gastric mucosa with special reference to the parietal cells. Scandinavian Journal of Gastroenterology 105(suppl):33–45.

Bloodworth L. L., Stevens P. E., Bury R. F., Arm J. P. and Rainford D. J. (1987) Emphysematous gastritis after acute pancreatitis. Gut 28:900–902.

Bloom R. A. (1981) Transient protein-losing enteropathy and enlarged gastric rugae. American Journal of Diseases of Children 135:29–33.

Bloom S. R. and Polak J. M. (1981) Gut Hormones. 2nd ed. Edinburgh: Churchill Livingstone.

Bodner E., Pointner R. and Glaser K. (1988) Natural history of early gastric cancer. Lancet 2:631.

Boger A. and Hort W. (1977) The importance of smooth muscle cells in the development of foam cells in the gastric mucosa: an electron microscopic study. Virchows Archiv (A) 372:287–297.

Bogomoletz W. V. (1984a) Early gastric cancer. American Journal of Surgical Pathology 8:381–391.

Bogomoletz W. V. (1984b) Eosinophilic gastroenteritis: a complex disease entity. Survey of Digestive Diseases 2:85–91.

Bogomoletz W. V., Molas G., Potet F., Qizilbash A. H. and Barge J. (1985) Pathological features and mucin histochemistry of primary gastric stump carcinoma associated with gastritis cystica polyposa. American Journal of Surgical Pathology 9:401–410.

Bonney G. E., Elston R. E., Correa P., Haenszel W., Zavala D. E., Zarama G., Collazos T. and Cuello C. (1986) Genetic etiology of gastric carcinoma. Genetic Epidemiology 3:213–224.

Boon M. E., Kurver P. J. H., Baak J. P. A. and Thompson H. T. (1981) The application of morphometry in gastric cytological diagnosis. Virchows Archiv (A) 393:159–164.

Borch K., Renvall H., Liedberg G. and Andersen B. N. (1986) Relations between circulating gastrin and endocrine cell proliferation in the atrophic gastric fundic mucosa. Scandinavian Journal of Gastroenterology 21:357–363.

Borchard F., Mittelstaedt A. and Kieker R. (1979) Incidence of epithelial dysplasia after partial gastric resection. Pathology, Research and Practice 164:282–293.

Bordi C., Ferrari C., D'Adda T., Pilato F., Carfagna G., Bertele A. and Missale G. (1986) Ultrastructural characterization of fundic endocrine cell hyperplasia associated with atrophic gastritis and hypergastrinaemia. Virchows Archiv (A) 409:335–347.

Bordi C. and Ravazzola M. (1979) Endocrine cells in the intestinal metaplasia of gastric mucosa. American Journal of Pathology 90:391–395.

Bordi C., Ravazzola M. and De Vita O. (1983) Pathology of endocrine cells in gastric mucosa. Annals of Pathology 3:19–28.

Borhan-Manesh F. and Farnum J. B. (1993) Study of *Helicobacter pylori* colonization of patches of heterotopic gastric mucosa (HGM) at the upper esophagus. Digestive Diseases and Sciences 38:142–146.

Boyd E. J. S., Hulks G., St. J. Thomas J., and McColl K. E. L. (1988) Hypertrophic gastritis associated with increased gastric mucosal prostaglandin E2 concentrations in a patient with the carcinoid syndrome. Gut 29:1270–1276.

Brooks A. M., Isenberg J. and Goldstein H. (1970) Giant thickening of the gastric mucosa with acid hyposecretion and protein-losing gastropathy. Gastroenterology 58:73–79.

Brooks J. J. and Enterline H. T. (1983) Gastric pseudolymphoma: its three subtypes and relation to lymphoma. Cancer 51:476–486.

Brooks W. S., Wenger J. and Hersh T. (1975) Bile reflux gastritis: analysis of fasting and postprandial gastric aspirates. American Journal of Gastroenterology 64:286–291.

Brousse N., Foldes C., Barge J., Molas G. and Potet F. (1983) Reliability of endoscopic biopsies in the diagnosis of malignant lymphomas of the stomach. Gastroenterologie Clinique et Biologique 7:145–149.

Brown R. C., Hardy G. J., Temperly J. M., Miloszewski K. J. A., Gowland G. and Losowsky M. S. (1981) Gastritis and cirrhosis: no association. Journal of Clinical Pathology 34:744–748.

Burke J. S., Sheibani K., Nathwani B. N., Winberg C. D. and Rappaport H. (1987) Monoclonal small (well-differentiated) lymphocytic proliferations of the gastrointestinal tract resembling lymphoid hyperplasia: a neoplasm of uncertain malignant potential. Human Pathology 18:1238–1245.

Burr M. L., Samloff I. M., Bates C. J. and Holliday R. M. (1987) Atrophic gastritis and vitamin C status in two towns with different stomach cancer death-rates. British Journal of Cancer 56:163–167.

Byrnes D. J., Young J. D., Chisholm D. T. and Lazarus L. (1970) Serum gastrin in patients with peptic ulceration. British Medical Journal ii:626–629.

Calam J., Krasner N. and Haqqani M. (1982) Extensive gastrointestinal damage following a saline emetic. Digestive Diseases and Sciences 27:936–940.

Cales P. (1993) Mucosal lesions of the digestive tract in cirrhosis. Acta Gastroenterologica Belgica 56:169–178.

Canioni D., Vassal G., Donadieu J. et al (1995) Toxicity induced by chemotherapy mimicking cytomegalovirus gastritis. Histopathology 26:473–475.

Carfagna G., Pilato F. P., Bordi C., Barsotti P. and Riva C. (1987) Solitary polypoid hamartoma of the oxyntic mucosa of the stomach. Pathology, Research and Practice 182:326–330.

Carneiro F., David L., Seruca R., Castedo S., Nesland J. M. and Sobrinho-Simões M. (1993) Hyperplastic polyposis and diffuse carcinoma of the stomach: a study of a family. Cancer 72:323–329.

Caruso R. A. and Famulari C. (1992) Neoplastic Paneth cells in adenocarcinoma of the stomach: a case report. Hepato-Gastroenterology 39:264–266.

Celik C., Ettinger D. and Satchidanand S. (1984) Massive bleeding in hypertrophic gastropathy (Menetrier's disease) due to arterio-venous malformation. Journal of Medicine 15:65–73.

Chakravorty R. C. and Schatzki P. F. (1975) Gastric cystic polyposis. American Journal of Digestive Disease 20:981–989.

Chambers L. A. and Clark W. E. (1986) The endoscopic diagnosis of gastroesophageal malignancy. Acta Cytologica 30:110–114.

Chan J. K. C. (1994) Antibiotic: responsive gastric lymphoma? Advances in Anatomic Pathology 1:33–37.

Chan T. O., Kuo Y. C., Chien R. N. Sheen I. S., Lin D. Y., Chu C. M., Chen P. C. and Wu C. S. (1992) Gastric adenocarcinoma simulating benign gastric ulcer. Chang Keng I Hsueh 15:59–63.

Chanarin I. and James D. (1974) Humoral and cell-mediated intrinsic-factor antibody in pernicious anaemia. Lancet i:1078–1080.

Cheli R., Perasso A. and Giacosa A. (1983) Dyspepsia and chronic gastritis. Hepato-Gastroenterology 30:21–23.

Cheng J., Ritchie W. P. Jr and Delaney J. (1969) Atrophic gastritis: an experimental model. Federation Proceedings 28:513.

Chinitz M. A., Brandt L. J., Frank M. S., Frager D. and Sablay L. (1985) Symptomatic sarcoidosis of the stomach. Digestive Diseases and Sciences 30:682–688.

Chlumsky J., Krtek V. and Chlumska A. (1985) Sarcoidosis of the stomach. Endoscopic diagnosis and possibilities of conservative treatment. Hepato-Gastroenterology 32:255–257.

Christ A. D., Meier R., Bauerfeind P., Wegmann W. and Gyr K. (1993) Simultaneous occurrence of lymphocytic gastritis and lymphocytic colitis with transition to collagenous colitis. Schweizerische Medizinische Wochenschrift 123:1487–1490.

Church J. M., McGannon E., Hull-Boiner S. Sivalc M. V., Van Stolk R., Jagelman D. G., Fazio V. W., Oakley J. R., Laver I. C. and Milsom J. W. (1992) Gastroduodenal polyps in patients with familial adenomatous polyposis. Diseases of the Colon and Rectum 35:1170–1173.

Churg J. and Strauss L. (1951) Allergic granulomatosis, allergic angiitis and periarteritis nodosa. American Journal of Pathology 27:277–294.

Cieslak T. J., Mullett C. T., Puntel R. A. and Latimer J. S. (1993) Menetrier's disease associated with cytomegalovirus infection in children: report of two cases and review of the literature. Pediatric Infectious Disease Journal 12:340–343.

Clark C. G., Fresini A. and Gledhill T. (1985) Cancer following gastric surgery. British Journal of Surgery 72:591–594.

Clarke A. C., Lee S. P. and Nicholson G. I. (1977) Gastritis varioliformis. American Journal of Gastroenterology 68:599–602.

Clarkson K. S. and West K. P. (1993) Gastric cancer and *Helicobacter pylori* infection. Journal of Clinical Pathology 46:997–999.

Coates A. G., Nostrant T. T., Wilson J. A. P., Dobbins W. O. and Agha F. P. (1986) Gastric xanthomatosis and cholestasis: a causal relationship. Digestive Diseases and Sciences 31:925–928.

Cocco A. E., Grayer D. I., Walker B. A. and Martyn L. J. (1969) The stomach in pseudoxanthoma elasticum. Journal of the American Medical Association 210:2381–2382.

Cocking J. B. and Grech P. (1973) Pyloric reflux and the healing of gastric ulcers. Gut 14:555–557.

Coghill N. F. (1960) The significance of gastritis. Postgraduate Medical Journal 36:733–742.

Coghill N. F. (1969) Chronic idiopathic gastritis: cause and effect. In: Fifth Symposium on Advanced Medicine. Edited by R. Williams. London: Pitman Medical, p 14.

Coghill N. F. and Williams A. W. (1958) Gastric mucosa in hypochromic anaemia. Proceedings of the Royal Society of Medicine 51:464.

Correa P. (1980) The epidemiology and pathogenesis of chronic gastritis: three etiologic entities. Frontiers of Gastrointestinal Research 6:98–108.

Correa P. (1982) Precursors of gastric and esophageal cancer. Cancer 50:2554–2565.

Correa P. (1988) Chronic gastritis: a clinico-pathological classification. American Journal of Gastroenterology 83:504–509.

Correa P. (1995) *Helicobacter pylori* and gastric carcinogenesis. American Journal of Surgical Pathology 19(suppl 1):S37–S43.

Correa P., Fox J., Fontham E., Ruiz B., Lin Y. P., Zavala D., Taylor N., Mackinleyy D., deLima E., Portilla H., et al. (1990) *Helicobacter pylori* and gastric carcinoma: serum antibody prevalence in populations with contrasting cancer risks. Cancer 66:2569–2574.

Correa P. and Yardley J. H. (1992) Grading and classification of chronic gastritis: one American response to the Sydney System. Gastroenterology 102:355–356.

Craanen M. E., Blok P., Dekker W. and Tytgat G. N. (1994) *Helicobacter pylori* and early gastric cancer. Gut 35:1372–1374.

Croft D. N. (1963) Aspirin and the exfoliation of gastric epithelial cells. Cytological and biochemical observations. British Medical Journal ii:897–901.

Cronkhite L. W. and Canada W. J. (1955) Generalized gastrointestinal polyposis: an unusual syndrome of polyposis, pigmentation, alopecia and onychotrophia. New England Journal of Medicine 252:1011–1015.

Croxon S., Chen K. and Davidson A. R. (1987) Sarcoidosis of the stomach. Digestion 38:193–196.

Cruveilhier J. (1862) Traite d'anatomie pathologique generale. Paris: Bailliere, p 484.

Cuello C., Lopez J., Correa P., Murray J., Zarama G. and Gordillo G. (1979) Histopathology of gastric dysplasias. Correlations with gastric juice chemistry. American Journal of Surgical Pathology 3:491–500.

Cunningham J. T. (1981) Gastric telangiectasias in chronic hemodialysis patients: a report of six cases. Gastroenterology 81:1131–1133.

Czerniak B., Herz F. and Koss L. G. (1987) DNA distribution patterns in early gastric carcinomas. Cancer 59:113–117.

Daibo M., Itabashi M. and Hirota T. (1987) Malignant transformation of gastric hyperplastic polyps. American Journal of Gastroenterology 82:1016–1025.

Daniel E. S., Ludwig S. L., Lewin K. J., Ruprecht R. M., Rajacich G. M. and Schwabe A. D. (1982) The Cronkhite-Canada syndrome: an analysis of clinical and pathologic features and therapy in 55 patients. Medicine 61:293–309.

Davenport H. W. (1967) Salicylate damage to the gastric mucosal barrier. New England Journal of Medicine 276:1307–1312.

Davenport H. W. (1968) Destruction of gastric mucosal barrier by detergents and urea. Gastroenterology 54:175–181.

Dawson I. (1970) The endocrine cells of the gastrointestinal tract. Histochemical Journal 2:527–549.

De Aizpurua H. J., Cosgrove L. J., Ungar B., and Toh B-H. (1983) Autoantibodies cytotoxic to gastric parietal cells in serum of patients with pernicious anemia. New England Journal of Medicine 309:625–629.

De Boer W. G. R. M., Forsyth A. and Nairn R. C. (1969) Gastric antigens in health and disease. Behaviour in early development, senescence, metaplasia and cancer. British Medical Journal iii:93–94.

De Boni M., De Bona M. and Cielo R. (1994) *Helicobacter pylori* and pre-neoplastic and neoplastic gastric lesions. Italian Journal of Gastroenterology 26(suppl 1):29–34.

Debray C., Hardouin J. P., Laumonier R., Housset P., Helie T. P. and Martin E. (1957) La gastrite ethylique sous le controle de la gastrobiopsie. Archives des maladies de l'appareil digestif et de la nutrition. 46:925–937.

De Escalante Yangüela B., Lacasa-Marzo J., Carrasquer Sese J. A., Oncins Torres R., Palazon Astiz R. and Sampedro Feliu J. A. (1993) Gastric ulcers: a rare manifestation of secondary syphilis. Anales de Medicina Interna 10:287–289.

De Giacomo C., Gianatti A., Negrini R. Perotti P., Bawa P., Maggiore G. and Fiocca R. (1994) Lymphocytic gastritis: a positive relationship with celiac disease. Journal of Pediatrics 124:57–62.

De Koster E., Buset M., Fernandes E. and Deltenre M. (1994) *Helicobacter pylori*: the link with gastric cancer. European Journal of Cancer Preview 3:247–257.

Delaney J. P., Cheng J. W. B., Butler B. A. and Ritchie W. P. (1970) Gastric ulcer and regurgitation gastritis. Gut 11:715–719.

D'Elia G. et al (1994) Gastric angiodysplasia: a rare cause of bleeding from the upper digestive tract. Giornale di Chirurgia 15:460–465.

DeSchryver-Kecskemeti K. and Clouse R. E. (1984) A previously unrecognized subgroup of "eosinophilic gastroenteritis." American Journal of Surgical Pathology 8:171–180.

Deutsch J. P., Mariette D., Moukarbel N., Pace R. and Tubiana J. M. (1994) Gastroduodenal intussusception secondary to Menetrier's disease. Abdominal Imaging 19:207–209.

Deviere J., Buset M., Dumonceau J-M., Rickaert F. and Cremer M. (1989) Regression of Barrett's epithelium with Omeprazole. New England Journal of Medicine 320:1497–1498.

Dewar P., Dixon M. F. and Johnston D. (1984) Bile reflux and degree of gastritis in patients with gastric ulcer: before and after operation. Journal of Surgical Research 37:277–284.

Dickey W., Collins J. S., Watson R. G., Sloan J. M. and Porter K. G. (1993) Secretor status and *Helicobacter pylori* infection are independent risk factors for gastroduodenal disease. Gut 34:351–353.

Di Gregorio C., Morandi P., Fante R. and De Gaetani C. (1993) Gastric dysplasia: a follow-up study. American Journal of Gastroenterology 88:1714–1719.

Dinoso V. P. Jr, Chey W. Y., Braverman S. P., Rosen A. P., Ottenberg D. and Lorber S. H. (1972) Gastric secretion and gastric mucosal morphology in chronic alcoholics. Archives of Internal Medicine 130:715–719.

Diss T. C., Peng H., Wotherspoon A. C., Pan L., Speight P. M. and Isaacson P. G. (1993) Single neoplastic clone in sequential biopsy specimens from a patient with primary gastric mucosa-associated lymphoid tissue lymphoma and Sjogren's syndrome. New England Journal of Medicine 329:172–175.

Dixon M. F. (1994) Pathophysiology of *Helicobacter pylori* infection. Scandinavian Journal of Gastroenterology 201(suppl):7–10.

Dixon M. F., O'Connor H. J., Axon A. T. R., King R. F. J. G. and Johnston D. (1986) Reflux gastritis: distinct histopathological entity? Journal of Clinical Pathology 39:524–530.

Dixon M. F., Wyatt J. I., Burke D. A. and Rathbone B. J. (1988) Lymphocytic gastritis: relationship to *Campylobacter pylori* infection. Journal of Pathology 154:125–132.

Doglioni C., Laurino L., Dei Tos A. P., De Boni M., Franzin G., Braidotti P. and Viale G. (1993) Pancreatic (acinar) metaplasia of the gastric mucosa: histology, ultrastructure, immunocytochemistry and clinico-pathologic correlations of 101 cases. American Journal of Surgical Pathology 17:1134–1143.

Dommellof L., Eriksson S., Helander H. F. and Janunger K.-G. (1977) Lipid islands in the gastric mucosa after resection for benign ulcer disease. Gastroenterology 72:14–18.

Dougherty St. H., Foster C. A. and Eisenberg M. M. (1982) Stomach cancer following gastric surgery for benign disease. Archives of Surgery 117:294–297.

Drude R. B., Balart L. A., Herrington J. P., Beckman E. N. and Burns T. W. (1982) Gastric xanthoma: histologic similarity to signet ring cell carcinoma. Journal of Clinical Gastroenterology 4:217–221.

Duggan J. M., Dobson A. J., Johnson H. and Fahey P. (1986) Peptic ulcer and non-steroidal anti-inflammatory agents. Gut 27:929–933.

Eastwood G. L. (1975) Effect of pH on bile salt injury to mouse gastric mucosa: a light and electron-microscopic study. Gastroenterology 68:1456–1465.

Eckardt V. F., Willems D., Kanzler G., Remmele W., Bettendorf U. and Paulus W. (1984) Eighty months persistence of poorly differentiated early gastric cancer. Gastroenterology 87:719–724.

Ectors N. L., Dixon M. F., Geboes K. J, Rutgeerts P. J., Desmet V. J. and Vantrappen G. (1993) Granulomatous gastritis: a morphological and diagnostic approach. Histopathology 23:55–61.

Edwards F. C. and Coghill N. F. (1966) Aetiological factors in chronic atrophic gastritis. British Medical Journal ii:1409–1415.

Edwards F. C. and Edwards J. H. (1956) Tea drinking and gastritis. Lancet ii:543–545.

Eidt S. and Stolte M. (1993a) Prevalence of lymphoid follicles and aggregates in *Helicobacter pylori* gastritis in antral and body mucosa. Journal of Clinical Pathology 46:832–835.

Eidt S. and Stolte M. (1993b) Antral and intestinal metaplasia in *Helicobacter pylori* gastritis. Digestion 55:13–18.

Eidt S. and Stolte M. (1994) Prevalence of intestinal metaplasia in *Helicobacter pylori* gastritis. Scandinavian Journal of Gastroenterology 29:607–610.

Eidt S., Stolte M. and Fischer R. (1994) *Helicobacter pylori* gastritis and primary gastric non-Hodgkin's lymphomas. Journal of Clinical Pathology 47:436–439.

Elkeles A. (1964) Gastric ulcer in the aged and calcified atherosclerosis. American Journal of Roentgenology 91:744–750.

Elsborg L., Anderson D., Myhre-Jansen O. and Bastrup-Madsen P. (1977) Gastric mucosal polyps in pernicious anaemia. Scandinavian Journal of Gastroenterology 12:49–52.

Elster K. (1974) A new approach to the classification of gastric polyps. Endoscopy 6:44–47.

Elster K. (1976) Histologic classification of gastric polyps. In: Current Topics in Pathology 63. Edited by B. C. Morson. Heidelberg: Springer-Verlag, pp 77–93.

Elster K., Carson W., Wild A. and Thomasko A. (1979) Evaluation of histological classification in early gastric cancer: (an analysis of 300 cases). Endoscopy 3:203–206.

Elta G. H., Fawaz K. A., Dayal Y., McLean A. M., Phillips E., Bloom S. M., Paul R. E. and Kaplan M. M. (1983) Chronic erosive gastritis: a recently recognized disorder. Digestive Diseases and Sciences 28:7–12.

Eras P., Goldstein M. J. and Sherlock P. (1972) *Candida* infection of the gastrointestinal tract. Medicine (Baltimore) 54:367–379.

Evans D. M. D., Craven J. L., Murphy F. and Cleary B. K. (1978) Comparison of "early gastric cancer" in Britain and Japan. Gut 19:1–9.

Faber K. (1935) Gastritis and Its Consequences. London: Oxford University Press.

Fahimi H. D., Deren J. J., Gottlieb L. S. and Zamcheck N. (1963) Isolated granulomatous gastritis: its relationship to disseminated sarcoidosis and regional enteritis. Gastroenterology 45:161–175.

Falkmer S. and Wilander E. (1995) The endocrine cell population. In: Gastrointestinal and Oesophageal Pathology, 2nd ed. Edited by R. Whitehead. Edinburgh: Churchill Livingstone, pp 63–71.

Farahat K., Hianaut P., Jamar F., Haot J. and Lambert M. (1993) Lymphocytic gastritis: an unusual cause of hypoproteinaemia. Journal of Internal Medicine 234:95–100.

Farinati F., Cardin F., Di Mario F., Vianello F., Battaglia G., agniini Pagnini C., Cannizzaro R., Sava G. A., Rugge M. and Naccarato R. (1987) Early and advanced gastric cancer during follow-up of apparently benign gastric ulcer: significance of the presence of epithelial dysplasia. Journal of Surgical Oncology 36:263–267.

Farinati F., Rugge M., Di Mario F., Valiante F. and Baffa R. (1993) Early and advanced gastric cancer in the follow-up of moderate and severe gastric dysplasia patients: a prospective study. Endoscopy 25:261–264.

Farinati F., Valiante F., Germana B., Della Lisera G., Batta R., Rugge M., Plebani M., Vianello F., DiMario F. and Naccarato R. (1993) Prevalence of *Helicobacter pylori* infection in patients with precancerous changes and gastric cancer. European Journal of Cancer Prevention 2:321–326.

Farini R., Leandro G., Farinati F., Di Mario F., Scalabrin G., Mazzucato B., Cecchetto A. and Naccarato R. (1981) Epithelial dysplasia in endoscopic gastric mucosal biopsies. Tumori 67:589–598.

Farrands P. A., Blake J. R. S., Ansell I. D., Cotton R. E. and Hardcastle J. D. (1983) Endoscopic review of patients who have had gastric surgery. British Medical Journal 286:755–758.

Farthing M. J. G., Fairclough P. D., Hegarty J. E., Swarbrick E. T. and Dawson A. M. (1981) Treatment of chronic erosive gastritis with prednisolone. Gut 22:759–762.

Fend F., Schwaiger A., Weyrer K., Propst A., Mairinger T., Umlauft F., Judmaier G. and Grünewald K. (1994) Early diagnosis of gastric lymphoma: gene rearrangement analysis of endoscopic biopsy samples. Leukemia 8:35–39.

Ferrer-Roca O. (1982) Primary gastric plasmacytoma with massive intracytoplasmic crystalline inclusions: a case report. Cancer 50:755–759.

Fertitta A. M., Comin U., Terruzzi V., Minoli G., Zambelli A., Canatelli G., Bodini P., Bertoli G., Negri R., Brunati S., et al (1993) Clinical significance of gastric dysplasia: a multicenter follow-up study. Endoscopy 25:265–268.

Filipe M. I. (1983) In: Histochemistry in Pathology. Edited by M. I. Filipe and B. D. Lake. Edinburgh: Churchill Livingston, p 128.

Filipe M. I. and Correia J. P. (1963) La valeur de la biopsie gastrique dans l'etude des lesions diffuses de l'estomac. Gastroenterologia 100:19–32.

Filipe M. I., Munoz N., Matko I., Kato I., Pompe-Kirn V., Juterselc A., Teuchmann S., Benz M. and Prijon T. (1994) Intestinal metaplasia types and the risk of gastric cancer: a cohort study in Slovenia. International Journal of Cancer 57:324–329.

Filipe M. I., Potet F., Bogomoletz W. V., Dawson P. A., Fabiani B., Chauveinc P., Fenzy A., Gazzard B., Goldfain D. and Zeegen R. (1985) Incomplete sulphomucin-secreting intestinal metaplasia for gastric cancer: preliminary data from a prospective study from three centres. Gut 26:1319–1326.

Fitzgibbons P. L., Dooley C. P., Cohen H. and Appleman M. D. (1988) Prevalence of gastric metaplasia, inflammation, and *Campylobacter pylori* in the duodenum of members of the normal population. American Journal of Clinical Pathology 90:711–714.

Flowers R. S., Kyle K. and Hoerr S. O. (1970) Post-operative hemorrhage from stress ulceration of the stomach and duodenum. American Journal of Surgery 119:632–639.

Fonde E. C. and Rodning C. B. (1986) Gastritis cystica profunda. American Journal of Gastroenterology 81:459–464.

Fontham E., Zavala D., Correa P., Rodriguez E., Hunter F., Haenszel W. and Tannenbaum S. R. (1986) Diet and chronic atrophic gastritis: a case control study. Journal of the National Cancer Institute 76:621–627.

Fortman L. M., Johanson J. F., Baskin W. N. and Greenlaw R. L. (1993) Eosinophilic ascites without eosinophilia: a unique presentation of serosal eosinophilic gastroenteritis. American Journal of Gastroenterology 88:1280–1281.

Fraile G., Rodriguez-Garcia J. L., Beni-Perez R. and Redondo C. (1994) Localized eosinophilic gastroenteritis with necrotizing granulomas presenting as acute abdomen. Postgraduate Medical Journal 70:510–512.

Franzin G., Manfrini C., Musola R., Rodella S. and Fratton A. (1984) Chronic erosions of the stomach. Endoscopy 16:1–5.

Franzin G., Muolo A. and Griminelli T. (1981) Cytomegalovirus inclusions in the gastroduodenal mucosa of patients after renal transplantation. Gut 22:698–701.

Franzin G., Musola R., Zamboni G. and Manfrini C. (1985) Gastritis cystica polyposa: a possible precancerous lesion. Tumori 71:13–18.

Franzin G. and Novelli P. (1981) Gastritis cystica profunda. Histopathology 5:535–547.

Fraser A. G., Koelmayer T., White A. C. and Nicholson G. I. (1992) Antral vascular ectasia: the watermelon stomach. New Zealand Medical Journal 105:338–339.

Freeman K., Anthony P. P., Miller D. S. and Warin A. P. (1985) Cronkhite-Canada syndrome: a new hypothesis. Gut 26:531–536.

Freise J., Hofmann R., Gebel M. and Huchzermeyer H. (1979) Follow-up study of chronic gastric erosions. Endoscopy 1:13–17.

Frommer D. J., Carrick J., Lee A. and Hazell S. L. (1988) Acute presentation of *Campylobacter pylori* gastritis. American Journal of Gastroenterology 83:1168–1171.

Fruin R. C., Littman M. S. and Littman A. (1963) Intragastric beta-irradiation with rutheniumrhodium 106 in patients with peptic ulcer and gastric neoplasm. Gastroenterology 45:34–42.

Fujimoto S., Takahashi M., Ohkubo H., Mutou T., Kure M., Masaoka H. and Kobayashi K. (1994) Comparative clinicopathologic features of early gastric cancer in young and older patients. Surgery 115:516–520.

Fujita S. (1978) Biology of early gastric carcinoma. Pathology, Research and Practice 163:297–309.

Fukuda T., Ohnishi Y., Nishimaki T., Ohtani H. and Tachikawa S. (1988) Early gastric cancer of the small cell type. American Journal of Gastroenterology 83:1176–1179.

Fung W. P., Foo K. T. and Lee Y. S. (1975) Gastric sarcoidosis presenting with haematemesis. Medical Journal of Australia 2:47–49.

Fyfe B., Poppiti R. J, Lubin J. and Robinson M. J. (1993) Gastric syphilis: primary diagnosis by gastric biopsy: report of four cases. Archives of Pathology and Laboratory Medicine 117:820–823.

Gabreau T., Delage Y., Conte-Marti J. and Bodin F. (1982) Menetrier's disease with normal gastric acid secretion: report of a patient treated with Cimetidine. Gastroenterologie Clinique et Biologique 6:38–42.

Gad A. (1986) Erosions: a correlative endoscopic histopathologic multicenter study. Endoscopy 18:76–79.

Gallagher C. G., Lennon J. R. and Crowe J. P. (1987) Chronic erosive gastritis: a clinical study. American Journal of Gastroenterology 82:302–306.

Gallagher P., Harris M., Turnbull F. W. A. and Turner L. (1984) Gastric sarcoidosis. Journal of the Royal Society of Medicine 77:837–839.

Gazzard B. G. (1988) HIV disease and the gastroenterologist. Gut 29:1497–1505.

Gear M. W. L., Truelove S. C. and Whitehead R. (1971) Gastric ulcer and gastritis. Gut 12:639–645.

Gear M. W. L., Truelove S. C., Gwyn Williams D., Massarella G. R. and Boddington M. M. (1969) Gastric cancer simulating benign gastric ulcer. British Journal of Surgery 56:739–742.

Genta R. M. and Hamner H. W. (1994) The significance of lymphoid follicles in the interpretation of gastric biopsy specimens. Archives of Pathology and Laboratory Medicine 118:740–743.

Genta R. M., Hamner H. W. and Graham D. Y. (1993) Gastric lymphoid follicles in *Helicobacter pylori* infection: frequency, distribution and response to triple therapy. Human Pathology 24:577–583.

Genta R. M., Huberman R. M. and Graham D. Y. (1994) The gastric cardia in *Helicobacter pylori* infection. Human Pathology 25:915–919.

Genta R. M., Lew G. M. and Graham D. Y. (1993) Changes in the gastric mucosa following eradication of *Helicobacter pylori*. Modern Pathology 6:281–289.

Genta R. M., Robason G. O. and Graham D. Y. (1994) Simultaneous visualization of *Helicobacter pylori* and gastric morphology: a new stain. Human Pathology 25:221–226.

Ghandur-Mnaymneh L., Paz J., Roldan E. and Cassady J. (1988) Dysplasia of nonmetaplastic gastric mucosa. American Journal of Surgical Pathology 12:96–114.

Giler S., Kadish U. and Urca I. (1976) Peroral staining method with toluidine blue as an aid in the diagnosis of malignant gastric lesions. American Journal of Gastroenterology 65:37–40.

Gill H. H. and Desai H. G. (1993) *Helicobacter pylori* and gastroduodenal disorders in India: lessons from epidemiology. Journal of Clinical Gastroenterology 16:6–9.

Glass G. B. (1965) The natural history of gastric atrophy: a review of immunologic aspects and possible links to endogenous inhibitors of gastric secretion. American Journal of Digestive Diseases 10:376–398.

Glass G. B. J. (1977) Immunology of atrophic gastritis. New York State Journal of Medicine 77:1697–1706.

Glass G. B. and Ishimori A. (1961) Passage of serum albumin into the stomach: its detection by paper electrophoresis of gastric juice in protein-losing gastropathies and gastric cancer. American Journal of Digestive Diseases 6:103–133.

Glass G. B., Speer F. D., Neiburgs H. E., Ishimori A., Jones E. L., Baker H., Schwartz S. A. and Smith R. (1960) Gastric atrophy, atrophic gastritis and gastric secretory failure: correlative study by suction biopsy and exfoliative cytology of gastric mucosa, paper electrophoretic and secretory assays of gastric secretion and measurements of intestinal absorption and blood levels of vitamin B_{12}. Gastroenterology 39:429–453.

Gledhill T., Leicester R. J, Addis B., Lightfoot N., Barnard J., Viney N., Darkin D. and Hunt R. H. (1985) Epidemic hypochlorhydria. British Medical Journal 290:1383–1386.

Glober G., Pena A. S., Whitehead G., Gear M. W. L., Roca M., Kerrigan G. and Truelove S. C. (1972) A. B. O. blood groups, rhesus factor and intestinal metaplasia of the stomach. British Journal of Cancer 26:420–422.

Goldgraber M. B., Rubin C. E., Palmer W. L., Dobson R. L. and Massey B. W. (1954) The early gastric response to irradiation, a serial biopsy study. Gastroenterology 27:1–20.

Goldman H., French S. and Burbige E. (1981) Kulchitsky cell hyperplasia and multiple metastasizing carcinoids of the stomach. Cancer 47:2620–2626.

Goldman H. and Ming S. C. (1968) Fine structure of intestinal metaplasia and adenocarcinoma of the human stomach. Laboratory Investigations 18:203–210.

Goldman R. L. (1964) Submucosal arterial malformation ("aneurysm") of the stomach with fatal haemorrhage. Gastroenterology 46:589–594.

Goldstein F., Kline T. S., Kline I. K., Thornton J. J., Abramson J. and Bell L. (1983) Early gastric cancer in a United States hospital. American Journal of Gastroenterology 78:715–719.

Gonzalez-Crussi F. and Hackett R. L. (1966) Phlegmonous gastritis. Archives of Surgery 93:990–995.

Gotlieb-Jensen K. and Andersen J. (1983) Occurrence of *Candida* in gastric ulcers. Gastroenterology 85:535–537.

Gottfried E. B., Korsten M. A. and Lieber C. S. (1978) Alcohol-induced gastric and duodenal lesions in man. American Journal of Gastroenterology 70:587–592.

Graem N., Fischer A. B., Hastrup N. and Povlsen C. O. (1981) Mucosal changes of the Billroth II resected stomach. Acta Pathologica, Microbiologica et Immunologica Scandinavica, Section A 89:227–234.

Graffner H. and Hesselvik M. (1987) Gastric pseudolymphoma. Acta Chirurgica Scandinavica 153:471–472.

Graham D. Y. (1989) *Campylobacter pylori* and peptic ulcer disease. Gastroenterology 96:615–625.

Graham D. Y., Agrawal N. M. and Roth S. H. (1988) Prevention of NSAID-induced gastric ulcer with Misoprostol: multicentre, double-blind, placebo-controlled trial. Lancet 2:1277–1280.

Graham D. Y. and Michaletz P. A. (1988) Should I search for *Campylobacter pylori* in my patients? Much ado about not much? American Journal of Gastroenterology 83:481–483.

Graham D. Y. and Smith J. L. (1986) Aspirin and the stomach. (review). Annals of Internal Medicine 104:390–398.

Green P. H. R., Fevre D. I., Barrett P. J., Hunt J. H., Gillespie P. E. and Nagy G. S. (1977) Chronic erosive (verrucous) gastritis: A study of 108 patients. Endoscopy 9:74–78.

Green P. H. R., O'Toole K. M., Weinberg L. M. and Goldfarb J. P. (1981) Early gastric cancer. Gastroenterology 81:247–256.

Greenson J. K., Trinidad S. B., Pfeil S. A., Brainard J. A., McBride P. T. Colijn H. O., Tesi R. J. and Lucas J. G. (1993) Gastric mucosal calcinosis. American Journal of Surgical Pathology 17:45–50.

Grigioni W. F., D'Errico A., Milani M., Villanacci V., Avellini C., Miglioli M., Mattioli S., Biasco G., Barbara L. and Possati L. (1984) Early gastric cancer: clinico-pathological analysis of 125 cases of early gastric cancer (EGC). Acta Pathologica Japonica 34:979–989.

Groisman G. M., George J., Berman D. and Harpaz N. (1994) Resolution of protein-losing hypertrophic lymphocytic gastritis with therapeutic eradication of *Helicobacter pylori*. American Journal of Gastroenterology 89:1548–1551.

Groisman G. M., Rosh J. R. and Harpaz N. (1994) Langerhans cell histiocytosis of the stomach: a cause of granulomatous gastritis and gastric polyposis. Archives of Pathology and Laboratory Medicine 118:1232–1235.

Guadagni S., Reed P. I., Johnston B. J., De Bernardinis G., Catarci M., Valenti M., di Orio F. and Carboni M. (1993) Early gastric cancer: follow-up after gastrectomy in 159 patients. British Journal of Surgery 80:325–328.

Guardia J., Mirada A., Moragas A., Armengol J. R. and Martinez-Vazquez J. M. (1980) Alpha chain disease of the stomach. Hepato-Gastroenterology 28:238–239.

Halbert R. E. (1982) Peutz-Jeghers syndrome with metastasizing gastric adenocarcinoma (report of a case). Archives of Pathology and Laboratory Medicine 106:517–520.

Halter F., Witzel L., Gretillat P. A., Scheurer U. and Keller M. (1977) Diagnostic value of biopsy, guided lavage, and brush cytology in esophagogastroscopy. American Journal of Digestive Diseases 22:129–131.

Hamilton S. R. and Yardley J. H. (1980) Endoscopic biopsy diagnosis of aspirin-associated chronic gastric ulcers. Gastroenterology 78:1178.

Haot J., Berger F., Andre C., Moulinier B., Mainguet P. and Lambert R. (1989) Lymphocytic gastritis versus varioliform gastritis: a historical series revisited. Journal of Pathology 158:19–22.

Haot J., Bogomoletz W. V., Jouret A. and Mainguet P. (1991) Menetrier's disease with lymphocytic gastritis: an unusual association with possible pathogenic implications. Human Pathology 22:379–386.

Haot J., Hamichi L., Wallez L. and Mainguet P. (1988) Lymphocytic gastritis: a newly described entity: a retrospective endoscopic and histological study. Gut 29:1258–1264.

Harned R. K., Buck J. L. and Sobin L. H. (1995) The hamartomatous polyposis syndromes: clinical and radiologic features. American Journal of Roentgenology 164:565–571.

Harris N. L. (1993) Low-grade B-cell lymphoma of mucous-associated lymphoid tissue and monocytoid B-cell lymphoma: related entities that are distinct from other low-grade B-cell lymphomas (editorial). Archives of Pathology and Laboratory Medicine 117:771–775.

Harvey B. C. H. (1907) A study of the structure of the gastric glands of dogs and the changes which they undergo after gastroenterostomy and occlusion of the pylorus. American Journal of Anatomy 6:207–243.

Hatfield A. R. W., Slavin G., Segal A. W. and Levi A. J. (1975) Importance of the site of endoscopic gastric biopsy in ulcerating lesions of the stomach. Gut 16:884–886.

Hattori T. (1985) Morphological range of hyperplastic polyps and carcinomas arising in hyperplastic polyps of the stomach. Journal of Clinical Pathology 38:622–630.

Henson D. (1972) Cytomegalovirus inclusion bodies in the gastrointestinal tract. Archives of Pathology 93:477–482.

Hermanek P. and Riemann J. F. (1982) The operated stomach: still a precancerous condition? Endoscopy 14:113–114.

Hernandez J. A. and Sheehan W. W. (1985) Lymphomas of the mucosa-associated lymphoid tissue: signet ring cell lymphomas presenting in mucosal lymphoid organs. Cancer 55:592–597.

Hirsch B. Z., Whitington P. F., Kirschner B. S., Black D. D., Bostwick D. G. and Yousefzadeh D. K. (1989) Isolated granulomatous gastritis in an adolescent. Digestive Diseases and Sciences 34:292–296.

Hizawa K., Iida M., Matsumoto T., Aoyagi K., Yao T. and Fujishima M. (1993) Natural history of fundic gland polyposis without familial adenomatosis coli: follow-up observations in 31 patients. Radiology 189:429–432.

Hizawa K., Iida M., Matsumoto T., Kohrogi N., Kinoshita H., Yao T. and Fujishima M. (1993) Cancer in Peutz-Jeghers syndrome. Cancer 72:2777–2781.

Hizawa K., Iida M., Matsumoto T., Kohrogi N., Suekane H., Yao T. and Fujishima M. (1994) Gastrointestinal manifestations of Cowden's disease: report of 4 cases. Journal of Clinical Gastroenterology 18:13–18.

Hoare A. M., Jones E. L., Alexander-Williams J. and Hawkins C. F. (1977) Symptomatic significance of gastric mucosal changes after surgery for peptic ulcer. Gut 18:295–300.

Hodges J. R., Isaacson P. and Wright R. (1981) Diffuse enterochromaffin-like (ECL) cell hyperplasia and multiple gastric carcinoids: a complication of pernicious anaemia. Gut 22:237–241.

Hoedemaeker P. J., Abels J., Wachters J. J., Adrends A. and Nieweg H. O. (1964) Investigations about the site of production of Castles' gastric intrinsic factor. Laboratory Investigation 13:1394–1399.

Hoftiezer J. W., O'Laughlin J. C. and Ivey K. J. (1982) Effects of 24 hours of aspirin, Bufferin, paracetamol and placebo on normal human gastroduodenal mucosa. Gut 23:692–697.

Hojgaard L., Matzen P. and Christoffersen P. (1987) Gastritis: a clinical entity? Scandinavian Journal of Gastroenterology 128 (suppl):90–93.

Holcombe C. (1992) *Helicobacter pylori*: the African enigma. Gut 33:429–431.

Holcombe C., Umar H., Lucas S. B. and Kaluba J. (1994) Low incidence of clinically significant gastroduodenal pathology despite a high incidence of *Helicobacter pylori* infection. Transactions of the Royal Society of Tropical Medicine and Hygiene 88:569–571.

Holt J. M., Gear M. W. L., and Warner G. T. (1970) The role of chronic blood loss in the pathogenesis of post-gastrectomy iron deficiency anaemia. Gut 11:847–850.

Honore L. H., Lewis A. S. and Ohara K. E. (1979) Gastric glandularis et cystica profunda: report of 3 cases with discussion of etiology and pathogenesis. Digestive Diseases and Sciences 24:48–52.

Houghton P. W. J., Mortensen N. J. McC., Thomas W. E. G., Cooper M. J., Morgan A. P. and Burton P. (1986) Intragastric bile acids and histological changes in gastric mucosa. British Journal of Surgery 73:354–356.

Hsing A. W., Hansson L. E., McLaughlin J. K., Nyren O., Blot W. J., Ekbom A. and Fraumeni J. F. Jr (1993) Pernicious anemia and subsequent cancer: a population-based cohort study. Cancer 71:745–750.

Hsiu J-G., Gamsey A. J, Ives C. E., D'Amato N. A. and Hiller A. N. (1986) Gastric anisakiasis: report of a case with clinical, endoscopic, and histological findings. American Journal of Gastroenterology 81:1185–1187.

Hyams J. S. and Treem W. R. (1993) Portal hypertensive gastropathy in children. Journal of Pediatric Gastroenterology and Nutrition 17:13–18.

Hyjek E. and Kelenyi G. (1982) Pseudolymphomas of the stomach: a lesion characterized by progressively transformed germinal centres. Histopathology 6:61–68.

Ida K., Hashimoto Y., Takeda S., Murakami K. and Kawai K. (1975) Endoscopic diagnosis of gastric cancer with dye scattering. American Journal of Gastroenterology 63:316–320.

Ignatius J. A., Armstrong C. D. and Eversole S. L. (1970) Multiple diffuse cystic disease of the stomach in association with carcinoma. Gastroenterology 59:610–614.

Iida F., Murata F. and Nagata T. (1978) Histochemical studies of mucosubstances in metaplastic epithelium of the stomach with special reference to the development of intestinal metaplasia. Histochemistry 56:229–237.

Iida M., Yao T., Itoh H., Watanabe H., Matsui T., Iwashita A. and Fujishima M. (1988) Natural history of gastric adenomas in patients with familial adenomatosis coli/Gardner's syndrome. Cancer 61:605–611.

Iida M., Yao T., Watanabe H., Imamura K., Fuyuno S. and Omae T. (1980) Spontaneous disappearance of fundic gland polyposis: report of three cases. Gastroenterology 79:725–728.

Ikeda K. and Murayama K. (1978) A case of amyloid tumor of the stomach. Endoscopy 10:54–58.

Ikkala E., Salmi H. J. and Siurala M. (1970) Gastric mucosa in iron deficiency anaemia. Results of a follow-up examination. Acta Haematologica 43:228–231.

Ikkala E. and Siurala M. (1964) Gastric lesion in iron deficiency anaemia. Acta Haematologica 31:313–324.

Imerslund O. (1960) Idiopathic chronic megaloblastic anaemia in children. Acta Paediatrica (suppl) 119:1–115.

Irvine W. J., Cullen D. R. and Mawhinney H. (1974) Natural history of autoimmune achlorhydric atrophic gastritis. A 1–15 year follow-up study. Lancet ii 482–485.

Isaacson P. G. (1992) Extranodal lymphomas: the MALT concept. Verhandlungen der Deutschen Gesellschaft für Pathologie 76:14–23.

Isaacson P. G. and Spencer J. (1987) Malignant lymphoma of mucosa-associated lymphoid tissue. Histopathology 11:445–462.

Isaacson P. G. and Spencer J. (1993). Is gastric lymphoma an infectious disease? Human Pathology 24:569–570.

Isaacson P. G., Spencer J. and Finn T. (1986) Primary B-cell gastric lymphoma. Human Pathology 17:72–82.

Isaacson P. G. and Wright D. H. (1983) Malignant lymphoma of mucosa-associated lymphoid tissue. Cancer 52:1410–1416.

Isaacson P. G. and Wright D. H. (1984) Extranodal malignant lymphoma arising from mucosa-associated lymphoid tissue. Cancer 53:2515–2524.

Isaacson P., Wright D. H, Judd M. A. and Mepham B. L. (1979) Primary gastrointestinal lymphomas: a classification of 66 cases. Cancer 43:1805–1819.

Ishido T. and Mori N. (1992) Primary gastric plasmacytoma: a morphological and immunohistochemical study of five cases. American Journal of Gastroenterology 87:875–878.

Itsuno M., Watanabe H., Iwafuchi M., Ito S., Yanaihara N., Sato K., Kikuchi M. and Akiyama N. (1989) Multiple carcinoids and endocrine cell micronests in type A gastritis: their morphology, histogenesis, and natural history. Cancer 63:881–890.

Iwasaki T. (1987) Alimentary tract lesions in cytomegalovirus infection. Acta Pathologica Japonica 37:549–565.

Jabbari M., Cherry R., Lough J. O., Daly D. S., Kinnear D. G. and Goresky C. A. (1984) Gastric antral vascular ectasia: the watermelon stomach. Gastroenterology 87:1165–1170.

Jablokow V. R., Aranha G. V. and Reyes C. V. (1982) Gastric stomal polypoid hyperplasia: report of four cases. Journal of Surgical Oncology 19:106–108.

Jaffe R., Wollman M. R., Kocochis S., Penchansky L. and Gilbert-Barness E. (1993) Pathological cases of the month: Langerhans' cell histiocytosis with gastrointestinal involvement. American Journal of Diseases of Children 147:79–80.

Jarvinen H., Nyberg M. and Peltokallio P. (1983) Upper gastrointestinal tract polyps in familial adenomatosis coli. Gut 24:333–339.

Jarvis L. R. and Whitehead R. (1980) Effects of nicotine on the morphology of the rat gastric mucosa. Gastroenterology 78:1488–1494.

Jarvis L. R. and Whitehead R. (1985) Morphometric analysis of gastric dysplasia. Journal of Pathology 147:133–138.

Jass J. R. (1983) A classification of gastric dysplasia. Histopathology 7:181–193.

Jass J. R. and Filipe M. I. (1979) A variant of intestinal metaplasia associated with gastric carcinoma: a histochemical study. Histopathology 3:191–199.

Jass J. R. and Filipe M. I. (1981) The mucin profiles of normal gastric mucosa, intestinal metaplasia and its variants and gastric carcinoma. Histochemical Journal 13:931–939.

Jeffries G. H. (1965) Recovery of gastric mucosal structure and function in pernicious anaemia during prednisolone therapy. Gastroenterology 48:371–378.

Jenkins D., Stephenson P. M. and Scott B. B. (1985) The Cronkhite-Canada syndrome: an ultrastructural study of pathogenesis. Journal of Clinical Pathology 38:271–276.

Johnson G. K., Soergel K. H., Hensley G. T., Dodds W. T. and Hogan W. J. (1972) Cronkhite-Canada: gastrointestinal pathophysiology and morphology. Gastroenterology 63:140–152.

Johnstone J. M. and Morson B. C. (1978a) Eosinophilic gastroenteritis. Histopathology 2:335–348.

Johnstone J. M. and Morson B. C. (1978b) Inflammatory fibroid polyp of the gastrointestinal tract. Histopathology 2:349–361.

Jones A. W., Kirk R. S. and Bloor K. (1970) The association between aneurysms of the abdominal aorta and peptic ulceration. Gut 11:679–684.

Joske R. A., Finckh E. S. and Wood I. J. (1955) Gastric biopsy: a study of 1,000 consecutive successful gastric biopsies. Quarterly Journal of Medicine 24:269–294.

Justrabo E., Guion L., Levillain P., Piard F. and Michiels R. (1987) Cystic glandular fundic polyps of the stomach: report on 12 cases and review of the literature. Annales de Pathologie 7:106–112.

Kahn L. B. (1963) Gastric mucormycosis: a report of a case with a review of the literature. South African Medical Journal 37:1265–1269.

Kalogeropoulos N. K. and Whitehead R. (1988) *Campylobacter* like organisms and *Candida* in peptic ulcers and similar lesions of the upper gastrointestinal tract: a study of 247 cases. Journal of Clinical Pathology 41:1093–1098.

Kamal M. F., Shaker K., Jaser N. and Leimoon B. A. (1985) Eosinophilic gastroenteritis with no peripheral eosinophilia. Annales Chirurgiae et Gynaecologiae 74:98–100.

Kamiya T., Morishita T., Asakura H., Munakata Y. and Miura S. (1981) Histoclinical long-standing follow-up study of hyperplastic polyps of the stomach. American Journal of Gastroenterology 75:275–281.

Karvonen A-L., Kekki M., Lehtola J., Sipponen P. and Ihamaki T. (1987) Prepyloric erosions: an entity of its own among erosive gastric lesions. Scandinavian Journal of Gastroenterology 22:1095–1101.

Karvonen A-L., Sipponen P., Lehtola J., and Ruokonen A. (1983) Gastric mucosal erosions. Scandinavian Journal of Gastroenterology 18:1051–1056.

Katayama Y., Kimura M. and Konn M. (1985) Cronkhite-Canada syndrome associated with a rectal cancer and adenomatous changes in colonic polyps. American Journal of Surgical Pathology 9:65–71.

Kath R., Donhuijsen K., Hayungs J. et al (1995) Primary gastric non-Hodgkin's lymphoma: a clinicopathological study of 41 patients. Journal of Cancer Research and Clinical Oncology 121:51–56.

Katz A. J. and Goldman H. and Grand R. J. (1977) Gastric mucosal biopsy in eosinophilic (allergic) gastroenteritis. Gastroenterology 73:705–709.

Katz S., Klein M. S., Winawer S. J. and Sherlock P. (1973) Disseminated lymphoma involving the stomach: correlation of endoscopy with directed cytology and biopsy. American Journal of Digestive Diseases 18:370–374.

Katzenstein A. L. and Maksem J. (1979) Candidal infection of gastric ulcers: histology, incidence, and clinical significance. American Journal of Clinical Pathology 71:137–141.

Kawai K., Shimamoto K., Misaki F., Murakami K. and Masuda M. (1970) Erosion of gastric mucosa: pathogenesis, incidence and classification of the erosive gastritis. Endoscopy 2:168–174.

Kaye M. D., Whorwell P. J. and Wright R. (1983) Gastric mucosal lymphocyte subpopulations in pernicious anemia and in normal stomach. Clinical Immunology and Immunopathology 28:431–440.

Kekki M., Hakkiluoto A. and Siurala M. (1976) Dynamics of atrophic gastritis in male and female subjects after partial gastric resection: an evaluation by stochastic analysis. Scandinavian Journal of Gastroenterology 11:597–601.

Kekki M., Saukkonen M., Sipponen P., Varis K. and Siurala M. (1980) Dynamics of chronic gastritis in the remnant after partial gastrectomy for duodenal ulcer. Scandinavian Journal of Gastroenterology 15:509–512.

Kekki M., Varis K., Pohjanpalo H., Isokoski M., Ihamaki T. and Siurala M. (1983) Course of antrum and body gastritis in pernicious anemia families. Digestive Diseases and Sciences 28:698–704.

Kekki M. and Villako K. (1981) Dynamic behaviour of gastritis in various populations and subpopulations. Annals of Clinical Research 13:119–122.

Kekki M., Villako K., Tamm A. and Siurala M. (1977) Dynamics of antral and fundal gastritis in an Estonian rural population sample. Scandinavian Journal of Gastroenterology 12:321–324.

Kenny F. D., Dockerty M. B. and Waugh J. M. (1954) Giant hypertrophy of gastric mucosa: a clinical and pathological study. Cancer 7:671–681.

Keshavarzian A., Saverymuttu S. H., Tai P-C., Thompson M., Barter S., Spry C. J. F. and Chadwick V. S. (1985) Activated eosinophils in familial eosinophilic gastroenteritis. Gastroenterology 88:1041–1049.

Kimura K. (1969) Gastric xanthelasma. Archives of Pathology 87:110–117.

Kimura K., Satoh K., Taniguchi Y., Ido K., Kihira K., Ohta Y. and Oshida Y. (1994) Some personal comments on the Sydney system for the classification of chronic gastritis. Journal of Gastroenterology 29(suppl):114–119.

Kinoshita Y., Tojo M., Yano T., Kitajima N., Itoh T., Nishiyama K., Inatome T., Fukuzaki H., Watanabe M.

and Chiba T. (1993) Incidence of fundic gland polyps in patients without familial adenomatous polyposis. Gastrointestinal Endoscopy 39:161–163.

Klein N. C., Hargrove R. L., Sleisenger M. H. and Jeffries G. H. (1970) Eosinophilic gastroenteritis. Medicine 49:299–319.

Kliems G., Paquet K. J., Lindstaedt H. and Miederen S. (1979) Atrophic gastritis after Billroth I gastrectomy. Endoscopy 2:127–130.

Kodama T., Fukuda S., Takino T., Omori Y. and Oka T. (1985) Gastroduodenal cytomegalovirus infection after renal transplantation: fiberscopic observations. Endoscopy 17:157–158.

Kojimahara K., Mukai M., Yamazaki K., Yamada T., Katayama T., Nakada K., Vematsu S., Umezano A. and Hosoda Y. (1993) Inflammatory pseudotumor of the stomach: report of a highly infiltrative case with electron microscopic and immunohistochemical studies. Acta Pathologica Japonica 43:65–70.

Konrad E. A. and Meister P. (1979) Fatal eosinophilic gastroenterocolitis in a two-year-old child. Virchows Archiv (A) 382:347–353.

Konturek S. J., Brzozowski T., Piastucki I., Dembinski A., Radecki T., Dembinska-Kiec A., Zmuda A. and Gregory H. (1981) Role of mucosal prostaglandins and DNA synthesis in gastric cyto-protection by luminal epidermal growth factor. Gut 22:927–932.

Korelitz B. I., Waye J. D., Kreuning J., Sommers S. C., Fein H. D., Beeber J. and Gelberg B. J. (1981) Crohn's disease in endoscopic biopsies of the gastric antrum and duodenum. American Journal of Gastroenterology 76:103–109.

Korman M. G., Soveney C. and Hansky J. (1971) Serum gastrin in duodenal ulcer. I: basal levels and effect of food and atropine. Gut 12:899–902.

Korman M. G., Soveney C. and Hansky J. (1972) Gastrin studies in gastric ulcer. Gut 13:166–169.

Krag E. (1966) Enlarged gastric and duodenal rugae: the prognostic significance of the radiological findings of coarse mucosal folds in the stomach and duodenum. Acta Medica Scandinavica 179:343–348.

Kraut J. R., Powell R., Hruby M. A. and Lloyd-Still J. D. (1981) Menetrier's disease in childhood: report of two cases and a review of the literature. Journal of Pediatric Surgery 16:707–711.

Krentz K. and Gohrband G. (1976) Klinik und Verlauf gastraler erosionen. Medizinische Klinik 71:156–162.

Kristensen M. and Nilsson T. (1985) Mucus secretion in hypertrophic, hypersecretory, protein-losing gastropathy. American Journal of Gastroenterology 80:77–81.

Kuipers F. C., Theil P. H. van and Roskam E. T. (1960) Eosinophilic phlegmon of the small intestine caused by a worm not adapted to the human body. Nederlands Tijdshrift Voor Geneeskunde 104:422–427.

Kundrotas L., Novak J., Kremzier J., Meenaghan M. and Hassett J. (1988) Gastric bleeding in pseudoxanthoma elasticum. American Journal of Gastroenterology 83:868–872.

Kuri K. and Lee M. (1994) Eosinophilic gastroenteritis manifesting with ascites. Southern Medical Journal 87:956–957.

Kwee W. S., Wils J. A., Schlangen J., Nuyens C. M. and Arends J. W. (1994) Gastric epithelial atypia complicating hepatic arterial infusion chemotherapy. Histopathology 24:151–154.

Lacy E. R. and Ito S. (1982) Microscopic analysis of ethanol damage in rat gastric mucosa after treatment with a prostaglandin. Gastroenterology 83:619–625.

Laine L. (1993) *Helicobacter pylori*, gastric ulcer and agents noxious to the gastric mucosa. Gastroenterology Clinics of North America 22:117–125.

Laine L. and Weinstein W. M. (1988a) Subepithelial hemorrhages and erosions of human stomach. Digestive Diseases and Sciences 33:490–503.

Laine L. and Weinstein W. M. (1988b) Histology of alcoholic hemorrhagic "gastritis": a prospective evaluation. Gastroenterology 94:1254–1262.

Lam S. K., Hui W. K. K., Ho J., Wong K. P., Rotter J. I. and Samloff I. M. (1983) Pachydermoperiostosis, hypertrophic gastropathy and peptic ulcer. Gastroenterology 84:834–839.

Lambert R., Andre C., Moulinier B. and Bugnon B. (1978) Diffuse varioliform gastritis. Digestion 17:159–167.

Lambert R., Moulinier B., Bugnon B. and Andre C. (1977) La gastrite hypertrophique superficielle (gastrite varioliforme). In: What's New in Endoscopy of the Upper Digestive Tract in Relation to Radiology and Surgery. Edited by M. Cremer. Brussels: Societe Belge d'Endoscopie Digestive.

Langhans P., Bues M. and Bunte H. (1984) Morphological changes in the operated stomach under the influence of duodenogastric reflux. Scandinavian Journal of Gastroenterology 19 (suppl 92):145–148.

Langman M. J. S. and Cooke A. R. (1976) Gastric and duodenal ulcer and their associated diseases. Lancet i:680–683.

Lanza F. L. (1984) Endoscopic studies of gastric and duodenal injury after the use of ibuprofen, aspirin and other nonsteroidal anti-inflammatory agents. American Journal of Medicine 77:19–24.

Larsen B., Tarp U. and Kristensen E. (1987) Familial giant hypertrophic gastritis (Menetrier's disease). Gut 28:1517–1521.

Lauren P. (1965) The two histological main types of gastric carcinoma: diffuse and so-called intestinal type carcinoma: an attempt at a histoclinical classification. Acta Pathologica Microbiologica et Immunologica Scandinavica 64:31–49.

Lawson H. H. (1988) Definition of gastroduodenal junction in healthy subjects. Journal of Clinical Pathology 41:393–396.

Leardi S., Valente A., Calvisi G., Risetti A. and Simi M. (1993) Menetrier's disease associated with a gastric ulcer: a clinical case report and review of the literature. Annali Italiani di Chirurgia 64:35–39.

Lee C. M., Changchien C. S., Chen P. C. Lin D. Y., Sheen I. S., Wang C. S., Tai D. I., Sheen-Chen S. M.,

Chen W. J., and Wu C. S. (1993) Eosinophilic gastroenteritis: 10 years experience. American Journal of Gastroenterology 88:70–74.

Lee J. G., Wilson J. A. and Gottfried M. R. (1994) Gastrointestinal manifestations of amyloidosis. Southern Medical Journal 87:243–247.

Lee R. G. and Burt R. W. (1986) The histopathology of fundic gland polyps of the stomach. American Journal of Clinical Pathology 86:498–503.

Lehnert T., Sternberg S. S., Sprossmann M. and DeCosse J. J. (1989) Early gastric cancer. American Journal of Surgery 157:202–207.

Leinbach G. E. and Rubin C. E. (1970) Eosinophilic gastroenteritis: a simple reaction to food allergens? Gastroenterology 59:874–889.

Leocata P., Gallo P., Chiominto A., Saltarelli S., Cioccocioppa R., Saltarelli P., Di Giacomo C. and Ventura L. (1993) Is early gastric cancer, diffuse type a forerunner of advanced gastric cancer. Tumori 79:108–111.

Lev R. (1966) The mucin histochemistry of normal and neoplastic gastric mucosa. Laboratory Investigations 14:2080–2100.

Lev R. and DeNucci T. D. (1989) Neoplastic Paneth cells in the stomach: report of two cases and review of the literature. Archives of Pathology and Laboratory Medicine 113:129–133.

Levine J. S. and Allen R. H. (1985) Intrinsic factor within parietal cells of patients with juvenile pernicious anemia. Gastroenterology 88:1132–1136.

Lewin K. J., Dowling F., Wright J. P. and Taylor K. B. (1976) Gastric morphology and serum gastrin levels in pernicious anaemia. Gut 17:551–560

Lin H-J., Lee F-Y., Tsai Y-T., Lee S-D., Lin C-Y., Tsay S-H. and Chiang H. (1989) Alimentary tract and pancreas: a prospective evaluation of biopsy site in the diagnosis of gastric malignancy: the margin or the base? Journal of Gastroenterology and Hepatology 4:137–141.

Lin J. T., Wu M. S., Wang J. T. et al (1994) Clinicopathologic study of 208 patients with early gastric cancer in Taiwan: a comparison between Eastern and Western contries. Journal of Hepatoenterology and Hepatology 9:344–349.

Lipkin M. (1981) Proliferation and differentiation of gastrointestinal cells in normal and diseased states. In: Physiology of the Gastrointestinal Tract. Edited by L. R. Johnson. New York: Raven Press, pp 145–167.

Lipper S. and Kahn L. B. (1977) Superficial cystic gastritis with alopecia. A forme fruste of the Cronkhite-Canada syndrome. Archives of Pathology and Laboratory Medicine 101:432–436.

Listrom M. B. and Fenoglio-Preiser C. M. (1987) Lymphatic distribution of the stomach in normal, inflammatory, hyperplastic, and neoplastic tissue. Gastroenterology 93:506–514.

Littler F. R. and Gleibermann E. (1972) Gastritis cystica polyposa. Cancer 29:205–209.

LiVolsi V. A. and Perzin K. H. (1975) Inflammatory pseudotumors (inflammatory fibrous polyps) of the small intestine: a clinicopathologic study. American Journal of Digestive Diseases 20:325–336.

Lopez J. A., Tamayo M. C., Mejia G. I., Trujillo H., Espinal O., Perez M. A. and Robledo J. A. (1993) Gastrospirillum hominis in a child with chronic gastritis. Pediatric Infectious Disease Journal 12:701–702.

Loux H. A and Zamcheck N. (1969) Cytological evidence for the long "quiescent" stage of gastric cancer in two patients with pernicious anaemia. Gastroenterology 57:173–184.

Lucak B. K., Sansaricq C., Snyderman S. E., Greco M. A., Fazzini E. P. and Bazaz G. R. (1982) Disseminated ulcerations in allergic eosinophilic gastroenterocolitis. American Journal of Gastroenterology 77:248–252.

Lundegardh G., Adami II-O., Helmick C., Zack M. and Meirik O. (1988) Stomach cancer after partial gastrectomy for benign ulcer disease. New England Journal of Medicine 319:195–200.

Lygidakis N. J. (1986) Histologic changes after elective surgery for duodenal ulcer. Acta Chirurgica Scandinavica 152:139–144.

Lynch H. T., Smyrk T. C., Lanspa S. J., Jenkins J. X., Lynch P. M., Cavalieri J. and Lynch J. F. (1993) Upper gastrointestinal manifestations in families with hereditary flat adenoma syndrome. Cancer 71:2709–2714.

Macartney J. C., Camplejohn R. S. and Powell G. (1986) DNA flow cytometry of histological material from human gastric cancer. Journal of Pathology 148:273–277.

MacDonald W. C. (1973) Correlation of mucosal histology and aspirin intake in chronic gastric ulcer. Gastroenterology 65:381–389.

MacDonald W. C. and Rubin C. E. (1967) Gastric biopsy: a critical evaluation. Gastroenterology 53:143–170.

McGuigan J. E. and Trudeau W. L. (1970) Serum gastrin concentrations in pernicious anaemia. New England Journal of Medicine 282:358–361.

McIntyre R. L. E., Irani M. S. and Piris J. (1981) Histological study of the effects of three anti-inflammatory preparations on the gastric mucosa. Journal of Clinical Pathology 34:836–842.

McKelvie P. A. and Fink M. A. (1994). A fatal case of emphysematous gastritis and esophagitis. Pathology 26:490–492.

McNulty C. A. M., Dent J. C., Curry A., Uff J. S., Ford G. A., Ger M. W. L. and Wilkinson S. P. (1989) New spiral bacterium in gastric mucosa. Journal of Clinical Pathology 42:585–591.

Magnus H. A. (1946) The pathology of simple gastritis. Journal of Pathology and Bacteriology 58:431–439.

Magnus H. A. (1952) Gastritis. In: Modern Trends in Gastroenterology. First series. Edited by F. H. Jones. London: Butterworth, p 323.

Magnus H. A. and Ungley C. C. (1938) The gastric lesion in pernicious anaemia. Lancet i:420–421.

Malfertheiner P. (1988) Role of infection in gastroduodenal pathology. Scandinavian Journal of Gastroenterology 23 (suppl 142):7–8.

Malhotra R. and Sheffield A. (1988) Cronkhite-Canada syndrome associated with colon carcinoma and adenomatous changes in C-C polyps. American Journal of Gastroenterology 83:772–776.

Mann N. S. (1976) Bile-induced acute erosive gastritis: its prevention by antacid, cholestyramine, and prostaglandin E$_2$. American Journal of Digestive Diseases 21:89–92.

Marano B. J. Jr, Smith F. and Bonanno C. A. (1993) *Helicobacter pylori* prevalence in acquired immunodeficiency syndrome. American Journal of Gastroenterology 88:687–690.

Marcheggiano A., Iannoni C., Agnello M., Paoluzi P. and Pallone F. (1987) *Campylobacter*-like organisms on the human gastric mucosa: relation to type and extent of gastritis in different clinical groups. Gastroenterologie Clinique et Biologique 11:376–381.

Marmaduke D. P., Greenson J. K., Cunningham I., Herderick E. E. and Cornhill J. F. (1994) Gastric vascular ectasia in patients undergoing bone marrow transplantation. American Journal of Clinical Pathology 102:194–198.

Marshall B. J. (1988) Should we now, routinely, be examining gastric biopsies for *Campylobacter pylori*? American Journal of Gastroenterology 83:479–481.

Marshall B. J., Armstrong J. A., McGechie D. B. and Glancy R. J. (1985) Attempt to fulfil Koch's postulates for pyloric *Campylobacter*. Medical Journal of Australia 142:436–444.

Mast A., Elewaut A., Mortier G., Quatacker J., Defloor E., Roels H. and Barbier F. (1976) Gastric xanthoma. American Journal of Gastroenterology 65:311–317.

Masugi J., Fukunaga H., Ochi F. et al (1994). Pigmentary retinopathy with nephrotic syndrome, Ménétrier's disease, and diabetes mellitus. Internal Medicine 33:644–648.

Mathis G., Dirschmid K. and Sutterlutti G. (1987) Tuberculous gastric ulcer. Endoscopy 19:133–135.

Matzinger M. A. and Daneman A. (1983) Esophageal involvement in eosinophilic gastroenteritis. Pediatric Radiology 13:35–38.

Meister H., Holubarsch C. H., Haverkamp O., Schlag P. and Herforth C. H. (1979) Gastritis, intestinal metaplasia and dysplasia versus benign ulcer in the duodenum and gastric carcinoma. Pathology, Research and Practice 164:259–269.

Ménétrier P. (1888) Des polyadenomes gastriques et de leurs rapports avec le cancer de l'estomac. Archives de Physiologie Normale et Pathologique 1:32–55 and 236–262.

Menke D. M., Kyle R. A., Fleming C. R., Wolfe J. T. 3rd, Kurtin P. J. and Oldenburg W. A. (1993) Symptomatic gastric amyloidosis in patients with primary systemic amyloidosis. Mayo Clinic Proceedings 68:763–767.

Metzger W. H., McAdam L., Bluestone R. and Guth P. H. (1976) Acute gastric mucosal injury during continuous or interrupted aspirin ingestion in humans. American Journal of Digestive Diseases 21:963–968.

Miller T. A. (1987) Mechanisms of stress-related mucosal damage. American Journal of Medicine 83(suppl 6A):8–14.

Ming S-C. (1977) The classification and significance of gastric polyps. In: The Gastrointestinal Tract. Edited by J. H. Yardley, B. C. Mason and M. R. Abell International Academy of Pathology Monograph 11. Baltimore: Williams & Wilkins, pp 149–175.

Ming S-C., Bajtai A., Correa P., Elster K., Jarvi O. H., Munoz N., Nagayo T. and Stemmerman G. N. (1984) Gastric dysplasia: significance and pathologic criteria. Cancer 54:1794–1801.

Mingazzini P., Carlei F., Malchiodi-Albedi F., Lezoche E., Covotta A., Speranza V. and Polak J. M. (1984) Endocrine cells in intestinal metaplasia of the stomach. Journal of Pathology 144:171–178.

Minoli G., Terruzi V., Butti G. C., Frigerio G. and Rossini A. (1982) Gastric candidiasis: an endoscopic and histological study in 26 patients. Gastrointestinal Endoscopy 28:59–61.

Minoli G., Terruzzi V., and Rossini A. (1979) Gastroduodenal candidiasis occuring without underlying diseases (primary gastroduodenal candidiasis). Endoscopy 1:18–22.

Misra R. C., Agarwal S. K., Prakash P., Saha M. M. and Gupta P. S. (1982) Gastric tuberculosis. Endoscopy 14:235–237.

Mitsufuji S., Tsuchihashi Y. and Kodama T. (1994) Histogenesis of hyperplastic polyps of the stomach in terms of cellular proliferation. Journal of Gastroenterology 29:559–568.

Mohri N. (1987) Primary gastric non-Hodgkin's lymphomas in Japan. Virchows Archiv (A) 411:459–466.

Monroe L. E., Boughton G. A. and Sommers S. C. (1964) The association of gastric epithelial hyperplasia and cancer. Gastroenterology 46:267–272.

Moore D., Lichtman S., Lentz J., Stringer D. and Sherman P. (1986) Eosinophilic gastroenteritis presenting in an adolescent with isolated colonic involvement. Gut 27:1219–1222.

Moreto M., Ojembarrena E., Zaballa M., Tanago J. G., Ibanez S. and Setien F. (1985) Retrospective endoscopic analysis of gastric xanthelasma in the non-operated stomach. Endoscopy 17:210–211.

Morgan A. G., McAdam W. A. F., Pyrah R. D. and Tinsley E. G. F. (1976) Multiple recurring gastric erosions (aphthous ulcers) Gut 17:633–639.

Mori K., Shinya H. and Wolff W. I. (1971) Polypoid reparative mucosal proliferation at the site of a healed gastric ulcer: sequential gastroscopic, radiological and histological observation. Gastroenterology 61:523–529.

Mori M., Kitagawa S., Iida M., Sakurai T., Enjoji M., Sugimachi K. and Ooiwa T. (1987) Early carcinoma of the gastric cardia. Cancer 59:1758–1766.

Morris A. and Nicholson G. (1987) Ingestion of *Campylobacter* pyloridis causes gastritis and raised fasting gastric pH. American Journal of Gastroenterology 82:192–199.

Morson B. C. (1955) Intestinal metaplasia of the gastric mucosa. British Journal of Cancer 9:365–376.

Morson B. C., Sobin L. H., Grundmann E., Johansen A., Nagayo T. and Serck-Hanssen A. (1980) Precancerous conditions and epithelial dysplasia in the stomach. Journal of Clinical Pathology 33:711–721.

Mosbech J. and Videbaek A. (1950) Mortality from and risk of gastric carcinoma among patients with pernicious anaemia. British Medical Journal ii:390–394.

Mosimann F., Burris B., Diserens H., Fontolliet C., Loup P. and Mosimann R. (1981) Enterogastric reflux: experimental and clinical study. Scandinavian Journal of Gastroenterology 16(suppl 67):149–152.

Mosimann F., Sorgi M., Wolverson R. L., Donovan I. A., Fielding J. W. L., Harding L. K., Alexander-Williams J. and Thompson H. (1984) Gastric histology and its relationship to entero-gastric reflux after duodenal ulcer surgery. Scandinavian Journal of Gastroenterology 19 (suppl 92):142–144.

Mosnier J. F., Flejou J. F., Amouyal G., Gayet B., Molas G., Henin D. and Potet F. (1991) Hypertrophic gastropathy with gastric adenocarcinoma: Menetrier's disease and lymphocytic gastritis? Gut 32:1565–1567.

Mountford R. A., Brown P., Salmon P. R., Alvarenga C., Neumann C. S. and Read A. E. (1980) Gastric cancer detection in gastric ulcer disease. Gut 21:9–17.

Mower G. A. and Whitehead R. (1986) Gastric hemorrhage due to ruptured arteriovenous malformation (Dieulafoy's disease). Pathology 18:54–57.

Mueller J., Kirchner T. and Mueller-Hermelink H. K. (1987) Gastric endocrine cell hyperplasia and carcinoid tumors in atrophic gastritis type A. American Journal of Surgical Pathology 11:909–917.

Murai N., Fukuzaki T., Nakamura T., Hayashida H., Okazaki M., Fujimoto K. and Hirai T. (1993) Cronkhite-Canada syndrome associated with colon cancer: report of a case. Surgery Today 23:825–829.

Muratani M., Nakamura T., Nakano G-I. and Mukawa K. (1989) Ultrastructural study of two subtypes of gastric adenoma. Journal of Clinical Pathology 42:352–359.

Myhre M. J. and Isaacson P. G. (1987) Primary B-cell gastric lymphoma: a reassessment of its histogenesis. Journal of Pathology 152:1–11.

Myren J. and Serck-Hanssen A. (1975) Gastroscopic observations related to bioptical histology in healthy medical students. Scandinavian Journal of Gastroenterology 10:353–355.

Nagayo T. (1972) Histological diagnosis of biopsied gastric mucosa with special reference to that of borderline lesions. Gann Monographs in Cancer Research 11:245–256.

Nakamura T. (1970) Pathohistologische Einteilung der Magenpolypen mit spezifischer Betrachtung ihrer malignen Entartung. Chirurg 41:122–130.

Nakamura T. and Nakano G-I. (1985) Histopathological classification and malignant change in gastric polyps. Journal of Clinical Pathology 38:754–764.

Nakanishi I., Kajikawa K., Migita S., Mai M., Akimoto R. and Mura T. (1982) Gastric plasmacytoma: an immunologic and immunohistochemical study. Cancer 49:2025–2028.

Nardelli J., Bara J., Bosa B. and Burtin P. (1983) Intestinal metaplasia and carcinomas of the human stomach. Journal of Histochemistry and Cytochemistry 31:366–375.

Nasrallah S. M., Johnston G. S., Gadacz T. R. and Kim K. M. (1987) The significance of gastric bile reflux seen at endoscopy. Journal of Clinical Gastroenterology 9:514–517.

Navab F., Kleinman M. S., Algazy K., Schenk E. and Turner M. D. (1972) Endoscopic diagnosis of eosinophilic gastritis. Gastrointestinal Endoscopy 19:67–69.

Naylor A. R. and Pollet J. E. (1985) Eosinophilic colitis. Diseases of the Colon and Rectum 28:615–618.

Nedenskov-Sorensen P., Bjorneklett A., Fausa O., Bukholm G., Aase S. and Jantzen E. (1988) Campylobacter pylori infection and its relation to chronic gastritis. Scandinavian Journal of Gastroenterology 23:867–874.

Nesland A. A. and Berstad A. (1985) Erosive prepyloric changes in persons with and without dyspepsia. Scandinavian Journal of Gastroenterology 20:222–228.

Nesland A. A., Berstad A. and Serck-Hanssen A. (1986) Histological findings in erosive prepyloric changes. Scandinavian Journal of Gastroenterology 21:239–245.

Nevin N. C., Eakins D., Clarke S. D. and Carson D. J. L. (1969) Acute phlegmonous gastritis. British Journal of Surgery 56:268–270.

Newbold K. M., MacDonald F. and Allum W. H. (1988) Undifferentiated columnar cells on the gastric interfoveolar crest: a previously undescribed observation. Journal of Pathology 155:311–316.

Niemela S., Karttunen T., Heikkila J. and Lehtola J. (1987) Characteristics of reflux gastritis. Scandinavian Journal of Gastroenterology 22:349–354.

Nonomura A., Ohta G., Ibata T., Shinozaki K. and Nishino T. (1980) Cronkhite-Canada syndrome associated with sigmoid cancer. Case report and review of 54 cases with the syndrome. Acta Pathologica Japonica 30:825–845.

O'Brien M. J., Burakoff R., Robbins E. A., Golding R. M., Zamcheck N. and Gottlieb L. S. (1985) Early gastric cancer: clinicopathologic study. American Journal of Medicine 78:195–202.

Oehlert W., Keller P., Henke M. and Strauch M. (1975) Die Dysplasien der Magenschleimhaut. Deutsche Medizinische Wochenschrift 100:1950–1956.

Oehlert W., Keller P., Henke M. and Strauch M. (1979) Gastric mucosal dysplasia: what is their clinical significance? Frontiers of Gastrointestinal Research 4:173–182.

Offerhaus G. J. A., Huibregtse K., De Boer J., Verhoeven T., Van Olffen G. H., Van De Stadt J. and Tytgat G. N. J. (1984a) The operated stomach: a premalignant condition? Scandinavian Journal of Gastroenterology 19:521–524.

Offerhaus G. J. A., VD Stadt J., Huibregtse K. and Tytgat G. N. J. (1984b) Endoscopic screening for malignancy in the gastric remnant: the clinical significance of dysplasia in gastric mucosa. Journal of Clinical Pathology 37:748–754.

Ohno F., Numata Y., Yamano T., Suzuki M. and Miyoshi K. (1982) Gastroscopic biopsy of the stomach for the diagnosis of amyloidosis. Gastroenterologica Japonica 17:415–421.

Ohta H., Noguchi Y., Takagi K., Nishi M., Kajitani T. and Kato Y. (1987) Early gastric carcinoma with special reference to macroscopic classification. Cancer 60:1099–1106.

Ohta J., Takeda J., Koufuji K., Kodama I., Tsuji V., Maruiwa M., Kumegawa H. and Kakegawa T. (1993) Early gastric cancer associated with synchronous multiple liver metastasis: two rare cases. Kurume Medical Journal 40:41–44.

Oi M., Oshida K. and Sugimura S. (1959) The location of gastric ulcer. Gastroenterology 36:45–56.

Oliva M. M., Lazenby A. J. and Perman J. A. (1993) Gastritis associated with gastrospirillum hominis in children: comparison with *Helicobacter pylori* and review of the literature. Modern Pathology 6:513–515.

Olivera P., Nobre-Leitao C. and Chaves P. (1992) Early gastric cancer: an analysis of 44 cases with emphasis on the prognostic significance of the macroscopic and microscopic growth patterns. Journal of Surgical Oncology 51:1218–121.

Olson A. D. and Fukui-Miner K. (1994) Eosinophilic mucosal infiltrate in infants with congenital gastrointestinal obstruction. American Journal of Gastroenterology 89:934–936.

Ona F. V. (1981) Gastric sarcoid. American Journal of Gastroenterology 75:286–288.

Ono H., Kondo H., Saito D., Yoshida S., Shirao K., Yamaguchi H., Yokota T., Hosokawa K., Fukuda H., Hayashi S., et al (1993) Rapid diagnosis of gastric malignant lymphoma from biopsy specimens: detection of immunoglobulin heavy chain rearrangement by polymerase chain reaction. Japan Journal of Cancer Research 84:813–817.

Ooi A., Nakanishi I. and Hashiba A. (1987) Gastric plasmacytoma: an early lesion diagnosed with the aid of immunoperoxidase and immunogold techniques. American Journal of Gastroenterology 82:572–578.

Orchard R., Reynolds K., Fox B., Andrews R., Parkins R. A. and Johnson A. G. (1977) Effect of lysolecithin on gastric mucosal structure and potential difference. Gut 18:457–461.

Ormiston M. C., Gear M. W. L. and Codling B. W. (1982) Five year follow-up study of gastritis. Journal of Clinical Pathology 35:757–760.

Ostertag H. and Georgii A. (1979) Early gastric cancer: a morphological study of 144 cases. Pathology, Research and Practice 164:294–315.

Ovaska J. T., Ekfors T. O., Havia T. V. and Kujari H. P. (1986) Endoscopic follow-up after resection for gastric or duodenal ulcer. Acta Chirurgica Scandinavica 152:289–295.

Overholt B. F. and Jeffries G. H. (1970) Hypertrophic, hypersecretory protein-losing gastropathy. Gastroenterology 58:80–87.

Owen D. A. (1986) Normal histology of the stomach. American Journal of Surgical Pathology 10:48–61.

Oyaizu N., Uemura Y., Izumi H., Morii S., Nishi M. and Hioki K. (1985) Eosinophilic gastroenteritis. Acta Pathologica Japonica 35:759–766.

Ozenc A. M., Ruacan S. and Aran O. (1988) Gastritis cystica polyposa. Archives of Surgery 123:372–373.

Palmer E. D. (1951) The morphologic consequences of acute exogenous (staphylococcic) gastroenteritis on the gastric mucosa. Gastroenterology 19:462–475.

Palmer E. D. (1954) Gastritis: a revaluation. Medicine 33:199–290.

Palmer E. D. (1958) Note of silent sarcoidosis of the gastric mucosa. Journal of Laboratory and Clinical Medicine 52:231–234.

Papazian A., Braillon A., Dupas J. L., Sevenet F. and Capron J. P. (1986) Portal hypertensive gastric mucosa: an endoscopic study. Gut 27:1199–1203.

Parks T. G., Bussey H. J. R. and Lockhart-Mummery H. E. (1970) Familial polyposis coli associated with extra colonic abnormalities. Gut 11:323–329.

Parl F. F., Lev R., Thomas E. and Pitchumoni C. S. (1979) Histologic and morphometric study of chronic gastritis in alcoholic patients. Human Pathology 10:45–56.

Pastore G., Schiraldi G., Fera G., Sforza E., and Schiraldi O. (1976) A bioptic study of gastrointestinal mucosa in cholera patients during an epidemic in Southern Italy. American Journal of Digestive Diseases 21:613–617.

Payen J. L. et al (1995) Severe portal hypertensive gastropathy and antral vascular ectasia are distinct entities in patients with cirrhosis. Gastroenterology 108:138–144.

Pearse A. G. E., Couling I., Weavers B. and Friesen S. (1970) The endocrine polypeptide cells of the human stomach, duodenum and jejunum. Gut 11:649–658.

Peart A. G., Sivak M. V., Rankin G. B., Kish L. S. and Steck W. D. (1984) Spontaneous improvement of Cronkhite-Canada syndrome in a postpartum female. Digestive Diseases and Sciences 29:470–474.

Pemberton R. E. and Strand L. J. (1979) A review of upper-gastrointestinal effects of the newer nonsteroidal antiinflammatory agents. Digestive Diseases and Sciences 24:53–64.

Peny M. O., Van Gossum A., Noel J. C., Capelli J. A., Lecocq E. and Haot J. (1994) Two cases of watermelon stomach and a review of the literature. Acta Gastroenterologica Belgica 57:166–170.

Petras R. E., Hart W. R. and Bukowski R. M. (1985) Gastric epithelial atypia associated with hepatic arterial infusion chemotherapy. Cancer 56:745–750.

Pickford I. R., Craven J. L., Hall R., Thomas G. and Stone W. D. (1984) Endoscopic examination of the gastric remnant 31–39 years after subtotal gastrectomy for peptic ulcer. Gut 25:393–397.

Pieterse A. S., Rowland R. and Labrooy J. T. (1985) Gastric xanthomas. Pathology 17:455–457.

Pinkerton H. and Iverson L. (1952) Histoplasmosis: three fatal cases with disseminated sarcoid-like lesions. Archives of Internal Medicine 90:456–467.

Pointner R., Schwab G., Konigsrainer A., Bodner E. and Schmid K. W. (1988) Early cancer of the gastric remnant. Gut 29:298–301.

Ponsot P., Theodore C., Julien P-E., Bard A., Molas G., Leymarios J. and Paolaggi J-A. (1983) Angiodysplasies gastriques et maladie de Rendu-Osler. Gastroenterologie Clinique et Biologique 7:321–322.

Pounder R. E., Hunt R. H., Stekelman M., Miton-Thompson G. J. and Misiewicz J. J. (1976) Healing of gastric ulcer during treatment with cimetidine. Lancet i:337–339.

Price A. B. (1988) Histological aspects of *Campylobacter pylori* colonisation and infection of gastric and duodenal mucosa. Scandinavian Journal of Gastroenterology 23 (suppl 142):21–24.

Price A. B. (1991) The Sydney System: histological division. Journal of Gastroenterology and Hepatology 6:209–222.

Pulimood B. M., Knudsen A. and Coghill N. F. (1976) Gastric mucosa after partial gastrectomy. Gut 17:463–470.

Publig W., Wustinger C. and Zandl C. (1994) Non-steroidal anti-inflammatory drugs (NSAID) cause gastrointestinal ulcers mainly in *Helicobacter pylori* carriers. Wiener Klinische Wochenschrift 106:276–279.

Queiroz D. M. M., Barbosa A. J. A., Mendes E. N., Rocha G. A., Cisalpino E. O., Lima G. F. and Oliveira C. A. (1988) Distribution of *Campylobacter pylori* and gastritis in the stomach of patients with and without duodenal ulcer. American Journal of Gastroenterology 83:1368–1370.

Quinn C. M., Bjarnason I. and Price A. B. (1993) Gastritis in patients on non-steroidal anti-inflammatory drugs. Histopathology 23:341–348.

Quintero E., Pique J. M., Bombi J. A., Bordas J. M., Sentis J., Elena M., Bosch J. and Rodes J. (1987) Gastric mucosal vascular ectasias causing bleeding in cirrhosis. Gastroenterology 93:1054–1061.

Rainsford K. D. and Willis C. (1982) Relationship of gastric mucosal damage induced in pigs by antiinflammatory drugs to their effects on prostaglandin production. Digestive Diseases and Sciences 27:624–638.

Ramesar K. C. R. B., Sanders D. S. A. and Hopwood D. (1987) Limited value of type III intestinal metaplasia in predicting risk of gastric carcinoma. Journal of Clinical Pathology 40:1287–1290.

Ramsey E. J., Carey K. V., Peterson W. L., Jackson J. J., Murphy F. K., Read N. W., Taylor K. B., Trier J. S. and Fordtran J. S. (1979) Epidemic gastritis with hypochlorhydria. Gastroenterology 76:1449–1457.

Rattan J., Arber N., Tiomny E., Moshkowitz M., Chapsky Y., Baratz M., Rosen P., and Gilat T. (1993) Gastric polypoid lesions: an eight year study. Hepatogastroenterology 40:107–109.

Rauws E. A. J., Langenberg W., Houthoff H. J., Zanen H. C. and Tytgat G. N. J. (1988) *Campylobacter pyloridis* associated chronic active antral gastritis. Gastroenterology 94:33–40.

Ravi S., Holubka J., Veneri R., Youn K. and Khatib R. (1993) Clofazimine-induced eosinophilic gastroenteritis in AIDS. American Journal of Gastroenterology 88:612–613.

Rees W. D. W. (1987) Mucus-bicarbonate barrier: shield or sieve? Gut 28:1553–1556.

Rees W. D. W. and Turnberg L. A. (1982) Mechanisms of gastric mucosal protection: a role for the "mucus-bicarbonate" barrier. Clinical Science 62:343–348.

Reisman T. N., Leverett F. L., Hudson J. R. and Kalser M. H. (1975) Syphilitic gastropathy. American Journal of Digestive Diseases 20:588–593.

Richter R. M. (1975) Massive gastric haemorrhage from submucosal arterial malformation. American Journal of Gastroenterology 64:324–326.

Ritchie W. P. (1984) Alkaline reflux gastritis: a critical reappraisal. Gut 25:975–987.

Ritchie W. P. (1986) Alkaline reflux gastritis: late results on a controlled trial of diagnosis and treatment. Annals of Surgery 203:537–544.

Ritchie W. Jr and Delaney J. (1968) Gastric ulcer: an experimental model. Surgical Forum 19:312–313.

Rodriguez J. M., Picardo A., Torres A. J., Garcia Calvo M., Ortega L., Martinez S., and Balibrea J. L. (1993) Peutz-Jeghers syndrome with malignization of hamartomatous polyp. Revista Española de Enfermedades Digestiva 84:56–59.

Roesch W. (1978) Erosions of the upper gastrointestinal tract. Clinics in Gastroenterology 7:623–634, Philadelphia: W.B. Saunders Co.

Roesch W., Demling L., and Elster K. (1975) Is chronic gastritis a reversible process? Follow-up study of gastritis by step-wise biopsy. Acta Hepato-Gastroenterologia 22:252–255.

Roesch W and Warnatz H. (1974) Immunofluoreszenzmikroskopische Untersuchungen bei Magenerosionen. In: Fortschritte in der gastroenterologischen Endoskopie. Edited by H. Lindner. Baden-Baden: Witzstrock, pp 194–251.

Ross D. A. and Vincenti A. C. (1994) Acute phlegmonous gastritis: a rare condition with a potentially common cause. British Journal of Hospital Medicine 52:115–116.

Roth S. H. and Bennett R. E. (1987) Nonsteroidal anti-inflammatory drug gastropathy: recognition and response. Archives of Internal Medicine 147:2093–2100.

Rubin W. (1969) Proliferation of endocrine-like (enterochromaffin) cells in atrophic gastric mucosa. Gastroenterology 57:641–648.

Rubin M., Tuthill R. J., Rosato E. F. and Cohen S. (1980) Cronkhite-Canada syndrome: report of an unusual case. Gastroenterology 79:737–741.

Rubio C. A. (1989) Paneth cell adenoma of the stomach. American Journal of Surgical Pathology 13:325–328.

Rubio C. A. and Kato Y. (1986) Ciliated metaplasia in the gastric mucosa: studies on Japanese patients. Japanese Journal of Cancer Research (Gann) 77:282–286.

Rubio C. A. and Kato Y. (1987) Classification of vacuolated cells in the gastric mucosa. Journal of Surgical Oncology 34:128–132.

Rubio C. A. and Kato Y. (1988) Six types of intraepithelial vacuoles in the human gastric mucosa. Pathology, Research and Practice 183:321–325.

Rubio C. A., Kato Y. and Kitagawa T. (1993) Atypical mitosis in gastric intestinal metaplasia in Japanese patients. Japanese Journal of Cancer Research 84:493–494.

Rubio C. A., Kato Y. and Kitagawa T. (1994) Frequency of atypical mitosis in intestinal metaplasia of the gastric mucosa in Japanese patients. Japanese Journal of Cancer Research 85:284–289.

Rubio C. A., Kato Y., Sugano H. and Kitagawa T. (1987) Intestinal metaplasia of the stomach in Swedish and Japanese patients without ulcers or carcinoma. Japanese Journal of Cancer Research (Gann) 78:467–472.

Rubio C. A. and Serck-Hanssen A. (1986) Ciliated metaplasia in the gastric mucosa II: in a European patient with gastric carcinoma. Pathology, Research and Practice 181:382–384.

Rubio C. A. and Slezak P. (1988) Foveolar cell vacuolization in operated stomachs. American Journal of Surgical Pathology 12:773–776.

Rugge M., Farinati F., Baffa R. et al (1994) Gastric epithelial dysplasia in the natural history of gastric cancer: a multicenter prospective follow-up study. Interdisciplinary Group on Gastric Epithelial Dysplasia. Gastroenterology 107:1288–1296.

Ruhl G. H., Schnabel R., Preiseler M. and Seidel D. (1994) Gastric antral vascular ectasia: a case report of a 10-year follow-up with special consideration of histo-pathological aspects. Zeitschrift für Gastroenterologie 32:160–164.

Rumans M. C. and Lieberman D. A. (1987) Eosinophilic gastroenteritis presenting with biliary and duodenal obstruction. American Journal of Gastroenterology 82:775–778.

Russell D. McR., Bhathal P. S. and St. John D. J. B. (1983) Complete remission in Cronkhite-Canada syndrome. Gastroenterology 85:180–185.

Saffos R. O. and Rhatigan R. M. (1977) Benign (nonpolypoid) mucosal changes adjacent to carcinomas of the colon: a light microscopic study of 20 cases. Human Pathology 8:441–449.

Sakita T., Oguro Y., Takasu S., Fukutomi H., Miwa T. and Yoshimori M. (1971) Observations on the healing of ulcerations in early gastric cancer. Gastroenterology 60:835–844.

Sano T., Kobori O. and Muto T. (1992) Lymph node metastasis from early gastric cancer: endoscopic resection of tumour. British Journal of Surgery 79:241–244.

Saraga E-P., Gardiol D. and Costa J. (1987) Gastric dysplasia: a histological follow-up study. American Journal of Surgical Pathology 11:788–796.

Saraga P., Hurlimann J. and Ozzello L. (1981) Lymphomas and pseudolymphomas of the alimentary tract: an immunohistochemical study with clinicopathologic correlations. Human Pathology 12:713–723.

Sarles H. E., Schenkein J. P., Hecht R. M., Sanowski R. A. and Miller P. (1984) Dieulafoy's ulcer: a rare cause of massive gastric hemorrhage in an 11-year-old girl: case report and literature review. American Journal of Gastroenterology 79:930–932.

Sasano N., Nakamuru K., Arai M. and Akazaki K. (1969) Ultrastructural cell patterns in human gastric carcinoma compared with non-neoplastic gastric mucosa: histogenetic analysis of carcinoma by mucin histochemistry. Journal of the National Cancer Institute 43:783–802.

Sassatelli R., Bertoni G., Serra L., Bedogni G. and Ponz de Leon M. (1993) Generalized juvenile polyposis with mixed pattern and gastric cancer. Gastroenterology 104:910–915.

Saukkonen M., Sipponen P., Varis K. and Siurala M. (1980) Morphological and dynamic behaviour of the gastric mucosa after partial gastrectomy with special reference to the gastroenterostomy area. Hepato-Gastroenterology 27:48–56.

Schade R. O. K. (1974) The borderline between benign and malignant lesions in the stomach. In: Early Gastric Cancer. Edited by E. Grundmann, H. Gruntze and S. Witte. Berlin: Springer Verlag, pp 45–53.

Schafer L. W., Larson D. E., Melton III L. J., Higgins J. A. and Zinsmeister A. R. (1985) Risk of development of gastric carcinoma in patients with pernicious anemia: a population-based study in Rochester, Minnesota. Mayo Clinic Proceedings 60:444–448.

Scharschmidt B. F. (1977) The natural history of hypertrophic gastropathy (Menetrier's disease): report of a case with 16-year follow-up and review of 120 cases from the literature. American Journal of Medicine 63:644–652.

Schindler R. (1947) Gastritis. London: Heinemann.

Schmidt-Wilcke H. A., Haake U. and Riecken E. O. (1974) Investigations on the relationship between maximal acid output and parietal cells in gastric mucosal biopsies with special reference to duodenal ulcer. Acta Hepato-Gastroenterologica 21:297–302.

Schrumpf E., Serck-Hanssen A., Stadaas J., Aune S., Myren J. and Osnes M. (1977) Mucosal changes in the gastric stump 20–25 years after partial gastrectomy. Lancet 2:467–469.

Schwartz J., Rozenfeld V., Stelian J., Leibovitz A., Rabinovitz H. and Habot B. (1993) Bleeding angiodysplasia of stomach associated with severe ischemic congestive cardiomyopathy: a case history. Angiology 44:584–586.

Scott B. B. and Jenkins D. (1982) Gastro-oesophageal candidiasis. Gut 23:137–139.

Searcy R. M. and Malagelada J-R. (1984) Menetrier's disease and idiopathic hypertrophic gastropathy. Annals of Internal Medicine 100:565–570.

Seifert E., Butke H., Gail K., Elster K. and Cote S. (1979) Diagnosis of early gastric cancer. American Journal of Gastroenterology 71:563–567.

Seo I. S., Binkley W. B., Warner T. F. C. S. and Warfel K. A. (1982) A combined morphologic and immunologic approach to the diagnosis of gastrointestinal lymphomas I: malignant lymphoma of the stomach (a clinicopathologic study of 22 cases). Cancer 49:493–501.

Seow-Choen F., Ho J. M., Wong J. and Goh H. S. (1992) Gross and histological abnormalities of the foregut in familial adenomatous polyposis: a study from a Southeast Asian Registry. International Journal of Colorectal Diseases 7:177–183.

Seppala K., Lehtola J., and Siurala M. (1976) The possible precancerous significance of abnormal cells in gastric cytology specimens: a follow-up study of 545 patients. Scandinavian Journal of Gastroenterology 11:513–515.

Sethi P., Banerjee A. K., Jones D. M., Eldridge J. and Hollanders D. (1987) Gastritis and gastric *Campylobacter*-like organisms in patients without peptic ulcer. Postgraduate Medical Journal 63:543–545.

Shah A. M. and Joglekar M. (1987) Eosinophilic colitis as a complication of the hypereosinophilic syndrome. Postgraduate Medical Journal 63:485–487.

Shabib S. M., Cutz E., Drumm B. and Sherman P. M. (1994) Association of gastric metaplasia and duodenitis with *Helicobacter pylori* infection in children. American Journal of Clinical Pathology 102:188–191.

Sherman M. P. and Cox K. L. (1982) Neonatal eosinophilic colitis. Journal of Pediatrics 100:587–589.

Shimer G. R. and Helwig E. B. (1984) Inflammatory fibroid polyps of the intestine. American Journal of Clinical Pathology 81:708–714.

Shiner M. and Doniach I. (1957) A study of x-ray negative dyspepsia with reference to histologic changes in the gastric mucosa. Gastroenterology 32:313–324.

Shousha S., Keen C. and Parkins R. A. (1989) Gastric metaplasia and *Campylobacter pylori* infection of duodenum in patients with chronic renal failure. Journal of Clinical Pathology 42:348–351.

Shousha S., el-Sherif A. M., el-Guncid A., Arnaort A. H. and Murray-Lyon I. M. (1993) *Helicobacter pylori* and intestinal metaplasia: comparison between British and Yemini patients. American Journal of Gastroenterology 88:1373–1376.

Shuster L. D., Cox G., Bhatia P. and Miner P. B. (1989) Gastric mucosal nodules due to cytomegalovirus infection. Digestive Diseases and Sciences 34:103–107.

Silen W. (1985) Pathogenetic factors in erosive gastritis. American Journal of Medicine (suppl 2C)79:45–48.

Silen W. (1987) The clinical problem of stress ulcers. Clinical and Investigative Medicine 10:270–274.

Silva S. and Filipe M. I. (1986) Intestinal metaplasia and its variants in the gastric mucosa of Portuguese subjects: a comparative analysis of biopsy and gastrectomy material. Human Pathology 17:988–995.

Sipponen P. (1994) Gastric cancer: a long term consequence of *Helicobacter pylori* infection? Scandinavian Journal of Gastroenterology (suppl)201:24–27.

Sipponen P. (1995) *Helicobacter pylori*: a cohort phenomenon. American Journal of Surgical Pathology (suppl 1)19:S30–S36.

Sipponen P. and Hyvarinen H. (1993) Role of *Helicobacter pylori* in the pathogenesis of gastritis, peptic ulcer and gastric cancer. Scandinavian Journal of Gastroenterology 196:3–6.

Sipponen P., Riihela M., Hyvarinen H. and Seppala K. (1994) Chronic nonatrophic ("superficial") gastritis increases the risk of gastric carcinoma: a case-control study. Scandinavian Journal of Gastroenterology 29:336–340.

Sirak H. D. (1954) Boeck's sarcoid of the stomach simulating linitis plastica: report of a case and comparison with twelve recorded cases. Archives of Surgery 69:769–776.

Siurala M. and Salmi H. J. (1971) Long-term follow-up of subjects with superficial gastritis or a normal gastric mucosa. Scandinavian Journal of Gastroenterology 6:459–463.

Siurala M. and Seppala K. (1960) Atrophic gastritis as a possible precursor of gastric carcinoma and pernicious anaemia: results of follow up examinations. Acta Medica Scandinavica 166:455–474.

Siurala M., Sipponen P. and Kekki M. (1985) Chronic gastritis: dynamic and clinical aspects. Scandinavian Journal of Gastroenterology (suppl 109)20:69–76.

Sjoblom S. M., Sipponen P. and Jarvinen H. (1993) Gastroscopic follow-up of pernicious anaemia patients. Gut 34:28–32.

Sjoblom S-M., Sipponen P., Karonen S-L. and Jarvinen H. J. (1989). Mucosal argyrophil endocrine cells in pernicious anaemia and upper gastrointestinal carcinoid tumours. Journal of Clinical Pathology 42:371–377.

Skillman J. J. and Silen W. (1972) Stress ulcers. Lancet 2:1303–1306.

Skinner J. M., Heenan P. J. and Whitehead R. (1975) Atrophic gastritis in gastrectomy specimens. British Journal of Surgery 62:23–25.

Smith J. M. B. (1969) Mycoses of the alimentary tract. Gut 10:1035–1040.

Snover D. C., Weisdorf S. A., Vercellotti G. M., Rank B., Hutton S. and McGlave P. (1985) A histopathologic study of gastric and small intestinal graft-versus-host disease following allogeneic bone marrow transplantation. Human Pathology 16:387–392.

Snyder J. D., Rosenblum N., Wershil B., Goldman H. and Winter H. S. (1987) Pyloric stenosis and eosinophilic gastroenteritis in infants. Journal of Pediatric Gastroenterology and Nutrition 6:543–547.

Sobala G. M., King R. F. G., Axon A. T. R. and Dixon M. F. (1990). Reflux gastritis in the intact stomach. Journal of Clinical Pathology 43:303–306.

Sobola G. M., O'Connor H. J., Dewar E. P., King R. F., Axon A. T. and Dixon M. F. (1993) Bile reflux and intestinal metaplasia in gastric mucosa. Journal of Clinical Pathology 46:235–240.

Sowa M., Kato Y., Onoda N., Kubo T., Maekawa H., Yoshikawa K., Nishimusa M., Nakanishi M., Maeda K., Chung Y. S. and Umeyama K. (1993) Early cancer of the gastric remnant with special reference to the importance of follow-up of gastrectomized patients. European Journal of Surgical Oncology 19:43–49.

Spiller R. C., Lovell D. and Silk D. B. A. (1988) Adult acquired cytomegalovirus infection with gastric and duodenal ulceration. Gut 29:1109–1111.

Spinelli P., Lo Gullo C. and Pizzetti P. (1980) Endoscopic diagnosis of gastric lymphomas. Endoscopy 12:211–214.

Stael von Holstein C., Hammar E., Eriksson S. and Huldt B. (1993) Clinical significance of dysplasia in gastric remnant biopsy specimens. Cancer 72:1532–1535.

Stalsberg H. and Taksdal S. (1971) Stomach cancer following gastric surgery for benign conditions. Lancet ii:1175–1177.

Stamm B. and Saremaslani P. (1989) Coincidence of fundic glandular hyperplasia and carcinoma of the stomach. Cancer 63:354–359.

Steele R. J. C., Mok S. D., Crofts T. J. and Li A. K. C. (1987) Two cases of eosinophilic enteritis presenting as large bowel perforation and small bowel haemorrhage. Australian and New Zealand Journal of Surgery 57:335–336.

Stemmermann G. N. (1967) Comparative study of histochemical patterns in non-neoplastic and neoplastic gastric epithelium: A study of Japanese in Hawaii. Journal of the National Cancer Institute 39:375–382.

Stemmermann G. N. (1994) Intestinal metaplasia of the stomach: a status report. Cancer 74:556–564.

Stemmermann G. N. and Hayashi T. (1979) Hyperplastic polyps of the gastric mucosa adjacent to gastroenterostomy stomas. American Journal of Clinical Pathology 71:341–345.

Stillman A. E., Sieber O., Manthei U., and Pinnas J. (1981) Transient protein-losing enteropathy and enlarged gastric rugae in childhood. American Journal of Diseases of Children 135:29–33.

Stolte M. and Eidt S. (1993) Healing gastric MALT lymphomas by eradicating H. pylori (editorial). Lancet 342:568.

Stolte M., Sticht T., Eidt S., Ebert D. and Finkenzeller G. (1994) Frequency, location, age and sex distribution of various types of gastric polyp. Endoscopy 26:659–665.

Strayer D. S., Phillips G. B., Barker K. H., Winokur T. and DeSchryver-Kecskemeti K. (1981) Gastric cytomegalovirus infection in bone marrow transplant patients. Cancer 48:1478–1483.

Strickland R. G., Bhathal P. S., Korman M. G. and Hansky J. (1971) Serum gastrin and the antral mucosa in atrophic gastritis. British Medical Journal iv:451–453.

Strickland R. G., Fisher J. M., Lewin K. and Taylor K. B. (1973) The response to prednisolone in atrophic gastritis: a possible effect on non-intrinsic factor-mediated vitamin B$_{12}$ absorption. Gut 14:13–19.

Strickland R. G. and Mackay I. R. (1973) A reappraisal of the nature and significance of chronic atrophic gastritis. Americal Journal of Digestive Diseases 18:426–440.

Stringel G., Mercer S., Sharpe D., Shipman R. and Jimenez C. (1984) Eosinophilic gastroenteritis. Canadian Journal of Surgery 27:182–183.

Subei I., Attar B., Schmitt G. and Levendoglu H. (1987) Primary gastric tuberculosis: a case report and literature review. American Journal of Gastroenterology 82:769–772.

Sue-Ling H. M., Johnston D., Martin I. G. et al (1993). Gastric cancer: a curable disease in Britain. British Medical Journal 307:591–596.

Sue-Ling H. M., Martin I., Griffith J. et al (1992) Early gastric cancer: 46 cases treated in one surgical department. Gut 33:1318–1322.

Suen K. C. and Burton J. D. (1979) The spectrum of eosinophilic infiltration of the gastrointestinal tract and its relationship to other disorders of angiitis and granulomatosis. Human Pathology 10:31–43.

Sugihara K., Muto T., Kamiya J., Konishi F., Sawada T. and Morioka Y. (1982) Gardner's syndrome associated with periampullary carcinoma, duodenal and gastric adenomatosis: report of a case. Diseases of the Colon and Rectum 25:766–771.

Sutton D. R., Baird I. M., Stewart J. S., and Coghill N. F. (1970) ''Free'' iron loss in atrophic gastritis, post-gastrectomy states, and adult coeliac disease. Lancet ii:387–389.

Suzuki S., Suzuki H., Endo M., Takemoto T., Kondo T. and Nakayama K. (1973) Endoscopic dyeing method for diagnosis of early cancer and intestinal metaplasia of the stomach. Endoscopy 5:124–129.

Takahashi S., Igarashi H., Ishiyama N., Nakamura K., Masubuchi N., Osaki M., Saito S., Aoyagi T., Koh T., and Hirata I. (1993) Is Helicobacter pylori a causal agent in gastric carcinoma? International Journal of Medical Microbiology, Virology, Parasitology and Infectious Diseases 280:144–149.

Takaki K. (1986) Lymphoid follicles appearing in gastric mucosa, especially in reactive lymphoid hyperplasia and malignant lymphoma. Acta Pathologica Japonica 36:1627–1641.

Takano Y., Kato Y. and Sugano H. (1994) Epstein-Barr virus–associated medullary carcinomas with lymphoid infiltration of the stomach. Journal of Cancer Research and Clinical Oncology 120:303–308.

Takechi K., Mihara M., Saito Y., Endo J., Maekawa H., Usui T., Moriwaki H. and Muto Y. (1992) A modified technique for endoscopic mucosal resection of small early gastric carcinomas. Endoscopy 24:215–217.

Talley N. J., Cameron A. J., Shorter R. G., Zinsmeister A. R. and Phillips S. F. (1988) Campylobacter pylori and Barrett's esophagus. Mayo Clinic Proceedings 63:1176–1180.

Talley N. J. and Phillips S. F. (1988) Non-ulcer dyspepsia: potential causes and pathophysiology. Annals of Internal Medicine 108:865–879.

Tanaka M., Saitoh A., Narita T., Hizawa Y., Nakazawa H., Narita N. and Kudo H. (1994) Gastrospirillum hominis–associated gastritis: the first reported case in Japan. Journal of Gastroenterology 29:199–202.

Tarpila S., Telkka A. and Siurala M. (1969) Ultrastructure of various metaplasias of the stomach. Acta Pathologica et Microbiologica Scandinavica 77:187–195.

Tatsuta M. and Okuda S. (1975) Location, healing, and recurrence of gastric ulcers in relation to fundal gastritis. Gastroenterology 69:897–902.

Tatsuta M., Okuda S., Tamura H. and Taniguchi H. (1982) Endoscopic diagnosis of early gastric cancer by the endoscopic Congo red-methylene blue test. Cancer 50:2956–2960.

Tedesco F. J., Huckaby C. B., Hamby-Allen M. and Ewing G. C. (1981) Eosinophilic ileocolitis: expanding spectrum of eosinophilic gastroenteritis. Digestive Diseases and Sciences 26:943–948.

Terruzzi V. and Minoli G. (1984) Gastric candidiasia revisited. Gastrointestinal Endoscopy 30:268–269.

Terruzzi V., Minoli G., Butti G. C. and Rossini A. (1980) Gastric lipid islands in the gastric stump and in non-operated stomach. Endoscopy 12:58–62.

Tokunaga O., Watanabe T. and Morimatsu M. (1987) Pseudolymphoma of the stomach. Cancer 59:1320–1327.

Tomenius J. (1950) Instrument for gastrobiopsies. Gastroenterology 15:498–504.

Tominaga K. (1975) Distribution of parietal cells in the antral mucosa of human stomachs. Gastroenterology 69:1201–1207.

Toner P. G. and Cameron C. H. S. (1995) The gastric mucosa. In: Gastrointestinal and Oesophageal Pathology, 2nd ed. Edited by R. Whitehead. Edinburgh: Churchill Livingstone, pp 15–32.

Torikata C., Mukai M. and Kawakita H. (1989) Ultrastructure of metaplastic ciliated cells in human stomach. Virchows Archiv (A) 414:113–119.

Torikata C., Mukai M., Kawakita H. and Kageyama K. (1986) Ciliated cells in human metaplastic gastric mucosa: a proposal of a new term: ciliated metaplasia. Proceedings of the XIth International Congress on Electron Microscopy, Kyoto 1986, pp 3549–3550.

Tosi P., Luzi P., Baak J. P. A., Miracco C., Vindigni C., Lio R. and Barbini P. (1987) Gastric dysplasia: a stereological and morphometrical assessment. Journal of Pathology 152:83–94.

Totten J., Burns H. J. G. and Kay A. W. (1983) Time of onset of carcinoma of the stomach following surgical treatment of duodenal ulcer. Surgery, Gynecology and Obstetrics 157:431–433.

Trounce J. Q. and Tanner M. S. (1985) Eosinophilic gastroenteritis. Archives of Disease in Childhood 60:1186–1188.

Tsuchikame N., Ishimaru Y., Ohshima S. and Takahashi M. (1993) Three familial cases of fundic gland polyposis without polyposis coli. Virchows Archiv (A) 422:337–340.

Tung K. T. and Millar A. B. (1987) Gastric angiodysplasia: a missed cause of gastrointestinal bleeding. Postgraduate Medical Journal 63:865–866.

Tytgat G. N., Grijm R., Dekker W., and Den Hartog N. A. (1976) Fatal eosinophilic enteritis. Gastroenterology 71:479–483.

Uemura Y., Tang X., Aihara H. and Tsutsumi Y. (1994) Mucosa associated lymphoid tissue (MALT) lymphoma of the stomach progressing to overt B cell malignancy. Pathology International 44:808–814.

Uemura Y., Tokunaga M., Arikawa J., et al (1994) A unique morphology of Epstein-Barr virus–related early gastric carcinoma. Cancer Epidemiology, Biomarkers and Prevention 3:607–611.

Uibo R. and Salupere V. (1981) Immunology of chronic gastritis. Annals of Clinical Research 13:130–132.

Utsunomiya J., Maki T., Iwama T., Matsunaga Y., Ichikawa S., Shimomura T., Hamaguchi E. and Aoki N. (1974) Gastric lesion of familial polyposis coli. Cancer 34:745–754.

Van den Heule B., Van Kerkem C. and Heimann R. (1979) Benign and malignant lymphoid lesions of the stomach. A histological reappraisal in the light of the Kiel classification for non Hodgkin's lymphomas. Histopathology 3:309–320.

Van Olmen G, Larmuseau M. F., Geboes K., Rutgeerts P., Penninckx F. and Vantrappen G. (1984) Primary gastric actinomycosis: a case report and review of the literature. American Journal of Gastroenterology 79:512–516.

Van Rensburg L. C. J., Keet A. C. and Adams G. (1986) Eosinophilic granuloma of the stomach. Journal of Surgical Oncology 31:143–147.

Varis K. (1981) Family behaviour of chronic gastritis. Annals of Clinical Research 13:123–129.

Varis O., Valle J. and Siurala M. (1993) Comparison between pernicious anaemia relatives and duodenal ulcer relatives. Scandinavian Journal of Gastroenterology 28:705–708.

Veldhuyzen Van Zanten S. J. O., Bartelsman J. F. W. M., Schipper M. E. I. and Tytgat G. N. J. (1986) Recurrent massive haematemesis from Dieulafoy vascular malformations: a review of 101 cases. Gut 27:213–222.

Vendelboe M. and Jespersen J, (1981) Hypertrophic protein-losing gastritis (Menetrier's disease) treated with Cimetidine. Acta Medica Scandinavica 209:125–127.

Vinograd I., Granot E., Ron N., Klin B., Tauber T. and Segal M. 1993. Chronic diffuse varioliform gastritis in a child: total gastrectomy for acute massive bleeding. Journal of Clinical Gastroenterology 16:40–44.

Voigt J-J., Cassigneul J., Pradere M, Vinel J-P., Carballido M. and Guiu M. (1983) Cystic glandular fundic polyps of the stomach. Gastroenterologie Clinique et Biologique 7:171–176.

Walker F. B. (1981) Spontaneous remission in hypertrophic gastropathy (Menetrier's disease). Southern Medical Journal 74:1273–1276.

Watanabe A., Nagashima H., and Motoi M. (1979) Familial juvenile polyposis of the stomach. Gastroenterology 77:148–151.

Watanabe H., Enjoji M., Yao T. and Ohsato K. (1978) Gastric lesions in familial adenomatosis coli. Human Pathology 9:269–283.

Watt I. A., McLean N. R., Girdwood R. W. A., Kissen L. H. and Fyfe A. H. B. (1979) Eosinophilic gastroenteritis associated with a larval anisakine nematode. Lancet 2:893–894.

Watt P. C. H., Sloan J. M. and Kennedy T. L. (1983) Changes in gastric mucosa after vagotomy and gastrojejunostomy for duodenal ulcer. British Medical Journal 287:1407–1410.

Watt P. C. H., Sloan J. M., Spencer A. and Kennedy T. L. (1983) Histology of the postoperative stomach before and after diversion of bile. British Medical Journal 287:1410–1412.

Wattel W. and Geuze J J. (1978) The cells of the rat gastric groove and cardia: an ultrastructural and carbohydrate histochemical study, with special reference to the fibrillovesicular cells. Cell and Tissue Research 186:375–391.

Wee A., Kang J. Y. and Teh M. (1992) Helicobacter pylori and gastric cancer: correlation with gastritis, intestinal metaplasia and tumour histology. Gut 33:1029–1032.

Weston A. P., Campbell D. R., McGregor D. H. and Cherian R. (1994) Endoscopic and histologic resolution of gastric pseudolymphoma (reactive lymphoid hyperplasia) following treatment with bismuth and oral antibiotics. Digestive Diseases and Sciences 39:2567–2574.

White R. M., Levine M. S., Enterline H. T. and Laufer I. (1985) Early gastric cancer: recent experience. Radiology 155:25–27.

Whitehead R. (1995). The classification of chronic gastritis: current status. J Clin Gastroenterol 21 (suppl):131–134.

Whitehead R., Truelove S. C. and Gear M. W. (1972) The histological diagnosis of chronic gastritis in fibreoptic gastroscope biopsy specimens. Journal of Clinical Pathology 25:1–11.

Widgren S. and Pizzolato G. P. (1987) Inflammatory fibroid polyp of the gastrointestinal tract: possible origin in myofibroblasts? Annales de Pathologie 7:184–192.

Wilander E. (1981) Achylia and the development of gastric carcinoids. Virchows Archiv (A) 394:151–160.

Williams A. W. (1956) The effects of alcohol on gastric mucosa. British Medical Journal i:256–259.

Winkler H., Zelikovski A., Gutman H., Mor C. and Reiss R. (1986) Inflammatory fibroid polyp of the jejunum causing intussusception. American Journal of Gastroenterology 81:598–601.

Witzel L., Halter F., Gretillat P. A., Scheurer U. and Keller M. (1976) Evaluation of specific value of endoscopic biopsies and brush cytology for malignancies of the oesophagus and stomach. Gut 17:375–377.

Wolf J. A. Jr and Spjut H. J. (1981) Focal lymphoid hyperplasia of the stomach preceding gastric lymphoma: case report and review of the literature. Cancer 48:2518–2523.

Wolfsen H. C., Carpenter H. A. and Talley N. J. (1993) Menetrier's disease: a form of hypertrophic gastropathy or gastritis? Gastroenterology 104:1310–1319.

Wood I. J., Doig R. K., Motteram R. and Hughes A. (1949) Gastric biopsy: report on 55 biopsies using new flexible gastric biopsy tubes. Lancet i:18–21.

Wotherspoon A. C., Doglioni C., Diss T. C., Pan L., Maschini A., de Boni M. and Isaacson P. G. (1993) Regression of primary low-grade B-cell gastric lymphoma of mucosa-associated lymphoid tissue type after eradication of *Helicobacter pylori*. Lancet 342:575–577.

Wotherspoon A. C., Ortiz-Hidalgo C., Falzon M. R. and Isaacson P. G. (1991) *Helicobacter pylori*–associated gastritis and primary B-cell gastric lymphoma. Lancet 338:1175–1176.

Wright R., Whitehead R., Wangel A. G., Salem S. N. and Schiller K. F. R. (1966) Autoantibodies and microscopic appearances of gastric mucosa. Lancet i:618–621.

Wu M. T., Pan H. B., Lai P. H., Chang J. M., Tsai S. H. and Wu C. W. (1994) CT of gastritis cystica polyposa. Abdominal Imaging 19:8–10.

Whatt J. I. (1995) Histopathology of gastroduodenal inflammation: the of *Helicobacter pylori*. Histopathology 26:1–15.

Wyatt J. I. and Dixon M. F. (1988) Chronic gastritis: a pathogenetic approach. Journal of Pathology 154:113–124.

Wyatt J. I., Shallcross T. M., Crabtree J. E. and Heatley R. V. (1992) *Helicobacter pylori*, gastritis and peptic ulceration in the elderly. Journal of Clinical Pathology 45:1070–1074.

Yamada M., Hatakeyama S. and Tsukagoshi H. (1985) Gastrointestinal amyloid deposition in AL (primary or myeloma-associated) and AA (secondary) amyloidosis. Human Pathology 16:1206–1211.

Yamashiro Y., Oguchi S., Otsuka Y., Nagata S. et al (1994) *Helicobacter pylori* colonization in children with gastritis and peptic ulcer I: the colonization rate and effects of colonization on mucin content and mucosal inflammation in the antrum. Acta Paediatrica Japonica 36:167–170.

Yeomans N. D. (1976) Electron microscopic study of the repair of aspirin-induced gastric erosions. American Journal of Digestive Diseases 21:533–541.

Zollinger R. M., and Moore F. T. (1968) Zollinger-Ellison syndrome comes of age. Journal of the American Medical Association 204:361–365.

Zora J. A., O'Connell E. J., Sachs M. I. and Hoffman A. D. (1984) Eosinophilic gastroenteritis: a case report and review of the literature. Annals of Allergy 53:45–47.

Zuckerman M. J., al-Samman M. and Boman D. A. (1994) Granulomatous gastroenteritis: case report with comparison to idiopathic isolated granulomatous gastritis. Digestive Diseases and Sciences 39:1649–1654.

Small Intestine Biopsy

III

10

NORMAL APPEARANCES IN SMALL INTESTINE BIOPSY SPECIMENS

Classic normal appearances are seen only in sections cut at right angles to the plane of the muscularis mucosa. Oblique sections produce a variable combination of two principal features: cross-sectioning of glands and cross-sectioning of villi. With technical care it is usually possible to produce correctly oriented sections, but an experienced pathologist generally can assess sections that are suboptimal in this respect. A possible source of misinterpretation is the presence of artefacts. A potential cause is the trauma of the suction used at biopsy. The superficial epithelium at the tips of villi may be lifted to produce subepithelial blebs (Fig. 10–1), or on occasion the villous tips are denuded. In people, ethanol ingested in quantities equivalent to moderate drinking seems to increase the incidence of this type of artefact (Millan et al 1980). In rats, alcohol temporarily destabilises the intercellular junction of the epithelium (Draper et al 1983), which could play a part in the production of this type of lesion. There is also some evidence that chronic ethanol ingestion in the rat reduces enterocyte turnover rates (Mazzanti and Jenkins 1987).

Figure 10–1. Small intestine suction biopsy shows a traumatic subepithelial bleb (H&E ×250).

This type of damage may also result from rough handling once the biopsy specimen has been obtained. Attempts to unroll a specimen in order to lay it flat or to remove adherent surface mucin so that a better dissecting microscope view can be obtained should be made with great care or avoided altogether. Sometimes tissue fluid or even blood appears under the surface epithelium and must be differentiated from oedema fluid or meaningful haemorrhage. These artefacts are not significantly hard for trained histopathologists to interpret because they are common to biopsy material from other areas. Clearly, however, every effort should be made to avoid them so that all possible information can be extracted from the tissue samples.

The mucosa of the small intestine has the same basic structure everywhere along its length. Villi project from a simple gland layer that lies on a muscularis mucosa (Fig. 10–2). Villi are approximately three times the length of the crypt in adults and about twice the length in children. Height of villi is also said to be slightly reduced in old age (Warren, Pepperman and Montgomery 1978). In normal adults finger-like villi predominate at all levels of the intestine (Baker 1973), but proximally and distally leaf-like forms and short ridges can be seen (Fig. 10–3) (Holmes, Hourihane and Booth 1961, Cocco, Dohrmann and Hendrix 1966, Stewart et al 1967). In addition leaf-like and ridge-like villi predominate in the proximal small intestine; the change occurs shortly after birth because in stillborn (Chacko et al 1969) and newborn infants, finger-like villi predominate (Phillips 1995). The villi are covered by a columnar epithelium that has a brush border with a distinct positive reaction to periodic acid–Schiff (PAS) stain. Sometimes in good preparations occasional minute PAS-positive granules, which are probably lysosomes, can be seen in the apical cytoplasm, and the faintly positive membranes of Golgi's apparatus just above the nucleus are visible. The villous epithelium is continuous with that lining the crypts, but the latter epithelium has a less distinct brush border. Whereas mitotic figures are frequently present in the crypt epithelium, they are never present in the villous epithelium. The crypt epithelium is the regenerative zone and, by a process of migration, is responsible for new cell types in the crypts and on the villous processes, the effete absorptive cells being lost from the villous tips.

At the base of the glands Paneth's cells are present. It is surprising that the functional significance of such a distinctive cell type should still be in doubt. Although goblet cells and Paneth's cells probably have a common precursor cell, and cells intermediate between the two occur (Montero and Erlandsen 1978), Paneth's cells usually do not migrate upward onto the villi. Sandow and Whitehead

Figure 10–2. Jejunal biopsy. Finger-like villi and a gland layer supported by a muscularis mucosa. Goblet cells, which appear as empty circular spaces, are obvious (H&E ×100).

Figure 10–3. Duodenal biopsy. The villi are shorter and broader and some forms are irregular. Note the Brunner's glands (H&E ×75).

(1979) and Trier and Madara (1981) extensively reviewed the structure and function of Paneth's cells; Mathan, Hughes and Whitehead (1987) studied their morphogenesis by immunocytochemical electron microscopy. In humans, the cells appear to rise away from the base of the crypts and then migrate toward the base as they mature. Occasional enterochromaffin cells are also scattered about in the crypts. These cells are only part of a much larger system of endocrine cells, the function of which has generated substantial research. Reviews by Rayford, Miller and Thompson (1976a and b), Buffa et al (1978), Buchan and Polak (1980), Solcia et al (1980), Bloom and Polak (1981), and Sjolund et al (1983) are testament to the complexity of the gut-associated endocrine system and the wide variety of tumours it can produce (Chejfec et al 1988).

PAS-positive goblet cells exist in the glands and among the surface absorptive cells, but they progressively decrease in number toward the villous tip, where they are scattered among the epithelial cells. Often appearing within a vacuole, which is probably a shrinkage artefact, it is usual to observe occasional intraepithelial lymphocytes; they were called theliolymphocytes by Fichtelius, Yunis and Good (1968). This is often shortened to theliocyte. They lie in the spaces between the epithelial cells after having passed through the basement membrane. They occur in a ratio of one for every six epithelial cells and form an integral part of the gut-associated lymphoid tissue along with the immunocytes of the lamina propria, the solitary lymphoid follicles, Peyer's patches, and mesenteric lymph nodes. There is evidence that the number of lymphoid follicles in the human large intestine has been greatly underestimated, Langman and Rowland (1986) having shown that there is an average density of 18.4 per cm^2 in the caecum, 15 per cm^2 in the colon, and as many as 25.4 per cm^2 in the rectum. This is far in excess of the 5 per cm^2 accepted as normal since the early study by Dukes and Bussey (1926).

Intraepithelial lymphocytes, or theliocytes, have been studied in detail in animals in an effort to establish their functional significance. In humans, Bartnick et al (1980), using a technique for producing isolates of lymphoid cells from intestinal mucosa, claimed that the theliocyte population contained approximately equal proportions of T, B, and null cells. Selby, Janossy and Jewell (1981), however, using frozen sections and lymphocyte antibodies in an immunofluorescent study, found that more than 95% of theliocytes were T cells, of which 85% were suppressor or cytotoxic phenotype and 15% were helper or inducer phenotype (Selby et al 1983). This is in keeping with the results of earlier observations in experimental animals.

Human intestinal intraepithelial lymphocytes, their origin and putative functions in relation to overall lymphoepithelial interactions and the mucosal immune system, have been reviewed (Dobbins 1986, Brandtzaeg et al 1988). In the jejunum there are usually 12–35 lymphocytes per 100 villous epithelial cells both in adults (Ferguson and Murray 1971) and in children (Phillips et al 1979); there are fewer in the ileum (Dobbins 1986). The exact functions of the lymphocytes are not known, but it has been suggested that they are involved in modulating local immune responses and may be involved in handling antigens (Cerf-Bensussan et al 1984).

Both in crypts and on villi, another cell type can be recognised by electron microscopy. It is called the caveolated cell or tuft cell (Nabeyama and Leblond 1974). It is pear-shaped with a narrow apex bearing long microvilli whose filamentous cores extend deep into the apical cytoplasm. Among the filaments are the caveoli, which appear as irregular vesicles occasionally in continuity with the apical plasma membrane. The function of these cells, which are also in the stomach and colon, is unknown.

Another cell type exists in the ileum. This is known as the M cell, and it can be seen only by means of an electron microscope. It always overlies Peyer's patches and other lymphoid follicles (Owen and Nemanic 1978, Jackson, Walker-Smith and Phillips 1982). The surface of the cell has low, anastomising convolutions, and its cytoplasm is attenuated around several lymphocytes although it maintains intercellular adhesion with neighbouring enterocytes. Owen (1977), using horseradish peroxidase as a tracer, demonstrated the M cell's capacity for macromolecular protein uptake. This allows the cell to function in the mechanisms for antigen absorption and processing.

In ordinary preparations the core of the villi and the rest of the lamina propria, that area between the crypts bounded externally by the muscularis mucosa, appear as delicate, loose connective tissue infiltrated by a small number of lymphocytes and occasional plasma cells, eosinophils, mast cells, and histiocytes. The importance of using the correct fixative (Carnoy's solution) in any study of mast cells in jejunal biopsies was stressed by Strobel, Busuttil and Ferguson (1983). The villi also contain a central blind-ending lacteal that is usually collapsed and often only recognisable as a parallel double row of flat endothelial nuclei in the villous core. A capillary plexus that lies beneath the basement membrane is more obvious, and the smooth muscle cells that extend upward from the muscularis mucosa can be recognised as they surround the central lacteal passing to the very tip of the villous process.

Brunner's glands, traditionally thought to be localised to the duodenum, have a marked variation of distribution often extending to the jejunum, particularly in children (Landboe-Christensen 1944). They occur on both sides of and between the elements of the muscularis mucosa, which thus appears split. Rarely, small groups of glands occur within the superficial epithelium (Fig. 10–4). Hyperplasia or undue prominence of Brunner's glands is often associated with obvious villous stunting. In the region of the duodenal papilla the villi are also short and stubby, and biopsies frequently include mucous glands and smooth muscle related to the termination of the duct system and mixing valve (see later). As the ileum is approached (Fig. 10–5), the ratio of goblet cells to absorptive cells increases, and the villi tend to become slightly broader and shorter than in the jejunum. Lymphoid aggregates that split the muscularis mucosa, being partially mucosal and partially submucosal, often show a central germinal centre. They increase in number in the more distal parts of the small intestine as solitary follicles, but they also increase in confluence in the ileum as Peyer's patches. Villi overlying lymphoid areas are often stubby or absent.

Villous architecture is determined in part by the depth of tissue obtained at biopsy. When the muscularis mucosa is present, the villi are taller and slimmer and lie more closely together than when this tethering layer is absent. Without a muscularis mucosa and with a measure of mucosal stretching due to too much handling of the biopsy specimen, the appearance produced, with broad-based, widely separated villi, can be distinctly abnormal (Fig. 10–6). It is also claimed that villi are shorter on the crests of mucosal folds than in the less exposed valleys between, and

Figure 10–4. Duodenal biopsy. A small group of Brunner's glands *(arrowhead)* is present within the epithelium (H&E ×225).

that increased trauma in the crests is the cause (Creamer 1967). This presupposes that such mucosal folds as may be seen at necropsy or in surgical specimens are fixed structures and reflect the living state. If the contours of the mucosal surface constantly change during life, as seems likely, this observation is possibly an artefact related to a terminal contracture of the bowel musculature.

Rare are the detailed studies of small-bowel mucosal morphology in a normal group rather than a control group of patients not suffering overtly from gastrointestinal disease, but it would appear that villous morphology varies in different ethnic groups. When compared with the villi in biopsy specimens from the English or North Americans, the villi of the Thai (Sprinz et al 1962), Africans (Banwell, Hutt and Tunnicliffe 1964), Indians (Baker et al 1962), South Vietnamese (Colwell et al 1968), Haitians (Brunser, Eidelman and Klipstein 1970), and Arabs (Shiner and Pearson 1981) are shorter and thicker and have an increased proportion of leaf-

Figure 10–5. Ileal mucosa. Villi are slightly shorter and broader than in the jejunum, and goblet cells are more obvious (H&E ×140).

Figure 10–6. Jejunal biopsy. The muscularis mucosa is absent, and the villi are more widely separated and appear somewhat shortened (H&E ×75).

shaped forms and short ridges, and the lamina propria contains proportionately more inflammatory cells. There has been debate whether these are true racial variations or simply reflections of altered intralumenal environment due to different standards of health and hygiene.

There is no doubt that alterations of gut flora in experimental animals have a profound effect on villous shape (Creamer 1967, King and Toskes 1979). In humans also, a range of jejunal mucosal abnormalities has been described in patients with parasitic infestations (Magalhaes, Trevisan and Pereira 1975), and the mild variations in small intestinal morphology that occur with age in infants younger than 5 years have been ascribed to the changing bacterial colonisation of the intestinal lumen (Walker-Smith 1972). The tendency for shorter villi and longers crypts to occur in children was verified in a morphological study by Penna et al (1981), but there is no evidence based on a morphometric study that the jejunal mucosal morphology varies in adult life; in particular, no reduction of surface area occurs with increasing age (Corazza et al 1986).

In a group of 21 volunteers from a normal population of white British people, jejunal biopsies showed finger-like villi as the sole or predominant villous feature (Pena, Truelove and Whitehead 1973). Fourteen of these showed one or more leaf-shaped villi that could be defined as two or three finger-like villi fused side by side. In addition to fingers and leaves, three specimens showed a small number of short ridges. Ridges resemble two or three leaves fused side by side. In the study of normal jejunal biopsies made by Burhol and Myren (1968), the histological appearances were divided into groups I and II. Group I had predominantly long and slender villi without an increased cellular infiltration of the lamina propria, and group II had predominantly branched and fused villi, also without increased cellular infiltration. These authors did not appear to have examined serial sections. In the normal cases examined by Pena, Truelove and Whitehead it was not possible to make a similar subdivision. Each biopsy specimen was examined in step serial sections, and appearances corresponding to groups I and II of Burhol and Myren were seen in different levels. In all specimens, most villi were tall, slender, and finger-like, but all specimens also showed a proportion of bifid (Fig. 10–7) and occasional trifid forms, and a few specimens showed fused or tongue-shaped villi with occasional mucosal bridges (Fig. 10–8). It is obvious that in any investigation involving morphology, anatomical and pathological variations will be minimised by standardising the biopsy site. It is the usual practice to secure jejunal biopsy specimens, for example, from a point just distal to Treitz's ligament under radiological control. Duodenal biopsies are being

Figure 10–7. Jejunal biopsy from a normal individual. Central villous process shows bifurcation (H&E ×128).

Figure 10–8. Jejunal biopsy from a normal individual. Fusion of villous tips and formation of mucosal bridges (H&E ×150).

performed under direct vision with the use of fibreoptic instruments and can be accurately located in relation to the anatomical landmarks. Comparisons should be made only with normal as opposed to control groups, and the normal cases should be selected from the same ethnic and environmental background as the test cases.

Even when all these criteria are fulfilled and there is meticulous care in the technical handling of the material, minor villous abnormalities still cause difficulties in interpretation. It is for this reason that several attempts were made to replace subjective by more objective, quantitative observations (Rubin et al 1960, Thurlbeck, Benson and Dudley 1960, Madanagopolan, Shiner and Rowe 1965, Stewart et al 1967, and many others). However, they were only partially successful because of the lack of proper normal control series and poor selection of abnormal material; e.g., Thurlbeck, Benson and Dudley (1960) compared tissue obtained at necropsy, at laparotomy, and by tube biopsy, all at unspecified sites. In addition, the methods used are open to criticism; e.g., the use of intersecting lines to assess villous surface area (Madanagopolan, Shiner and Rowe 1965) without relating this to volume results in gross underestimates if there is any amount of villous separation due to an absent muscularis mucosa or a stretching artefact. Measurements of villous height and depth of glands are only approximate because in the majority of biopsies most of the villi are bent over to some extent. The point at which a villus ends and a crypt begins cannot be standardised, and when there is a severe degree of total villous atrophy it becomes impossible. Accurate measurements of epithelial cell height in the normal case are feasible, but on the surface epithelium of a flat mucosa of severe gluten-sensitive enteropathy it becomes virtually impossible because of the palisading of cells and the irregularity of basement membranes and brush border.

It is doubtful if these insensitive quantitative methods gave any better idea of minor morphological changes than a simple visual assessment by an experienced interpreter, and some researchers (Rubin and Dobbins 1965) have thus resorted to the so-called method of blind review. The complexity of a mathematically accurate method of quantitation of the small intestine was described by Hennig (1956). He shows that in order to obtain absolutely accurate information the mucosa must be sectioned and quantitated in three different planes, and the method includes a very large number of observations and therefore its value for the easy application to human jejunal biopsy tissue is limited.

Dunnill and Whitehead (1972), however, devised a simple method of quantitating the surface area to volume ratio in jejunal biopsies. This method, based on the point-counting principle (Chaukley 1943) for volume determination combined with the linear intercept principles (Short 1950) for surface area measurement, is free from the errors of earlier simple methods and, although it does not give absolute information, it allows a relative comparison of one biopsy with another. A template of 15 lines of equal length (Fig. 10–9) is drawn according to the specifications of Weibel (1963) in such a way that each line joins the vertices of a regular hexagonal point network. Weibel states that this avoids bias and allows for an even distribution. The jejunal biopsy specimen to be examined is projected onto the template by a Leitz's projector fitted with a xenon lamp (Fig. 10–10). The magnification is kept constant, and the section is cast at random onto the template. On each occasion, the number of times, c, the lines cut the mucosal surface and the number of end points of the lines, h, that fall on the tissue above, but not including, the muscularis mucosa, are counted. The greater the number of fields cast on the template, the more accurate is the final result, but in practice it was found to be sufficient if the value for h was about 200. If the biopsy specimen is large, it is possible to superimpose the grid on more than one field in a single section; if this is so, it is usually sufficient to make counts on two or three sections. For small biopsy specimens a larger number of serial sections must be examined, perhaps six or eight. If l is the length of the line used, the ratio $c{:}lh$ gives an index of the complexity of the villous pattern and of the surface-to-volume ratio. The length of the line used must always be stated in order that the ratio $c{:}lh$ can be compared between different centres of investigation. Providing the magnification is also kept constant during the examination, the mean

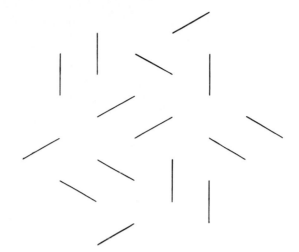

Figure 10–9. The template of 15 lines of equal length drawn according to Weibel (1963).

number of hits per field on the mucosa, h, for each specimen is proportional to the mucosal volume. It is thus possible to compare not only the state of the villi but also the mucosal volumes between specimens.

In this way an assessment of the efficacy of treatment in sequential follow-up studies (Pena et al 1972, Pena, Truelove and Whitehead 1972) can be carried out, and an easy comparison of information arising in different centres of study can be made. There have been several attempts to apply morphological techniques for the measurement of other histological components. The sources of inaccuracy and the rationale for acceptable methods are discussed by Skinner and Whitehead (1976). With increasingly sophisticated computerised image analysis, with systems such as described by Slavin et al (1980) minor abnormalities in jejunal morphology can now be routinely objectively measured. Even with the method of Dunnill and Whitehead (1972) significant subjective inter-observer variation has been convincingly demonstrated (Corazza et al 1982). There have also been applications of morphometric

Figure 10–10. The template in Figure 10–9 superimposed on a normal jejunal biopsy specimen. The end points of the lines lying on the mucosa are counted as hits. The places where the lines cut the mucosal surface are counted as cuts (H&E ×150).

techniques in the determination of numbers of lamina propria cell types (Dhesi et al 1984). The principles involved in mathematically accurate determination are outlined by Skinner and Whitehead (1976). A comprehensive publication by Aherne and Dunnill (1982) is recommended to those wishing to employ a variety of morphometric methods in the study of small intestine diseases, but it is of interest that Corazza et al (1985), who compared computer-aided microscopy, linear measurement, and stereology in the assessment of jejunal biopsy specimens, concluded that the last technique employing a simple eye-piece graticule was the method of choice.

11

SMALL INTESTINE BIOPSY IN DISEASE

The preservation of the morphological form of the small intestine mucosa is the result of a balance between the rate of cell loss from the villous surface and the rate of cell production in the crypts. There is some experimental evidence that this is controlled by a feedback mechanism operating from the surface to the crypts (Galjaard, van der Meer-Fieggen and Giesen 1972, Rijke et al 1976). Williamson (1982) summarised the situation concerning the many factors involved in the maintenance of small intestine morphology. Acceleration of cell renewal, for example, is triggered by a variety of stimuli. Notably, intestinal resection and hyperphagia both result in an increase in the volume of the small intestine mucosa. Jejunal bypass causes overall mucosal hyperplasia and can even result in changes in the type of mucins produced (Olubuyide et al 1984). The importance of oral food intake in maintaining intestinal mucosal morphology has even been demonstrated in humans (Biasco et al 1984). Alkaline phosphatase activity is increased locally and produces a rise in serum levels following intestinal resection (Delgado et al 1986). Not surprisingly hypophagia, or deprival of the mucosa of contact with the lumenal contents, results in a decrease in the mucosa's mass. The trophic effects are mediated in part by bile and pancreatic juice (Hauer-Jensen et al 1988), but there are numerous and complex neurovascular and humoral influences the precise nature of which are yet to be determined.

The other aspects of small bowel morphology, such as the lamina propria lymphoid tissue, the lacteal system, and the Brunner's gland, are also known to be dependent for their form and maintenance on equally complex controlling systems. The range of abnormalities that results when these controls are disturbed by disease processes is very wide. Nevertheless, because of functional physiological differences and the pathological problems that result when these differences are compromised by disease, abnormalities in the small intestine mucosa are best considered on a regional basis. The morphologist should never forget that disease and malfunction of one segment of the gastrointestinal tract can affect the histological appearances in another. An example of this is the effect of vitamin B_{12} deficiency on nuclear morphology in areas of the gut other than the stomach.

BIOPSIES FROM THE DUODENAL BULB

Bulbitis

Biopsy specimens taken from the proximal duodenum in that part known as the bulb frequently show villous abnormalities, even allowing for the increased number of leaf-shaped forms and short ridges that are normal in this zone. Inflammatory infiltration and other morphological abnormalities are also encountered fairly commonly (Takahashi 1994). Abnormalities in the duodenal bulb may, but do not necessarily, reflect the remainder of the upper small intestine. Because of this fact, the practice of precisely located jejunal biopsy arose for the investigation of malabsorption states. However, this was before the era of fibreoptic endoscopes; with their increased use and the ability to perform biopsies on more distal parts of the duodenum, it became plain that there was often no necessity to sample the small intestine in the investigation of malabsorptive and other states at a site beyond the Teitz's ligament (Granot et al 1993, Maurino et al 1993). However, small bowel biopsy is still regarded as the gold standard for the diagnosis of coeliac disease (Carroccio et al 1993), provided that fibreoptic endoscopes equipped with "jumbo" biopsy forceps are used (Ladas et al 1994). The duodenal bulb is the usual site of duodenal ulcer disease, and the inflammatory lesion that precedes this is known as bulbitis or ulcer-associated duodenitis. One of the difficulties in defining the criteria for diagnosing significant bulbitis is the wide variations seen in biopsies from this site, even in the absence of a specific cause (Triadafilopoulos 1993). Furthermore, some doubt has been cast on the concept that duodenitis and ulcer disease are uncommon in the mucosa beyond the bulb (Rao and Murthy 1993). The changes range from a simple excess of plasma cells and lymphocytes in the lamina propria to increasing inflammatory infiltrate and progressive villous deformity and atrophy (Figs. 11–1 to 11–6). The surface epithelium shows degenerative changes and loses its characteristic appearances, assuming a flatter simple type, with nuclear hyperchromasia, cytoplasmic basophilia, and sometimes a syncytial appearance (Fig. 11–7). Frank metaplasia to a surface gastric epithelium is seen, as are all apparent stages in between (Fig. 11–8). Sometimes a more acute inflammatory cell component is superimposed on the lymphocyte and plasma cell population, and the picture is one of acute disease superimposed on chronic disease. Surface erosions (Figs. 11–9 and 11–10), produced when the loss of superficial epithelium exceeds the regenerative process of repair, are seen in the most severe stage. From the pathologist's point of view there is every indication that the changes constitute a readily recognisable lesion. The precise significance of these changes, however, has been the subject of a variety of interpretations. One of the difficulties has been the failure to recognise that the theliocytes and the other white blood cells of the lamina propria as part of

Figure 11–1. Duodenal biopsy specimens (Figs. 11–1 to 11–6) show progressive increase in inflammatory changes with distortion and effacement of villous processes. The Brunner's glands on the lumenal side of the muscularis mucosa become more obvious (H&E ×140).

Figure 11–2. Duodenal biopsy specimen. See Figure 11–1.

Figure 11–3. Duodenal biopsy specimen. See Figure 11–1.

Figure 11–4. Duodenal biopsy specimen. See Figure 11–1.

Figure 11–5. Duodenal biopsy specimen. See Figure 11–1.

the gut-associated lymphoid tissue may react as part of the whole system when the stimulus to react occurs in a site distant from the duodenum. This may occur in viral, bacterial, or parasitic infections or in other circumstances of antigenic stimulation such as protein intolerance or when the duodenum is involved in a specific disease process such as Crohn's disease. The duodenum may also exhibit changes in cellularity of the lamina propria as the result of its involvement in a "field" change due to lesions in neighbouring organs, such as the stomach, pancreas, or bile ducts. Lev et al (1980) showed, for example, that mononuclear cell counts in duodenal biopsies are elevated in the presence of chronic gastritis. When these considerations are made, there can be little doubt that duodenitis or nonspecific duodenitis as first described by Baudin (1837) exists as a specific entity. Konjetzny (1924) recognised duodenitis in the mucosa adjacent to duodenal ulcer, and MacCarty (1924) showed

Figure 11–6. Duodenal biopsy specimen. See Figure 11–1.

Figure 11–7. Superficial epithelium in duodenitis. Degenerative changes and transformation into syncytial masses (H&E ×300).

that identical appearances were sometimes seen in operation specimens from patients with typical duodenal ulcer history but no ulcer. Thus, a relationship between this form of duodenitis (bulbitis) and duodenal ulcer was proposed (Judd and Nagel 1927). With the advent of flexible tube biopsy procedures, the evidence of a diathesis comprising hyperchlorhydria and proximal duodenitis proceeding to duodenal ulcer has been strengthened (Rhodes 1964, Beck et al 1965, Rhodes et al 1968, Gear and Dobbins 1969, Whitehead, Roca and Truelove 1972, Cotton et al 1973, Thomson et al 1977, Paoluzi et al 1982, Schmitz-Moormann et al 1984, Jenkins et al 1985, Scott et al 1985, Sircus 1985, Venables 1985).

Other researchers (Doniach and Shiner 1957, Aronson and Norfleet 1962, Gear and Dobbins 1969, Cheli, Aste and Ciancamerla 1973, Gregg and Garabedian 1974,

Figure 11–8. Superficial epithelium in duodenitis. Stages of progressive metaplasia visible from left to right. Process on right is covered by almost normal gastric superficial epithelium (H&E ×300).

Figure 11–9. Superficial epithelial erosions in duodenitis (H&E ×210).

Gelzayd, Biederman and Gelfand 1975, Cheli 1985, Lawson 1987) regard duodenitis as a lesion not closely related to duodenal ulcer, which may or may not have clinical manifestations. These discordant results are due to a variety of factors. In earlier studies, cases were selected on the basis of radiological findings, and biopsies were blind and localised fluoroscopically. Since the use of fibreoptic instruments, cases have been selected on the basis of directly viewed mucosal appearances. Nevertheless, there has been no standardisation of the endoscopic appearance of duodenitis, and different authors may be studying different groups of patients. It is becoming plain, however, that a reddened duodenal mucosa is not necessarily inflamed and that the appearances are likely to be the result of vasomotor phenomena. Over the years, varying histological criteria were used in defining duodenitis. These have now been refined because of the need in the light of endoscopic and clinical parameters to arrive at a decision as to their likely significance, a point made by Jeffers and Hourihane (1993) in a paper concerning the shared histological features of coeliac disease and peptic duodenitis.

The grading of histological features seen in duodenal biopsies first proposed by Whitehead et al (1975) and later modified (Whitehead 1979) is still regarded as an

Figure 11–10. Superficial epithelial erosions in duodenitis (H&E ×210).

essential base protocol in their interpretation (Table 11–1). Each main histological parameter of the mucosa is considered in turn.

(a) *Villous processes.* The villous processes of the duodenum are less regular and shorter than those in the jejunum and tend to be even more stubby or absent over lymphoid follicles or prominent mucosal Brunner's glands. There is, however, a progressive villous obliteration that is related to increasing inflammation of the mucosa, and in its severest form this leads to a flat mucosal surface.

(b) *Superficial epithelium.* The superficial epithelium may appear flatter than normal and shows nuclear hyperchromasia and increased basophilia of the diminished cytoplasm. The brush border becomes progressively less distinct, and the cells may come to appear stratified with nuclei at different levels. Sometimes bud-like syncytial masses are formed that project from the surface. The increased cellularity of the epithelium is associated with occasional mitotic figures, and there is an additional increase in the number of intraepithelial lymphocytes and invading polymorphs. When polymorph invasion is marked, epithelial erosions also occur. These epithelial changes clearly reflect a change in mucosal dynamics and cell turnover. Mitotic activity in the crypts is increased, and the tendency for immature cells to occupy the surface is apparent with a decrease in the goblet cell population. Another distinctive superficial epithelial feature is metaplastic transformation focally or more widespread into an epithelium of gastric surface mucin-secreting type. This change is most easily appreciated in the section stained by the periodic acid–Schiff (PAS) technique. The change is most common in the more severe degrees of inflammation (Whitehead, Roca and Truelove 1972), but with increasing experience it has been appreciated that focal areas may be present when inflammation is relatively slight or even absent.

(c) *Crypts.* The crypts are involved in the inflammatory degenerative and regenerative changes only in the most severe examples of duodenitis. The ducts of Brunner's glands may also be involved as they enter the base of the crypts, but as most of the glands are beneath the muscularis mucosa, they are usually spared. Sometimes, however, glands also occur internal to and among the fibres of the muscularis mucosa, so they may also be involved.

(d) *Lamina propria.* The lamina propria shows a variable increase in inflammatory cells including lymphocytes, plasma cells, and polymorphs. Neutrophil polymorphs occur in increased numbers, especially in the more severe grades of epithelial damage, and may be accompanied by vascular dilatation and oedema. Lymphoid aggregates occur normally in approximately 20% of normal duodenal biopsics, but in duodenitis they are seen in increased numbers.

The least severe amount of recognizable change is designated grade 1. There

Table 11–1. Histological Grading of Duodenitis (Bulbitis)

Grade of Change	Distinguishing Histological Features		General Histological Features
0	Normal		
1	Superficial epithelium and general morphology normal; Increased cellularity of lamina propria	Increasing cellularity of lamina propria and loss of the villous pattern	Neutrophil polymorph infiltration + or −
2	Abnormality of the surface epithelium		Gastric superficial epithelial metaplasia
3	Erosion of the surface epithelium		+ or −

are no significant alterations in general morphology, and the superficial epithelium is normal in height but may contain an excess of lymphocytes. The principal histological feature is an excessive cellularity of the lamina propria, with or without lymphoid aggregates. It is obvious that there is some difficulty in differentiating those biopsies with a minimal increase of cells from those that are normal, and with increasing experience it is becoming apparent that this type of abnormality may constitute the upper end of the normal range.

The next grade of severity is grade 2. In addition to increased cellularity of the lamina propria, there are abnormalities of the superficial epithelium; this is the critical feature. Sometimes there is also deformity of the villous architecture, with shortening of the processes.

Grade 3, the most severe, is characterised by the critical feature of erosion of the abnormal epithelium. This is invariably associated with complete effacement and loss of the villous processes and the greatest amount of inflammatory cell infiltration.

When there is a polymorph component in the inflammatory infiltrate, it may be associated with vascular dilatation and some oedema. The presence of polymorphs can be recorded as a separate feature because, although they are usually found in the severe group, this is not always so, and it might be of significance in terms of activity of the inflammatory process as has been suggested to be the case in chronic gastritis (Whitehead 1973). It should be noted that the blood vessel changes that accompany acute inflammation, namely dilatation and congestion, are notoriously difficult to assess in histological preparations unless polymorph margination is seen. Dilatation may well disappear during the fixation procedure and subsequent tissue processing with its attendant tissue shrinkage. As a consequence there is poor correlation between histological inflammation and erythema seen at endoscopy (MacKinnon, Willing and Whitehead 1982). Reddening with erosion and petechiae, however, correlates well with severe histological duodenitis.

The presence of gastric surface epithelial metaplasia should also be recorded. This is an entity distinct from gastric heterotopia that occurs as slightly raised isolated islands of gastric mucosa composed of superficial epithelium, crypts, and specialised glands usually containing parietal cells but occasionally also chief cells (see Fig. 14–24). The capacity of this ectopic mucosa to secrete acid has been demonstrated at endoscopy by using Congo red after pentagastrin stimulation (Ikeda et al 1982). The occurrence of this mucosa is not as rare as was once thought. Shousha, Spiller and Parkins (1983) found it in 10% of duodenal biopsies from patients with dyspepsia, but it can also occur in coeliac disease and Crohn's disease. Another fact that requires emphasis is that the pyloroduodenal junction is frequently not well demarcated. Biopsies from the transitional zone can easily be misinterpreted as duodenal mucosa showing gastric metaplasia and vice versa. This probably accounts in part for the very high incidence of "gastric metaplasia" reported in a normal population by Kreuning et al (1978). Indeed, if gastric surface epithelium is seen in the absence of significant duodenal inflammation, the biopsy site is probably from a broader than usual transitional zone between pylorus and duodenum. Gastric metaplasia is extensive only in biopsy specimens that show a severe grade of duodenitis. Focal areas can also be seen in grade 2 changes and rarely in grade 1 changes but hardly ever if the biopsy specimen is entirely normal. In normal circumstances it is rarely seen except in the first part of the duodenum. Johansen and Hansen (1973) and Patrick, Denham and Forrest (1974) showed that there is a statistically significant correlation between prevalence of metaplasia and gastric acid output. Indeed, metaplasia can be induced in cats by stimulating hypersecretion of hydrochloric acid (Rhodes 1964). The metaplastic epithelium has the same histochemical profile as the identical epithelium in the stomach (Johansen 1974). Hara et al (1988) suggested that it is important as one of the pathophysiological mechanisms involved in the recurrence of duodenal ulcer. This is of interest in view of the proposal that colonisation of the metaplastic epithelium by *Helicobacter pylori* is related to a mucosal defence weakness and the genesis of duodenal ulcer (Goodwin 1988).

This basic grading of duodenal change was shown to be accurate by Whitehead et al (1975) by comparing the results of subjective examination of duodenal biopsies with those obtained by two morphometric methods. One method estimated the surface-to-volume ratio of the mucosa, and the other method estimated the number of cells in the lamina propria. By the use of this or similar classifications, it is becoming increasingly plain that changes of grade 2 or 3 are a significant cause of duodenal ulcer-like symptoms. Grade 1 change, which corresponds to the "interstitial duodenitis" of Cheli, Aste and Ciancamerla (1973), is likely to represent a variation of normal or a lesion associated with neighbouring pathological problem or be the result of a generalised stimulation of the gut-associated immune system. Indeed, grade 1 change has been reported to exist in normal subjects (Roca, Truelove and Whitehead 1975). It is now the consensus view that duodenitis most commonly affecting the bulb corresponding to grades 2 and 3 is always part of the duodenal ulcer diathesis at least at some time (Walan 1981, Paoluzi et al 1982, Hasan et al 1983).

Brunner's Gland Hyperplasia

Some patients with the clinical picture of non-ulcer dyspepsia and duodenal ulcer disease have radiological evidence of coarse duodenal folds, and in the past it was postulated that this may be due to Brunner's gland hyperplasia. There are obvious difficulties in assessing Brunner's gland mass in endoscopic biopsies, but some studies claimed that Brunner's gland hyperplasia may well be associated with duodenitis (Maratka et al 1979). In an autopsy study made by Feyrter (1934) enlargement of Brunner's glands was classified as circumscribed nodular hyperplasia, diffuse nodular hyperplasia, and adenomatous hyperplasia. It is not clear why the first form was not regarded as an earlier stage of the third. Ten years later Landboe-Christensen (1944) claimed that Brunner's gland hyperplasia was almost always associated with signs of inflammation, lymphoid hyperplasia, or scarring of the duodenum. This suggested that there is an association between duodenitis, previous ulceration, and Brunner's gland hyperplasia, and these findings are perhaps more significant when it is realised that cases with obvious ulcers or larger scars were excluded from the study. Cases showing hyperplasia of Brunner's glands that did not have evidence of inflammation or ulceration were also observed, and thus evidence for two varieties of Brunner's gland enlargement, focal and diffuse, strengthened. Currently, most researchers recognise a diffuse form associated with duodenitis or duodenal ulcer and a localised form presenting as a tumour. The latter has been called a Brunneroma (Bastlein et al 1988) and regarded as an adenoma (Major and Brandt 1976, Nakanishi et al 1984), whereas others argue that it is a hamartoma (Skellenger, Kinner and Jordan 1983, Rufenacht et al 1986).

The author has experience of one case of Brunner's gland enlargement great enough to present on radiological examination as pyloric obstruction and a multiple duodenal polyposis. The extent of the lesion would almost certainly not have been revealed by endoscopic biopsy and became apparent only when an open surgical biopsy was examined subsequently. This showed not only the Brunner's gland nature of the polypoidal lesions but also a diffuse duodenitis and superficial gastric epithelial metaplasia. Thus in some instances a diffuse nodular Brunner's hyperplasia associated with duodenitis may give rise to more massive focal hyperplasia/adenoma, and this would parallel the situation that occurs in other glandular tissues. Certainly, the diffuse multinodular lesion would appear to be more common. Matsui and Kitagawa (1993) found that Brunner's gland hyperplasia was a relatively common cause of polypoidal nodularity of the duodenum, accounting for up to 10% of cases studied by endoscopy and biopsy. Franzin et al (1985) described 206 cases of nodular hyperplasia in association with hyperacidity, of which more than 80% had coexisting duodenitis. They stressed that a biopsy indication of Brunner's hyperplasia in these circumstances is for the glands to appear consistently extending up to the surface mucosa, which is frequently avillous and flattened (Fig. 11–11). There is also some

Figure 11–11. Duodenitis with a prominent extension of Brunner's glands into the lamina propria above the muscularis mucosa, which is seen at the bottom of the field (H&E ×75).

evidence that the nodular duodenitis that is frequently seen in patients with end-stage renal disease (Zukerman et al 1983, Mangla, Pereira and Bhargava 1985) is often characterised by Brunner's gland hyperplasia (Paimela et al 1984). In Feyrter's autopsy study, 55% of cases showing Brunner's hyperplasia had had uraemia. On a physiological note, a reactive hyperplasia of Brunner's glands driven by hyperchlorhydria would be explicable on the basis of its neutralising bicarbonate secretion and the production of urogastrone, an inhibitor of gastric secretion (Stolte, Schwabe and Prestele 1981).

Lymphoid Hyperplasia

Hyperplasia of the mucosal lymphoid elements may be so marked as to cause irregularity of the duodenal mucosa, and this should be clearly evident in a duodenal biopsy specimen. This type of lymphoid hyperplasia is distinct from that associated with gammaglobulin abnormalities (see Chapter 14), and it is almost always associated with the changes of duodenitis (Jepsen et al 1994), so that at least sometimes it is probably similar to that which occurs in the stomach affected by chronic gastritis or in the colon affected by chronic ulcerative colitis. Why it occurs in some cases and not in others that otherwise show the same morphological features is not known. Apart from Brunner's gland hyperplasia, some of the nodular appearances seen in uraemic patients also seem to be due to lymphoid nodular hyperplasia as part of the coexisting duodenitis (Zukerman et al 1983). Some cases of duodenal lymphoid hyperplasia, however, are not associated with any significant inflammatory features of duodenitis; it is assumed that they represent a reactive phenomenon triggered by a different mechanism, such as a viral infection.

BIOPSIES BEYOND THE BULB

Biopsies on the duodenum are being done more and more frequently in circumstances other than when duodenitis or peptic ulcer is present. Most endoscopists can produce biopsy specimens from well into the third part of the duodenum and beyond. Mucosal irregularities often sampled prove to be ectopic gastric body mucosa or isolated lymphoid nodules.

Most islands of ectopic gastric body mucosa are small and barely raised, but some are frankly polypoidal (Tsadilas 1984, Tsubone et al 1984, Kundrotas et al 1985, Jepsen et al 1994). It is claimed that sometimes such islands of gastric mucosa show hyperplastic change and give rise to polyps similar to the lesions that occur in the stomach (Rosch and Hoer 1983). Franzin, Novelli and Fratton (1983) also described a hyperplastic polyp with characteristics similar to the common lesion of the colon, with villi and crypts lined by serrated hyperplastic epithelium. In this author's experience, this type of hyperplastic polyp is not so uncommon. It is composed of irregular villous or cystic formations covered by simple cuboidal epithelium that shows a variable amount of gastric superficial epithelial metaplasia and residual small bowel–type epithelium usually with scanty goblet cells. Frequently, some Brunner's glands are incorporated and halfway stages between Brunner's-type gland cells, undifferentiated crypt cells, and gastric epithelial mucous cells can be seen. These lesions are almost certainly the result of a hyperplastic response to mucosal injury or an erosion that is sometimes also revealed in the biopsy. The lamina propria in relation to these hyperplastic polyps is frequently inflamed (Figs. 11–12 to 11–17).

More rarely small lymphangiomas (Salata et al 1984), haemangiomas, or vascular hamartomas are recognised. Duodenal varices (Nakayama et al 1983, Gushurst and Lesesne 1984, Sukigara et al 1987) and Dieulafoy's aneurysm (McClave et al 1988) are described, but only rarely are biopsies done on vascular lesions (Fig. 11–18).

With the increasing use of endoscopy in the investigation of jaundice, a wider range of lesions of the papilla is being seen. Small villous adenomas or early carcinomas that are most commonly located at this site cause little problems in interpretation (Figs. 11–19 to 11–21) because they are essentially similar to their much more common colonic counterparts (Blackman and Nash 1985). When the adenomatous change involves the duct system in the region of the ampulla, the abnormal glands have a very close relationship to the muscle bundles in that region;

Text continued on page 200

Figure 11–12. Hyperplastic duodenal polyp. Note the branched irregular mucosal projections covered by metaplastic epithelium with only scattered goblet cells *(arrows)* and the irregular configuration of the Brunner's glands (H&E ×75).

Figure 11–13. Showing the character of the gastric superficial epithelial metaplasia and the residual goblet cells in Figure 11–12 (H&E ×300).

Figure 11–14. Hyperplastic duodenal polyp. The Brunner's gland component shows a focal cystic change (H&E ×75).

Figure 11–15. Detail of Figure 11–14. The epithelium varies between small intestinal type and gastric superficial epithelial type, and there are interspersed goblet cells (H&E ×300).

Figure 11–16. Hyperplastic duodenal polyp with only a minor Brunner's gland component. The configuration is bizarre and bears no resemblance to a normal duodenum. The gastric metaplasia is widespread and is easily seen in this preparation (PAS ×75).

Figure 11–17. This hyperplastic polyp could be easily misinterpreted as tubulovillous adenoma, but the epithelium, although metaplastic (shown to best effect at left), is not in any way dysplastic (PAS ×75).

Figure 11–18. A small submucosal vascular abnormality of predominantly cavernous type. The superficial duodenal mucosa has eroded and caused significant haemorrhage (H&E ×150).

Figure 11–19. Small tubulovillous adenoma of duodenal papilla (H&E ×75).

Figure 11–20. Detail of Figure 11–19. The dysplastic nature of the epithelium is clearly different from that of metaplastic polyps (compare with Figs. 11–13 and 11–15) (H&E ×400).

Figure 11–21. Mainly villous adenoma of duodenum. This lesion has a rich Paneth's cell population visible even in an H&E preparation *(arrows)* (H&E ×400).

this can make differentiation between adenoma and adenocarcinoma quite difficult. Cytological features and the absence of convincing desmoplasia have to be relied on to resolve this (Fig. 11–22). In a similar fashion, regenerative and reactive changes that occur in the epithelium of the collecting tubules of the ampullary valve can cause similar problems in interpretation; the same guidelines are advocated in reaching a diagnosis (Figs. 11–23 and 11–24). Sometimes, however, a small biopsy specimen of a larger villous lesion may not reveal the malignant nature in another area of the same lesion (Ryan, Schapiro and Warshaw 1986). It has been accepted

Figure 11–22. Adenomatous change involving the duct system and epithelial elements of the mixing value at the ampulla. The atypical glandular formations are surrounded by normal smooth muscle elements (H&E ×350).

Figure 11–23. Duodenal biopsy in the region of the papilla, following an episode of biliary colic. Note the duct-like structures beneath the muscularis (H&E ×125).

Figure 11–24. Detail of Figure 11–23. The duct-lining cells exhibit reactive atypia. Note the normal appearance of the surrounding smooth muscle (H&E ×400).

that carcinomas of the ampullary region arise, as in the colon, through an adenoma-carcinoma sequence (Talbot et al 1988), and some examples are notably rich in Paneth's cells (London et al 1988). Adenomas seem to be especially common in patients with familial adenomatous polyposis (Noda et al 1992, Penna et al 1993, Nugent et al 1994), and there is much debate concerning their clinical management and the role of endoscopic removal in the prevention of adenocarcinoma. There is some evidence that the risk of malignancy in these duodenal adenomas may be as high as that for their colonic counterpart. Duodenal adenomas are frequently accompanied by a conspicuous argyrophil and argentaffin endocrine cell populations (Morgensen, Bulow and Hage 1989, Morgensen, Hage and Bulow 1989). Mixed glandular and carcinoid differentiation is also occasionally seen in tumours arising in nonpolyposis patients (Jones, Griffith and West 1989).

The interpretation of other biopsy specimens from the ampullary region in the investigation of jaundice can be more difficult. This is in part due to the complexity of the glands, muscle bundles, and epithelial folds that make up the mixing valve at this end of the duct system. Stones passed cause inflammatory fibrosis and regenerative epithelial changes that can exhibit marked atypia suggesting invasive malignancy, especially because of their close relationship to the muscle bundles in the vicinity. Malformations or hamartomas of this area also are occasionally seen (Fig. 11–25); no doubt, with increasing numbers of biopsies of the area, dysplasia and the earlier lesions of malignancy will be identified.

Biopsies beyond the papilla are used in the evaluation of malabsorption and other lesions for which jejunal mucosa was once preferred. This is discussed in further detail in the consideration of the lesion of villous atrophy, which immediately follows. Duodenal biopsy also may reveal diagnostic information in Crohn's disease, amyloidosis, giardiasis, storage diseases, and other conditions. As for Crohn's disease,

Figure 11–25. Biopsy excision of a small duodenal nodule that is clearly a small hamartoma of pancreatic or bile ducts (H&E ×1250).

it is argued that the biopsy specimens are too small for there to be a significant diagnostic yield. In the absence of granulomas, a range of nonspecific findings may occur (Schuffler and Chaffee 1979), but these can be of importance in diagnosis when seen in the context of other clinical, radiological, endoscopic, and biopsy findings. As in the stomach, ulceration and gross epithelial atypia in duodenal biopsies easily misinterpreted as malignant have been described in patients receiving hepatic arterial infusion chemotherapy (Schuger et al 1988).

DUODENAL BIOPSY IN THE INVESTIGATION OF MALABSORPTION

Use of the distal duodenal biopsy in the investigation of malabsorption has been accepted (Mee et al 1985, Achkar et al 1986, Sanfilippo et al 1986). The procedure has lent itself to large screening procedures for the detection of coeliac disease in both normal populations (Catassi et al 1994) and as a follow-up procedure for patients with reticulin and gliadin antibodies but a normal small bowel mucosa. The changes that occur in the bulb in peptic ulcer disease in association with hyperchlorhydria do not affect the distal duodenum, except in rare instances of hypergastrinaemia, such as in the Zollinger-Ellison syndrome. Furthermore, it is possible to suspect coeliac disease by endoscopic appearances alone. Brocchi et al (1988) described markedly decreased or absent duodenal Kerckring's folds and recommended biopsy when this sign is present, even if the patient has minimal transient or seemingly unrelated symptomatology. Other endoscopic abnormalities that have been described are mosaic patterns, scalloped folds, and visibility of the underlying blood vessels (Maurino et al 1993).

Detailed morphological observations coupled with an increasing knowledge of cell turnover have resulted in the recognition of two types of villous atrophy: one associated with hyperplasia of the crypts and one with hypoplasia of the crypts.

Crypt Hyperplastic Villous Atrophy

In this type the villi are atrophic or absent, but the overall thickness of the mucosa is normal or only slightly decreased, and the crypts are clearly hyperplastic and elongated. The absorptive epithelium shows a variable amount of damage manifested by an apparent increase in intraepithelial lymphocytes between the surface cells, which themselves may show hyperchromasia and palisading of nuclei that often appear pyknotic. There is blurring of the cytoplasmic boundaries so that in PAS preparations the normally distinct brush borders of the enterocytes appear frayed and ragged. Since the paper by Ferguson and Murray (1971), has been frequently stated that the number of theliocytes per unit of epithelium in the coeliac mucosa is increased. The increase has been credited with diagnostic importance (Holmes et al 1974, Lancaster-Smith et al 1976a). This increase, however, is a function of the method of quantitating the theliocytes in that the coeliac lesion is characterised by a marked decrease in epithelial surface per unit length of muscularis mucosa. If expressed as number of theliocytes per unit length of mucosa, a normal number will therefore appear as an increase. If quantitated per unit of muscularis mucosa that is not altered by the disease process, it has been shown that the number of intraepithelial lymphocytes is either normal (Guix, Skinner and Whitehead 1979) or slightly decreased (Marsh 1980, Corazza, Franzzoni and Gasbarrini 1984). The role of intraepithelial lymphocytes is still being debated (Marsh 1985), and much of this may be caused by claims based on faulty methodology.

There is the claim that blast transformation and an increased mitotic rate occur in the intraepithelial lymphocytes in coeliac disease (Marsh 1982, Marsh and Haeney 1983) and that these can be used to differentiate a coeliac mucosa from a flat mucosa due to other causes. The method of determining the mitotic index in each specimen necessitates observation of lymphocyte metaphase figures in a population of 3,000 epithelial cells located between the mouths of crypts. Another claim is made that an index in excess of 0.2% is indicative of gluten-sensitive enteropathy and that it excludes other causes of a flat mucosa, namely, immunodeficiency, lymphoma, or Crohn's disease. It has not been this author's experience that this diagnostic criterion is useful. First, lymphocyte mitoses are clearly uncommon. Second, recognising them is difficult in ordinary paraffin sections because the heaped and palisaded superficial epithelium contains a large proportion of degenerating cells with pyknotic nuclei. Third, in a light microscope examination it is unclear how to ascertain that in a flat mucosa a mitotic figure is located in a lymphocyte as opposed to an epithelial cell at the top of a crypt that is not in the plane of sectioning. Marsh also advocated the counting of only metaphase-anaphase figures, and this is a further restriction of the method. Resin-embedded semithin sections lend themselves better to this type of examination, but the pursuit of this diagnostic phenomenon is probably not justified on the evidence. Ferguson and Ziegler (1986) claimed that the presence of intraepithelial lymphocyte mitoses is a nonspecific phenomenon that can be seen when the jejunal mucosa is otherwise normal. It has also been claimed that subjects who do not have coeliac disease but who have raised alpha-gliadin antibody titres also have raised intraepithelial lymphocyte counts (O'Farrelly et al 1987). The lymphocytes are known to be T cells of both suppressor/cytotoxic and helper/inducer type and supposedly increase significantly in number in treated coeliacs subjected to a gluten challenge (Freedman et al 1987). However, because the lymphocytes tend to return to normal levels on gluten exclusion, it has been suggested that these changes are the result of a stimulation of the mucosal immune mechanisms and do not imply a primary pathogenetic role (Kelly et al 1987). Epithelial lymphocyte numbers in rectal mucosa have been said to increase in treated coeliacs following instillation of gluten enemas (Austin and Dobbins 1988). There is also some evidence that an adenovirus protein may have a role in the pathogenesis of coeliac disease and that there is immunological cross-reactivity between antigens shared by the virus and alpha-gliadins (Kagnoff et al 1987).

The lamina propria contains an increased number of lymphocytes, plasma cells, some eosinophils, histiocytes, and mast cells. Whether mucosal mast cells in coeliac disease are increased or decreased has been the subject of dispute, even in quantitative studies (Strobel, Busuttil and Ferguson 1983, Kosnai et al 1984). Marsh and Hinde (1985), however, have concluded that there is an increase in mast cells, eosinophils, and basophils that is gluten-dependent and probably the result of a cell-mediated effector mechanism concerned in the pathogenesis of the disease. A similar claim has been made for neutrophils (Hallgren et al 1989). The crypts contain an increased number of cells in mitosis. Paneth's cells and enterochromaffin cells, which normally are also found in the crypts, may appear numerically increased. This was substantiated by Polak et al (1973), Challacombe and Robertson (1977), and Sjolund et al (1979). Wheeler and Challacombe (1984) showed that the enterochromaffin cells were producing mainly serotonin. Furthermore, Pietroletti et al (1986) demonstrated that the increase in endocrine cells demonstrated by a chromagranin monoclonal antibody is abolished by successful treatment with a gluten-free diet. In about one third of cases with severe changes, collagen deposition may be seen immediately beneath the surface epithelium (this is referred to in some detail in Chapter 12).

In its severest form this type of villous atrophy is seen in gluten-sensitive enteropathy, and in the untreated case the mucosa either shows a severe amount of villous effacement or is wholly devoid of villous processes (Figs. 11–26 and 11–27). Villous atrophy appears to be the direct result of ingestion of gluten in the diet and a toxic action on the mucosa that results in increased cell loss from the villous surface (Croft, Loehry and Creamer 1968, Pink, Croft and Creamer 1970). Similar appearances are produced by chronic trauma to the small intestine mucosa in abnormal situations, e.g., in jejunum transplanted as an artificial oesophagus (personal observation), at ileostomy stomas, in urinary ileal conduits, or immediately neighbouring areas of

Figure 11–26. Jejunal mucosa in severe untreated gluten-sensitive enteropathy. Extent of villous atrophy corresponds to convoluted mucosa seen in the dissecting microscope (H&E ×100).

ulceration. It has been produced experimentally by the repeated instillation of acid into the jejunum of dogs (Townley, Cass and Anderson 1964) and in jejunum explanted to the anterior abdominal wall in rats (Loehry and Grace 1974). Wright et al (1973a, b) and Watson, Appleton and Wright (1982) showed a threefold expansion of the mass of proliferating and maturing cells with a halving of the cell cycle time, thus resulting in a sixfold increase in the crypt cell production rate. Coupled with a pathologically rapid cell loss from the mucosal surface, this forms the basis of the change in mucosal morphology.

In earlier descriptive accounts of this type of mucosal lesion, the terms "partial villous atrophy" and "subtotal villous atrophy" (Doniach and Shiner 1957) were used and are still in use. They correspond roughly to the dissecting microscopic appearances of convoluted and flat types, respectively (Fig. 11–28). In practice, however, there is a continuum of appearances from normal to a completely flat-surfaced mucosa without villous projections. This is paralleled stereoscopically by an

Figure 11–27. Jejunal mucosa in severe untreated gluten-sensitive enteropathy. Extent of villous atrophy corresponds to the flat or mosaic type seen in the dissecting microscope (H&E ×100).

Figure 11–28. Dissecting microscope appearances. Jejunal biopsies show *(A)* normal, *(B)* convoluted.

Figure 11–28 *Continued (C)* mosaic, and *(D)* flat biopsies (H&E ×20).

increasing number of leaf-shaped villi and short then long ridges that anastomose, form convolutions, and become progressively lower, sometimes passing through a mosaic phase, to finally end up completely flat. It is clear that the two descriptive terms do not satisfactorily cover the possible histological range. A better but not ideal terminology, therefore, is "crypt hyperplasia with total villous atrophy" when there are no villous projections from the surface, and "mild, moderate, or severe partial villous atrophy" when there are. Assessment of partial villous atrophy is best accomplished, however, by the simple quantitative method already outlined. There is another extremely important consideration in the diagnosis of coeliac disease, the length of the small bowel mucosa that is involved. If limited to the duodenum and proximal jejunum, overt gastrointestinal symptoms and steatorrhoea may be absent. Clinical manifestations may be limited to iron and folate malabsorption (Trier 1993).

There is a long list of case reports of disease states said to be associated with a jejunal mucosal lesion identical to that in untreated gluten-sensitive enteropathy (childhood and adult coeliac disease), i.e., crypt hyperplasia with total or severe partial villous atrophy. In coeliac disease the causal agent has been identified. There is a disparity between the histological findings and the extent of malabsorption of individual dietary factors. This accounts for the diverse clinical presentations of the disease, not the least of which is an apparent onset in adult life. Usually there is a clinical improvement on gluten withdrawal, and the jejunal mucosa reverts to normal morphologically (Pollack et al 1970) and histochemically (Riecken 1970). However, the extent of clinical improvement may not parallel the improvement in mucosal appearances (Kumar et al 1979). More specifically, if there is a subsequent gluten challenge, damage to the mucosa is reestablished, and within a few hours of the dose, changes can be seen by electron microscope and by immunocyte counts, suggestive of an immune reaction (Shiner and Shmerling 1970, Shiner 1973, Holmes et al 1974, Lancaster-Smith et al 1976a, b, Baklien, Brandtzaeg and Fausa 1977). A similar series of changes can be demonstrated by using subfractions of Frazer III on duodenal mucosal explants from patients with coeliac disease (Fluge et al 1994) or when used in challenge experiments on patients (Dissanayake et al 1973, Anand et al 1981). Further evidence for a role of the immune system in mucosal injury in this condition is provided by the depleted circulating thymus-dependent lymphocytes in coeliacs that return to normal after dietary gluten exclusion (O'Donoghue et al 1976). It is perhaps of some importance, therefore, that prednisolone administered to coeliac patients has the same effect on the mucosa as gluten withdrawal (Wall et al 1970). Nevertheless doubt is raised as to the role of B cells in the pathogenesis of coeliac disease by the occurrence of gluten-sensitive enteropathy in hypogammaglobulinaemia (Webster et al 1981). As Kelly et al (1987) indicated, many of the immune phenomena observed in this intriguing disease may be secondary. Davidson and Bridges (1988) made an analysis of the aetiological possibilities and argued a strong case for investigating a possible fault in the intralumenal phase of the in vivo processing of dietary gluten.

A group of cases with morphological lesions otherwise identical to those in adult coeliac disease apparently fail to respond to gluten withdrawal, and when the patient has also had another disease at the same time it has been implied that the malabsorption is secondary to this disease and in some way responsible for it. Failure of a clinical response is not an adequate criterion for assessing gluten sensitivity. A clinical response is difficult to assess, because when it does occur it can be extremely variable. Failure of a morphological response of the mucosa is a much more objective measurement, although this too is extremely variable, especially in adults. Kluge et al (1982), for example, failed to achieve a complete restitution of the mucosa in any of 18 patients on a strict gluten diet although, in an analysis of their study, only three of these gave no history of occasional lapses. However, in a similar study (Bardella et al 1985), a quarter of the cases subject to rebiopsy had mild partial villous atrophy even when the diet was strictly controlled.

The longer the disease state has been present, the more likely it is that secondary factors may be having an additional effect. Some secondary factors, such as vitamin deficiency or protein depletion, may be the direct result of the malabsorption syndrome itself, but there may be many others. It is not surprising that gluten withdrawal results in a much slower recovery of the mucosa when the disease has been untreated for many years, and in general the longer it has gone untreated the slower is the response once treatment is instituted, although age at time of diagnosis does not seem to be a factor (Dissanayake, Truelove and Whitehead 1974). However, it has been claimed that challenge in some childhood cases, by using a normal diet, may not provoke severe morphological changes even after weeks or months (Lebenthal and Branski 1981), and it has also been suggested that susceptibility to gluten damage may vary in severity between individuals and in the same individual with time (McNeish 1980).

This is highlighted by the report of Paerregaard et al (1988), who showed that in some cases of adults with coeliac disease, even with a flat mucosa and evidence of biochemical malabsorption there was no evidence of clinical disease or growth retardation. These patients had been treated in early childhood for presumed gluten sensitivity, but biopsies had not been done. Variation in susceptibility to mucosal damage and malabsorption is well established and, perhaps surprisingly, healthy siblings of coeliac patients do not show mucosal sensitivity to damage by diets containing large supplements of gluten (Polanco et al 1987).

The situation concerning gluten sensitivity and response to gluten exclusion is far from clear in view of the findings that in adults mucosal recovery may be incomplete even as long as 4 years on a gluten-free diet (Grefte et al 1988). The quality of the gluten-free control is, however, a factor difficult to ascertain, especially in adults, and the failure of some patients to respond is often due to an inadvertent or unadmitted gluten ingestion (Pink and Creamer 1967). Some children who seem to be progressing satisfactorily on a gluten-free diet often exhibit mucosal abnormalities on biopsy (Congdon et al 1981), and this is more common in adults (Kluge et al 1982). Relatively small quantities of gluten can produce marked mucosal change, and only a week's lapse is needed to perpetuate the mucosal damage. Consequently, for a proper diagnosis sequential morphological studies should be performed during a strict period of gluten withdrawal, preferably in a hospitalised patient, and this should be followed by a gluten challenge. Until a better and simpler method is available, this should be the minimum requirement for a strict diagnosis of gluten-sensitive enteropathy before a patient, especially a child, is subjected to a lifelong gluten-free diet. Only when such a method is employed will it be possible to categorise other forms of enteropathy and so determine whether some cases are aetiologically independent of gluten. Holmes et al (1974) suggested that mucosal lamina propria cell counts may prove of value in the accurate diagnosis of gluten-sensitive enteropathy, but Macromichalis et al (1976) found considerable overlap of lamina propria cell counts in patients with coeliac disease, cow's milk protein intolerance, giardiasis, and intractable diarrhoea. The value of theliocyte counts and theliocyte mitosis has already been referred to in this regard.

It is pertinent that the malabsorption syndrome so often associated with dermatitis herpetiformis has been shown to be of gluten-sensitive type (Marks et al 1968). In fact, there is evidence that all patients, given a big enough gluten load, will develop small intestine mucosal abnormalities (Andersson et al 1984, Reunala et al 1984, Kosnai et al 1986, Ferguson, Blackwell and Barnetson 1987). Furthermore, if a sufficient number of biopsy specimens are examined, almost all cases of dermatitis herpetiformis will show some intestinal mucosal abnormalities (Brow et al 1971). This implication of a patchy distribution of the abnormality led to multiple biopsy studies in coeliac disease, and some patchiness was observed in these also (Scott and Losowsky 1976). Variation in the amount of damage in coeliacs is slight, however, although the extent of abnormality decreases proceeding distally down the bowel. Degrees of gluten sensitivity as exhibited in patients with dermatitis herpetiformis may suggest a possible reason why some coeliacs present in childhood and others apparently in adult life. The remission that seems to occur in the teen years might also suggest a varying sensitivity, although Weir and Hourihane (1974) showed persistent flat mucosa even in teenagers who had wholly remitted clinically. The acquisition of gluten sensitivity, e.g., following gastroenteritis, has also been postulated, and transient gluten sensitivity is also described (see the following section on postinfective malabsorption syndrome). The author has personal experience of one female patient, age 28 years with a flat mucosa and proven gluten sensitivity by strict criteria, who had been investigated for iron deficiency anemia 2 years previously and was found to have normal jejunal biopsy results. An almost identical case was reported by Egan-Mitchell, Fottrell and McNicholl (1981) but in a much younger patient. In patients with recurrent aphthous stomatitis but no evidence of malabsorption, it is not unusual to find mild small bowel morphological abnormalities, and some 16% have been shown to have reversible gluten-sensitive villous atrophy (Veloso and Saleiro 1987).

Similarly, those cases of malabsorption in diabetes that have a coeliac-like mucosal lesion are gluten-sensitive (Rubin and Dobbins 1965). The coeliac-like mucosal atrophy seen occasionally in patients with carcinoma outside the bowel (Creamer 1964) has also been shown in some cases to be gluten-sensitive (Pollack et al 1970). The concurrence of gluten-sensitive enteropathy with inflammatory bowel disease (Gillberg, Dotevall and Ahren 1982) is probably more common than has been suspected. Of 42 patients with coeliac disease who underwent rectal biopsy, 14 had inflammation of varying severity, and in 3 it was compatible with a diagnosis of ulcerative colitis. Furthermore, the diarrhoea in these three cases persisted despite a gluten-free diet (Breen et al 1987). An association between coeliac disease and systemic sarcoidosis has also been claimed (Douglas et al 1984). Primary biliary cirrhosis coincident with coeliac disease (Olsson, Kagevi and Rydberg 1982) is also well documented. It has become evident that the group of patients with malabsorption syndrome and a jejunal lesion typical of that seen in coeliac disease who are not gluten-sensitive is certainly very much smaller than earlier papers (e.g., Cooke et al 1963) have suggested. It is becoming clear that coeliac disease occurs in association with a wide range of other pathological conditions (Collins et al 1994) and occurs in association with autoimmune disease and sarcoidosis more frequently than can be accounted for by chance (Collins et al 1994, Papadopoulos, Hornblad and Hallengren 1994). The use of antibody screening for antireticulin, antigliadin, and antiendomysial antibodies (Unsworth and Brown 1994, Vogelsang et al 1995) has shown that coeliac disease has been significantly underdiagnosed. Critical diagnostic tests in the future may reduce this number even further, but it seems likely that gluten-induced damage over a long period or of a severe amount may reach a state from which recovery is impossible. This would certainly seem to apply to those cases of longstanding gluten-sensitive enteropathy that develop malignant lymphoma (see Chapter 12).

There is an even longer list of conditions said to be associated with minor amounts of crypt hyperplastic villous atrophy (Rubin and Dobbins 1965, Whitehead 1968b). Poor histological technique, inexperienced interpretation, and lack of proper controls account for many of the reports that have led to conflicting results and much controversy (Shidrawi et al 1994). Marks and Shuster (1970), for example, showed that the so-called mucosal abnormalities described in association with eczema, psoriasis, and rosacea are fictitious. Until evaluated in much more critical fashion, the previously reported non–gluten-sensitive jejunal abnormalities said to be associated with cirrhosis of the liver other than the primary biliary type, postgastrectomy states, iron deficiency anaemia, scleroderma, neomycin administration, Crohn's disease not involving the site of small bowel biopsy or neighbouring bowel, ulcerative colitis, chronic pancreatitis, and sarcoidosis must remain the subject of doubt. The validity of the observations of villous abnormalities in various generalised virus infections (Sheehy, Artenstein and Green 1964) must also be questioned until reinvestigated in a more critical manner using sequential biopsies during and after recovery from the illness. Soltoft and Soeberg (1972a), however, showed an increase in cells containing the immunoglobulins A and D (IgA and IgD) in the lamina propria of patients with viral hepatitis when compared with normal control subjects.

The authors did not follow up these patients in an attempt to show reversal to normal on recovery from the illness. The jejunal mucosal morphology in more specific gastroenteritides is discussed in the next section on postinfective malabsorption syndrome. Schlossberg et al (1984) described a case of crypt hyperplastic villous atrophy that resulted in diarrhoea in a patient with relapsing secondary syphilis. Although the lamina propria contained an excess of plasma cells, spirochaetes were not demonstrated. The mucosal morphology returned to normal following therapy, and the symptoms subsided.

In tropical sprue, the morphological abnormality varies from "normal" to "very abnormal" (Baker and Mathan 1970), bearing in mind that the normal has to be defined with reference to the local population. Brunser, Eidelman and Klipstein (1970) showed, for example, that in rural Haitians there are no qualitative differences in jejunal morphology between those with and those without tropical sprue, but in the latter the changes were more severe. With a few exceptions, the most severe lesion is a crypt hyperplastic partial villous atrophy (Fig. 11–29) with chronic inflammatory cell infiltration of the lamina propria and surface epithelial changes similar to but milder than those seen in gluten-sensitive enteropathy. Schenk, Samloff and Klipstein (1965) claimed that when frozen sections of biopsy tissue in both tropical sprue and glute-sensitive enteropathy are stained with oil red O, the appearances in tropical sprue are distinctive. Neutral lipid is said to be found in the epithelial cell cytoplasm and in the basement membrane in tropical sprue but only in the supranuclear cytoplasm of epithelial cells in gluten-sensitive enteropathy. Electron microscopy studies suggest faults in fat transport (Mathan, Mathan and Baker 1975), but this cannot be regarded as specific for tropical sprue. In practice, as total villous atrophy seldom if ever occurs in tropical sprue, differentiation from untreated coeliac disease causes little difficulty.

Sequential biopsy studies after treatment with vitamin B_{12} or folic acid (Swanson, Wheby and Bayless 1966) show somewhat variable results, although it is perhaps pertinent that both agents produce maximum effect in the cases with the severest mucosal lesions. Guerra, Wheby and Bayless (1965) demonstrated marked histological improvement after tetracycline therapy, and more than half of their cases had already shown resistance to folic acid and vitamin B_{12}. This introduced the possibility of an infectious aetiology, and Tomkins, Drasar and James (1975) isolated enterobacteria from cases of tropical sprue and showed that after specific treatment with tetracycline, which eliminated the organisms, there was a clinical and biochemical cure. Klipstein and Schenk (1975) tested the enterotoxins of certain coliform organisms isolated from tropical sprue patients for their effects on the ileal mucosa of rats. The mucosa showed a direct toxic effect manifested as a mucosal damage

Figure 11–29. Jejunal mucosa in tropical sprue. There is crypt hyperplasia and villous atrophy (H&E ×75).

similar to that in tropical sprue, and it was independent of the presence or absence of the organisms themselves. The upper-intestinal colonisation by enterobacteria, which is so frequent in sprue, could be responsible for mucosal damage via an enterotoxin-induced or other cytopathic effect. In addition, Baker et al (1982) described sprue patients with a chronic enterocyte infection by coronavirus. Both phenomena are compatible with the view that the syndrome has a complex aetiology involving several agents. This is expressed in an editorial review of tropical malabsorption by Tomkins (1981), who concluded that it is unlikely that a single "sprue agent" will be found that is common to all cases in different parts of the world. Whatever these agents are, it appears that they produce their effect on the mucosa via a direct action on the epithelium rather than on the lymphoid tissue, which nevertheless appears to be involved in a cell-mediated immune reaction. This was the conclusion reached by Marsh, Mathan and Mathan (1983), who showed that the epithelial changes characterised more critically in a further study (Mathan, Ponniah and Mathan 1986) actually precede the changes in the epithelial lymphoid population. This view is in accord with the hypothesis that initial enterocyte damage and resultant release of enteroglucagon cause a slowing of intestinal transit and further bacterial overgrowth, which perpetuates the initial injury. This cycle of events with its consequent folic acid deficiency explains the favourable response to antibiotics, particularly if folic acid supplements are also used (Cook 1984). There is no doubt that tropical sprue is becoming more commonly reported from countries not hitherto regarded as risk areas, e.g., Egypt (Martinez-Salmeron et al 1994), Peru (Frisancho et al 1994), and Guadeloupe (Cnudde et al 1994).

There are further conditions with which crypt hyperplastic villous atrophy is associated. Ament and Rubin (1972) described a case in which soy protein ingestion was associated with a rapidly developing jejunal mucosal lesion indistinguishable from that seen in gluten-sensitive enteropathy. There are also infants who have a milk-protein intolerance (Fontaine and Navarro 1975, Shiner et al 1975), and Walker-Smith (1978) showed that acute symptoms can be precipitated by challenging with milk after a period of milk exclusion, and the morphology of the jejunal mucosa is adversely affected (Vitoria, Camarero and Solaguren 1979, de Sousa et al 1986). Jejunal biopsy may show obvious villous atrophy (Fig. 11–30). Shiner, Ballard and Smith (1975) demonstrated that following milk challenge, there is also evidence of deposition of IgG and complement on basement membranes and connective tissue and a degranulation of mast cells with increase in the number of IgM plasma cells in the lamina propria. These findings were interpreted as indicative of several

Figure 11–30. Jejunal mucosa in milk protein intolerance (H&E ×180).

simultaneous immune reactions occurring in the intestinal mucosa. In a quantitative study, Maluenda et al (1984) claimed that the principal change seen in cow's milk–sensitivity enteropathy is increase in intraepithelial eosinophils but not those of the lamina propria. There was also a decrease in overall mucosal thickness during active disease despite milk withdrawal; thickness returned to normal when the condition resolved. The authors concluded that in this condition there is a limitation of the capacity of crypt cells to respond to and compensate for the loss of villous epithelium. One of the characteristics of the mucosal lesion in cow's milk protein intolerance is said to be its patchy distribution (Variend, Phillips and Walker-Smith 1984), although this is difficult to explain unless the intolerance is secondary to focal damage produced by another agent. It is of some interest that there is a poor correlation between cow's milk protein intolerance and the presence of IgE serum antibodies for milk and the presence of mucosal IgE plasma cells (Schrander et al 1993). Of some interest in this regard is the demonstration in some cases of rotavirus particles in the epithelial cells (Phillips et al 1985). There is evidence that, commonly, other infections precede cow's milk protein, soy protein, and other intolerance states in infants (Iyngkaran et al 1988a, Iyngkaran et al 1989). Cow's milk intolerance or sensitivity may manifest itself by primarily involving other parts of the gastrointestinal tract such as the stomach and upper duodenum (Coello-Ramirez and Larossa-Haro 1984) or the colon. Although cow's milk protein intolerance is normally a self-limiting condition lasting a few months or a year, there is a likelihood that these patients retain an atopic tendency throughout childhood (Businco et al 1985). Vitoria et al (1982) described an essentially similar enteropathy associated with the ingestion of fish, rice, and chicken protein. Unlike gluten enteropathy, all these protein-intolerant states are transient, and this is true even in the rare event of combined cow's milk protein and gluten-induced enteropathy (Watt, Pincott and Harries 1983). There is some evidence that in gluten-sensitive enteropathy, coexisting dietary soy protein sensitivity may adversely influence the response to gluten withdrawal (Haeney et al 1982). It is thus becoming clear that diet may have a significant role in the clinical course and management of protein intolerance states that frequently follow gastroenteritis in infancy (Iyngkaran et al 1988a, b).

In view of the experimental evidence of mucosal damage to the jejunum of dogs following the instillation of acid (Townley, Cass and Anderson 1964), it is not surprising that patchy jejunal atrophy and microulceration are described in Zollinger-Ellison syndrome with hyperchlorhydria (Singleton, Kern and Waddell 1965). The mucosa, however, shows a much more obvious polymorphonuclear leukocytic infiltrate than is seen in the coeliac lesion. There are also some severe degenerative changes in the surface epithelium, which may show erosions and almost invariably exhibits superficial gastric epithelial metaplasia or so-called antralisation with the acquisition of pyloric-type mucous glands. However, extensive villous atrophy may be present in some cases. Kingham, Levison and Fairclough (1981) described two patients with Zollinger-Ellison syndrome who presented with steatorrhoea and who responded to treatment with histamine$_2$ antagonists. In stasis or blind loop syndrome, there is bacterial colonisation of parts of the small intestine where normally there is only a transient population. Sometimes the mucosa related to this abnormal bacterial proliferation shows morphological changes. This is usually patchy in distribution and of only moderate severity, i.e., a crypt hyperplasia with slight to moderate villous atrophy. The small intestine mucosa also shows a villous atrophy in association with mural infiltration by malignancy (see Fig. 12–1). Whether this is also related to stasis caused by mechanical interference or secondary to the infiltration or due to lymphatic obstruction is not known.

Postinfective Malabsorption Syndrome

Bacterial and viral gastroenteritis are known to cause reversible small intestine mucosal damage (Burke, Kerry and Anderson 1965, Soltoft and Soeberg 1972b,

Davidson and Barnes 1979, Ulshen and Rollo 1980), but until recently small bowel biopsy has played little if any part in diagnosis or management. The mucosa, however, may show crypt hyperplastic villous atrophy and cellular infiltration of the lamina propria that is usually only mildly or moderately severe, although of 31 cases described by Barnes and Townley (1973) 5 had severe mucosal lesions comparable to those seen in gluten-sensitive enteropathy. One of the characteristics of the infective lesions is its more obviously acute inflammatory nature. One may see hyperaemia and oedema with polymorph margination of capillaries. Polymorphs can also be seen traversing the epithelium of the crypts to form so-called crypt abscesses. In adults, the acute lesion is not as marked. Montgomery et al (1973), describing 13 adult cases, stressed the absence of severe mucosal lesions and the similarity of the clinical features to tropical sprue. Walker-Smith (1970) described an infant who appeared to develop typical biopsy-positive gluten-sensitive enteropathy following an episode of *Salmonella* enteritis. After a dramatic response to a gluten-free diet that was continued for a year, the child was given a normal diet, and a subsequent biopsy proved to be normal. It should be pointed out, however, that the gluten-free diet may have coincided with the recovery phase of the intestinal infection and that the question of transient gluten intolerance is still open. Gracey (1993) also drew attention to the fact that more favourable outcomes for persistent diarrhoea following infection with enteric pathogens relate to better clinical management and the recognition that impaired immune mechanisms may be at fault.

Postinfective malabsorption syndromes may be preceded by bacterial or viral gastroenteritis. Patients give a clear history of gastroenteritis of acute onset and typical symptomatology. In contrast to the usual course of events, the diarrhoea continues, weight loss occurs, and on investigation a malabsorption syndrome has clearly developed. Jejunal biopsy usually shows crypt hyperplasia and partial villous atrophy of mild to moderate degree (Fig. 11–31). There is a striking increase in round cells of lymphocyte and plasma cell type in the lamina propria and an apparent increase of those in the intraepithelial zone. Histiocytes sometimes containing haematoxylphilic debris in their cytoplasm may also be seen, and the appearance of the mucosa is distinctly abnormal. Montgomery and Shearer (1974) drew attention to the similarity of the cell population in the mucosal lesion to that in gluten-sensitive enteropathy and tropical sprue. Indeed, when folic acid deficiency is

Figure 11–31. Jejunal biopsy appearance in postinfective malabsorption. Note the heavy inflammatory infiltrate in the lamina propria (H&E ×175).

the main clinical feature, such cases are reported as acute nontropical or temperate sprue (Drummond and Montgomery 1970). Why reaction to an infection should take this form in some persons and not others is not known, but Gracey postulated (1993) that reaction may be related to subtle differences in individual immune mechanisms. Clearly, the condition needs further study. Halliday, Edmeades and Shepherd (1982), in a prospective analysis of 32 cases of postenteritis diarrhoea in children, identified persisting pathogenic agents and carbohydrate intolerance or milk-protein intolerance in slightly more than half the cases. In the remainder no significant cause for persisting diarrhoea could be ascertained. There is some evidence that selective deficiency of IgA plasma cells in the lamina propria may determine a susceptibility to gastroenteritis in patients with protein-energy malnutrition (Green and Heyworth 1980). Protracted diarrhoea associated with varying amounts of villous atrophy and crypt hyperplasia has recently been ascribed to infection by a coccidia-like body (Connor et al 1993).

Intractable (Protracted) Diarrhoea of Early Infancy

Most of the chronic diarrhoeas in infancy can be diagnosed with precision; they are short-lived and can be managed effectively. Avery et al (1968) characterised a subgroup in patients younger than 3 months of age in which the diarrhoea was without apparent cause, refractory to treatment, and frequently fatal. In a biopsy study Rossi et al (1980) established that the condition was usually associated with a mucosal abnormality. Total villous atrophy with crypt hyperplasia was described by Stern, Gruttner and Krumbach (1980), whereas Davidson et al (1978) and Fisher, Boyle and Holtzapple (1981) reported cases with villous atrophy and crypt hypoplasia. In the large series published by Candy et al (1981), both types of lesions were observed. Shwachman et al (1973) commented on the striking eosinophil infiltration of the lamina propria in some patients and the occasional presence of lymphangiectasia. With the advent of intravenous alimentation, it would appear that fewer cases end in death and complete recovery is possible. The true nature of this condition is unknown, but both Davidson et al and Candy et al described a tendency for cases to occur on a familial basis. Booth et al (1982) described an association with severe combined immunodeficiency and drew attention to the presence of large PAS–positive macrophages in the jejunal mucosa in such cases.

By the early 1980s it was apparent that this clinical entity was probably the manifestation of several different forms of mucosal injury. An initial mucosal insult and resultant malnutrition could then cause disturbances in immune function and sensitisation to ingested proteins, making the mucosa susceptible to further damage. Thus the morphological appearances of the small intestine mucosa could be expected to vary, and it has been claimed that there is often a disparity between the clinical course of the illness and the biopsy findings (Goldgar and Vanderhoof 1986, Orenstein 1986). Nevertheless, there seems to be emerging at least two recognisable morphological subgroups within the range of changes in this condition.

The first of these has been called microvillous inclusion disease. These patients have persistent intractable diarrhoea from birth or shortly afterward. There is evidence that the diarrhoea is secretory (Candy et al 1981), and at least some cases are inherited in an autosomal recessive manner (Davidson et al 1978, Howard et al 1981). The mucosa is hypoplastic with stunted villi and no elongation of the crypts; inflammatory changes are not a feature. The condition can be demonstrated by ordinary light microscopy using a histochemical method for alkaline phosphatase because the brush border inclusions are strongly positive for this enzyme and can be clearly visualised in the apical enterocyte cytoplasm (Lake 1988). PAS-positive material also accumulates in surface enterocytes as does carcinoembryonic antigen, which can be demonstrated by immunostaining (Groisman et al 1993). Electron microscopic examination reveals relatively normal crypts, but surface cells are shorter and have few stunted microvilli, increased lysosomal and cytolysosomal bodies, and characteristic membrane-bound bodies containing obvious microvilli. These mucosal microvillous inclusions are regarded as the diagnostic feature of this condition (Phillips et al 1985). Phillips et al (1993) have provided evidence that the disorder is believed to arise because of a transport defect that prevents exocytosis of brush border–related material and enzymes. In colonic mucosa that otherwise appears normal the typical inclusions may also be seen. It seems that the intestinal mucosa is inherently abnormal in this disease, and oral feeding after birth precipitates a secretory diarrhoea that is usually fatal.

A group larger than that due to microvillous inclusion disease is created by two other forms of intractable diarrhoea of infancy. This second group usually has a later onset outside the neonatal period, but generally within the first few months of life. The small bowel biopsy in this case is somewhat variable, which accounts for the reports already mentioned in which both crypt hyperplastic and crypt hypoplastic villous atrophy were described. In some patients, however, the enteropathy may have an autoimmune basis, and circulating antibodies to gut enterocytes have been demonstrated (Walker-Smith et al 1982, Savage et al 1985); thus a second variant can be defined. The jejunal morphology is said to vary from near normal to one that is completely flat. Mirakian et al (1986) proposed that a positive test for enterocyte antibody is diagnostic for this condition and that a persisting high titre indicates a poor prognosis.

The categorisation of intractable diarrhoea is still evolving. Kanof et al (1987), for example, described a case with diarrhoea from birth due to secretory diarrhoea; further evidence that some cases may have a secretory basis comes from the occasional beneficial effect of somatostatin (Bisset et al 1993). In the case reported by Kanof et al (1987), there was histological evidence of both acute and chronic inflammation of the small bowel, an avillous mucosa, and submucosal fibrosis. Of interest, however, was the concomitant involvement by the inflammatory and fibrosing process in the colon; concomitant colitis was present in the group of cases described by Girault et al (1994), although these patients also had a number of other features in common such as facial dysmorphism, hypertelorism, and wooly, easily removable hair, coupled with immune abnormalities. It is possible therefore that microvillous inclusion disease and the autoimmune variety of the intractable diarrhoea of childhood are the first two of several possible definable subgroups. Certainly the morphological appearances show a good deal of variation from case to case (Figs. 11–32 to 11–34 and 11–35 to 11–37). Varying amounts of villous atrophy, crypt hyperplasia and hypoplasia, some or no inflammatory component, increase or decrease in goblet cells, and a range of ultrastructural abnormalities have been described (Fagundes-Neto et al 1985, Orenstein 1986). This disorder clearly presents a continuing challenge for further research as outlined by Walker-Smith (1994).

Crypt Hypoplastic Villous Atrophy

This lesion has not received a great deal of attention. It is characterised by shortening of the crypts, which show a reduced mitotic rate, and a varying amount of villous atrophy so that the overall thickness of the mucosa is decreased. Creamer (1967) was the first to draw attention to it, and the lesion has been likened to hypoplastic anaemia in that a decreased cell production, rather than an increased loss, seems to be involved. It appears, however, that a simple hypoplasia of the crypts may not be the full explanation as experimental reduction of the crypt mitotic rate in humans with methotrexate (Trier 1962) did not produce villous abnormalities. Moreover, the appearances in animals and people following irradiation, which produces reduction of the crypt cell mitosis rate and a collapse of the villous architecture (Wiernik, Shorter and Creamer 1962, Wiernik 1966), are not identical to those of crypt hypoplastic villous atrophy. It is, nevertheless, clear that manoeuvres that decrease cell turnover (Creamer 1967) in the small intestine may greatly influence villous shape and crypt length, and the closest approximation to crypt hypoplastic

Figure 11–32. Duodenal endoscopic biopsy in intractable diarrhoea in a child 3 months of age. The first biopsy (see also Figs. 11–33 and 11–34) shows partial villous atrophy with slight crypt hyperplasia (H&E ×70).

Figure 11–33. Follow-up biopsy 2 weeks after that in Figure 11–32. The infiltrate is denser, villi are absent, and the crypts are hypoplastic (H&E ×250).

Figure 11–34. Further biopsy of the same case as in Figures 11–32 and 11–33. The avillous mucosa now has virtually no crypts. The patient died (H&E ×250).

villous atrophy as it occurs in humans is seen in Rhesus monkeys after protein malnutrition (Deo and Ramalingaswami 1965).

Malnutrition in children, however, may result in a jejunal lesion similar to that in gluten-sensitive enteropathy (Shiner, Redmond and Hansen 1973). One might expect a crypt hypoplastic villous atrophy such as occurs in hypophagic animals (Robinson 1972), but it is likely that lesions seen in kwashiorkor have multiple causes. Green and Heyworth (1980), for example, showed a decrease in IgA plasma cells of the lamina propria in children with protein-energy malnutrition, and this might predispose to recurrent infection and alteration in villous morphology secondary to inflammatory damage to the mucosa.

Crypt hypoplasia and villous atrophy in association with intractable diarrhoea of

Figure 11–35. Jejunal biopsy in intractable diarrhoea from a child 1 month of age (see also Fig. 11–36). The lamina is expanded by oedema and cellular infiltrate, but the villi and crypts are atrophic. Note the superficial epithelium is not greatly abnormal (H&E ×250).

Figure 11–36. Biopsy 1 week later. Even more atrophy and increased cellularity of the lamina propria are evident. The superficial epithelium is more abnormal (H&E ×250).

Figure 11–37. Detail of Figure 11–36. The lamina propria is occupied by a very prominent histiocyte population, especially noticeable nearer the lumen *(arrow)* (H&E ×500).

Figure 11–38. Jejunal mucosa showing crypt hypoplastic villous atrophy associated with malabsorption not responding to a gluten-free diet (H&E ×70).

infancy have already been referred to, but it should be noted that normal or hyperplastic crypts and villous atrophy create the more usual lesion.

In adults, crypt hypoplastic villous atrophy has been described in association with malignancy (Creamer 1964), with Paneth's cell deficiency (Pink and Creamer, 1967), with hypopituitarism (Riecken 1970), and with some cases of coeliac disease at a time when the patients no longer respond to a gluten-free diet (Fig. 11–38).

It has been demonstrated that the jejunal mucosa shows varying amounts of crypt hypoplastic villous atrophy in untreated pernicious anaemia (Pena et al 1972) (Fig. 11–39). The crypt and superficial epithelial cells show typical megalocytic changes (Foroozan and Trier 1967) characterised by large round and pale nuclei (Fig. 11–40). The superficial epithelium may otherwise appear relatively normal but, in those cases more severely affected, slight nuclear palisading, distortion of the cells, and lack of definition of the brush border in PAS preparations are seen. Mitotic figures are decreased in number, and there are fewer Paneth's cells, which are often poorly granulated. The lamina propria shows a mixed inflammatory infiltrate of varying density with a high lymphocytic preponderance. In some cases, the inflammatory infiltrate is more marked (Fig. 11–41). Another abnormality occasionally observed consists of colonies of bacteria within the lumen, but the significance of this is not known. All the observed changes revert to normal if vitamin B_{12} is given (Figs. 11–42 and 11–43), and in treated pernicious anaemia they are absent. It is tempting to assume that the hypoplastic villous appearance is related to the disturbances of desoxyribonucleic acid metabolism induced by vitamin B_{12} deficiency.

Such an explanation might account for some of the cases of crypt hypoplastic

Figure 11–39. Jejunal mucosa in untreated pernicious anaemia showing crypt hypoplastic villous atrophy (H&E ×70).

Figure 11–40. Detail of superficial epithelium in Figure 11–39. The nuclei vary in size and are "megalocytic" in type (H&E ×350).

villous atrophy seen in malignancy, and it is of interest that in Creamer's case 5 (1964) there was a carcinoma of the stomach, although vitamin B_{12} levels were not measured, and in case 4, which was associated with carcinoma of the bronchus, there was vitamin B_{12} deficiency. It is known that the latter is often present in some cases of coeliac disease. Because vitamin B_{12} is absorbed in the ileum, it is not surprising that Stewart et al (1967) showed a better correlation between abnormality of vitamin B_{12} absorption and ileal rather than jejunal mucosal atrophy. Ileal involvement is more common in the severe or longstanding untreated disease, and a delayed poor-quality response to gluten withdrawal may in part be due to the vitamin B_{12} deficiency that is tending to produce crypt hypoplasia. In addition to the superficial absorptive cells, proliferative activity of the crypt cells also gives rise to Paneth's cells and goblet cells. A crypt hypoplasia induced by vitamin B_{12} deficiency might thus result in Paneth's cell deficiency, and this could have secondary deleterious effects on the

Figure 11–41. Jejunal mucosa in pernicious anaemia shows heavy cellular infiltration of the lamina propria (H&E ×140).

Figure 11–42. Jejunal mucosa in the same patient as in Figure 11–39 1 week after treatment with vitamin B_{12} (H&E ×105).

mucosa. Creamer (1967) postulated a sustentacular role for Paneth's cell, its secretions helping to support the rest of the mucosa.

Swanson and Thomassen (1965) described a tendency toward "atrophy" of the mucosa in severe tropical sprue. This is associated with a fall in the mitosis count and a decrease in crypt length and number of argentaffin cells. Whatever the agent primarily responsible for the mucosal damage in coeliac disease, tropical sprue, or any other malabsorption syndrome, when the disorder is well established one or more additional factors may begin to influence the morphology of the mucosa. The situation is complex; Davidson and Townley (1977) described four infants with nutritional folic acid deficiency who showed villous shortening in the jejunal biopsy but elongation of the crypts. The enterocytes showed macrocytic characteristics.

Figure 11–43. Detail of Figure 11–42 shows reversion of nuclear appearance to normal; compare with Figure 11–40 (H&E ×350).

Other Abnormalities

It is likely that villous atrophy will occur not only in association with crypt hyperplasia and hypoplasia but also with all stages in between. An unusual association with villous atrophy is the generalised growth failure that occurs in the syndrome accompanied by ring chromosome 15 (Kosztolanyi and Pap 1986).

Pinkerton et al (1982) reported a fall in the crypt mitotic index and degenerative changes in Paneth's cells and crypt enterocytes following methotrexate therapy for childhood leukaemia. These changes have also been seen following the administration of other chemotherapeutic agents in animals and humans (Moore 1984, Cunningham et al 1985). The question of whether they can induce villous atrophy is not settled. Nevertheless, it is sensible that the overall mucosal structure seen in such circumstances will depend on the balance between cell loss and cell production so that one might expect that villous atrophy could occur. It is claimed that the fat stains may be an aid in the interpretation of minor amounts of villous atrophy (Variend, Phillips and Walker-Smith 1984). Fine granular fat globules are seen in surface cells in normal and abnormal mucosa, but deep mucosal fat is seen in normal mucosa. Large fat globules, however, are seen only in surface cells in coeliac mucosa and cow's milk protein enteropathy, and this may relate to the extent of villous atrophy. However, in cow's milk sensitivity large globules were also present in the surface cells even when the villous atrophy was minimal. Similarly, an increased cell proliferation in the crypts and a normal rate of surface loss would be expected to result in villous hypertrophy. Gleeson et al (1970) described villous enlargement in humans occurring in association with a renal tumour. Villous atrophy has also been reported as the result of a pancreatic glucagonoma (Jones et al 1983, Stevens et al 1984).

Mucosal hyperplasia is well recognised in experimental animals (Dowling 1967, Fenyo et al 1976, Obertop et al 1977), and it occurs in humans following jejunal resection or jejuno-ileal bypass operations for intractable obesity (Solhaug 1976). It is also well recognised that experimental hyperthyroidism in animals results in intestinal villous hyperplasia (Wall et al 1970) and that hypothyroidism has the reverse effect (Blanes et al 1977). The author, however, knows of no reports of villous alterations in thyroid disease in humans.

ILEAL BIOPSY

In gastroenterological practice, a preferential biopsy is rarely done on the ileum with the expectation of a diagnostic yield. It is clearly possible to obtain tissue via an ileostomy stoma, and biopsy specimens are frequently obtained through the ileocaecal valve at colonoscopy.

Most of the pathological processes that may affect the small intestine mucosa diffusely along its length, such as Whipple's disease, the storage diseases, lymphangiectasia, and so on, will be diagnosed with greater facility in upper intestinal biopsy tissue. Some pathological processes, however, are characteristically located at the terminal ileum or ileocaecal region. Consequently, on occasion, a tissue diagnosis of Crohn's disease can be made in an ileal biopsy by finding epithelioid granulomas when colonic mucosal tissues are unproductive. Indeed, Coremans et al (1984) claimed ileoscopy and biopsy as valuable procedures in the diagnosis of ileal disease. Even ileoscopic removal of inflammatory polyps has been described in Crohn's disease (Corless et al 1984). However, biopsy of other lesions may also reveal characteristic features. It is possible, for example, that the typical sulphur granules composed of colonies of actinomycosis organisms may be seen, although it is usually diagnosed in resection specimens (Mahant et al 1983). The same could be said to apply to the recognition of the tissue reaction in ileocaecal tuberculosis and the demonstration of acid-fast bacilli. Lesions of *Yersinia enterocolitica* infections of the ileocaecal region also may rarely provide diagnostic biopsy tissue (Fig. 11–44).

Figure 11–44. Biopsy of terminal ileal ulceration in *Yersinia* infection. Note the granuloma with central necrosis (H&E ×300).

Figure 11–45. Ileal mucosa in a patient investigated for diarrhoea. Subsequent investigation indicated a salmonella infection. Note the mild acute enteritis with polymorph invasion of the surface epithelium (H&E ×500).

Characteristically, pathological conditions have been described in resection specimens (Gleason and Patterson 1982), and biopsy specimens of the aphthoid ulcers that occur in hyperplastic lymphoid follicles might reveal the typical central microabscess and peripheral palisade of histiocytes. However, some difficulty would be experienced in differentiating these appearances from Crohn's disease if epithelioid granulomas were absent. Sometimes amoebic infection occurs as a mass lesion in the ileocaecal region, but in chronic cases vegetative organisms are few and likely to be deep-seated. It is nevertheless possible that a colonoscopic ileal or ileocaecal biopsy would prove diagnostic. Rarely does an ileal biopsy specimen show evidence of acute inflammation in patients being investigated for diarrhoea; presumably, this is sometimes due to infection (Fig. 11–45).

In the mucosa of ileal reservoirs constructed in the treatment of colonic diseases such as familial adenomatous polyposis and ulcerative colitis, a variety of pathological changes have been observed. Chronic inflammation and varying amounts of villous atrophy are common. Pyloric metaplasia of the pouch is less common as are acute inflammation and ulceration, or "pouchitis," which more commonly occurs in association with ulcerative colitis (Fig. 11–46) (Shepherd et al 1993). Despite a vast research effort, the aetiology of pouchitis remains obscure (Kmiot et al 1993, Rothenberger and Wiltz 1993, Hallak et al 1994, McLeod et al 1994, Ruseler van Embden, Schouten and van Lieshout 1994). There appears to be no relationship between the presence of backwash ileitis and the subsequent complication of pouchitis in ulcerative colitis patients treated by ileal pouch anal anastomosis (Gustavsson, Weiland and Kelly 1987). Furthermore, in histochemical studies there is a change from small to large bowel mucin type (Shepherd et al 1987) together with acquisition of colonic antigens (Campbell et al 1994). However, there does not

Figure 11–46. Ileal biopsy from a case of stomal ileitis in an ulcerative colitis patient. Note the marked inflammation and crypt abscess formation *(arrow)* (H&E ×200).

appear to be any predictive criteria as to which patients with ileal reservoirs in ulcerative colitis will get the most severe degree of pouchitis (Setti-Carraro, Talbot and Nicholls 1994). Johnson and White (1988) described not only colonic metaplasia but also the formation of adenomatous polyps. Seemingly, even metaplastic colonic mucosa in such patients is prone to neoplastic change. In ileal mucosa chronically exposed to urine in reservoirs created following total cystectomy, changes vary from villous blunting and crypt hyperplasia to more severe atrophy of villi and crypts, decreased epithelial height, and even ulceration (Hockenstrom et al 1986, Chen, Chen and Chang 1993).

Halphen et al (1989) described a curious case of idiopathic villous atrophy of the ileum. The proximal half of the small intestine was quite normal. Accompanying the ileal lesion there was a vascular abnormality consisting of mucosal and submucosal glomeruloid collections of capillaries that contained occasional hyaline thrombi.

12

LYMPHOMA IN COELIAC DISEASE; UNRESPONSIVE, COLLAGENOUS, AND ULCERATIVE COELIAC DISEASE; MEDITERRANEAN LYMPHOMA

LYMPHOMA IN COELIAC DISEASE

The association of abdominal lymphadenopathy and steatorrhoea has long been recognised and has been extensively reviewed (Kent 1964, Eidelman, Parkins and Rubin 1966). There seems no doubt that a generalised lymphoma with involvement of the bowel and/or abdominal lymph nodes can be associated with steatorrhoea (Sleisenger, Almy and Barr 1953) and that at least in some areas the mucosa shows the same histological lesion as in gluten-sensitive enteropathy (Selby and Gallagher 1979). This is probably nonspecific, because a flat coeliac-like mucosa is sometimes, but not always, also seen in the intestine when there is lymphatic infiltration by other forms of malignancy (Figs. 12–1 to 12–3). Nevertheless, the view has been expressed that because of the marked variation in the clinical manifestations of gluten-sensitive enteropathy, the development of lymphoma may cause the patient to present for the first time with malabsorption (Cooper, Holmes and Cooke 1982). If there is still some doubt that primary abdominal lymphoma can cause mucosal atrophy and a malabsorption, there can be no doubt that longstanding gluten-sensitive enteropathy may be complicated by bowel or abdominal lymph node sarcoma (Austad et al 1967, Harris et al 1967, Swinson et al 1983). This was characterised as a reticulosarcoma by Whitehead (1968a), but in today's terminology it includes any large-cell lymphoma. The characterisation of this lesion in terms of actual subtype has been the subject of debate, and various claims have been made according to the methods used for typing the cells. Taylor (1976) included a number of the cases originally examined by Whitehead in a study that aimed to determine whether or not the cells of these lymphomas had surface immunoglobulins. All were positive, and it was thought to indicate that the tumour possibly originated in B-type lymphocytes. This was of interest because of the claim that the development of the lymphoma could be traced to the cellular elements of the lamina propria of the bowel wall and the regional lymph nodes and that the lymphoma emerged through a stage of progressive hyperplasia (Whitehead 1968a). This process was seemingly characterised by a

Figure 12–1. Flat jejunal mucosa overlying an infiltrating adenocarcinoma of colonic origin (H&E ×75).

deterioration in the clinical picture associated with recurrence of diarrhoea, a reversal of the response to gluten withdrawal, fever, weight loss, abdominal pain, and finger clubbing. In some cases, there was a sustained rise in serum immunoglobulin A (IgA) levels, which occurred independently of whether there were disturbances in immunoglobulins (Hobbs et al 1969) before the gluten-free diet was instituted earlier in the disease. Interestingly, two cases of lymphadenopathy associated with coeliac disease that regressed on a gluten-exclusion diet have been described (Simmonds and Rosenthal 1981). The account of the histological appearances was, unfortunately, poor and thus it is difficult to know if the lymphadenopathy was comparable to the progressive hyperplasia described by Whitehead (1968a), but it raised the possible reversibility of the condition should early diagnosis and treatment be instituted. Kavin et al (1981) described a patient with coeliac disease complicated by nonspecific ulceration of the small and large intestine and pronounced nonspecific mesenteric lymphoid hyperplasia. The concept of a malignancy arising in hyperplasia is not new, as the neoplastic process is generally accepted as being a gradual step-wise alteration in the genome. Nevertheless, some part of the apparent lymphoid hyperplasia could conceivably be the result of a reactive infiltrate stimulated by the emerging malignant cells such as is postulated in Hodgkin's lymphoma. It is of interest that in a retrospective electron microscopic examination of five patients with presumed coeliac disease that proved fatal and in three with a terminal lymphoma, occasional abnormal cells with features suggestive of malignancy were described (Horowitz and Shiner 1981).

Isaacson and Wright (1978) and Isaacson (1981) outlined claims that the lesion was a malignant histiocytosis based on polyclonality of the cells for immunoglobulins

Figure 12–2. Detail of Figure 12–1. The epithelial surface is not greatly abnormal, and there is a dilated lacteal centrally containing lymphocytes and histiocytes, which is an indication of lymphatic obstruction by the tumor infiltration (H&E ×600).

Figure 12–3. Duodenal mucosa with extensive lacteal permeation by malignant melanoma cells (H&E ×200).

and their possession of markers for histiocytes, particularly alpha$_1$-antitrypsin. Other researchers did not support this claim (Otto et al 1981) and classified the tumour as of B-lymphocyte origin and of immunoblastic type. The assertion that the lesion was a malignant histiocytosis prevailed for some time owing to the insistence of Isaacson et al (1982). However, there was evidence that malignant large-cell lymphomas could be polyclonal (Curran and Jones 1979, Robinson et al 1980, Warnke et al 1980), and clonal switch from IgM to IgG synthesis by lymphoma has been described (Gordon and Smith 1980). On general grounds, it seemed reasonable that the gene derepression that occurs as part of the malignant process could account for many of the apparently contradictory phenomena observed in these tumours, especially as by ordinary standards they appear poorly differentiated. Whereas a well-differentiated B cell tumour composed of plasma cells might predictably be monoclonal, a poorly differentiated B cell tumour might be polyclonal, and similar arguments could easily explain the loss or the acquisition of other proteins such as alpha$_1$-antitrypsin, which might lead to argument as to the histiocytic nature of the cells. However, despite having classified the tumour as malignant histiocytosis, Isaacson et al (1985) provided evidence for a T cell origin based on the tumour's reaction with monoclonal antibodies against T lymphoid cell lines and a rearrangement of genes for the beta chain of the T-cell antigen receptor. Despite this and arguably to the detriment of the subject, this tumour was still being referred to as malignant histiocytosis long after 1985 (Mead et al 1987, Spencer et al 1989). There is evidence for a T cell origin from other researchers (Loughran, Kadin and Deeg 1986, Spencer et al 1988), but others have suggested that it is more likely a centroblastic B cell tumour (Nash, Gradwell and Day 1986), and some authors (Van der Valk, Lindeman and Meijer 1988) believed that the lymphoma complicating coeliac disease might be B cell, T cell, or histiocytic phenotype. It seems likely that, as is being appreciated more widely in tumour biology generally, the more that tumours are examined by increasing numbers of different antibodies, the more diverse their antigen expression becomes apparent. This probably reflects only the different amounts of alteration of the genome that is integral to the neoplastic process; it also underlines the claim that, increasingly, phenotyping needs to be based on the use of large panels of antisera so that patterns rather than single antigen expression can be recognised (Norton and Isaacson 1989a, b). The two aspects of this lesion that are clear are its malignant character and the fact that in coeliac patients it may arise not only in the small bowel in multifocal fashion (Freeman and Chiu 1986a) and related nodes but also elsewhere in the gastrointestinal tract, including the stomach (Roehrkasse et al 1986). The malignancy is now known as enteropathy-associated T-cell lymphoma, and a full account of its pathology has been given by Isaacson and Wright (1995).

From a diagnostic point of view, the jejunal biopsy may show features that together with the clinical and biochemical abnormalities, allow a diagnosis to be strongly suspected. The usual finding is a flat mucosa with total villous atrophy and crypt hyperplasia that exhibits an obviously dense cellular infiltrate of the lamina propria (Fig. 12–4). The mucosa may be slightly thicker than normal, but it is the infiltrate that may be of diagnostic importance (Fig. 12–5). Especially in those cases with an increased serum IgA level, there is a plasma cell component in obvious excess of that seen in an ordinary coeliac mucosa. Most plasma cells are in no way cytologically abnormal, and they occur in the company of lymphocytes and eosinophils. Eosinophils are always more obvious in the deeper layers of the lamina and may be very conspicuous so that they constitute a striking feature of the histological picture (Shepherd et al 1987). There will be a variable number of abnormal cells suggesting they are malignant because of the cytological features that early in the course of this complication of coeliac disease may be found only with difficulty. This was confirmed by Isaacson (1980), who advocated multiple biopsies and that serial sections of the tissues be obtained. Later, the collections of cells are obvious and show a range of abnormality varying from enlarged normal to frankly atypical and malignant. A characteristic feature is the tendency for these cells to invade the epithelium of glands in small groups. These cells subsequently increase in number

Figure 12–4. Jejunal biopsy in longstanding gluten-sensitive enteropathy in the stage of progressive hyperplasia. Note the elongated crypts, total villous atrophy, and extremely dense cellular infiltrate in the lamina propria (H&E ×75).

at the expense of other cell types to produce the sarcomatous appearance. At this stage or even earlier in the disease, surface ulceration may occur not only in the jejunum but also in other areas of the gastrointestinal tract. The cellular infiltrate often extends below the muscularis mucosa, a feature that may be of value in biopsy material (Fig. 12–6). This infiltrate is frequently composed of cells similar to those in the nonmalignant areas of the bowel, especially early in the disease when the frankly malignant cells are hard to find. Later, however, there is a clear malignant infiltration of the deeper aspects of the bowel mucosa.

The time that elapses between the stage of progressive hyperplasia and the development of sarcoma seems to vary from a few months to many years. In the

Figure 12–5. Detail of cellular infiltrate in Figure 12–4. Large lymphoid cells are obvious, and some appear abnormal *(arrowheads)* (H&E ×450).

Figure 12–6. Jejunal biopsy in longstanding gluten-sensitive enteropathy in the stage of progressive hyperplasia. Note extension of the infiltrate through the muscularis mucosa (H&E ×75).

cases seen by the author, the longest was 8 years. There is no doubt that many patients die in the phase of progressive hyperplasia from perforation of ulcers or intercurrent infection. In the case described by Kavin (1981), death followed an episode of intravascular coagulation. Infections are frequently of fungal type and probably reflect a disturbed immunological state as postulated by Hobbs et al (1969). A suggestion that poor dietary control might increase the incidence of sarcoma was at first not substantiated by Holmes et al (1976). These authors reviewed all their 292 patients with coeliac disease and found that of the 43 deaths one third were caused by "reticulosarcoma." After a longer follow-up, however, Holmes et al (1989) reported that a gluten-free diet protects against lymphoma and other malignancies to which coeliac patients seem prone, e.g., cancers of the mouth, pharynx, and oesophagus. There is also an association between coeliac disease, splenic atrophy, and cavitation of enlarged mesenteric nodes (Matuchansky et al 1984, Burrell et al 1994). The so-called cavitation is in fact a hyaline or necrotic central area with peripheral nodal remains that are often hyperplastic. The association of splenic atrophy and small bowel lymphoma in coeliacs is well recognised (O'Grady, Stevens and McCarthy 1985), and a case of lymphoma, splenic atrophy, and lymph node cavitation is also on record (Freeman and Chiu 1986b). This author postulates that these are all manifestations of the complex immune disturbance involved in longstanding gluten-sensitive enteropathy that involves lymphoid hyperplasia and subsequent atrophy or progression to sarcoma.

UNRESPONSIVE COELIAC DISEASE, MUCOSAL COLLAGENISATION, AND ULCERATION

Weinstein et al (1970) described a case with typical jejunal morphology showing an initial response to dietary gluten exclusion but subsequent relapse. This was followed by a steady deterioration despite a rigid gluten-free regimen and was associated with severe jejunal mucosal atrophy and deposition of collagen in the immediately subepithelial zone of the lamina propria. The authors called this lesion "collagenous sprue" and thought it was possibly a new and distinct entity. It seems more likely that it represented an end stage of gluten-sensitive enteropathy at a time when the mucosa can no longer respond to gluten exclusion.

Deposition of collagen under the enterocyte basement membrane is common in mucosal biopsies showing severe partial or total villous atrophy. This deposition

Figure 12–7. Jejunal biopsy in longstanding gluten-sensitive enteropathy. There is a thin layer of subepithelial collagen (H&E ×245).

has been discussed in some of the earliest observations on the jejunal morphology associated with steatorrhoea (Cooke et al 1963, Houriihane 1963). It is this author's experience that it must be extremely rare in young children with gluten-sensitive enteropathy and is seen only in adults, especially those with a long history of disease (Fig. 12–7). Sometimes it is barely perceptible, but at other times it is obvious, and in sequential biopsies it may be seen to progress (Figs. 12–8 and 12–9). When collagen deposition is marked, the mucosa shows a crypt hypoplastic appearance and sometimes Paneth's cell deficiency, but the latter is not invariable. However, one thing common to all these cases is the much worse prognosis when compared with uncomplicated gluten-sensitive enteropathy. This was the conclusion of Bossart et al (1975), who, in a large series of 146 coeliac patients, noted subepithelial

Figure 12–8. Progression (Figs. 12–8 and 12–9) in the deposition of subepithelial collagen in the jejunal mucosa of a patient with gluten-sensitive enteropathy who became gradually resistant to treatment. This biopsy was taken 3 months before that in Figure 12–9 (H&E ×280).

Figure 12–9. This biopsy was taken 3 months after that in Figure 12–8 (H&E ×140).

collagen in 36% and concluded that, although its presence when severe might indicate a poor prognosis, it did not represent a separate clinical entity.

Some cases give a clear history of gluten-sensitive disease becoming refractory, but others are unresponsive to gluten-exclusion diets at the time they present (Jarmay, Varkonyi and Hajnal-Papp 1993). This does not necessarily mean that they are fundamentally different. If, as many believe, gluten-sensitive enteropathy is an immune-mediated disease, an analogy with Hashimoto's disease of the thyroid can be drawn. Low-grade nongoitrous Hashimoto's disease may first present as hypothyroidism at a time when the autoimmune process is no longer active and the thyroid is a tiny fibrous remnant showing marked epithelial atrophy. Low-grade or subclinical gluten-sensitive disease likewise may first present at a time when the mucosa is so atrophic that it can no longer respond to gluten-exclusion diets. Whatever the aetiology, ulceration may supervene, and when it does there is usually a fatal outcome because, although evidence of healing may be seen in surgical or autopsy material, the ulceration is always recurrent.

An interesting association of collagenous colitis and severe partial duodenal villous atrophy with subepithelial collagen deposition has also been described (Eckstein, Dowsett and Riley 1988). It is probably too early to speculate that there is some form of relationship between collagenous colitis and gluten-sensitive enteropathy.

Some cases referred to as chronic ulcerative jejunitis (Bayless et al 1967, Jeffries, Steinberg and Sleisenger 1968, Moritz, Moran and Patterson 1971, Gouffier et al 1977) are also considered by some to be related to coeliac disease, although the position is far from clear. Although ulceration can occur in proven coeliac disease (Thompson 1976), it is less certain whether chronic ulcerative jejunitis exists as a separate entity comparable to nonspecific ileal ulceration in patients who do not have coeliac disease or some other primary disease, e.g., a vasculitis. One of the four cases described by Jeffries, Steinberg and Sleisenger developed a "reticulosarcoma" of the bowel and elsewhere after the excision of an ulcerated segment of small bowel. In a case reported by Chatti et al (1994), the authors speculated that collagenous enterocolitis may be related to the use of nonsteroidal anti-inflammatory drugs.

The case reported by Barry, Morris and Read (1970) associated with hyperglobulinaemia and the cases of Hourihane and Weir (1970) associated with focal intestinal lymphoma, although not gluten-sensitive at the time of presentation, suggest that these and similar cases represent an end stage in a complex immune-mediated disease. This is manifested by a failure to maintain the structure of the intestinal mucosa and leads to ulceration and, as in other longstanding immune-mediated disease, sarcoma may develop. The view that ulceration is always a manifestation of early lymphoma development is held by Isaacson (1980), but Kavin (1981) described a case in which the ulceration seemed to have occurred at the stage of lymphoid hyperplasia. This author has experience of similar cases in which at presentation the patient has a flat mucosa with a dense lymphoplasmacytic infiltrate that is not cytologically malignant (Figs. 12–10 and 12–11). There are multiple ulcers of the mucosa, and the lesion is nonresponsive to a gluten-free diet. It could be argued that this represents a clinical presentation of occult gluten-sensitive enteropathy due to ulceration at a time when the disease is no longer responsive to gluten exclusion. However, in a study of eight cases Robertson et al (1983) concluded that small bowel ulceration of this type is a spectrum of disorders with an inconsistent relationship to gluten sensitivity and small intestine lymphoma; Jewell (1983) reached the same conclusion. Isaacson and Wright (1995), however, believe that ulcerative jejunitis occurring in patients with coeliac disease is invariably a manifestation of enteropathy-associated T-cell lymphoma, but in the patient reported by De Thomas et al (1994) intestinal resection of histologically benign ulcerated segments of jejunum was followed, in the short term at least, by weight gain and a good recovery in nutritional state.

However, it is only in sequential jejunal biopsies over many years in all patients with proven coeliac disease, and in particular those with a recent change in clinical picture, that early diagnosis of these conditions will be possible, and a better understanding of the exact relationships between gluten-sensitive enteropathy, so-called chronic ulcerative jejunitis, and intestinal lymphoma complicating steatorrhoea will be gained. It seems possible that at least some of these cases are more closely related to immunoproliferative small intestinal disease. The doubts that some have of the relationship of these lymphomas to preexisting coeliac disease have led them to

Figure 12–10. Jejunal biopsy in a patient nonresponsive to a gluten-exclusion diet at time of presentation. Multiple mucosal ulcers were also present. Note the density of the infiltrate (H&E ×150).

Figure 12–11. Detail of base of an ulcer in the case in Figure 12–10. Apart from lymphocytes and plasma cells there are scattered immunoblasts with central nucleoli *(arrows)*, but there are no definitive indications of malignancy (H&E ×500).

suggest that it is the lymphoma that causes the mucosal changes (Hall et al 1988). Thus, the term enteropathy-associated T-cell lymphoma may be the best terminology for such lesions (Isaacson and Spencer 1987).

MEDITERRANEAN LYMPHOMA (ALPHA-CHAIN DISEASE)

Non-Ashkenazi Jews and Israeli Arabs were shown to be particularly prone to the development of a primary small intestine and regional node lymphoma associated with a malabsorption syndrome (Eidelman, Parkins and Rubin 1966). The disease was characterised by the youth of the patients and by the more or less diffuse nature of the intestinal involvement. Later, it became clear that the disease also occurred in many other parts of the world. In a study of five new cases and a review of previous literature, Doe et al (1972) commented that the disease was seen not only in the Middle East and North Africa but also in Colombia, Argentina, Cambodia, South Africa, Bangladesh, Greece, Pakistan, and Iran; however, it is still extremely rare in Western countries. Solidoro et al (1993) referred to it as a disease of underdevelopment; in a review of mucosa-associated lymphoid tissue neoplasms, Isaacson (1994) commented on its restricted geographical distribution.

It has been suggested that intestinal infection, possibly parasitic, may be the common factor in these patients, providing a stimulus for the excessive proliferation of IgA-synthesising plasma cells (Seligmann, Mihaesco and Frangione 1971). Doe et al (1972) used electron microscopy to confirm that most cells in the infiltrate were plasma cells, but in one of their cases the cells were intermediate between plasma cells and lymphocytes. The cytoplasmic features were typical of the former, but the nuclei were typical of the latter. In another ultrastructural study (Crow and Asselah 1984), the early stages of the disease were found to be characterised by immature plasma cells, whereas later the cells had immunoblastic features. In some of the

Figure 12–12. Multiple distal duodenal biopsies show clear evidence of a nodular lymphoid lesion (H&E ×50).

patients reported, excessive amounts of the heavy chains of IgA were identified in the blood, urine, and intestinal juice (Rambaud et al 1968, Doe et al 1972). The condition has thus come to be known as alpha-chain disease and does not appear to be related to gluten-sensitive enteropathy. Further evidence (Brouet et al 1977) confirmed that the condition is basically an immunoblastic lymphoma, and that a proportion of cases are associated with specific globulin synthesis and secretion. In some cases, the same pathological condition is not accompanied by secretion of IgA-heavy chains. The term immunoproliferative small intestinal disease (IPSID) was coined (World Health Organization meeting report 1976). However, the alpha chain may be present in jejunal juice or at a cellular level, even if it does not circulate (Hibi et al 1982, Asselah et al 1983, Rambaud et al 1983, Salem et al 1987). Khojasteh, Haghshenass and Haghighi (1983) claimed that the production of the alpha-heavy chain protein is more likely to occur in the earlier, better differentiated stages of the disease, although Gilinsky et al (1985) concluded that not all cases of IPSID elaborate detectable alpha-heavy chains or evolve into a lymphoma. McDonald et al (1985) described a similar group of cases whose clinical course was characterised by intestinal pseudo-obstruction. Galian et al (1977) recognised three stages in its development: stage A is morphologically plasmacytic; stage C is an immunoblastic sarcoma; and stage B is a transitional stage between A and C. All stages arise from the same clone of cells, but the development of the stages is not synchronous for the different sites of involvement, and the authors therefore proposed a staging laparotomy in order to determine the best form of treatment. The importance of jejunal biopsy in the diagnosis of this disorder has been stressed (Nasr et al 1976, Helmy 1980), and areas involved show a dense cellular infiltrate of the lamina propria with cells distinctly plasmacytic or less characteristically so and sometimes appearing as large undifferentiated cells. These cells may dominate the histological picture, especially late in the course of the disease. The villous pattern is also abnormal, but this is probably secondary to the cellular infiltration. The pattern takes the form of shortening of villi, which appear bloated and deformed, and the epithelial abnormalities seen in gluten-sensitive enteropathy are usually absent. The cellular infiltrate is so dense that it also alters the crypt pattern, tending to push the villi further apart. In the later stages the villous pattern is lost more or less completely as the lamina becomes packed with cellular elements and more or less serious

Figure 12–13. Detail of lymphoid nodules shows atypical morphological forms of the malignant lymphoid cells (H&E ×500).

malabsorption ensues (Martin and Aldoori 1994). Although recovery following treatment has been described (Manousos et al 1974, Doe 1975, Gilinsky, Chaimowitz and Van Staden 1986), complete or prolonged remission probably occurs only in the early plasmacytic stage of the disease (Galian et al 1977, Monges et al 1975, 1980), and cases refractory to treatment on presentation are not uncommon (Kaufmann, Schmitt and Seib 1994). The diagnostic value of upper intestinal fibreoptic endoscopy in this disease has already been demonstrated (Halphen et al 1986), and there is hope that flow cytometric measurement of proliferation-associated nuclear antigen P105 and DNA content of the abnormal cells might provide prognostic information in individual patients with this disease (Demirer et al 1995). A distinct condition is multiple lymphomatous polyposis (Figs. 12–12 and 12–13). This is another B cell neoplasm that has also been diagnosed by endoscopic biopsy (Fernandes, Amato and Goldfinger 1985, Stessens et al 1986).

13

PARASITIC DISEASES

GIARDIASIS

Although there is some controversy over the actual pathogenicity of *Giardia lamblia,* it has long been recognised that a heavy infestation can cause disturbance of intestinal function (Petersen 1972, Raizman 1976). When there is a sufficient number of organisms so that they can be seen in a jejunal biopsy specimen, infestation can be presumed to be heavy, and in such a circumstance they are capable of producing both diarrhoea and malabsorption. Population groups that are not normally exposed to infection may exhibit an illness of epidemic proportions on first contact with the organism (Lancet 1974), and giardiasis is a well-recognised complication of hypogammaglobulinaemia (Webster 1980). Kamath and Murugasu (1974), in a study comparing four different methods of identifying *Giardia,* found examination of biopsy impression smears to be superior to examination of stool, duodenal aspirations, and processed and sectioned jejunal specimens. Eastham, Douglas and Watson (1976), however, found examination of biopsy specimens to be superior to examination of mucosal imprints. Individual expertise in recognising the organisms in either preparation probably plays a part in the success rate. A technique applied to tissue sections utilising the immunoperoxidase method and specific antisera has also been used (Fleck, Hames and Warhurst 1985). The further evaluation of an immunofluorescent test is indicated, using patients' sera and *Giardia lamblia* cysts as antigen (Ridley and Ridley 1976).

In ordinary hematoxylin and eosin (H&E) preparations, the vegetative forms appear as grey, flattened, pear-shaped structures (Fig. 13–1) that are bilaterally symmetrical and 10–18 μm in length. The organism has two nuclei, which can be identified at light microscope level when seen "en face." Eight flagella are arranged in pairs, and ventrally the organism has a sucking disc, but these and others of its finer structures can be appreciated only by electron microscopy (Fig. 13–2). Claims that the protozoon can invade the surface epithelium (Morecki and Parker 1967) and the lamina propria (Brandborg et al 1967) have not been substantiated by other researchers, and the author has never seen this invasion in human or in experimental animal material, despite a careful search in serial preparations stained by the method advocated by Brandborg et al or in material examined by electron microscopy. The latest claim purporting to have demonstrated mucosal invasion is by Saha and Ghosh (1977). A careful appraisal of their illustrations does not reveal convincing proof. Two of the photomicrographs show parasites in close proximity to discharging goblet cells; this has been misinterpreted as evidence of invasion. In one photomicrograph, the collapsed goblet cell is identified as an intramucosal parasite, and a further parasite tail-on to the discharging mucin is identified as being in the process of entering the track made by the first. It is pertinent that Saha and Ghosh find no tissue reaction to the so-called invasive *Giardia,* and their interpretation is regarded by this author as fanciful. However, remnants of *Giardia muris* have been described

Figure 13–1. Jejunal biopsy shows vegetative *Giardia lamblia* (H&E ×525).

in macrophages within Peyer's patches in a mouse experimental model of giardiasis (Owen, Allen and Stevens 1981).

Even in the heaviest of infestations, the small bowel mucosa shows only a minimal amount of villous atrophy of crypt hyperplastic type, with a slight but definite increase in inflammatory cells in the lamina (Fig. 13–3). A high proportion of these are often eosinophil polymorphs (Abbas et al 1994). In a quantitative study,

Figure 13–2. Electron micrograph of *Giardia lamblia*. Note the two nuclei, the dorsal phagocytic vesicles, and the ventral sucking disc with which the organism probably attaches itself to the microvillous layer (×7,000).

Figure 13–3. Jejunal biopsy in heavy *Giardia* infestation. There is slight villous atrophy with crypt hyperplasia. *Giardia* organisms are just visible in the intervillous spaces (H&E ×75).

Wright and Tomkins (1978) showed a correlation between decrease in surface area and impairment of absorptive functions; Randhawa et al (1994) showed that a heavy trophozoite count is also related to the more severe morphological changes but only partial villous atrophy is ever encountered. If *Giardia* organisms are seen in association with a villous atrophy comparable to that in untreated gluten-sensitive enteropathy, a coexisting pathological condition should be suspected (see Chapter 14), although it occurs only rarely. Rosekrans, Lindeman and Meijer (1981) stressed that increased numbers of immunoglobulin A (IgA) cells as opposed to IgM plasma cells that occur in coeliac disease, are of differential diagnostic importance.

Several theories have been postulated to explain how *Giardia* organisms exert their deleterious effect on the intestinal mucosa. It has been suggested that they damage the microvilli of absorptive epithelial cells of the mucosa (Balazs and Szatloczky 1978), or that there is a significant nutritional competition between host and parasite. The evidence for the assertion that *Giardia* organisms damage the epithelial cells is not convincing (Owen, Nemanic and Stevens 1979), but when present in large numbers they may cause a mechanical blockade of the mucosa (Barbieri et al 1970). The parasite attaches itself to the microvillous surface of the absorptive cells by means of its ventral suction disc and feeds through its dorsal surface. As the microvillous layer is the site of most of the digestive enzymes, it is feasible that in heavy infestation enough of the microvillous layer of the small intestine is covered by parasites to prevent interaction of digestive enzymes and lumenal substrate.

The mechanism of malabsorption in giardiasis was also studied by Tandon et al (1977), who showed that steatorrhoea and D-xylose malabsorption in infected patients correlated significantly with evidence of jejunal bacterial overgrowth and that the malabsorption was related to bile-salt deconjugation as in the stagnant loop syndrome (Gorbach and Tabaqchali 1969). Anand et al (1980), using an experimental model in rats, concluded that *Giardia* trophozoites in some way interfere with the active transport mechanisms of the enterocytes; Gillon, Thamery and Ferguson (1982), in another mouse model, postulated a direct toxic or irritant effect of the parasite on the brush border of the enterocyte.

In a review of the pathogenesis of the diarrhoea and malabsorption secondary to giardiasis, Halliday and Farthing (1986) listed the mucosal damage, bacterial overgrowth, and both bile salt uptake and deconjugation by the organism as the important factors. However, Inge, Edson and Farthing (1988) later demonstrated that *Giardia* organisms possess a surface membrane mannose-binding lectin. There are appropriate binding sites on intestinal epithelial cells, at least in the rat; thus having attached to the cells, the *Giardia* organisms are set to interfere with the cells' function.

HOOKWORM DISEASE

Ankylostomiasis is caused by two hookworms, *Ankylostoma duodenale* and *Necator americanus.* The adult worm lives in the intestine, and the eggs that are passed develop in soil into infective filariform larvae. These invade the venous system by penetrating the skin and lodge in the lungs. They then migrate via the trachea and oesophagus to the intestine, where they mature into adults attaching themselves to the mucosa, where each worm consumes as much as 0.5 mL of blood daily (Meyers, Naefie and Connor 1976). In developing countries, infestation is fairly common. Chavalittamrong and Jirapinyo (1984), for example, found infestation in 2% of a paediatric population investigated for diarrhoea in Thailand, but it is also still a problem in aboriginal communities in otherwise developed Australia (Prociv and Luke 1995).

In addition to causing iron deficiency anaemia, it is claimed that hookworm infestation can also result in a malabsorption syndrome with steatorrhoea (Sheehy et al 1962) and in hypoproteinaemia (Jensenius 1995). Disturbance of small intestine function probably occurs only with an extremely heavy infestation. It is only in this group that morphological abnormalities occur. In the author's experience, these have consisted of crypt hyperplasia and mild to moderate villous atrophy characterised by stunted, branched, and leaf-shaped villi and few ridges. Exactly how much of this abnormality is related to the infestation and how much is simply a reflection of, for example, racial variation will be determined only on follow-up studies on patients who have been treated successfully. Occasionally, circular spaces in the mucosa are observed (Fig. 13–4); these represent the channels in which the adult worms lie, and there may be erosions of the superficial epithelium, which are presumably the sites where the worms attach themselves to the mucosa by means of their mouth parts. In the lamina propria, it is usual to see an increase in inflammatory cells, and particu-

Figure 13–4. Jejunal biopsy in heavy hookworm infestation. Note the cellular infiltrate, mild villous atrophy, and crypt hyperplasia and the obvious circular channel in the mucosa (H&E ×75).

larly in relation to the circular channels and erosions there is often a conspicuous eosinophil leukocyte element.

STRONGYLOIDIASIS

Strongyloides stercoralis has a life cycle similar to that of the hookworm, but the eggs hatch in the bowel, and some undergo a metamorphosis into infective larvae and penetrate the gut wall so that an endogenous cycle is established. This is called autoinfestation and accounts for the persistence of the parasite even when the patient has left the area where the infestation was acquired; it also accounts for the hyperinfestation syndrome.

Diarrhoea and malabsorption syndrome are frequent complications of *S. stercoralis* infestation, although it is more usually symptomless (de Paola, Dias and da Silva 1962). The infestation invariably results in a transient duodenojejunitis, but rarely is the whole bowel involved in severe cases due to autoinfection. An uncommon complication is paralytic ileus (Cookson et al 1972). Secondary gram-negative septicaemia and *Escherichia coli* meningitis also have been described (Smallman et al 1986). A jejunal biopsy may reveal crypt hyperplasia and a varying amount of villous atrophy associated with an inflammatory infiltrate of the lamina propria. Distortion of crypts and erosions of the epithelium can be clearly related to the presence of adult worms, rhabditiform larvae, and ova (Figs. 13–5 to 13–7). The ova characteristically embed themselves in the crypt walls, and within the lumen of the crypts the larval forms can be seen. The jejunal morphology appears to be the direct result of the presence of parasites, because in treated cases the villous pattern returns to normal (Bras et al 1964), and Da Costa (1971) showed a high turnover rate of intestinal epithelial cells in this condition. Hyperinfection with *S. stercoralis* may also occur in states of altered immunity such as malignant lymphoma (Adam et al 1973)

Figure 13–5. Strongyloidiasis. Adult worms (H&E ×120).

Figure 13–6. Strongyloidiasis. Rhabditiform larvae (H&E ×300).

and other forms of immunosuppression, including acquired immunodeficiency syndrome (Haque et al 1994). Strongyloidiasis is a rare cause of biliary obstruction due to stenotic involvement of the duodenal papilla (Delarocque-Astagneau et al 1994). Humans are the main hosts for *S. stercoralis*; a second species, *Strongyloides fulleborni*, is a natural parasite of monkeys, humans being secondarily infected. *S. fulleborni* more commonly affects infants than adults.

CAPILLARIASIS

Whalen et al (1969) described a human infestation of epidemic proportions by a species of the roundworm *Capillaria*. Occurring first in the Philippines, the disease has since been described in Korea (Lee et al 1993, Hong et al 1994). The disease takes the form of severe painful diarrhoea associated with protein-losing enteropathy and malabsorption. Jejunal biopsies show moderate to severe mucosal abnormalities with villous atrophy and inflammatory infiltration of the lamina propria. These

Figure 13–7. Strongyloidiasis. Egg in jejunal mucosa (H&E ×300).

changes, however, were no more marked than in control groups. In about half the cases examined, *Capillaria* worms were found to have penetrated beneath the superficial mucosa. In postmortem material from one of the original epidemic cases, which was made available to the author by Professor Marcial-Rojas of the Puerto Rico Medical School, eggs were found after a search within the small intestine crypts, but in contrast to those in strongyloidiasis they do not appear to embed themselves in the mucosa (Fig. 13–8).

COCCIDIOSIS

Reviewing the literature and describing six new cases, Brandborg, Goldberg and Breidenbach (1970) produced evidence that human infection with the protozoon *Isospora belli* may produce diarrhoea and steatorrhoea. There is a simple, direct transmission cycle in humans, but a related organism, *Isospora hominis,* produces a similar illness and has humans as the definitive hosts and the cow or pig as the obligative intermediate hosts (Knight and Wright 1978). The jejunal biopsy changes apparently vary from slight villous abnormality with clubbing to a flat mucosa with an increased cellular infiltrate of the lamina propria.

Parasites in all stages of endogenous development are observed within the epithelial cells, but rarely in the lamina propria and submucosa. Ingested oocysts penetrate the epithelial cells and undergo progressive cyclical development. Recognition of the merozoites, schizonts, and gametocytes is facilitated using a combination of staining procedures, including Giemsa, in addition to H&E. In a guinea pig model of the disease, the cellular localisation and the structural analysis of the absorptive cell–parasite membrane interactions were described in detail in an electron microscopic study (Marcial and Madara 1986). These authors also describe that, in the guinea pig at least, although *Cryptosporidium* organisms are confined to the apex of absorptive cells in the region of Peyer's patches, they can be seen in macrophages subjacent to overlying M cells. This suggests that cryptosporidial antigens may be sampled by the lymphoid cells in these sites.

Figure 13–8. Capillariasis. Eggs in jejunal crypt (H&E ×375).

Human coccidiosis has been considered rare, but it may be responsible for many cases of undiagnosed malabsorption. Connor et al (1993), for example, reported biopsy changes characterised by acute and chronic inflammation, surface epithelial degeneration, and a variable villous atrophy in nine patients with protracted diarrhoea who had coccidia-like organisms in the stool, although the authors were not able to demonstrate organisms in the mucosa. However, there is a distinct possibility that the parasitisation in some cases is coincidental. For example, Henry, Bird and Doe (1974) reported a single case of coccidiosis arising in association with alpha-chain disease. The organisms were identified by electron microscopy and occurred within the epithelial cell cytoplasm.

Human infection with a related organism in the coccidia group, *Cryptosporidium*, has also been recorded (Nime et al 1976), and sometimes it has occurred as a complication of hypogammaglobulinaemia (Meisel et al 1976, Lasser, Lewin and Ryning 1979). Weinstein et al (1981) described coexisting cryptosporidiosis and cytomegalovirus infection. Tzipori et al (1982) transferred cryptosporidiosis from an adult human to newborn lambs using faecal extracts. Current et al (1983) claimed that infection of immunocompetent humans with *Cryptosporidium* may be more common than suspected, especially those in contact with infected animals. A case was made for the screening of all patients with acute diarrhoea for the organism (Biggs et al 1987), and in developing countries *Cryptosporidium* appears to be a major pathogen being isolated from 13.5% of children hospitalised for diarrhoea (Sallon et al 1988). The incidence in countries with a higher standard of living, however, is very low, and the disease seems to be limited largely to the immunocompromised (Marshall et al 1987). At light microscope level, the organisms appear as round or oval bodies 2–3 μm in diameter applied to the surface of the epithelial cells. They are weakly basophilic in H&E preparations and are better demonstrated in Giemsa preparations. A periodic acid–Schiff stain demonstrates the cyst wall. With electron microscopy, the organisms appear to be incorporated into the apex of the cell and are covered by the surface membrane. In this site various stages in the life cycle of the parasite can be recognised (Bird and Smith 1980).

SCHISTOSOMIASIS

There are sporadic reports of schistosomal *(Schistosoma mansoni)* involvement of the upper small intestine (Sadek 1965, Sherif 1970). The organism most likely to affect the small intestine is *Schistosoma japonicum.* Ova and a secondary inflammatory infiltration occur in the mucosa (Contractor et al 1988), but whether these changes are always or ever associated with malabsorption seems not to have been ascertained. The jejunal mucosa was examined in detail in 100 patients with schistosomiasis (Castro et al 1971). Light microscopy sections and mucosal crush preparations for the identification of schistosomal elements showed that the villous pattern did not differ from that seen in a comparable control group. They also revealed that the mucosal crush preparations were superior to routine histological section procedures in the study of involvement of the small intestine in schistosomiasis. Jejunal biopsy specimens are poor indicators of schistosomal infestation in patients excreting eggs (Halstead, Sheir and Raasch 1969), although occasional cases have been recorded (Witham and Mosser 1979) in which upper small bowel biopsy specimens showed eggs when they were not found in the faeces.

LEISHMANIASIS

In a study of jejunal function and morphology in visceral leishmaniasis, Muigai et al (1983) described mucosal abnormalities. In heavy infestation, crypt hyperplasia and partial villous atrophy were seen, but the striking feature was the presence of parasites, both free and within histiocytes in the lamina propria, especially in the tips of villi. They were also seen in the submucosa.

14

MISCELLANEOUS CONDITIONS

IMMUNE DEFICIENCY

The morphological abnormalities that may occur in the jejunum of patients with immune deficiency syndromes are reviewed by Doe (1979) and Ament (1985). These are distinct from the wide range of morphological abnormalities that may be associated with lymphopenia and low levels of gamma globulin and albumin due to excessive loss from the intestine or urinary tract (Waldmann 1970). Sometimes the level of serum immunoglobulin G (IgG) is low when those of IgA and IgM are normal, which reflects its considerably slower rate of synthesis. Small bowel biopsy may prove helpful in the diagnosis of these states of immune deficiency if the lesion is diffuse or if it involves a sufficient length of the small intestine. In intestinal lymphangiectasia and Whipple's disease (see the section on Whipple's disease), for example, the biopsy sample shows typical features, and the low levels of IgM (Hobbs and Hepner 1968) and IgA (Crabbe and Heremans 1967) that can occur in gluten-sensitive enteropathy are associated with the morphological abnormalities that are usual for that condition. Malignancy, especially the lymphomas and myeloma, may decrease the competency of the immune mechanism as may steroid and cytotoxic therapy. Whenever this occurs, the gastrointestinal tract is likely to be the site of lesions produced by an increased susceptibility to infections by a wide spectrum of pathogens, bacterial, fungal, and viral. Clearly, small bowel biopsy may be helpful in the diagnosis of these.

There is no doubt that diarrhoea and a malabsorption syndrome can complicate primary hypogammaglobulinaemia of the congenital and acquired types (Barandun, Riva and Spengler 1968), and it varies in severity from case to case. This in part may be due to the variation that occurs between local concentrations of immunoglobulin and those circulating in the serum. Another factor is the compensatory expansion in secretory IgM capacity in some patients (Nagura, Kohler and Brown 1979). The classification of the immunodeficiencies given by Good et al (1968) has been expanded considerably, and there are increasing reports of gastrointestinal disturbances associated with immunological deficiency in the paediatric age group.

B Lymphocyte Abnormalities

In infantile X-linked hypogammaglobulinaemia (Bruton's type), small intestine biopsy usually shows only sparsity or absence of lamina propria plasma cells (Fudenberg et al 1970), and the mucosa-associated lymphoid tissue lacks germinal centres (Huber, Zegers and Schuurman 1992). Clinically acute gastrointestinal infection is often the clinical presentation, but chronic infection is less common, although rotavirus infection and giardiasis can result in malabsorption (Ament, Ochs and Davis 1973, Ross and Asquith 1979, Ament 1985, Lederman and Winkelstein 1985). Villous architecture is usually normal, but Rhee et al (1975) described a case with villous atrophy and intramucosal bacteria. In X-linked immunodeficiency with elevated or normal IgM level apart from oesophageal candidiasis, intestinal cryptosporidiosis is described (Vanderhoof et al 1977). Ament (1985) also recorded moderate to severe crypt hyperplastic villous atrophy in immunodeficiency associated with hyperglobulinaemia. There was a noticeable increase in lamina propria plasma cells, and rotavirus infection was the putative cause. Common variable hypogammaglobulinaemia is usually sporadic, but some familial cases appear to be inherited in an autosomal recessive manner, and it forms a heterogeneous group. Small intestine abnormalities in this condition are common. Some have abnormality of brush border enzymes comparable to those that occur in tropical malabsorption syndrome (Dawson et al 1986). A minority show crypt hyperplastic villous atrophy and may have a severe coexisting *Giardia* infestation. *Giardia* infestation is fairly common in the absence of villous changes but may be associated with disaccharidase deficiencies (Ament, Ochs and Davis 1973). When villous abnormality and giardiasis coexist, an improvement in villous architecture is said to follow specific anti–*Giardia lamblia* therapy (Ament and Rubin 1972). In those patients with a serious mucosal lesion comparable to that seen in coeliac disease, the lesion is only rarely responsive to a gluten exclusion diet (Frexinos et al 1979). Webster et al (1981), however, described another such case, with relapse of the mucosal lesion following gluten challenge. Whatever the state of the villous pattern in this condition, the lamina propria contains few or no plasma cells, the predominant cell type being a small lymphocyte (Fig. 14–1). Ulcerative jejunitis and protein-losing enteropathy may also

Figure 14–1. Duodenal biopsy in a patient with acquired hypogammaglobulinaemia. There is crypt hyperplastic villous atrophy and an absence of plasma cells in the lamina propria. Note that the superficial epithelium is relatively normal. No *Giardia* organisms were present (H&E ×250).

occur (Corlin and Pops 1972). Nodular lymphoid hyperplasia also occurs in a proportion of these patients (see later in this chapter), and there is sometimes coexisting Crohn's disease or ulcerative colitis (Ross and Asquith 1979).

In selective IgA deficiency, which is the most common primary immunodeficiency in humans, the majority of patients suffer no significant disability. This may reflect the fact that the lack of IgA is compensated for by an increase in secretory IgM, although in some cases serum levels of IgA may not reflect either the mucosal levels or their functional capacity. Diarrhoea and steatorrhoea are the most common intestinal manifestations and may be due to cow's milk intolerance, disaccharidase deficiency, giardiasis, or gluten-sensitive enteropathy. The frequency of coeliac disease in selective IgA deficiency is 10 times that in the population at large. The mucosal lesion is identical to that seen in the usual form of the disease, except that cells containing IgA as demonstrated by immunohistochemical methods are either few or absent. It has been suggested that in the absence of local IgA, bowel antigens enter the intestine unimpeded and thus predispose to the acquisition of gluten sensitivity. There is also an increase in the incidence of Crohn's disease in isolated IgA deficiency and a greater risk of malignancies, especially B-cell lymphomas (Cunningham-Rundles 1988).

In transient IgA deficiency and isolated secretory piece deficiency, diarrhoea is a frequent complication. It is probably the result of intestinal infection, and it could be predicted that the mucosa in such circumstances would show nonspecific inflammatory changes and villous atrophy. In a study by Perlmutter et al (1985), some 50% of 55 infants with low IgG levels and chronic diarrhoea showed a crypt hyperplastic villous atrophy varying from mild to severe.

T Lymphocyte Abnormalities

In congenital thymic aplasia (DiGeorge's syndrome), the lamina propria of the small intestine is devoid of all lymphoid cells (Dubois et al 1970), and any follicular collections are atrophic and have no germinal centres. Diarrhoea may occur, but it is rarely severe and is sometimes due to lactose deficiency (Ament, Ochs and Davis 1973).

In chronic mucocutaneous candidiasis no distinctive intestinal lesion is described, but oesophageal involvement may lead to strictures.

Combined B and T Lymphocyte Abnormalities

In infants suffering from severe combined immunodeficiency, T and B lymphocyte functions are compromised. The jejunal mucosa may reveal stunting of villi, absence of plasma cells, and lymphocytes and oedema of the lamina propria; the striking feature is the presence of microphages in the lamina propria (Horowitz et al 1974, Doe 1979) that stain positive in the periodic acid–Schiff (PAS) test. They are not unlike the macrophages seen in Waldenstein's macroglobulinaemia (see later section). Death results early from respiratory and alimentary tract infection and malnutrition.

Diarrhoea and malabsorption may be a clinical feature in Nezelof's syndrome, ataxia telangiectasia, the short-limbed dwarfism syndrome, and Wiskott-Aldrich syndrome. In Nezelof's syndrome, small bowel biopsy may show blunting of villi with increased markers of plasma cells and polymorphs in the lamina propria (Ament 1975, Ross and Asquith 1979).

Bare Lymphocyte Syndrome

This syndrome has an autosomal recessive pattern of inheritance and is characterised by the absence of class I or class II major histocompatibility complex molecules. Clinical manifestations are immunodeficiency combined with oral candidiasis, *Pneumocystis carinii* pneumonia, and repeated persistent viral gastrointestinal infections (Touraine et al 1992).

Chronic Granulomatous Disease

In this disease, there is an inherited defect of neutrophil and macrophage functions so that they are unable to kill catalase-positive organisms. Diarrhoea and steatorrhoea commonly occur, and intestinal biopsy shows a normal villous structure with PAS-positive macrophages at the tips of villi. Ament and Ochs (1973) recorded the presence of lipofuscin in some of the macrophages and noted there is a generalised reticuloendothelial hyperplasia in this disease. Some cases have a chronic noncaseating granulomatous enteritis somewhat similar to Crohn's disease (Werlin et al 1982).

Nodular Lymphoid Hyperplasia

Hypogammaglobulinaemia and nodular lymphoid hyperplasia, first described in detail by Hermans et al (1966), is characterised by very low or absent IgA and IgM levels and a decreased IgG level. There is a susceptibility to infections, particularly in the respiratory tract; diarrhoea, which may or may not be associated with steatorrhoea; and nodular hyperplasia of the lymphoid elements of the small and sometimes the large intestine. The small intestine also invariably harbours the parasite *G. lamblia*. Ajdukiewicz, Youngs and Bouchier (1972), describing a patient, also reviewed the related literature, which to the time of their report accounted for 22 other cases. Since then, several other cases have been described (Brindicci et al 1993, Castaneda-Romero et al 1993, Daniel, Debonne and Klotz 1993, Rodriguez-Maria 1994). The jejunal biopsy specimen (Figs. 14–2 and 14–3) may show a nodular mucosal appearance visible to the unaided eye. The nodules vary from 1 to 4 mm, and histologically they are composed of normal immature cells and scattered pale histiocytes containing nuclear debris. The case illustrated here did not reveal an increased mitotic rate in the follicles, although this was reported by Hermans et al (1966). The margin of the germinal centre is characterised by an abrupt edge next to a very thin layer

Figure 14–2. Jejunal biopsy. Nodular lymphoid hyperplasia with hypogammaglobulinaemia (H&E ×43).

Figure 14–3. Detail of Figure 14–2. Note the germinal centre, its clean-cut margin bounded by small lymphocytes and *Giardia* organisms *(arrow)* just discernible in the intervillous space (H&E ×175).

of compressed small lymphocytes. Beyond the follicles, the cellular component of the lamina propria shows a virtual absence of plasma cells, but a very painstaking search may reveal occasional examples. Although not reported by Hermans et al in their material, the lamina propria shows a patchy and slight increase in eosinophil polymorphonuclear leukocytes. The villous pattern remains basically normal except over the follicles, where the villi are stunted or absent (as is usual even over normal follicles), and even in the biopsy tissues most cases show numerous vegetative *G. lamblia* both in relation to the surface epithelium and in the crypts.

It has been postulated (Webster et al 1977) that nodular lymphoid hyperplasia is a secondary phenomenon in association with hypogammaglobulinaemia and represents a local immune response to antigens originating in the gut lumen. Macroscopically similar lymphoid hyperplasia also occurs in the small intestine unassociated with hypogammaglobulinaemia. It is probably a reactive phenomenon and has been seen by the author associated with caecal carcinoma. Atwell, Burge and Wright (1985) ascribed its occurrence in infants to echovirus and adenovirus infection. Shaw and Hennigar (1974) described its occurrence as a nonspecific benign entity and in association with lymphoma in other parts of the lymphoid system.

As more cases are described, it is becoming clear that nodular lymphoid hyperplasia is not a distinct clinical entity. As a benign condition, it is seen as an apparent reaction to small intestine malignant lymphoma in the absence of hypogammaglobulinaemia (Matuchansky et al 1980) or in association with it (Lamers et al 1980, Chiaramonte and Glick 1994) and in patients with coexisting giardiasis who have normal immunoglobulins (Ward et al 1983). It is to be distinguished from malignant lymphoid polyposis, which is a true lymphoma of B cells (Isaacson, MacLennan and Subbuswamy 1984, Isaacson 1985, Zuckerman et al 1986).

Waldenström's Macroglobulinaemia

Diarrhoea and steatorrhoea are uncommon manifestations of Waldenström's macroglobulinaemia. Cabrera, de la Pava and Pickren (1964) reported an infiltration of the lamina propria by large foamy histiocytes in Waldenström's macroglobulinaemia. Some of the cells were positive on PAS staining, and similar homogeneous material giving the same staining reaction was also seen in the lamina propria, both in an extracellular situation and distending the lymphatics (Fig. 14–4). Villous abnormalities, when present, are slight and appear as simple deformities secondary to the infiltration. The tips of villi often are most severely involved, and this imparts a distinctive club-like appearance so that the diagnosis may be suspected at endoscopy (Parrish, Hemming and Matthewson 1994). The material has been shown by means of immunofluorescence stains to be monoclonal IgM macroglobulin (Pruzanski et al 1973). The material also stains for fat (Brandt et al 1981), which suggests that its presence may interfere with the absorption of fat so that fat is held up in the lamina propria before entering the lymphatics. Hoang et al (1985) described a case with the additional feature of lymphangiectasia to which they ascribed a coexisting protein-losing enteropathy. Lymphangiectasia and malabsorption were the features presented by the patient described by Tait et al (1993), who were also able to demonstrate a lupus anticoagulant activity by the paraprotein.

ACANTHOCYTOSIS (ABETALIPOPROTEINAEMIA, BASSEN-KORNZWEIG SYNDROME)

This is a syndrome (Bassen and Kornzweig 1950) comprising acanthocytosis of red cells, retinitis pigmentosa, central nervous system manifestations, absence of beta lipoproteins, and steatorrhoea. The jejunal biopsy reveals no significant abnormality in villous shape, but the absorptive cells of the superficial epithelium show typical vacuolation of the apical cytoplasm (Salt et al 1960, Lamy et al 1962). This is seen even in the fasting state and is known to be due to accumulation of lipid (Figs. 14–5 to 14–7). Dobbins (1966) showed in an electron microscopic study that, in this

Figure 14–4. Jejunal mucosa in Waldenström's macroglobulinaemia. The lamina propria is filled with PAS-positive immunoglobin (PAS ×550).

Figure 14–5. Jejunal biopsy in abetalipoprotein-aemia. There is a normal villous pattern, but the enterocytes appear vacuolated (H&E ×300).

syndrome, free fatty acids and monoglycerides enter the absorptive cell and are re-esterified in normal fashion. However, Golgi's vacuoles do not subsequently become distended with lipid nor is there chylomicron formation, and the re-esterified lipid accumulates in the cells to be seen as apical vacuolation in light microscopic preparations. These findings support the concept that the absorptive defect is concerned with the exit of fat from the absorptive cell and that this is the result of impaired chylomicron formation with which beta lipoproteins are intimately concerned (Isselbacher et al 1964).

Treatment with low-fat diets does not significantly alter the histological appearances (Greenwood 1976). Although the disease is generally fatal in childhood, Lazaro et al (1986) described a male patient 29 years of age. There is some evidence (Scott, Miller and Losowsky 1979) that there may be a broader spectrum of beta lipoprotein abnormality than hitherto appreciated. Lesser degrees of the beta lipoprotein deficiency may be associated with milder and less complete forms of the disease. For example, steatorrhoea with fat-filled enterocytes is also a classic feature of homozygous hypobetalipoproteinaemia (Cottrill et al 1974). There is an absence of apolipoprotein B in their plasma, and it cannot be demonstrated histochemically in small intestine absorptive cells (Green et al 1982, Herbert et al 1982). A similar clinical syndrome with fat-filled enterocytes, decreased plasma apolipoprotein B, and apolipoprotein A-I, but increased enterocyte apolipoprotein B, was described by Roy et al (1987). This recessively transmitted condition differs from abetalipoproteinaemia and the homozygous form of hypobetalipoproteinaemia but is also caused by a defect in the final assembly of chylomicrons or in the mechanism by which they leave the enterocyte. This type of defect may also explain the familial cases described

Figure 14–6. Detail of absorptive epithelium. Note normal brush border and vacuolated apical cytoplasm. Occasional cells show nuclear reversion *(arrows)* (H&E ×500).

Figure 14–7. Electron micrograph of the apical cytoplasm of the enterocytes showing neutral fat accumulation. Artefacts are due to prior formalin fixation (H&E ×4,580).

by Strich et al (1993) in which three of the offspring of related parents exhibited the intestinal morphology identical to that seen in Bassen-Kornzweig syndrome.

WHIPPLE'S DISEASE

Except for the PAS positivity of the macrophages and recent electron microscopic observations, little has been added to the morphological descriptions of this condition since it was first described by Whipple (1907). However, it is now known that it is a systemic disease and, apart from the gastrointestinal tract, may have manifestations due to involvement of the joints, skin, nervous system, eye, skeletal muscle, heart, serosal membranes, lung, kidney, liver, spleen, and lymph nodes (Feldman 1986, Fleming, Wiesner and Shorter 1988, Gaist and Ladefoged 1993, Labenz et al 1993, Schrenk et al 1994). The small intestine is almost always involved, and biopsy is the method of choice as a diagnostic procedure (Hendrix and Yardley 1970). Because the duodenum beyond the bulb is usually involved, duodenal endoscopic biopsy examination usually provides a diagnosis. In the case described by Meier et al (1994), duodenal biopsy examination results were negative, and this was so in 6 of 18 cases described by Geboes et al (1992). The dissecting microscope reveals several low, bulging, bloated villi of white or yellow appearance. Histologically, the villous pattern is distorted by a mucosal infiltrate of large macrophages (Fig. 14–8) with a basophilic, stippled cytoplasm. The macrophages surround empty spaces and are PAS-positive diastase-resistant (Fig. 14–9), which is due to cytoplasmic inclusions of rods and granules. Similar particles also occur outside the macrophages lying free in the lamina propria. In preparations stained for iron, macrophages containing haemosiderin are frequently located deep in the lamina propria, and the muscularis mucosal cells may contain lipofuscin.

Electron microscopic studies (Watson and Haubrich 1969, Silva, Macedo and Nunes 1985) have confirmed Whipple's original suggestion that the basophilic macrophages might contain organisms. These appear as bacilliform bodies that may be seen in the lumen of the bowel in between the epithelial cells as well as in and between macrophages in the mucosa and submucosa. In addition to more or less well-preserved intracellular forms, there are others within lysosomes that show various stages of intracellular digestion. There are also granular and membranous dense

Figure 14–8. Jejunal biopsy in untreated Whipple's disease (H&E ×75).

Figure 14–9. Whipple's disease. PAS-positive macrophages surround the empty spaces. Occasional granules appear to be extracellular (PAS ×600).

bodies that represent the end products of this digestion and that are the counterpart of the PAS-positive granules seen with the light microscope. Dobbins and Kawanishi (1981), in a more extensive study, also described bacilli in epithelial cells, lymphatic and capillary endothelium, polymorphs, plasma cells, lymphocytes, and mast cells. Degranulation of mast cells has been described as a prominent feature in Whipple's disease, and it has been suggested that there may be cooperation between macrophage and mast cell in the defence against Whipple's bacillus (Veloso and Saleiro 1982).

Dobbins and Kawanishi also stressed the unique nature of the outer membrane external to the cell wall of the organism, and they expressed the view that this may be related to difficulty in culturing the organism in vitro. Attempts to culture the organisms in Whipple's disease have not given any consistent results to date. Recognised bacteria include *Klebsiella, Haemophilus, Nocardia, Corynebacterium,* and several strains of *Streptococcus,* some of which have shown cell wall deficiency. Evans and Ali (1985) used immunohistochemistry to demonstrate the presence of a rhamnose polysaccharide antigen in Whipple's bacilli. It is known that this sugar is found in many bacterial polysaccharides, notably those in streptococci, lactobacilli, shigellae, and corynebacteria. Gupta et al (1986) also demonstrated that the reaction between circulating antibodies and the characteristic material in Whipple's macrophages can be blocked by rhamnose. It has been postulated, therefore, that more than one organism may be responsible and that there is a basic immunological defect in the patient. Dobbins (1981) argued the case for an abnormality in the cellular immune system, and Kwitko et al (1980) favoured an underlying defect in intestinal antigen exclusion. This appears to be substantiated by later work by Ectors et al (1992), who demonstrated an abnormal phagocytic capacity, an increased number of intraepithelial lymphocytes, a decreased C4/C8 ratio, and IgM plasma cells outnumbering IgA-positive cells in the lamina propria. Earlier researchers (Tytgat et al 1977, Clancy et al 1975), however, demonstrated a return to normal of the decreased cell-mediated immunity that was present before treatment had been given, and this has been substantiated (Veloso et al 1981). Together with the apparent antigenic similarity of the agent in three different cases of Whipple's disease described by Keren et al (1976), the evidence so far seems to favour a previous claim by Charache et al (1966) that organisms with an unusual cell wall are responsible and that any immunological deficit is secondary, although there is clearly scope for further investigation. The fact that Whipple's disease is rare in acquired immunodeficiency syndrome is probably in favour of this (Donaldson 1992). Antibiotic therapy is certainly effective in treatment. The disease is no longer inevitably fatal.

The circular spaces in the lamina propria and elsewhere in the other tissues involved contain neutral fat, but exactly how they form is in dispute. Some believe that they are dilated lymphatics, but others deny this, pointing out that the spaces are not lined by endothelium, but by macrophages. Endothelium, however, has the capacity to convert into macrophages, but lymphatic obstruction has not been demonstrated, and there seems to be no good reason why fat should accumulate in dilated lymphatic spaces. The reason for the presence of the lipid deposits is that they form as the result of a disturbance in fat absorption, but this hardly explains why they are also seen in sites other than the bowel and mesenteric nodes.

The changes that occur in the mucosa following antibiotic treatment have been reported in detail by Maizel, Ruffin and Dobbins (1970) and Denholm, Mills and More (1981). The gradual disappearance of the organisms and PAS-positive macrophages (Figs. 14–10 and 14–11) and the slow return of the mucosa to normal are further evidence that the various features of the disease are manifestations of an infection. Antibiotics are widely used, often in repeated regimens of treatment for a variety of disease states. Under these conditions, the classic clinicopathological picture of Whipple's disease may be modified, and this should be borne constantly in mind if the diagnosis is not to be missed (Figs. 14–12 and 14–13). Atypical forms exist, and the case described by Moorthy, Nolley and Hermos (1977), in which intestinal lesions were minimal, bears this out. A morphological feature in treated Whipple's disease not stressed by other authors was reported by Oliva et al (1972). They described lymphohistiocytic granulomas in the lamina propria. Centrally there is a necrotic cell, probably a degenerate histiocyte, and this is surrounded by a cuff of lymphocytes. These granulomas were seen when the jejunal biopsy was otherwise almost normal after nearly 10 years of intermittent antibiotic therapy. Babaryka, Thorn and Langer (1979) also described sarcoid-like epithelioid granulomas in an untreated case of Whipple's disease. Sometimes a sarcoid-like systemic disease proves to be Whipple's disease when the typical bacilliform bodies are demonstrated in noncaseating granulomas in the lymph nodes or other tissues affected (Cho et al 1984, Wilcox et al 1987). Aloy-Duch et al (1993) listed colonic obstruction due to mesenteric retraction secondary to lymph node enlargement as a rare complication. Whipple's disease has also been listed as a rare cause of amyloidosis (Leidig et al 1994).

Figure 14–10. Jejunal mucosa in Whipple's disease shows partial recovery of villous pattern with fewer macrophages and absence of fat spaces (H&E ×150).

Figure 14-11. Treated Whipple's disease shows marked decrease in PAS-positive histiocytes (PAS ×800).

INTESTINAL LYMPHANGIECTASIA

Small bowel biopsy plays an important role in the diagnosis of protein-losing enteropathy because many of the 70 or more conditions associated with protein loss from the gastrointestinal tract may be associated with morphological abnormalities.

Among these are coeliac disease, tropical sprue, hookworm infestation, giardiasis, Crohn's disease, and numerous other inflammatory and neoplastic lesions. (For a comprehensive list, see Waldmann 1970.) It is being increasingly recognised that protein-losing enteropathy and lymphopenia are the sole presenting features of a morphologically distinct condition known as intestinal lymphangiectasia. This

Figure 14-12. Jejunal mucosa in a patient who had for years received several courses of antibiotics for bronchiectasis. Note the absence of lipid spaces (H&E ×75).

Figure 14–13. Same case as in Figure 14–12. A diagnosis of Whipple's disease modified by previous therapy was made after a PAS stain was obtained (PAS ×75).

abnormality of lymphatics usually involves the small intestine (Fox and Lucani 1993, Won et al 1993, Heresbach et al 1994). It is unusual for the colon to be involved and even rarer for the condition to be confined to the large intestine only (Asakura et al 1986). This designation should probably be reserved for those cases showing villi with oedematous tips, giving the mucosa a pebble-like appearance as seen in the dissecting microscope. Histologically, there is oedema of the lamina propria, submucosa, and the absorptive cells of the surface epithelium. The latter is said to push the nucleus away from its basal position toward the lumenal surface (Mistilis, Skyring and Stephen 1965), an appearance also seen in relation to the suction trauma of biopsy. The mucosal lymphatics within the tips of the villi are dilated (Fig. 14–14), but the villi are only slightly distorted, and there is no villous atrophy. The lamina propria contains foamy macrophages and an occasional multinucleated giant cell. The macrophages, which are only weakly PAS-positive (Fig. 14–15), also contain neutral fat. Fat as chilomicrons can also be demonstrated between epithelial cells and in the lamina propria, and there is dilation of the interepithelial cell spaces—especially noticeable on electron microscopy (Asakura et al 1981, Bujanover et al 1981, Riemann and Schmidt 1981).

The intestinal lymphatic dilation is frequently part of a more widespread congenital abnormality. Pomerantz and Waldmann (1963) and Mistilis, Skyring and Stephen (1965) showed ectasia of some and absence of other lymphatics in lower extremity lymphangiograms in patients with intestinal lymphangiectasia. Intestinal lymphangiectasia should always be suspected in childhood or adolescent onset of bilateral leg oedema (Gallo-Van Ess, Strasburger and Turetsky 1986). A generalised lymphangiectasia involving intestine, lung, and lymph nodes was accompanied by thymic hypoplasia in the case described by Sorensen et al (1985). It is also claimed that any lymphatic obstruction, whether due to malignancy, fibrosis (Rubin and Dobbins 1965, Belaiche et al 1980), or simply congestive cardiac failure (Waldmann 1970), may produce a similar picture. Lymphangiectasia is said to occur in Behçet's disease (Asakura et al 1973), but the illustrations in that report are far from convincing; an electron microscopic abnormality that they describe was present in only 1 of 16

Figure 14–14. Jejunal biopsy in intestinal lymphangiectasia. Bloated villous tip with dilated lymphatic vessels (PAS ×280).

Figure 14–15. Jejunal biopsy in intestinal lymphangiectasia to show PAS-positive macrophages around the lymphatic spaces (PAS ×280).

cases. None of the patients had hypoproteinaemia. The coexistence of intestinal lymphangiectasia and the nephrotic syndrome (de Sousa et al 1968) also requires further investigation, but the association with macroglobulinaemia (Harris, Burton and Scarffe 1983) seems more than fortuitous. The increased viscosity of the lymph as a consequence on its high IgM content may be important in the pathogenesis. Bolton, Cotter and Losowsky (1986) also described an association with impaired neutrophil function, and the condition has been reported as a consequence of combined radiotherapy and chemotherapy (Rao, Dundas and Holdsworth 1987). Chemotherapy for coexisting lymphoma, conversely, has been shown to cause remission of the gastrointestinal effects of congenital lymphangiectasia (Shpilberg et al 1993). The condition occasionally complicates autoimmune disease (Bereket et al 1995) but is rarely a cause of acute ileus (Lenzhofer et al 1993). Intestinal lymphangiectasia must be distinguished from lymphangiectatic cysts (Shilken, Zerman and Blackwell 1968), which usually have no clinical significance. These occur particularly in the jejunum in 20% of necropsies, usually in patients older than 55 years of age (Aase and Gundersen 1983). The cysts are up to 1 cm in diameter and often multiple; biopsy specimens may be taken during life (Fig. 14–16). The dilated lymphatic spaces are large and irregular, and they usually affect the submucosa. Sometimes the villi are involved, but in contrast to lymphangiectasia, several adjacent villi appear distorted by large and irregular lymphatic spaces, whereas their neighbours are entirely normal. There may be lipid-containing histiocytes, found not in the lamina propria but within the lymphatic spaces. The spaces frequently contain pink inspissated lymph rich in neutral fat. A further contrast with diffuse intestinal lymphangiectasia is that lipofuscinosis is not seen. However, lymphangiectatic cysts have also been described in otherwise characteristic lymphangiectasia (Barnes and DeRidder 1993), but it is of interest that, despite the claim, laboratory studies failed to show coincidental fat and protein loss from the bowel, casting some doubt on the validity of the observation.

Figure 14–16. Lymphangiectatic cyst in jejunum. Large irregular spaces distort the villous pattern and contain coagulated lymph and macrophages. The villi adjacent to the lesion are normal (PAS ×17).

ALLERGIC GASTROENTEROPATHY AND FOOD ALLERGY

A condition that requires more precise definition is allergic gastroenteropathy (Waldmann et al 1967). These authors described a protein-losing enteropathy occurring in children who also show anaemia, eosinophilia, and growth retardation. The jejunum had a normal villous architecture or minor abnormalities, but there was an eosinophilic infiltration in the lamina propria. Sometimes there was associated asthma, eczema, and rhinitis. An allergy to ingested milk protein was suggested; further claims for such an entity were made by Businco et al (1985) and Challacombe, Wheeler and Campbell (1986). One of the problems is to decide where in the spectrum of food allergy in general the condition of allergic gastroenteropathy as a specific entity occurs. Urticarial reactions, oedema, eczema, and asthmatic attacks may be precipitated by certain foodstuffs (Walker-Smith 1978, Lancet 1979). Van Spreeuwel et al (1984) also claimed that allergy to foodstuff may be reflected in an increase in IgE plasma cells in the mucosa of the upper gastrointestinal tract. The relationship of so-called allergic gastroenteropathy to milk protein intolerance needs clarification. The evidence suggests they are related but that they possibly differ in magnitude. Advances in immunology in the last few years and a greater understanding of the immediate hypersensitivity reaction have opened up a new and vast field for further investigation. It could be suggested, for example, that the effects of parasitic infestations, the mechanisms of some causes of protein-losing enteropathy, and such diseases as pylorospasm, colonic spasm, "idiopathic" diarrhoea and proctitis, nausea, and upper abdominal pain are all mediated through the mechanism of local anaphylaxis. The morphological features of hyperaemia, oedema, eosinophil leukocyte and lymphocyte infiltration, and degranulation of basophils, among other conditions, need only be transient, and biopsy examination carried out when major symptoms have subsided would be normal.

The problem of allergic gastroenteropathy was put into perspective by the report of Cooper et al (1980) describing eight adult patients with abdominal pain and diarrhoea. The only abnormalities in jejunal morphology were an increase in plasma cells, a decrease in lymphocytes in the lamina propria, and an increase in intraepithelial lymphocytes. These patients had their symptoms greatly relieved by a gluten-free diet, but there was a return of symptoms when gluten was reintroduced.

The problem of food allergy is probably greater in children and often involves several food substances in the same patients. The jejunal biopsy is usually reported as normal (Minford, MacDonald and Littlewood 1982). There are abdominal symptoms, and eczema, urticaria, oedema, and asthma may occur. There is some evidence that patients with eczema and food allergy have an abnormally increased molecular permeability of their bowel wall (Jackson et al 1981). Thus, it is of interest that atopic children without gastrointestinal symptoms often show eosinophil infiltration and minor villous abnormalities on jejunal biopsy (Kokkonen, Simila and Herva 1980). In children with mucosal abnormalities in cow's milk protein intolerance and in adults with a variety of food allergies, Rosekrans et al (1980) claimed to show an increase in plasma cells containing IgE in the lamina propria. More research to establish a morphological or physiological basis for allergic reaction in relation to food substances is needed. Kikindjanin et al (1985), for example, described a case of recurrent urticaria and diarrhoea in which impaired intestinal mucosal immunity could be implicated. Allergic gastroenteropathy has also been described in association with the inhalation of mites in household dust (Toyoshima et al 1994). Moon and Kleinman (1995) concluded that the symptoms may be those of classic allergy or may include diarrhoea, malabsorption, and protein-losing enteropathy but that the immunopathogenesis is still not clearly understood. The author of this book has seen significant changes in small bowel morphology in association with putative food allergy, and these changes and symptomatology have resolved when the allergen was removed from the diet. There is minor villous stunting, increased cellularity of the lamina propria, and a pronounced eosinophil component that sometimes occurs as microabscesses in the epithelium of the crypts (Figs. 14–17 to 14–19).

Figure 14–17. Jejunal biopsy in allergic enteropathy. There is obvious hypercellularity of the lamina propria (H&E ×150).

LIPOFUSCINOSIS

In any case of hypoalbuminaemia, the muscularis mucosae and occasional histiocytes in the lamina propria and submucosa of the jejunal biopsy may show lipofuscin pigmentation (Fig. 14–20). It is probably found in these sites only when pigmentation of other smooth muscle is fairly heavy. The muscularis propria of the bowel wall is usually heavily infiltrated, so much so that the bowel is obviously discoloured macroscopically. The condition is sometimes called brown-bowel syndrome. The pigment is PAS-positive, autofluorescent in ultraviolet light, can be

Figure 14–18. Detail of Figure 14–17. Eosinophil leukocytes are present in the epithelium (H&E ×250).

Figure 14–19. Eosinophils are sometimes present as intraepithelial microabscesses *(arrowhead)* (H&E ×250).

stained by Sudan black, and is usually acid-fast with Ziehl-Neelsen stain. The significance of the pigmentation is not fully understood but is thought to be related to vitamin E deficiency (Ansanelli and Lane 1957, Tofler, Hukill and Spiro 1963, Binder et al 1965, Hosler, Kimmel and Moeller 1982) and hypoalbuminaemia (Richards 1959). In human jejunal biopsy material, when lipofuscin pigmentation is seen, hypoalbuminaemia is almost always present; this is probably explained by the close interrelationship between vitamin E and protein metabolism (Fox 1967). Lipofuscin production is thought to be the result of a progressive oxidation of various cellular

Figure 14–20. Jejunal biopsy in hypoalbuminaemia due to gluten-sensitive enteropathy. The muscularis mucosal cells contain lipofuscin pigment *(arrowheads)* (H&E ×300).

constituents (Lancet 1970), and it is seen in a variety of body tissues as a normal concomitant of aging. Deficiency of a potent antioxidant such as vitamin E might therefore be expected to contribute to an accelerated and excessive production of this pigment. Certainly, cases are recorded of disappearance of the pigment following vitamin E supplements (Lee and Nicholson 1976). In an ultrastructural study, Foster (1979) compared the abnormalities in smooth muscle with skeletal muscle changes in myopathies of mitochondrial origin and proposed that lipofuscinosis be considered a smooth muscle myopathy. These mitochondrial changes seen by electron microscopy have been confirmed (Horn et al 1985). However, in most instances the condition appears to be secondary to a systemic disease, sometimes in the bowel itself (Gallager 1980), and is regularly described in association with coeliac disease (Connolly et al 1994). In coeliac disease, the underlying vitamin E deficiency has been linked with the increased susceptibility in this condition to gastrointestinal malignancy (Reynaert et al 1993). There is doubt whether the pigmentation interferes significantly with muscle function (Stamp and Evans 1987), although claims for this are still being made (Ruchti, Eisele and Kaufmann 1990, Narvaez-Rodriguez et al 1993). Lin et al (1993) described two cases presenting as intestinal pseudo-obstruction.

DISACCHARIDASE DEFICIENCIES

In isolated disaccharidase deficiency, no detectable abnormality of the jejunal mucosa can be demonstrated in the light microscope or by conventional electron microscopy. Where there are morphological abnormalities in the jejunal biopsies, all the disaccharidases measured (lactase, maltase, and sucrase) are depressed. Results of estimating villous surface area by relating it to volume indicate that depression of disaccharidase levels is a sensitive index of decrease in villous surface area, i.e., villous atrophy. For example, the depression of enzymes in the jejunal mucosa in pernicious anaemia is much less than in untreated coeliac disease. Moreover, in coeliac disease during treatment by gluten-exclusion diet, the enzyme level corresponds closely with the extent of persistent villous atrophy, returning to normal only when the villous pattern is normal (Pena et al 1972, Pena, Truclove and Whitehead 1972). In an electron microscopic study Phillips et al (1980) showed that in secondary disaccharidase deficiency there is a correlation between enzyme levels and the surface area of the microvilli. This is what might be predicted because the enzymes are located in that site. It has been shown that disaccharidases can be demonstrated on light microscopy in resin-embedded sections, whereas in the past frozen sections were advocated (Hand 1987). In a retrospective assessment of the clinical value of disaccharidase analysis, it has been shown that the measurement should be reserved for the investigation of sucrase-alpha-dextrinase deficiency (Duncan et al 1994).

RADIATION INJURY

This is discussed more fully in the section on irradiation colitis in Chapter 17. The small intestine, however, is more sensitive than the colon to the effects of irradiation, but from external sources it receives better protection from the body wall. The lesions parallel those described in the colon, with an early phase of mucosal degeneration followed by recovery and, later, more chronic reaction with persistent ulceration, scarring, and fistula formation. In the acute phase, the features of which were described by Trier and Browning (1966), a reduction in crypt mitoses is the first change, and then cell damage becomes evident. The dividing cells in the crypts are most severely affected and are shed into the lumen. The decreased production of cells results in shortening of crypts and villi, and Paneth's cells are reduced in number. The goblet cells and absorptive cells are shorter than normal, and there may be an increase in nuclear size and abnormalities of shape. Lymphocytes in the lamina propria disappear and plasma cells increase in number. An infiltrate of polymorphs in response to cell damage occurs, and cell debris and neutrophils occupy some of the crypts. These changes take place in the 3 weeks after exposure and revert to normal if exposure ceases over the next 2 weeks. Late changes develop and cause symptoms any time from 2 months to 20 years after exposure. In some instances, the chronic changes are responsible for malabsorption (Tankel, Clark and Lee 1965), which probably has a varied range of causes. In the event of strictures and intestinal stasis, the defect has the same cause as other stagnant loop syndromes and is related to bacterial colonisation of the bowel. This leads to disturbances in bile salt deconjugation and the deleterious effect that this has on fat absorption (Tabaqchali and Booth 1970). Malabsorption, however, may also be related to residual mucosal damage, and changes may be seen in small intestine biopsy material. The features of old irradiation injury that may be seen include a varying amount of villous atrophy, in the extreme case so severe as to produce a flat mucosa. There may also be an increase in round cells in the lamina propria, but a striking feature is the fibrosis than can occur in this zone (Fig. 14–21). This is often accompanied by hypoplasia and distortion due to atrophy of the crypts, and in the submucosa typical small vessel hyalinisation is present.

STORAGE DISEASES

Owing to an increasing sophistication of biochemical and electron microscope technology, there is a rapidly growing list of inborn errors of metabolism that result in the excessive formation and storage of a number of different substances. Usually the genetic disorder results in excessive accumulation of a normal metabolite owing to a defect in an enzyme involved in its metabolism, or there is similar accumulation of an abnormal substance produced as the result of the unsuccessful operation of an alternative biochemical pathway. The enzymes involved are frequently lysosomal, and the disorders are sometimes collectively known as lysosomal storage disorders. They have been grouped together according to certain similarities that have traditionally been described under such headings as "glycogen storage diseases," "glycogenoses," "lipoidoses," and "mucopolysaccharidoses," according to the

Figure 14–21. Jejunal mucosa shows villous atrophy and fibrosis of the lamina propria due to irradiation (H&E ×113).

group of macromolecular substances that accumulate. These storage abnormalities are responsible for the distention and vacuolation of affected cells, and different combinations of tissue and organ involvement have allowed reasonably specific clinical subgroups to be defined. These are the subject of a comprehensive review by Glew et al (1985), who classified lysosomal storage disease into the sphingolipidoses, glycoproteinoses, mucolipidoses, mucopolysaccharidoses, and others such as cystinosis, Pompe's disease, Wolman's disease, and cholesterol ester storage disease. Not all these subtypes are associated with involvement of the gastrointestinal tract, but when it is involved, the abnormality may be recognised in biopsy tissues. When there is colonic involvement, a rectal biopsy is obviously preferred, but small bowel involvement interferes with function and may lead to a small biopsy procedure. There is a modern trend, however, for biochemical determination of the diagnosis of lysosomal storage disease in samples of chorionic villi obtained early in pregnancy (Kerr 1984). This allows termination of pregnancy and thus avoids the birth of babies with devastating physical and mental defects for which there is currently no therapy.

Malabsorption is rarely due to small intestine involvement in Fabry's disease, an X-linked disorder of lipid metabolism caused by a deficiency of ceramide trihexosidase. Flynn et al (1972) reported a case with jejunal biopsy appearances characterised by a normal villous pattern but with abnormalities of the blood vessels, submucosal neurones, and muscularis mucosae. The neurones were enlarged and vacuolated; they stained positively with Sudan black and Luxol fast blue; and the blood vessels and muscularis mucosae contained birefringent deposits of sudanophilic material that stained positively with Luxol fast blue. This material is the sphingolipid ceramide trihexose. In an electron microscope study, O'Brien et al (1982) ascribed the diarrhoea that may occur in these cases to secondary intestinal bacterial overgrowth This is the consequence of stasis secondary to the neural and muscle deposits. Sheth et al (1981) noted a high rate of occurrence of gastrointestinal symptoms in the 50 patients in their series, and Jardine et al (1994) described frank small bowel ischaemia due to the small vessel changes. Ganglion cell involvement also occurs in Niemann-Pick disease. Dinari et al (1980) also described lipid-filled histiocytes in the lamina propria in jejunal biopsies in this condition and suggested the intestinal involvement is more frequent than hitherto recognised in the type A disease. Involvement of the lamina propria by histiocytes swollen with lipid is recognised in the small as well as the large intestine in cholesterol ester storage disease, Tangier disease, and Wolman's disease. Dincsoy et al (1984) also described nonbirefringent autofluorescent granules within histiocytes in the duodenum in cholesterol ester storage disease. Electron microscopic changes were described by Partin and Schubert (1969) and Tylki-Szymanska et al (1987). It is likely that as this group of diseases becomes more frequently recognised and investigated, intestinal involvement will be described more commonly.

CYSTINOSIS

Morecki, Paunier and Hamilton (1968) reported changes in jejunal biopsy tissues in a case of cystinosis. In ordinary hematoxylin and eosin–stained sections of formalin-fixed, paraffin-embedded material, no abnormalities were present, but in 1-μm sections of epoxy resin–embedded material, changes were present that were later confirmed by electron microscopy. Angular spaces corresponding to the shape of cystine crystals were prominent in the lamina propria and located in an intracellular site within histiocytes. A proportion of the surface absorptive cells contained vacuoles. Some of these were small and basally situated in a subnuclear position, but others were large and appeared in a supranuclear site in the region of Golgi's apparatus.

ACRODERMATITIS ENTEROPATHICA

This is a rare familial disorder with autosomal recessive inheritance. Chronic dermatitis of the oro-anal regions and the extremities, along with baldness, are associated with diarrhoea and failure to thrive. No consistent abnormality of the jejunal mucosa is seen on light microscopy. Electron microscopy, however, reveals abnormal inclusion bodies in Paneth's cells. These resemble abnormal granules but could represent lysosomes, although they have been shown to be acid phosphatase–negative. In view of the high zinc content of normal Paneth's cells and the response of this disease to zinc therapy, it has been postulated that a Paneth's cell abnormality is concerned in its aetiology. Bohane et al (1977), however, examined Paneth's cells before and after treatment and showed that the lysosome-like inclusions or altered granules disappear following therapy. Accordingly, the authors claimed that Paneth's cell abnormalities could be caused by a primary zinc deficiency.

METAPLASIA

The intestinal crypts on occasion may be replaced by simple mucous glands of pyloric type (Fig. 14–22). These always occur above the muscularis mucosa, and because of this the change is often referred to as pyloric gland metaplasia rather than Brunner's gland metaplasia. It is simply a manifestation of the marked metaplastic potential of the epithelium of the gastrointestinal tract as a whole. This metaplasia rarely, if ever, occurs unless there is or has been ulceration in the vicinity, and this is clearly of diagnostic importance when seen in jejunal or other small intestine biopsy material.

As already mentioned in the section dealing with the duodenum, the superficial epithelium of the small intestine undergoes metaplasia to a type that is typical of the superficial gastric epithelium (Fig. 14–23). It is seen in the duodenum or jejunum in conditions of high gastric acid secretion (James 1964, Rhodes 1964), but like pyloric metaplasia it may also appear near areas of ulceration, and both are particularly frequent as part of the histological spectrum of Crohn's disease of the small intestine. It is an easy matter to distinguish these appearances from those seen when true heterotopic gastric mucosa (Fig. 14–24) occurs in the small intestine.

Figure 14–22. Jejunal biopsy near ulceration due to Crohn's disease. There is crypt hyperplasia and villous atrophy with pyloric gland metaplasia *(arrow)* (H&E ×75).

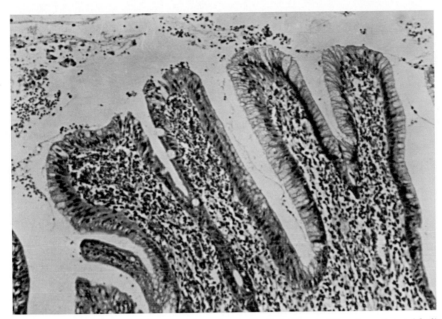

Figure 14–23. Jejunal biopsy near ulceration due to Crohn's disease. The absorptive epithelium was replaced largely by metaplastic gastric superficial epithelium (H&E ×375).

HAEMOSIDERIN PIGMENTATION

Frequently the lamina propria in the tips of villi contain groups of macrophages filled with haemosiderin granules (Fig. 14–25). This occurs normally but is much more frequent after oral or parenteral iron administration. In transfusional haemosiderosis, the appearances are accentuated and sometimes pigmented macrophages appear to be traversing the epithelium. The epithelial cells themselves do not contain iron, in contrast to the appearances in haemochromatosis (Astaldi, Meardi and Lisino 1966). In addition to the epithelial haemosiderin, the pattern of distribution

Figure 14–24. Ectopic gastric mucosa (left) in the duodenum (right) (H&E ×38).

Figure 14–25. Jejunal villous tip containing macro-phages *(arrowheads)* filled with haemosiderin (Perls's ×500).

of the pigment macrophages is also different. In haemochromatosis the pattern tends to be more diffusely scattered throughout the lamina propria and around vessels, a distribution similar to that shown by the iron-containing macrophages in Whipple's disease. A rare case of haemosiderosis of the ileum has been described (Ghadially, Boone and Walley 1994).

PSEUDOMELANOSIS DUODENI

Since its recognition in the early days of fibreoptic endoscopy (Bisordi and Kleinman 1976), there have been several case reports of this curious pigmentation of the duodenal mucosa. It affects the bulb and often the second part. The mucosa has a speckled dark-brown or black appearance that is due to pigment accumulation in the lysosomes of lamina propria macrophages at the tips of villi (Fig. 14–26). The pigment has been analysed by electron probe and shown to contain iron and sulphur as ferric sulphide (Pounder et al 1982, Kang et al 1987, Rex and Jersild 1988). It usually, but not always, stains positively with Perls's and the PAS method and occasionally with Masson-Fontana as does true melanin. The condition has been ascribed to the ingestion of a variety of drugs, and there is an association with hypertension and renal failure. It is apparently more common in black females, but it has been described in Asians and whites (Yamase, Norris and Gillies 1985, Gupta and Weinstock 1986, Lee, O'Donnell and Keren 1987, Castellano et al 1988, Kuo and Wu 1988, Lin et al 1988, West 1988).

MEASLES GIANT CELLS AND CYTOMEGALOVIRUS INCLUSIONS

Giant cells may occur in the jejunal mucosa during the prodromal phase of measles, as they may in other lymphoid tissues, and thus can be seen on occasion in biopsy tissues from all areas of the gastrointestinal tract. Watson and Parkin (1970) illustrated these cells as an incidental finding in a patient who was subjected to

Figure 14–26. Duodenal appearance in pseudomelanosis. The pigment is much more prominent and blacker than the brown colour of haemosiderin pigmentation in routine H&E sections (H&E ×500).

biopsy as part of the investigation for a malabsorption syndrome. The patient had a typical flat mucosa, characteristic of gluten-sensitive enteropathy, and measles giant cells in the lamina propria. The rash ensued 4 days after the biopsy was performed.

Cytomegalovirus inclusions in the epithelial cells of the stomach have already been mentioned. The increasing number of patients receiving immunosuppressive therapy has led to an increase in secondary cytomegalovirus infection in adults, and involvement of the gastrointestinal tract is common (Henson 1972). Primary cytomegalovirus infection of the small bowel is distinctly uncommon (Dent et al 1975). The typical inclusions are intranuclear and separated from the nuclear membrane by a clear halo. Less frequently, PAS-positive intracytoplasmic inclusions occur. Inclusions may be located in lamina propria fibroblasts and capillary endothelial cells as well as the epithelial cells.

GRANULOMAS

The significance of granulomas in jejunal biopsy material poses the same problem as when they occur in other areas of the gastrointestinal tract. As already discussed in the section concerning gastric sarcoidosis (see Chapter 9), granulomas usually prove to be a manifestation of generalised sarcoidosis, of Crohn's disease, or of some other chronic granulomatous disease, e.g., tuberculosis. Hermos et al (1970) reported two patients in whom the diagnosis of Crohn's disease of the upper small intestine was verified by finding granulomas in peroral duodenal biopsy specimens. Rarely, however, are granulomas found in biopsies that are otherwise normal (Fig. 14–27); sometimes they are found in biopsies showing the apparently unrelated lesions of gluten-sensitive enteropathy (Fig. 14–28). Their presence in these circumstances defies adequate explanation, although Bjorneklett et al (1977) described disappearance of the granulomas in response to gluten exclusion in a similar case.

HISTOPLASMOSIS

Involvement of the gastrointestinal tract in this fungal disease is discussed in more detail in Chapter 17. Predominant involvement of the small intestine, although

Figure 14–27. Jejunal biopsy is normal except for an epithelioid and giant cell granuloma in the lamina propria (H&E ×280).

Figure 14–28. Jejunal biopsy in a patient who responded later to a gluten-free diet. The mucosa shows a crypt hyperplastic type of villous atrophy with an epithelioid and giant cell granuloma in the lamina propria (H&E ×105).

Figure 14–29. Jejunal involvement in histoplasmosis. Pale foamy histiocytes, some with rounded cytoplasmic inclusions (H&E ×450).

rare, does occur, and a jejunal biopsy diagnosis is thus possible. Sometimes a malabsorption syndrome (Orchard, Luparello and Brunskill 1979) or a protein-losing enteropathy (Bank et al 1965) results. In a single case seen by the author, diagnosis was a simple matter once the condition was considered. There was total villous atrophy and lateral separation of the crypts due to an inflammatory infiltrate and the presence of typical histiocytes containing the organisms that displayed a pronounced PAS-positive capsule (Figs. 14–29 and 14–30). The histopathology of

Figure 14–30. Detail of histiocytes to show numerous encapsulated yeast forms of histoplasmosis (PAS ×850).

Langerhans's cell histiocytosis was reviewed (Favara and Jaffe 1994) and Beverley and Abbas (1994) discussed its pathophysiology.

MASTOCYTOSIS

The literature concerning mastocytosis and mast cell involvement of the small intestine was reviewed by Scott, Hardy and Losowsky (1975). They described a case and discussed its relationship to gluten-sensitive enteropathy, which appears to be more than fortuitous. In addition to mast cell infiltration of the lamina propria, there may be a crypt hyperplastic villous atrophy that reverts to normal following gluten exclusion. Blunting and shortening of villi with crypt hyperplasia, however, may be seen in mastocytosis of the jejunum in the absence of gluten sensitivity (Belcon et al 1980, Braverman, Dollberg and Shiner 1985). Cases with a simple increase in lamina propria mast cells and otherwise normal jejunal morphology have also been described (Reisberg and Oyakawa 1987). The whole subject of gastrointestinal dysfunction in mastocytosis, including hyperchlorhydria and either duodenitis or duodenal ulcer, was reviewed by Cherner et al (1988).

HISTIOCYTOSIS X

Keeling and Harries (1973) reported an infant with unequivocal evidence of intestinal malabsorption associated with histiocytic involvement of the small intestine lamina propria. They also examined autopsy tissues from 11 fatal cases that revealed small intestine involvement in almost 50%.

MYELOID METAPLASIA

The gut is rarely the site of extramedullary haematopoiesis. Schreibman et al (1988) described small bowel involvement in a patient with myelofibrosis.

SYPHILITIC ENTERITIS

Syphilitic involvement of the gastrointestinal tract usually involves the rectum. Schlossberg et al (1984) described a seemingly unique example of symptomatic small bowel relapsing secondary syphilis characterised by partial villous atrophy, crypt hyperplasia, and pronounced plasma cell infiltration of the lamina propria. The mucosa returned to normal following 2 months of antisyphilitic therapy.

EFFECT OF CYTOTOXIC DRUGS

In humans (Cunningham et al 1985) and in experimental animals (Moore 1984), cytotoxic drugs used in the therapy of cancer have been shown to cause damage to intestinal crypt cells. Whereas mature epithelium is unaffected, immature cells in the crypts show vacuolation on light microscopy; on electron microscopy they were seen to be due to large secondary lysosomes containing partially degraded fragments of damaged crypt cells.

INFANTILE SYSTEMIC HYALINOSIS

Hyaline material is deposited in the skin, gastrointestinal tract, adrenals, bladder, skeletal muscles, thymus, parathyroids, and other sites in this presumed autosomal recessive disease. The hyaline material is characteristically laid down in lamina propria and submucosa of the stomach and intestine. It leads to intractable diarrhoea and malabsorption and is usually fatal within the first 2 years of life (Landing and Nodorra 1986). A recent review of this rare disorder, including electron microscopic observations and report of a case in a black infant, was given by Sahn et al (1994).

ATHEROMATOUS EMBOLI

Rarely, small intestine biopsy reveals evidence of small vessel embolisation by atheromatous material. Socinski et al (1984) described a case of a patient diagnosed on jejunal biopsy who presented with diarrhoea.

REFERENCES—SECTION THREE: SMALL INTESTINE BIOPSY

Aase S. and Gundersen R. (1983) Submucous lymphatic cysts of the small intestine. Acta Pathologica, Microbiologica et Immunologica Scandinavica 91:191–194.

Abbas Z., Qureshi A.A., Sheikh H., Jafri S.M. and Khan A.H. (1994) Peculiar histopathological features of giardiasis in distal duodenal biopsies. Journal of the Pakistani Medical Association 44:206–209.

Achkar E., Carey W.D., Petras R., Sivak M.V. and Revta R. (1986) Comparison of suction capsule and endoscopic biopsy of small bowel mucosa. Gastrointestinal Endoscopy 32:278–281.

Adam M., Morgan O., Persaud C. and Gibbs W.N. (1973) Hyperinfection syndrome with strongyloides stercoralis in malignant lymphoma. British Medical Journal 1:264–266.

Aherne W.A. and Dunnill M.S. (1982) Morphometry. London: Edward Arnold.

Ajdukiewicz A.B., Youngs G.R. and Bouchier I.A.D. (1972) Nodular lymphoid hypoplasia with hypogammaglobulinaemia. Gut 13:589–595.

Aloy-Duch A., Callejero Baguena A., Murcia Mesa C., Leal Perez J.R., Fernandez Rosaenz H., Paz Pachon R. and Bombi Latorre J.A. (1993) Colonic obstruction in Whipple's disease. Revista Espānola de Enfermedades Digestivas 84:263–266.

Ament M.E. (1975) Immunodeficiency syndromes and gastro-intestinal disease. Pediatric Clinics of North America 22:807–825.

Ament M.E. (1985) Immunodeficiency syndromes of the gut. Scandinavian Journal of Gastroenterology 20 (suppl 114):127–135.

Ament M.E. and Ochs H. (1973) Gastrointestinal manifestations of chronic granulomatous disease. New England Journal of Medicine 288:382–387.

Ament M.E., Ochs H.D. and Davis S.D. (1973) Structure and function of the gastrointestinal tract in primary immunodeficiency syndromes. Medicine 52:227–248.

Ament M.E. and Rubin C.E. (1972) Soy protein—another cause of the flat intestinal lesion. Gastroenterology 62:227–234.

Anand B.S., Kumar M., Chakravarti R.N., Sehgal A.K. and Chhuttani P.N. (1980) Pathogenesis of malabsorption in Giardia infection: an experimental study in rats. Transactions of the Royal Society of Tropical Medicine and Hygiene 74:565–569.

Anand B.S., Piris J., Jerrome D.W., Offord R.E. and Truelove S.C. (1981) The timing of histological damage following a single challenge with gluten in treated coeliac disease. Quarterly Journal of Medicine 197:83–94.

Andersson H., Bjorkman A-C., Gillberg R., Kastrup W., Mobacken H. and Stockbrugger R. (1984) Influence of the amount of dietary gluten on gastrointestinal morphology and function in dermatitis herpetiformis. Human Nutrition: Clinical Nutrition 38C:279–285.

Ansanelli V. Jr and Lane N. (1957) Lipochrome (ceroid) pigmentation of the small intestine. Annals of Surgery 146:117–123.

Aronson A.R. and Norfleet R.G. (1962) The duodenal mucosa in peptic ulcer disease: a clinical pathological correlation. American Journal of Digestive Diseases 7:506–514.

Asakura H., Miura S., Morishita T., Aiso S., Tanaka T., Kitahora T., Tsuchiya M., Enomoto Y. and Watanabe Y. (1981) Endoscopic and histopathological study on primary and secondary intestinal lymphangiectasia. Digestive Diseases and Sciences 26:312–320.

Asakura H., Morita A., Morishita T., Tsuchiya M., Watanabe Y. and Enomoto Y. (1973) Histopathological and electron microscopic studies of lymphangiectasia of the small intestine in Behçet's disease. Gut 14:196–203.

Asakura H., Tsuchiya M., Katoh S., Kobayashi K., Yonei Y., Yoshida T., Hamada Y., Miura S., Morita A., Kuramochi S. and Teramoto T. (1986) Pathological findings of lymphangiectasia of the large intestine in a patient with protein-losing enteropathy. Gastroenterology 91:719–724.

Asselah F., Slavin G., Sowter G. and Asselah H. (1983) Immunoproliferative small intestinal disease in Algerians: light microscopic and immunochemical studies. Cancer 52:227–237.

Astaldi G., Meardi G. and Lisino T. (1966) The iron content of jejunal mucosa obtained by Crosby's biopsy in haemochromatosis and haemosiderosis. Blood 28:70–82.

Atwell J.D., Burge D. and Wright D. (1985) Nodular lymphoid hyperplasia of the intestinal tract in infancy and childhood. Journal of Pediatric Surgery 20:25–29.

Austad W.I., Cornes J.S., Gough K.R., McCarthy C.F. and Read A.E. (1967) Steatorrhea and malignant lymphoma. American Journal of Digestive Diseases 12:475–490.

Austin L.L. and Dobbins W.O. (1988) Studies of the rectal mucosa in coeliac sprue: the intraepithelial lymphocyte. Gut 29:200–205.

Avery G.B., Villavicencio O., Lilly J.R. and Randolph J.G. (1968) Intractable diarrhea in early infancy. Pediatrics 41:712–722.

Babaryka I., Thorn L. and Langer E. (1979) Epithelioid cell granulomata in the mucosa of the small intestine in Whipple's disease. Virchows Archiv A 382:227–235.

Baker S.J. (1973) Geographical variations in the morphology of the small intestinal mucosa in apparently healthy individuals. Pathologia et Microbiologia 39:222–237.

Baker S.J., Ignatius M., Mathan V.I., Vaish S.K. and Chacko C.C. (1962) Intestinal Biopsy. Edited by G.E. Wolstenholme and M.P. Cameron (Study Group No. 14). London: Ciba Foundation, p 184.

Baker S.J. and Mathan V.I. (1970) In: Modern Trends in Gastroenterology. Volume 4. Edited by W.I. Card and B. Creamer. London: Butterworth, p 198.

Baker S.J., Mathan M., Mathan V.I., Jesudoss S. and Swaminathan S.P. (1982) Chronic enterocyte infection with coronavirus: one possible cause of the syndrome of tropical sprue? Digestive Diseases and Sciences 27:1039–1043.

Baklien K., Brandtzaeg P. and Fausa O. (1977) Immunoglobulins in jejunal mucosa and serum from patients with adult coeliac disease. Scandinavian Journal of Gastroenterology 12:149–159.

Balazs M. and Szatloczky E. (1978) Electron microscopic examination of the mucosa of the small intestine in infection due to *Giardia lamblia*. Pathology Research and Practice 163:251–260.

Bank S., Trey C., Gans I., Marks I.N. and Groll A. (1965) Histoplasmosis of the small bowel with "giant" intestinal villi and secondary protein-losing enteropathy. American Journal of Medicine 39:492–504.

Banwell J.G., Hutt M.S.R. and Tunnicliffe R. (1964) Observations on jejunal biopsy in Ugandan Africans. East African Medical Journal 41:46–54.

Barandun D., Riva G. and Spengler G.A. (1968) Immunological deficiency diseases in man. In: Birth Defects. Original article series IV, 1. Edited by D. Bergsma and R.A. Good. New York: The National Foundation—March of Dimes, p 40.

Barbieri D., de Brito T., Hoshino S., Nasciemento O.B., Martins-Campos J.V., Quarentei G. and Marcondes E. (1970) Giardiasis in childhood: absorption tests and biochemistry, histochemistry, light, and electron microscopy of jejunal mucosa. Archives of Disease in Childhood 45:466–472.

Bardella M.T., Molteni N., Quatrini M., Velio P., Ranzi T. and Bianchi P.A. (1985) Clinical, biochemical and histological abnormalities in adult celiac patients on gluten-free diet. Gastroenterologie Clinique et Biologique 9:787–789.

Barnes G.L. and Townley R.R.W. (1973) Duodenal mucosal damage in 31 infants with gastroenteritis. Archives of Disease in Childhood 48:343–349.

Barnes R.E. and DeRidder P.H. (1993) Fat absorption in patients with functional intestinal lymphangiectasia and lymphangiectic cysts. American Journal of Gastroenterology 88:887–890.

Barry R.E., Morris J.S. and Read A.E.A. (1970) A case of small intestinal mucosal atrophy. Gut 11:743–747.

Bartnick W., ReMine S.G., Chiba M., Thayer W.R. and Shorter R.G. (1980) Isolation and characterization of colonic intraepithelial and lamina proprial lymphocytes. Gastroenterology 78:976–985.

Bassen F.A. and Kornzweig A.L. (1950) Malformation of the erythrocytes in a case of atypical retinitis pigmentosa. Blood 5:381–387.

Bastlein C., Decking R., Voeth C. and Ottenjann R. (1988) Giant Brunneroma of the duodenum. Endoscopy 20:154–155.

Baudin J.B. M.D. thesis, University of Paris, 1837. Ostow J.D. and Resnick R.H. (1959) Annals of Internal Medicine: 51, 1303.

Bayless T.M., Kapelowitz R.F., Shelley W.M., Ballinger W.F. and Hendrix T.R. (1967) Intestinal ulceration—a complication of coeliac disease. New England Journal of Medicine 276:996–1002

Beck I.T., Kahn D.S., Lacerte M., Solymar J., Callegarini U. and Geokas M.C. (1965) Chronic duodenitis. Gut 6:376–383.

Belaiche J., Vesin P., Chaumette M.T., Julien M. and Cattan D. (1980) Lymphangiectasies intestinales et fibrose des ganglions mesenteriques. Gastroenterologie Clinique et Biologique 4:52–58.

Belcon M.C., Collins S.M., Castelli M.F. and Qizilbash A.H. (1980) Gastrointestinal hemorrhage in mastocytosis. Cancer Medical Association Journal 122:311–314.

Bereket A., Lowenheim M., Blethen S.L., Kane P. and Wilson T.A. (1995) Intestinal lymphangiectasia in a patient with autoimmune polyglandular disease type I and steatorrhea. Journal of Clinical Endocrinology and Metabolism 80:933–935.

Beverley P.C. and Abbas A.K. (1994) The scientific challenge of Langerhans cell histiocytosis. British Journal of Cancer (suppl 23):s61–s63.

Biasco G., Callegari C., Lami F., Minarini A., Miglioli M. and Barbara L. (1984) Intestinal morphological changes during oral refeeding in a patient previously treated with total parenteral nutrition for small bowel resection. Americal Journal of Gastroenterology 79:585–588.

Biggs B-A., Megna R., Wickremesinghe S. and Dwyer B. (1987) Human infection with *Cryptosporidium* spp.: results of a 24-month survey. Medical Journal of Australia 147:175–177.

Binder H.J., Herting D.C., Hurst V., Finch S.C. and Spiro H.M. (1965) Tocopherol deficiency in man. New England Journal of Medicine 273:1289–1297.

Bird R.G. and Smith M.D. (1980) Cryptosporidiosis in man: parasite life cycle and fine structure pathology. Journal of Pathology 132:217–233.

Bisordi W.M. and Kleinman M.S. (1976) Melanosis duodeni. Gastrointestinal Endoscopy 23:37–38.

Bisset W.M., Jenkins H., Booth I., Smith V. and Milla P.J. (1993) The effect of somatostatin on small intestinal transport in intractable diarrhoea of infancy. Journal of Pediatric Gastroenterology and Nutrition 17:169–175.

Bjorneklett A., Fausa O., Refsum S.B., Torsvik H. and Sigstad H. (1977) Jejunal villous atrophy and granulomatous inflammation responding to gluten-free diet. Gut 18:814–816.

Blackman E. and Nash S.V. (1985) Diagnosis of duodenal and ampullary epithelial neoplasms by endoscopic biopsy. Human Pathology 16:901–910.

Blanes A., Martinez A., Bujan J., Ramon Y., Cajal S. and Carballido S.M. (1977) Intestinal mucosal changes following induced hypothyroidism in the developing rat. Virchows Archiv A 375:233–239.

Bloom S.R. and Polak J.M. (1981) Gut Hormones. London: Churchill Livingstone.

Bohane T.D., Cutz E., Hamilton J.R. and Gall D.G. (1977) Acrodermatitis enteropathica, zinc, and the Paneth cell: a case report with family studies. Gastroenterology 73:587–592.

Bolton R.P., Cotter K.L. and Losowsky M.S. (1986) Impaired neutrophil function in intestinal lymphangiectasia. Journal of Clinical Pathology 39:876–880.

Booth I.W., Chrystie I.L., Levinsky R.J., Marshall W.C., Pincott J. and Harries J.T. (1982) Protracted diarrhoea, immunodeficiency and viruses. European Journal of Pediatrics 138:271–272.

Bossart R., Henry K., Booth C.C. and Doe W.F. (1975) Subepithelial collagen in intestinal malabsorption. Gut 16:18–22.

Brandborg L.L., Goldberg S.B. and Breidenbach W.C. (1970) Human coccidiosis—a possible cause of malabsorption. New England Journal of Medicine 283:1306–1313.

Brandborg L.L., Tankersley C.B., Gottlieb S., Barancik M. and Sartor V.E. (1967) Histological demonstration of mucosal invasion by Giardia lamblia in man. Gastroenterology 52:143–150.

Brandt L.J., Davidoff A., Bernstein L.H., Biempica L., Rindfleisch B. and Goldstein M.L. (1981) Small intestinal involvement in Waldenstrom's macroglobulinemia: case report and review of the literature. Digestive Diseases and Sciences 26:174–180.

Brandtzaeg P., Sollid L.M., Thrane P.S., Kvale D., Bjerke K., Scott H., Kett K. and Rognum T.O. (1988) Lymphoepithelial interactions in the mucosal immune system. Gut 29:1116–1130.

Bras G., Richards R.C., Irvine R.A., Milner P.F.A. and Ragbeer M.M.S. (1964) Infection with Strongyloides stercoralis in Jamaica. Lancet ii:1257–1260.

Braverman D.Z., Dollberg L. and Shiner M. (1985) Clinical, histological and electron microscopic study of mast cell disease of the small bowel. American Journal of Gastroenterology 80:30–37.

Breen E.G., Coughlan G., Connolly C.E., Stevens F.M. and McCarthy C.F. (1987) Coeliac proctitis. Scandinavian Journal of Gastroenterology 22:471–477.

Brindicci D., Grimaldi F., Fracella M.R. and Abrusci M.R. (1993) Radiologic evaluation and prognosis of lymphoid nodular hyperplasia of the mesenteric intestine. Radiologia Medica 86:622–625.

Brocchi E., Corazza G., Caletti G., Treggiari E.A., Barbara L. and Gasbarrini G. (1988) Endoscopic demonstration of loss of duodenal folds in the diagnosis of celiac disease. New England Journal of Medicine 319:741–744.

Brouet J.C., Mason D.Y., Danon F., Preud'homme J.L., Seligmann M., Reyes F., Navab F., Galian A., Rene E. and Rambaud J.C. (1977) Alpha-chain disease: evidence for common clonal origin of intestinal immunoblastic lymphoma and plasmacytic proliferation. Lancet i:861.

Brow J.R., Parker F., Weinstein W.M. and Rubin C.E. (1971) The small intestinal mucosa in dermatitis herpetiformis: severity and distribution of the small intestinal lesion and associated malabsorption. Gastroenterology 60:355–361.

Brunser O., Eidelman S. and Klipstein F.A. (1970) Intestinal morphology in rural Haitians: a comparison between overt tropical sprue and asymptomatic subjects. Gastroenterology 58:655–668.

Buchan A.M.J. and Polak J.M. (1980) The classification of the human gastroenteropancreatic endocrine cells. Investigative and Cell Pathology 3:51–71.

Buffa R., Capella C., Fontana P., Usellini L. and Solcia E. (1978) Types of endocrine cells in the human colon and rectum. Cell and Tissue Research 192:227–240.

Bujanover Y., Liebman W.M., Goodman J.R. and Thaler M.M. (1981) Primary intestinal lymphangiectasia: case report with radiological and ultrastructural study. Digestion 21:107–114.

Burhol P.G. and Myren T. (1968) Jejunal biospy findings in healthy young men. Scandinavian Journal of Gastroenterology 3:346–350.

Burke V., Kerry K.R. and Anderson C.M. (1965) The relationship of dietary lactose to refractory diarrhoea in infancy. Australian Paediatric Journal 1:147–152.

Burrell H.C., Trescoli C., Chow K. and Ward M.J. (1994) Care report: mesenteric lymph node cavitation, an unusual complication of coeliac disease. British Journal of Radiology 67:1139–1140.

Businco L., Benincori N., Cantani A., Tacconi L. and Picarazzi A. (1985) Chronic diarrhea due to cow's milk allergy. A 4 to 10 year follow-up study. Annals of Allergy 55:844–847.

Cabrera A., de la Pava S. and Pickren J.W. (1964) Intestinal localisation of Waldenstrom's disease. Archives of Internal Medicine 114:399–407.

Campbell A.P., Merrett M.N., Kettlewell M., Mortensen N.J. and Jewell D.P. (1994) Expression of colonic antigens by goblet and columnar epithelium cells in ileal pouch mucosa: their association with inflammatory change and faecal stasis. Journal of Clinical Pathology 47:834–838.

Candy D.C.A., Larcher C.F., Cameron D.J.S., Norman A.P., Tripp J.H., Milla P., Pincott J.R. and Harries J.T. (1981) Lethal familial protracted diarrhea. Archives of Disease in Childhood 56:15–23.

Carroccio A., Iacono G., Montalto G., Cavataio F., Soresi M., Kazmierska I. and Notarbartolo A. (1993) Immunologic and absorptive tests in celiac disease: can they replace intestinal biopsies? Scandinavian Journal of Gastroenterology 28:673–676.

Castãneda-Romero B., Díaz-Caldeza L., Galván-Guerra E., Sixtos S., Arista J. and Uscanga L. (1993) Intestinal lymphoid nodular hyperplasia in a patient with acquired dysgammaglobulinemia, chronic diarrhea and bacterial overgrowth syndrome. Revista de Gastroenterologia de Mexico 58:225–228.

Castellano G., Canga F., Lopez I., Colina F., Gutierrez J., Costa R. and Solis-Herruzo J.A. (1988) Pseudomelanosis of the duodenum. Journal of Clinical Gastroenterology 10:150–154.

Castro L., de P., Dani R., Alvarenga R.J., Chamone D. de A.F. and de Oliveira C.A. (1971) A peroral biopsy study of the jejunum in human schistosomiasis mansoni. Review of the Insitute of Tropical Medicine, Sao Paulo 13:103–109.

Catassi C., Rätsch I.M., Fabiani E., Rossini M., Bordicchia F., Candela F., Coppa G.V. and Giorgi P.L. (1994) Coeliac disease in the year 2000: exploring the iceberg. Lancet 343:200–203.

Cerf-Bensussan N., Quaroni A., Kurnick J.T. and Bhan A.K. (1984) Intraepithelial lymphocytes modulate Ia expression by intestinal epithelial cells. Journal of Immunology 132:2244–2252.

Chacko C.J., Paulson A.K., Mathan V.I. and Baker S.J. (1969) The villous architecture of the small intestine in the tropics: a necropsy study. Journal of Pathology 98:146–151.

Challacombe D.N. and Robertson K. (1977) Enterochromaffin cells in the duodenal mucosa of children with coeliac disease. Gut 18:373–376.

Challacombe D.N., Wheeler E.E. and Campbell P.E. (1986) Morphometric studies and eosinophil cell counts in the duodenal mucosa of children with chronic nonspecific diarrhoea and cow's milk allergy. Journal of Pediatric Gastroenterology and Nutrition 5:887–891.

Charache P., Bayless T.M., Shelley W.M. and Hendrix T.R. (1966) Atypical bacteria in Whipple's disease. Transactions of the Association of American Physicians 79:399–408.

Chatti S., Haouet S., Ourghi H. et al (1994) Collagenous enterocolitis: apropos of a case and review of the literature. Archives D'Anatomie et de Cytologie Pathologiques 42:149–153.

Chaukley H.W. (1943) Method for the quantitative morphological analysis of tissues. Journal of the National Cancer Institute 4:47–53.

Chavalittamrong B. and Jirapinyo P. (1984) Intestinal parasites in pediatric patients with diarrhoeal diseases in Bangkok. Southeast Asian Journal of Tropical Medicine and Public Health 15:385–388.

Chejfec G., Falkmer S., Askensten U., Grimelius L. and Gould V.E. (1988) Neuroendocrine tumours of the gastrointestinal tract. Pathology, Research and Practice 183:143–154.

Cheli R. (1985) Is duodenitis always a peptic disease? American Journal of Gastroenterology 80:442–444.

Cheli R., Aste H. and Ciancamerla G. (1973) Histological follow-up of duodenitis. Endoscopy 5:135–139.

Chen K.K., Ho D.M., Chen M.T. and Chang L.S. (1993) Histopathological changes in Kock pouch. British Journal of Urology 72:433–440.

Cherner J.A., Jensen R.T., Dubois A., O'Dorisio T.M., Gardner J.D. and Metcalfe D.D. (1988) Gastrointestinal dysfunction in systemic mastocytosis. Gastroenterology 95:657–667.

Chiaramonte C. and Glick S.N. (1994) Nodular lymphoid hyperplasia of the small bowel complicated by jejunal lymphoma in a patient with common variable immune deficiency syndrome. American Journal of Roentgenology 163:1118–1119.

Cho C., Linscheer W.G., Hirschkorn M.A. and Ashutosh K. (1984) Sarcoidlike granulomas as an early manifestation of Whipple's disease. Gastroenterology 87:941–947.

Clancy R.L., Tomkins W.A.F., Muckle T.J., Richardson H. and Rawls W.E. (1975) Isolation and characterisation of an aetiological agent in Whipple's disease. British Medical Journal 3:568–570.

Cnudde F., Boulard F., Teron-Aboud B. and Chevallier J. (1994) Tropical sprue: diagnostic difficulties. Apropos of 2 cases in Guadeloupe. Annales de Gastroenterologie et D' Hepatologie 30:163–165.

Cocco A.E., Dohrmann M.J. and Hendrix T.R. (1966) Reconstruction of human jejunal biopsies: three dimensional histology. Gastroenterology 51:24–31.

Coello-Ramirez P. and Larrosa-Haro A. (1984) Gastrointestinal occult hemorrhage and gastroduodenitis in cow's milk protein intolerance. Journal of Pediatric Gastroenterology and Nutrition 3:215–218.

Collins P., Reunala T., Pukkala E., Laippala P., Keyrilainen O. and Pasternack A. (1994) Coeliac disease—associated disorders and survival. Gut 35:1215–1218.

Colwell E.J., Welsh J.D., Legters L.J. and Proctor R.F. (1968) Jejunal morphological characteristics in South Vietnamese residents. Journal of the American Medical Association 206:2273–2276.

Congdon P., Mason M.K., Smith S., Crollick A., Steel A. and Littlewood J. (1981) Small-bowel mucosa in asymptomatic children with celiac disease. Mucosal changes with gluten-free diets. American Journal of Diseases in Children 135:118–121.

Connolly C.E., Kennedy M., Stevens F.M. and McCarthy C.F. (1994) Brown bowel syndrome occurring in coeliac disease in the west of Ireland. Scandinavian Journal of Gastroenterology 29:91–94.

Connor B.A., Shlim D.R., Scholes J.V., Rayburn J.L., Reidy J. and Rajah R. (1993) The pathological changes in the small bowel in nine patients with diarrhoea associated with a coccidia-like body. Annals of Internal Medicine 119:377–382.

Contractor Q.Q., Benson L., Schulz T.B., Contractor T.Q. and Kasturi N. (1988) Duodenal involvement in *Schistosoma mansoni* infection. Gut 29:1011–1012.

Cook G.C. (1984) Aetiology and pathogenesis of postinfective tropical malabsorption (tropical sprue). Lancet i:721–723.

Cooke W.T., Fone D.J., Cox E.V., Meynell M.J. and Gaddie R. (1963) Adult coeliac disease. Gut 4:279–291.

Cookson J.B., Montgomery R.D., Morgan H.V. and Tudor R.W. (1972) Fatal paralytic ileus due to strongyloidiasis. British Medical Journal 4:771–772.

Cooper B.T., Holmes G.K.T. and Cooke W.T. (1982) Lymphoma risk in coeliac disease of later life. Digestion 23:89–92.

Cooper B.T., Holmes G.K.T., Ferguson R., Thompson R.A., Allan R.N. and Cooke W.T. (1980) Gluten-sensitive diarrhea without evidence of celiac disease. Gastroenterology 79:801–806.

Corazza G.R., Bonvicini F., Frazzoni M., Gatto M. and Gasbarrini G. (1982) Observer variation in assessment of jejunal biopsy specimens. Gastroenterology 83:1217–1222.

Corazza G.R., Frazzoni M., Dixon M.F. and Gasbarrini G. (1985) Quantitative assessment of the mucosal architecture of jejunal biopsy specimens: a comparison between linear measurement, stereology, and computer aided microscopy. Journal of Clinical Pathology 38:765–770.

Corazza G.R., Frazzoni M. and Gasbarrini G. (1984) Jejunal intraepithelial lymphocytes in coeliac disease: are they increased or decreased? Gut 25:158–162.

Corazza G.R., Frazzoni M., Gatto M.R.A. and Gasbarrini G. (1986) Ageing and small-bowel mucosa: a morphometric study. Gerontology 32:60–65.

Coremans G., Rutgeerts P., Geboes K., Van den Oord J., Ponette E. and Vantrappen G. (1984) The value of ileoscopy with biopsy in the diagnosis of intestinal Crohn's disease. Gastrointestinal Endoscopy 30:167–172.

Corless J.K., Tedesco F.J., Griffin J.W. and Panish J.K. (1984) Giant ileal inflammatory polyps in Crohn's disease. Gastrointestinal Endoscopy 30:352–354.

Corlin R.F. and Pops M.A. (1972) Nongranulomatous ulcerative jejunoileitis with hypogammaglobulinaemia. Gastroenterology 62:473–478.

Cotton P.B., Price A.B., Tighe J.R. and Beales J.S.M. (1973) Preliminary evaluation of duodenitis by endoscopy and biopsy. British Medical Journal 3:430–433.

Cottrill C., Glueck C.J., Lauba V., Millet F., Pupprione D. and Brown M.V. (1974) Familial homozygous hypobetalipoproteinemia. Metabolism 23:779–791.

Crabbe P.A. and Heremans J.F. (1967) Selective IgA deficiency with steatorrhea. American Journal of Medicine 42:319–326.

Creamer B. (1964) Malignancy and the small intestinal mucosa. British Medical Journal 2: 1435–1436.

Creamer B. (1967) The turnover of the epithelium of the small intestine. British Medical Bulletin 23:226–230.

Croft D.N., Loehry C.A. and Creamer B. (1968) Small bowel cell loss and weight loss in the coeliac syndrome. Lancet ii:68–70.

Crow J. and Asselah F. (1984) Immunoproliferative small intestinal disease in Algerians. Cancer 54:1908–1913.

Cunningham D., Morgan R.J., Mills P.R., Nelson L.M., Toner P.G., Soukop M., McArdle C.S. and Russell R.I. (1985) Functional and structural changes of the human proximal small intestine after cytotoxic therapy. Journal of Clinical Pathology 38:265–270.

Cunningham-Rundles C. (1988) Selective IgA deficiency and the gastrointestinal tract. Immunological Allergy Clinic of North America 8:435–449.

Curran R.C. and Jones E.L. (1979) Non-Hodgkin's lymphomas: an immunohistochemical and histological study. Journal of Pathology 129:179–190.

Current W.L., Reese N.C., Ernst J.V., Bailey W.S., Heyman M.B. and Weinstein W.M. (1983) Human cryptosporidiosis in immunocompetent and immunodeficient persons. New England Journal of Medicine 308:1252–1257.

Da Costa L.R. (1971) Small intestinal cell turnover in patients with parasitic infections. British Medical Journal 3:281–283.

Daniel R., Debonne J.M. and Klotz F. (1993) Common variable hypogammaglobulinemia: a rare cause of chronic diarrhea: a case. Presse Medicale 22:1696–1698.

Davidson A.G.F. and Bridges M.A. (1988) Coeliac disease: an analysis of aetiological possibilities and re-evaluation of the enzymopathic hypothesis. Medical Hypotheses 26:155–160.

Davidson G.P. and Barnes G.L. (1979) Structural and functional abnormalities of the small intestine in infants and young children with rotavirus enteritis. Acta Paediatrica Scandinavica 68:181–186.

Davidson G.P., Cutz E., Hamilton J.R. and Gall D.G. (1978) Familial enteropathy: a syndrome of protracted diarrhea from birth, failure to thrive, and hypoplastic villus atrophy. Gastroenterology 75:783–790.

Davidson G.P. and Townley R.R.W. (1977) Structural and functional abnormalities of the small intestine due to nutritional folic acid deficiency in infancy. Journal of Paediatrics 90:590–594.

Dawson J., Bryant M.G., Bloom S.R. and Peters T.J. (1986) Jejunal mucosal enzyme activities, regulatory peptides and organelle pathology of the enteropathy of common variable immunodefiency. Gut 27:273–277.

Delarocque-Astagneau E., Hadengue A., Degott C., Vilgrain V., Erlinger S. and Benhamou J.P. (1994) Biliary obstruction resulting from *Strongyloides stercoralis* infection: report of a case. Gut 35:705–706.

Delgado M.J., Moreno J., Murillo M.L., Bolufer J. and Lopez-Campos J.L. (1986) Histophysiologic aspects of the remnant intestine of rats subjected to partial resection of the small intestine. Revista Espānola de Fisiologia 42:205–212.

Demirer T., Uzunalimoglu O., Anderson T. et al (1995) Flow cytometric measurement of proliferation-associated nuclear antigen P105 and DNA content in immuno-proliferative small intestinal disease (IPSID). Journal of Surgical Oncology 58:25–30.

Denholm R.B., Mills P.R. and More I.A.R. (1981) Electron microscopy in the long-term follow-up of Whipple's Disease. American Journal of Surgical Pathology 5:507–516.

Dent D.M., Duys P.J., Bird A.R. and Birkenstock W.E. (1975) Cytomegalic virus infection of bowel in adults. South African Medical Journal 49:669–672.

Deo M.G. and Ramalingaswami V. (1965) Reaction of the small intestine to induced protein malnutrition in Rhesus monkeys—a study of cell population kinetics in the jejunum. Gastroenterology 49:150–157.

de Paola D., Dias L.B. and da Silva J.R. (1962) Enteritis due to *Strongyloides stercoralis:* a report of five fatal cases. American Journal of Digestive Diseases 7:1086–1098.

de Sousa J.S., da Silva A., Pereira M.V., Soares J. and Ramalho P.M. (1986) Cow's milk protein-sensitive enteropathy: number and timing of biopsies for diagnosis. Journal of Pediatric Gastroenterology and Nutrition 5:207–209.

de Sousa J.S., Guerreiro O., Cunha A. and Araujo J. (1968) Association of nephrotic syndrome with intestinal lymphangiectasia. Archives of Disease in Childhood 43:245–248.

De Thomas J., Munoz-Calero A., Gonzalez-Lara V. et al (1994) Ulcerative jejunitis: a complication of celiac disease. Revista Espānola de Enfermedades Digestivas 86:761–763.

Dhesi I., Marsh M.N., Kelly C. and Crowe P. (1984) Morphometric analysis of small intestinal mucosa. Virchows Archiv A 403:173–180.

Dinari G., Rosenbach Y., Grunebaum M., Zahavi I., Alpert G. and Nitzan M. (1980) Gastrointestinal manifestations of Neimann-Pick disease. Enzyme 25:407–412.

Dincsoy H.P., Rolfes D.B., McGraw C.A. and Schubert W.K. (1984) Cholesterol ester storage disease and mesenteric lipodystrophy. American Journal of Clinical Pathology 81:263–269.

Dissanayake A.S., Truelove S.C., Offord R.E. and Whitehead R. (1973) Nature of toxic component of wheat gluten in coeliac disease. Lancet ii:709–710.

Dissanayake A.S., Truelove S.C. and Whitehead R. (1974) Jejunal mucosal recovery in coeliac disease in relation to adherence to a gluten free diet. Quarterly Journal of Medicine 170:161–185.

Dobbins W.O. III (1966) An ultrastructural study of the intestinal mucosa in congenital B-lipoprotein deficency with particular emphasis upon the intestinal absorptive cell. Gastroenterology 50:195–210.

Dobbins W.O. III (1981) Is there an immune deficit in Whipple's disease? Digestive Diseases and Sciences 26:247–252.

Dobbins W.O. III (1986) Human intestinal intraepithelial lymphocytes. Gut 27:972–985.

Dobbins W.O. III and Kawanishi H. (1981) Bacillary characteristics in Whipple's disease: an electron microscopic study. Gastroenterology 80:1468–1475.

Doe W.F. (1975) Alpha chain disease: clinicopathological features and relationship to so-called Mediterranean lymphoma. British Journal of Cancer 31 (suppl II):350–355.

Doe W.F. (1979) An overview of intestinal immunity and malabsorption. The American Journal of Medicine 67:1077–1084.

Doe W.F., Henry K., Hobbs J.R., Avery Jones F., Dent C.E. and Booth C.C. (1972) Five cases of alpha chain disease. Gut 13:947–957.

Donaldson Jr R.M. (1992) Whipple's disease: rare malady with uncommon potential. New England Journal of Medicine 327:346–348.

Doniach D. and Shiner M. (1957) Duodenal and jejunal biopsies. Gastroenterology 33:71–86.

Douglas J.G., Gillon J., Logan R.F.A., Grant I.W.B. and Crompton G.K. (1984) Sarcoidosis and coeliac disease: an association. Lancet ii:13–14.

Dowling R.H. (1967) Compensatory changes in intestinal absorption. British Medical Bulletin 23:275–278.

Draper L.R., Gyure L.A., Hall J.G. and Robertson D. (1983) Effect of alcohol on the integrity of the intestinal epithelium. Gut 24:399–404.

Drummond M.B. and Montgomery R.D. (1970) Acute sprue in Britain. British Medical Journal 2:340–341.

Dubois R.S., Roy C.C., Fulginiti V.A., Merrill D.A. and Murray R.L. (1970) Disaccharidase deficiency in children with immunologic deficits. Journal of Pediatrics 76:337.

Dukes C. and Bussey H.J.R. (1926) The number of lymphoid follicles of the human large intestine. Journal of Pathology and Bacteriology 29:111–116.

Duncan A., Park R.P., Lee F.D. and Russell R.I. (1994) A retrospective assessment of the clinical value of jejunal disaccharidase analysis. Scandinavian Journal of Gastroenterology 29:1111–1116.

Dunnill M.S. and Whitehead R. (1972) A method for the quantitation of small intestinal biopsy specimens. Journal of Clinical Pathology 25:243–246.

Eastham E.J., Douglas A.P. and Watson A.J. (1976) Diagnosis of *Giardia lamblia* infection as a cause of diarrhoea. Lancet ii:950–951.

Eckstein R.P., Dowsett J.F. and Riley J.W. (1988) Collagenous enterocolitis: a case of collagenous colitis with involvement of the small intestine. American Journal of Gastroenterology 83:767–771.

Ectors N., Geboes K., De Vos R., Heidbuchel H., Rutgeerts P., Desmet U. and Vantrappen G. (1992) Whipple's disease: a histobiological immunocytochemical and electron microscopic study of the immune response in the small intestinal mucosa. Histopathology 21:1–12.

Eidelman S., Parkins R.A. and Rubin C.E. (1966) Abdominal lymphoma presenting as malabsorption. Medicine 45:111–137.

Egan-Mitchell B., Fottrell P.F. and McNicholl B. (1981) Early or pre-coeliac mucosa: development of gluten enteropathy. Gut 22:65–69.

Evans D.J. and Ali M.H. (1985) Immunocytochemistry in the diagnosis of Whipple's disease. Journal of Clinical Pathology 38:372–374.

Fagundes-Neto U., Wehba J., Viaro T., Machado N.L. and Patricio F.R. (1985) Protracted diarrhea in infancy: clinical aspects and ultrastructural analysis of the small intestine. Journal of Pediatric Gastroenterology and Nutrition 4:714–722.

Favara B.E. and Jaffe R. (1994) The histopathology of Langerhans cell histiocytosis. British Journal of Cancer (suppl 23):s17–s23.

Feldman M. (1986) Whipple's Disease. (Southern Internal Medicine Conference). American Journal of Medical Sciences 291:56–67.

Fenyo G., Hallberg D., Soda M. and Roos K.A. (1976) Morphological changes in the small intestine following jejuno-ileal shunt in parenterally fed rats. Scandinavian Journal of Gastroenterology 11:635–640.

Ferguson A., Blackwell J.N. and Barnetson R. St. C. (1987) Effects of additional dietary gluten on the small-intestinal mucosa of volunteers and of patients with dermatitis herpetiformis. Scandinavian Journal of Gastroenterology 22:543–549.

Ferguson A. and Murray D. (1971) Quantitation of intraepithelial lymphocytes in human jejunum. Gut 12:988–994.

Ferguson A. and Ziegler K. (1986) Intraepithelial lymphocyte mitosis in a jejunal biopsy correlates with intraepithelial lymphocyte count, irrespective of diagnosis. Gut 27:675–679.

Fernandes B.J., Amato D. and Goldfinger M. (1985) Diffuse lymphomatous polyposis of the gastrointestinal tract. Gastroenterology 88:1267–1270.

Feyrter F. (1934) Über wucherungen der brunnerschen drusen. Virchows Archiv A 293:509–520.

Fichtelius K.E., Yunis J.E. and Good R.A. (1968) Occurrence of lymphocytes within the gut epithelium of normal and neonatally thymectomised mice. Proceedings of the Society for Experimental Biology 128:185–188.

Fisher S.E., Boyle J.T. and Holtzapple P. (1981) Chronic protracted diarrhoea and jejunal atrophy in an infant: cimetidine-associated stimulation of jejunal mucosal growth. Digestive Diseases and Sciences 26:181–186.

Fleck S.L., Hames S.E. and Warhurst D.C. (1985) Detection of *Giardia* in human jejunum by immunoperoxidase method: specific and non-specific results. Transactions of the Royal Society of Tropical and Medical Hygiene 79:110–113.

Fleming J.L., Wiesner R.H. and Shorter R.G. (1988) Whipple's disease: clinical, biochemical and histopathologic features and assessment of treatment of 29 patients. Mayo Clinic Proceedings 63:539–551.

Fluge O., Sletten K., Fluge G., Aksnes L. and Elsayed S. (1994) In vitro toxicity of purified gluten peptides tested by organ culture. Journal of Pediatric Gastroenterology and Nutrition 18:186–192.

Flynn D.M., Lake B.D., Boothby D.B. and Young E.P. (1972) Gut lesions in Fabry's disease without a rash. Archives of Disease in Childhood 47:26–33.

Fontaine J.L. and Navarro J. (1975) Small intestinal biopsy in cow's milk protein allergy in infancy. Archives of Disease in Childhood 50:357–362.

Foroozan P. and Trier J.S. (1967) Mucosa of the small intestine in pernicious anaemia. New England Journal of Medicine 277:553–559.

Foster C.S. (1979) The brown bowel syndrome: a possible smooth muscle mitochondrial myopathy? Histopathology 3:1–17.

Fox B. (1967) Lipofuscinosis of the gastrointestinal tract in man. Journal of Clinical Pathology 20:806–813.

Fox U. and Lucani G. (1993) Disorders of the intestinal mesenteric lymphatic system. Lymphology 26:61–66.

Franzin G., Musola R., Ghidini O., Manfrini C. and Fratton A. (1985) Nodular hyperplasia of Brunner's glands. Gastrointestinal Endoscopy 31:374–378.

Franzin G., Novelli P. and Fratton A. (1983) Hyperplastic and metaplastic polyps of the duodenum. Gastrointestinal Endoscopy 29:140–142.

Freedman A.R., Macartney J.C., Nelufer J.M. and Ciclitira P.J. (1987) Timing of infiltration of T lymphocytes induced by gluten into the small intestine in coeliac disease. Journal of Clinical Pathology 40:741–745.

Freeman H.J. and Chiu B.K. (1986a) Multifocal small bowel lymphoma and latent celiac sprue. Gastroenterology 90:1992–1997.

Freeman H.J. and Chiu B.K. (1986b) Small bowel malignant lymphoma complicating celiac sprue and the mesenteric lymph node cavitation syndrome. Gastroenterology 90:2008–2012.

Frexinos J., Pudebat M., Duffaut M., Rumeau J-L. and Arlet P. (1979) Hypogammaglobulemie globale et atrophie villositaire sensible au regime sans gluten. Gastroenterologie Clinique et Biologique 8:893–898.

Frisancho O., Ulloa V., Ruiz W. et al (1994) Megaloblastic anemia associated with chronic diarrhea: a prospective and multicentre study in Lima. Revista de Gastroenterologia del Peru 14:189–195.

Fudenberg H.H., Good R.A., Hitzig W., Kunkel H.G., Roitt I.M., Rosen F.S., Rowe D.S., Seligmann M. and Soothill J.R. (1970) Classification of the primary immunodeficiencies: W.H.O. recommendation. New England Journal of Medicine 283:656.

Gaist D. and Ladefoged K. (1993). Whipple Disease. Ugeskrift for Laeger 155:3394–3396.

Galian A., Lecestre M-J., Scott J., Bognel C., Matuchansky C. and Rambaud J-C. (1977) Pathological study of alpha-chain disease, with special emphasis on evolution. Cancer 39:2081–2101.

Galjaard H., van der Meer-Fieggen W. and Giesen J. (1972) Feedback control by functional villus cells on cell proliferation and maturation in intestinal epithelium. Experimental Cell Research 73:197–207.

Gallager R.L. (1980) Intestinal ceroid deposition—"brown bowel syndrome": a light and electron microscopic study. Virchows Archiv A 389:143–151.

Gallo-Van Ess D.M., Strasburger V.C. and Turetsky R.A. (1986) Intestinal lymphangiectasia in an adolescent. Journal of Adolescent Health Care 7:259–264.

Gear E.V. and Dobbins W.O. (1969) The histologic spectrum of proximal duodenal biopsy in adult males. The American Journal of Medical Science 257:90–99.

Geboes K., Ectors N., Heidbuchel H., Rutgeerts P., Desmet V. and Vantrappen G. (1992) Whipple's disease: the value of upper gastrointestinal endoscopy for the diagnosis and follow-up. Acta Gastroenterologica Belgica 55:209–219.

Gelzayd E.A., Biederman M.A. and Gelfand D.W. (1975) Changing concepts of duodenitis. American Journal of Gastroenterology 64:213–216.

Ghadially F.N., Boone S.A. and Walley V.M. (1994) Melanosis (haemosiderosis) ilei. Journal of Submicroscopic Cytology and Pathology 26:461–465.

Gilinsky N.H., Chaimowitz G. and Van Staden M.C. (1986) Immunoproliferative small-intestinal disease with lymphoma: diagnostic difficulties and pitfalls. South African Medical Journal 69:260–262.

Gilinsky N.H., Mee A.S., Beatty D.W., Novis B.H., Young G., Price S., Purves L.R. and Marks I.N. (1985) Plasma cell infiltration of the small bowel: lack of evidence for a non-secretory form of alpha-heavy chain disease. Gut 26:928–934.

Gillberg R., Dotevall G. and Ahren C. (1982) Chronic inflammatory bowel disease in patients with coeliac disease. Scandinavian Journal of Gastroenterology 17:491–496.

Gillon J., Thamery D.A. and Ferguson A. (1982) Features of small intestinal pathology (epithelial cell kinetics, intraepithelial lymphocytes, disaccharidases) in a primary *Giardia muris* infection. Gut 23:498–506.

Girault D., Goulet O., Le Deist F., Brousse N., Colomb V., Césarini J.P., de Potter S., Canioni D., Griscelli

C., Fischer A., et al (1994) Intractable infant diarrhea associated with phenotypic abnormalities and immunodeficiency. Journal of Pediatrics 125:36–42.

Gleason T.H. and Patterson S.D. (1982) The pathology of *Yersinia enterocolitica* ileocolitis. American Journal of Surgical Pathology 6:347-355.

Gleeson M.H., Bloom S.R., Polak J.M., Henry K. and Dowling R.H. (1970) An endocrine tumour in kidney affecting small bowel structure, motility, and function. (Abstract) Gut 11:1066.

Glew R.H., Basu A., Prence E.M. and Remaley A.T. (1985) Lysosomal storage diseases. Laboratory Investigation 53:250–269.

Goldgar C.M. and Vanderhoof J.A. (1986) Lack of correlation of small bowel biopsy and clinical course of patients with intractable diarrhea of infancy. Gastroenterology 90:527–531.

Good R.A. Peterson R.D.A., Percy D.Y., Finstad J. and Cooper M.D. (1968) Immunological deficiency diseases in man. In: Birth Defects. Original article series IV, 1. Edited by D. Bergsma and R.A. Good. New York: The National Foundation—March of Dimes, p 17.

Goodwin C.S. (1988) Duodenal ulcer, *Campylobacter pylori,* and the leaking roof concept. Lancet ii: 1467–1469.

Gorbach S.L. and Tabaqchali S. (1969) Bacteria, bile and the small bowel. Gut 10:963–972.

Gordon J. and Smith J.L. (1980) Immunoglobulin synthesis by neoplastic cells: models of a clonal transition from IgM to IgG synthesis. Journal of Clinical Pathology 33:539–554.

Gouffier E., Phan A., Paraf A., Boddaert A. and Chevrel J-P. (1977) Recurrent ulcerative jejuno-ileitis: report of a case with operative and endoscopic observations. Gastroenterologie Clinique et Biologique 1.545–552.

Gracey M. (1993) Bacterial diarrhoea. Annals of Tropical Paediatrics 13:107–119.

Granot E., Goodman-Weill M., Pizov G. and Sherman Y. (1993) Histological comparison of suction capsule and endoscopic small intestinal mucosal biopsies in children. Journal of Pediatric Gastroenterology and Nutrition 16:397–401.

Green F. and Heyworth B. (1980) Immunoglobulin-containing cells in jejunal mucosa of children with protein-energy malnutrition and gastroenteritis. Archives of Diseases in Childhood 55:380–383.

Green P.H.R., Lefkowitch J.H., Glickman R.M., Riley J.W., Quinet F. and Blum C.B. (1982) Apoprotein localization and quantitation in the human intestine. Gastroenterology 83:1223–1230.

Greenwood N. (1976) The jejunal mucosa in two cases of A-beta-lipoproteinemia. American Journal of Gastroenterology 65:160 162.

Grefte J.M.M., Bouman J.G., Grond J., Jansen W. and Kleibeuker J.H. (1988) Slow and incomplete histological and functional recovery in adult gluten-sensitive enteropathy. Journal of Clinical Pathology 41:886–891.

Gregg J.A. and Garabedian M. (1974) Duodenitis. American Journal of Gastroenterology 61:177–184.

Groisman G.M., Ben-Izhak O., Schwersenz A., Berant M. and Fyfe B. (1993) The value of polyclonal carcinoembryonic antigen immunostaining in the diagnosis of microvillous inclusion disease. Human Pathology 24:1232–1237.

Guerra R., Wheby M.S. and Bayless T.M. (1965) Long-term antibiotic therapy in tropical sprue. Annals of Internal Medicine 63:619–634.

Guix M., Skinner J.M. and Whitehead R. (1979) Measuring intraepithelial lymphocytes, surface area, and volume of lamina propria in the jejunal mucosa of coeliac patients. Gut 20:275–278.

Gupta S., Pinching A.J., Onwubalili J., Vince A., Evans D.J. and Hodgson H.J.F. (1986) Whipple's disease with unusual clinical, bacteriologic and immunologic findings. Gastroenterology 90.1286–1289.

Gupta T.P. and Weinstock J.V. (1986) Duodenal pseudomelanosis associated with chronic renal failure. Gastrointestinal Endoscopy 32:358–360.

Gushurst T.P. and Lesesne H.R. (1984) Isolated duodenal varix: an unusual cause of gastrointestinal hemorrhage. Southern Medical Journal 77:915–918.

Gustavsson S., Weiland L.H. and Kelly K.A. (1987) Relationship of backwash ileitis to ileal pouchitis after ileal pouch-anal anastomosis. Diseases of the Colon and Rectum 30:25–28.

Haeney M.R., Goodwin B.J.F., Barratt M.E.J., Mike N. and Asquith P. (1982) Soya protein antibodies in man: their occurrence and possible relevance in coeliac disease. Journal of Clinical Pathology 35:319–322.

Hall P.A., Jass J.R., Levison D.A., Morson B.C., Shepherd N.A., Sobin L.H. and Stansfeld A.G. (1988) Classification of primary gut lymphomas. Lancet ii:958.

Hallak A., Baratz M., Santo M., Halpern Z., Rabau M., Werbin N., Gilat T. (1994) Ileitis after colectomy for ulcerative colitis or carcinoma. Gut 35:373–376.

Hallgren R., Colombel J.F., Dahl R., Fredens K., Kruse A., Jacobsen N.O., Venge P. and Rambaud J.C. (1989) Neutrophil and eosinophil involvement of the small bowel in patients with celiac disease and Crohn's disease: studies on the secretion rate and immunohistochemical localisation of granulocyte granule constituents. American Journal of Medicine 86:56–64.

Halliday C.E.W. and Farthing M.J.G. (1986) Giardiasis. Gastroenterology 5:3–7.

Halliday K., Edmeades R. and Shepherd R. (1982) Persistent post-enteritis diarrhoea in childhood: a prospective analysis of clinical features, predisposing factors and sequelae. Medical Journal of Australia 1:18–20.

Halphen M., Galian A., Certin M., Ink F., Filali A. and Rambaud J-C. (1989) Clinicopathological study of a patient with idiopathic villous atrophy and small vessel alterations of the ileum. Digestive Diseases and Sciences 34:111–117.

Halphen M., Najjar T., Jaafoura H., Cammoun M. and Tufrali G. (1986) Diagnostic value of upper intestinal fiber endoscopy in primary small intestinal lymphoma. Cancer 58:2140–2145.

Halstead C.H., Sheir S. and Raasch F.O. (1969) The small intestine in human schistosomiasis. Gastroenterology 57:622–623.

Hand N.M. (1987) Enzyme histochemistry on jejunal tissue embedded in resin. Journal of Clinical Pathology 40:346–352.

Haque A.K., Schnadig V., Rubin S.A. and Smith J.H. (1994) Pathogenesis of human strongyloidiasis: autopsy and quantitative parasitological analysis. Modern Pathology 7:276–288.

Hara M., Harasawa S., Tani N., Miwa T. and Tsutsumi Y. (1988) Gastric metaplasia in duodenal ulcer. Acta Pathologica Japonica 38:1011–1018.

Harris M., Burton I.E. and Scarffe J.H. (1983) Macroglobulinaemia and intestinal lymphangiectasia: a rare association. Journal of Clinical Pathology 36:30–36.

Harris O.D., Cooke W.T., Thompson M. and Waterhouse J.A.H. (1967) Malignancy in adult celiac disease and idiopathic steatorrhea. American Journal of Medicine 42:899–912.

Hasan M., Hay F., Sircus W. and Ferguson A. (1983) Nature of the inflammatory cell infiltrate in duodenitis. Journal of Clinical Pathology 36:280–288.

Hauer-Jensen M., Poulakos L., Milani F.X. and Osborne J.W. (1988) Effects of exocrine pancreatic secretions on hyperthermic injury of rat small intestine. International Journal of Hyperthermia 4:417–426.

Helmy I. (1980) Endoscopic diagnosis of immunoproliferative small intestinal disease (IPSID) Endoscopy 12:114–116.

Hendrix T.R. and Yardley J.H. (1970) Modern Trends in Gastroenterology. Volume 4. Edited by W.I. Card and B. Creamer. London: Butterworth, p 229.

Hennig A. (1956) Inhalt einer aus papilleu oder zotten gebildeten fläche. Mikroscopie 11:206–213.

Henry K., Bird R.G. and Doe W.F. (1974) Intestinal coccidiosis in a patient with alpha-chain disease. British Medical Journal 1:542–543.

Henson D. (1972) Cytomegalovirus inclusion bodies in the gastrointestinal tract. Archives of Pathology 93:477–482.

Herbert P.N., Assmann G., Gotto A.M. and Fredrickson D.S. (1982) Familial lipoprotein deficiency: abetalipoproteinemia, hypobetalipoproteinemia and Tangier disease. In: The metabolic Basis of Inherited Disease. Edited by J.B. Stanbury, J.B. Wyngaarden, and D.S. Fredrickson. 4th ed. New York: McGraw-Hill, pp 589–621.

Heresbach D., Raoul J.L., Genetet N., Noret P., Siproudhis L., Ramée M.P., Bretagne J.F. and Gosselin M. (1994) Immunological study in primary intestinal lymphangiectasia. Digestion 55:59–64.

Hermans P.E., Huizenga K.A., Hoffman H.N., Brown A.L. and Markowitz H. (1966) Dysgammaglobulinemia associated with nodular lymphoid hyperplasia of the small intestine. American Journal of Medicine 40:78–79.

Hermos J.A., Cooper H.L., Kramer P. and Trier J.S. (1970) Histological diagnosis by peroral biopsy of Crohn's disease of the proximal intestine. Gastroenterology 59:868–873.

Hibi T., Asakura H., Kobayashi K., Munakata Y., Kano S., Tsuchiya M., Teramoto T. and Uematsu Y. (1982) Alpha heavy chain disease lacking secretory alpha chain, with cobblestone appearance of the small intestine and duodenal ulcer demonstrated by endoscopy. Gut 23:422–427.

Hoang C., Halphen M., Galian A., Brouet J-C., Marsan C., Leclerc J-P. and Rambaud J-C. (1985) Small bowel involvement and exudative enteropathy in Waldenstrom's macroglobulinemia. Gastroenterologie Clinique et Biologique 9:444–448.

Hobbs J.R. and Hepner G.W. (1968) Deficiency of gamma-M-globulin in coeliac disease. Lancet i:217–220.

Hobbs J.R., Hepner G.W., Douglas A.P., Crabbe P.A. and Johansson S.G.O. (1969) Immunological mystery of coeliac disease. Lancet ii:649–650.

Hockenstrom T., Kock N.G., Norlen L.J., Ahren C. and Philipson B.M. (1986) Morphologic changes in ileal reservoir mucosa after long-term exposure to urine. Scandinavian Journal of Gastroenterology 21:1224–1234.

Holmes G.K.T., Asquith P., Stokes P.L. and Cooke W.T. (1974) Cellular infiltrate of jejunal biopsies in adult coeliac disease in relation to gluten withdrawal. Gut 15:278–283.

Holmes G.K.T., Prior P., Lane M.R., Pope D. and Allan R.N. (1989) Malignancy in coeliac disease: effect of a gluten-free diet. Gut 30:333–338.

Holmes G.K.T., Stokes P.L., Sorahan T.M., Prior P., Waterhouse J.A.H. and Cooke W.T. (1976) Coeliac disease, gluten-free diet and malignancy. Gut 17:612–619.

Holmes R., Hourihane D. O'B., Booth C.C. (1961) Dissecting microscope appearances of jejunal biopsy specimens from patients with idiopathic steatorrhoea. Lancet 1:81–83.

Hong S.T., Kim Y.T., Choe G., Min Y.I., Cho S.H., Kim J.K., Kook J., Chai J.Y. and Lee S.H. (1994) Two cases of intestinal capillariasis in Korea. Korean Journal of Parasitology 32:43–48.

Horn T., Svendsen L.B., Johansen A. and Backer O. (1985) Brown bowel syndrome. Ultrastructural Pathology 8:357–361.

Horowitz A. and Shiner M. (1981) The recognition of premalignant change in jejunal mucosal biopsies of patients with malabsorption. Journal of Submicroscopic Cytology 13:423–443.

Horowitz S., Lorenzsonn V.W., Olsen W.A. et al (1974) Small intestinal disease in T cell deficiency. Journal of Pediatrics 85:457–462.

Hosler J.P., Kimmel K.K. and Moeller D.D. (1982) The "brown bowel syndrome": a case report. American Journal of Gastroenterology 77:854–855.

Hourihane D.O'B. (1963) Diarrhoea of small bowel origin: the histology of small intestinal biopsies. Proceedings of the Royal Society of Medicine 56:1073–1077.

Hourihane D.O'B. and Weir D.G. (1970) Malignant celiac syndrome: report of two cases with malabsorption and microscopic foci of intestinal lymphoma. Gastroenterology 59:130–139.

Howard F.M., Carter C.O., Candy D.C.A. and Harries J.T. (1981) A family study of protracted diarrhea in infancy. Journal of Medical Genetics 18:81–86.

Huber J., Zegers B.J.M. and Schuurman H-J. (1992) Pathology of congenital immunodeficiencies. Seminars in Diagnostic Pathology 9:31–62.

Ikeda K., Sannohe Y., Murayama H., Ikeda R. and Inutsuka S. (1982) Heterotopic gastric mucosa in the duodenum: reaction to congo red under fiberscopic observation. Endoscopy 14:168–170.

Inge P.M.G., Edson C.M. and Farthing M.J.G. (1988) Attachment of *Giardia lamblia* to rat intestinal epithelial cells. Gut 29:795–801.

Isaacson P. (1980) Malignant histiocytosis of the intestine: the early histological lesion. Gut 21:381–386.

Isaacson P. (1981) Primary gastrointestinal lymphoma. Virchows Archiv A 391:1–8.

Isaacson P.G. (1985) B-cell lymphomas of the gastrointestinal tract. American Journal of Surgical Pathology 9 (suppl):117–128.

Isaacson P.G. (1994) Gastrointestinal lymphoma. Human Pathology 25:1020–1029.

Isaacson P.G., Jones D.B., Sworn M.J. and Wright D.H. (1982) Malignant histiocytosis of the intestine: report of three cases with immunological and cytochemical analysis. Journal of Clinical Pathology 35:510–516.

Isaacson P.G., MacLennan K.A. and Subbuswamy S.G. (1984) Multiple lymphomatous polyposis of the gastrointestinal tract. Histopathology 8:641–656.

Isaacson P.G., O'Connor N.T., Spencer J., Bevan D.H., Connolly C.E., Kirkham N., Pollock D.J., Wainscoat J.S., Stein H. and Mason D.Y. (1985) Malignant histiocytosis of the intestine: a T-cell lymphoma. Lancet ii:688–691.

Isaacson P.G. and Spencer J. (1987) Malignant lymphoma of mucosa-associated lymphoid tissue. Histopathology 11:445–462.

Isaacson P.G. and Wright D.H. (1978) Malignant histiocytosis of the intestine: its relationship to malabsorption and ulcerative jejunitis. Human Pathology 9:661–677.

Isaacson P.G. and Wright D.H. (1995) Gut-associated lymphoid tumours. In: Gastrointestinal and Oesophageal Pathology. Edited by R. Whitehead. Edinburgh: Churchill Livingstone, pp 755–775.

Isselbacher K.J., Scheig R., Plotkin G.R. and Caulfield J.B. (1964) Congenital b-lipoprotein deficiency: a hereditary disorder involving a defect in the absorption and transport of lipids. Medicine 43:347–361.

Iyngkaran N., Yadav M., Boey C.G., Kamath K.R. and Lam K.L. (1989) Causative effect of cow's milk protein and soy protein on progressive small bowel mucosal damage. Journal of Gastroenterology and Hepatology 4:127–136.

Iyngkaran N., Yadav M., Boey C.G., Meng L.L., Puthucheary S.D. and Lam K.L. (1988a) Effect of diet on the clinical course and repair of the small bowel mucosa in infantile gastroenteritis. Journal of Gastroenterology and Hepatology 3:337–344.

Iyngkaran N., Yadav M., Looi L.M., Boey C.G., Lam K.L., Balabaskaran S., and Puthucheary S.D. (1988b) Effect of soy protein on the small bowel mucosa of young infants recovering from acute gastroenteritis. Journal of Pediatric Gastroenterology and Nutrition 7:68–75.

Jackson D., Walker-Smith J.A. and Phillips A.D. (1982) M cells in rat and childhood follicle associated epithelium in the small intestine. Gut 23:A923.

Jackson P.G., Lessof M.H., Baker R.W.R., Ferrett J. and MacDonald D.M. (1981) Intestinal permeability in patients with eczema and food allergy. Lancet i:1285–1286.

James A.H. (1964) Gastric epithelium in the duodenum. Gut 5:285–294.

Jardine D.L., Fitzpatrick M.A., Troughton W.D. and Tie A.B. (1994) Small bowel ischaemia in Fabry's disease. Journal of Gastroenterology and Hepatology 9:201–204.

Jarmay K., Varkonyi T. and Hajnal-Papp R. (1993) Collagenous sprue—a rare form of celiac disease in adulthood. Zeitschrift für Gastroenterologie 31:144–146.

Jeffers M.D. and Hourihane D.O. (1993) Coeliac disease with histological features of peptic duodenitis: value of assessment of intraepithelial lymphocytes. Journal of Clinical Pathology 46:420–424.

Jeffries G.H., Steinberg H. and Sleisenger M.H. (1968) Chronic ulcerative (nongranulomatous) jejunitis. American Journal of Medicine 44:47–59.

Jenkins D., Goodall A., Gillet F.R. and Scott B.B. (1985) Defining duodenitis: quantitative histological study of mucosal responses and their correlations. Journal of Clinical Pathology 38:1119–1126.

Jensenius M. (1995) Hookworm disease: a differential diagnosis in iron deficiency anemia. Tidsskrift for den Norske Laegeforening 115:367–369.

Jepsen J.M., Persson M., Jakobsen N.O., Christensen T., Skoubo-Kristensen E., Funch-Jensen P., Kruse A. and Thommesen P. (1994) Prospective study of prevalence and endoscopic and histopathologic characteristics of duodenal polyps in patients submitted to upper endoscopy. Scandinavian Journal of Gastroenterology 29:483–487.

Jewell D.P. (1983) Ulcerative enteritis. British Medical Journal 287:1740–1741.

Johansen A. (1974) Enzyme histochemical investigations of heterotopic gastric epithelium in the duodenum. Acta Pathologica et Microbiologica Scandinavica 82:613–617.

Johansen A. and Hansen O.H. (1973) Heterotopic gastric epithelium in the duodenum and its correlation to gastric disease and acid level. Acta Pathologica et Microbiologica Scandinavica 81:676–680.

Johnson C.D. and White H. (1988) Colonic metaplasia with colonic-type polyps on an ileostomy stoma in polyposis coli. Diseases of the Colon and Rectum 31:405–407.

Jones B., Fishman E.K., Bayless T.M. and Siegelman S.S. (1983) Villous hypertrophy of the small bowel in a patient with glucagonoma. Journal of Computer Assisted Tomography 7:334–337.

Jones M.A., Griffith L.M. and West A.B. (1989) Adenocarcinoid tumor of the periampullary region: a novel duodenal neoplasm presenting as biliary tract obstruction. Human Pathology 20:198–200.

Judd E.S. and Nagel W.G. (1927) Duodenitis. Annals of Surgery 85:380.

Kagnoff M.F., Paterson Y.J., Kumar P.J., Kasarda D.D., Carbone F.R., Unsworth D.J. and Austin R.K. (1987) Evidence for the role of a human intestinal adenovirus in the pathogenesis of coeliac disease. Gut 28:995–1001.

Kamath K.R. and Murugasu R. (1974) A comparative study of four methods for detecting *Giardia lamblia* in children with diarrheal disease and malabsorption. Gastroenterology 66:16–21.

Kang J.Y., Wu A.Y.T., Chia J.L.S., Wee A., Sutherland I.H. and Hori R. (1987) Clinical and ultrastructural studies in duodenal pseudomelanosis. Gut 28:1673–1681.

Kanof M.E., Rance N.E., Hamilton S.R., Luk G.D. and Lake A.M. (1987) Congenital diarrhea with intestinal inflammation and epithelial immaturity. Journal of Pediatric Gastroenterology and Nutrition 6:141–146.

Kaufmann H.P., Schmitt W. and Seib H.J. (1994) Alpha-heavy chain disease: Mediterranean lymphoma. Leber, Magen, Darm 24:32–35.

Kavin H. (1981) Celiac disease complicated by chronic nongranulomatous ulcerative enterocolitis, nodular lymphoid hyperplasia, and disseminated intravascular coagulation. Digestive Diseases and Sciences 26:73–80.

Keeling J.W. and Harries J.T. (1973) Intestinal malabsorption in infants with histiocytosis X. Archives of Disease in Childhood 48:350–354.

Kelly J., O'Farrelly C., O'Mahony C., Weir D.G. and Feighery C. (1987) Immunoperoxidase demonstration of the cellular composition of the normal and coeliac small bowel. Clinics of Experimental Immunology 68:177–188.

Kent T.H. (1964) Malabsorption syndrome with malignant lymphoma. Archives of Pathology 78:97–103.

Keren D.F., Weisburger W.R., Yardley J.H., Salyer W.R., Arthur R.R. and Charache P. (1976) Whipple's disease: demonstration by immunofluorescence of similar bacterial antigens in macrophages from three cases. Johns Hopkins Medical Journal 139:51–59.

Kerr C. (1984) Diagnosis of lysosomal storage disorders. Medical Journal of Australia 140:188–189.

Khojasteh A., Haghshenass M. and Haghighi P. (1983) Immunoproliferative small intestinal disease: a ''third-world lesion.'' New England Journal of Medicine 308:1401–1405.

Kikindjanin V., Vukavic T., Opric M. and Novakov G. (1985) Local immunodeficiency of the intestinal mucosa: a contribution to etiopathogenesis of recurrent urticaria and diarrhoea. Allergie et Immunologie 31:183–188.

King C.E. and Toskes P.P. (1979) Small intestinal bacterial overgrowth. Gastroenterology 76:1035–1055.

Kingham J.G., Levison D.A. and Fairclough P.D. (1981) Diarrhoea and reversible enteropathy in Zollinger-Ellison syndrome. Lancet ii:610–612.

Klipstein F.A. and Schenk E.A. (1975) Enterotoxigenic intestinal bacteria in tropical sprue: effect of the bacteria and their enterotoxins on intestinal structure. Gastroenterology 68:642–655.

Kluge F., Koch H.K., Grosse-Wilde H., Lesch R. and Gerok W. (1982) Follow-up of treated adult celiac disease: clinical and morphological studies. Hepato-gastroenterology 29:17–23.

Kmiot W.A., Youngs D., Tudor R., Thompson H. and Keighley M.R. (1993) Mucosal morphology, cell proliferation and faecal bacteriology in acute pouchitis. British Journal of Surgery 80:1445–1449.

Knight R. and Wright S.G. (1978) Progress report intestinal protozoa. Gut 19:940–953.

Kokkonen J., Simila S. and Herva R. (1980) Gastrointestinal findings in atopic children. European Journal of Pediatrics 134:249–254.

Konjetzny G.E. (1924) Zur pathologie und chirurgischen behandlung des ulcus duodeni. Deutche Zeitschrift der Chirurgie 184:85.

Kosnai I., Karpati S., Savilahti E., Verkasalo M., Bucsky P. and Torok E. (1986) Gluten challenge in children with dermatitis herpetiformis: a clinical, morphological and immunohistological study. Gut 27:1464–1470.

Kosnai I., Kuitunen P., Savilahti E. and Sipponen P. (1984) Mast cells and eosinophils in the jejunal mucosa of patients with intestinal cow's milk allergy and celiac disease of childhood. Journal of Pediatric Gastroenterology and Nutrition 3:368–372.

Kosztolanyi G. and Pap M. (1986) Severe growth failure associated with atrophic intestinal mucosa and ring chromosome 15. Acta Paediatrica Scandinavica 75:326–331.

Kreuning J., Bosman F.T., Kuiper G., v.d. Wal A.M. and Lindeman J. (1978) Gastritis and duodenal mucosa in ''healthy'' individuals: an endoscopic and histopathological study of 50 volunteers. Journal of Clinical Pathology 31:69–77.

Kumar P.J., O'Donoghue D.P., Stenson K. and Dawson A.M. (1979) Reintroduction of gluten in adults and children with treated coeliac disease. Gut 20:743–749.

Kundrotas L.W., Camara D.S., Meenaghan M.A., Montes M., Wosick W.F. and Weiser M.M. (1985) Heterotopic gastric mucosa: a case report. American Journal of Gastroenterology 80:253–256.

Kuo Y-C. and Wu C-S. (1988) Duodenal melanosis. Journal of Clinical Gastroenterology 10:160–164.

Kwitko A.O., Shearman D.J.C., McKenzie P.E., La Brooy J.T., Rowland R. and Woodroffe A.J. (1980) Whipple's disease: a case with circulating immune complexes. Gastroenterology 79:1318–1323.

Labenz J., Peitz U., Madeya S., Wieczorek M., Erdelkamp J. and Börsch G. (1993) Arthralgia, weight loss and polyserositis as chief symptoms of Whipple's disease (clinical conference). Medizinische Klinik 88:427–431, 448.

Ladas S.D., Tsamouri M., Kouvidou C. and Raptis S.A. (1994) Effect of forceps size and mode of orientation on endoscopic small bowel biopsy evaluation. Gastrointestinal Endoscopy 40:51–55.

Lake B.D. (1988) Microvillus inclusion disease: specific diagnostic features shown by alkaline phosphatase histochemistry. Journal of Clinical Pathology 41:880–882.

Lamers C.B.H.W., Wagener D.J.T., Assmann K.J.M. and Van Tongeren J.H.M. (1980) Jejunal lymphoma in a patient with primary adult-onset hypogammaglobulinemia and nodular lymphoid hyperplasia of the small intestine. Digestive Diseases and Sciences 25:553–557.

Lamy M., Frezal J., Polonovski J., Druez G. and Rey J. (1962) Congenital absence of beta-lipoproteins. Paediatrics 31:277–289.

Lancaster-Smith M., Packer S., Kumar P.J. and Harries J.T. (1976a) Cellular infiltrate of the jejunum after re-introduction of dietary gluten in children with treated coeliac disease. Journal of Clinical Pathology 29:587–591.

Lancaster-Smith M., Packer S., Kumar P.J. and Harries J.T. (1976b) Immunological phenomena in the jejunum and serum after re-introduction of dietary gluten in children with treated coeliac disease. Journal of Clinical Pathology 29:592–597.

Landboe-Christensen E. (1944) The duodenal glands of Brunner in man, their distribution and quantity. Acta Pathologica et Microbiologica Scandinavica 52 (suppl):240.

Landing B.H. and Nadorra R. (1986) Infantile systemic hyalinosis. Pediatric Pathology 6:55–79.

Langman J.M. and Rowland R. (1986) The number and distribution of lymphoid follicles in the human large intestine. Journal of Anatomy 194:189–194.

Lasser K.H., Lewin K.J. and Ryning F.W.(1979) Cryptosporidial enteritis in a patient with congenital hypogamma-globulinemia. Human Pathology 10:234–240.

Lawson H.H. (1987) Is duodenitis related to duodenal ulceration as gastritis is to gastric ulceration? South African Journal of Surgery 25:85–86.

Lazaro R.P., Dentinger M.P., Rodichok L.D., Barron K.D. and Satya-Murti S. (1986) Muscle pathology in Bassen-Kornzweig syndrome and vitamin E deficiency. American Journal of Clinical Pathology 86:378–387.

Leading Article. (1970) A new line on age pigment? Lancet ii:451–452.

Leading Article. (1974) Epidemic giardiasis. Lancet ii:1493.

Leading Article. (1979) Food allergy. Lancet i:249–250.

Lebenthal E. and Branski D. (1981) Childhood celiac disease: a reappraisal. Journal of Pediatrics 98:681–690.

Lederman H.M. and Winkelstein J.A. (1985) X-linked agamma-globulinaemia: an analysis of 96 patients. Medicine 64:145–156.

Lee H.H., O'Donnell D.B. and Keren D.F. (1987) Characteristics of melanosis duodeni: incorporation of endoscopy, pathology and etiology. Endoscopy 19:107–109.

Lee S.H. et al (1993) A case of intestinal capillariasis in the Republic of Korea. American Journal of Tropical Medicine and Hygiene 48:542–546.

Lee S.P. and Nicholson G.I. (1976) Ceroid enteropathy and vitamin E deficiency. New Zealand Medical Journal 83:318–320.

Leidig P., Stolte M., Krakamp B. and Storkel S. (1994) Whipple's disease: a rare cause of secondary amyloidosis. Zeitschrift für Gastroenterologie 32:109–112.

Lenzhofer R., Lindner M., Moser A., Berger J., Schusnigg C. and Thurner J. (1993) Acute jejunal ileus in intestinal lymphangiectasia. Clinical Investigations 71:568–571.

Lev R., Thomas E., Parl F.F. and Pitchumoni C.S. (1980) Pathological and histomorphometric study of the effects of alcohol on the human duodenum. Digestion 20:207–213.

Lin C.N., Huang A.H., Hsu S.I., Lee C., Liang A.I., Kuo C.I. and Chuang S.S. (1993) Brown bowel syndrome: report of two cases. Journal of the Formosan Medical Association 92:1090–1094.

Lin H-J., Tsay S-H., Chiang H., Tsai Y-T., Lee S-D., Yeh Y-S. and Lo G-H. (1988) Pseudomelanosis duodeni. Journal of Clinical Gastroenterology 10:155–159.

Loehry C.A. and Grace R. (1974) The dynamic structure of a flat small intestinal mucosa studied on the explanted rat jejunum. Gut 15:289–293.

London N.J.M., Leese T., Bingham P., O'Reilly K. and Self J.B. (1988) Invasive Paneth cell-rich adenocarcinoma of the duodenum. British Journal of Hospital Medicine 40:222–223.

Loughran T.P., Kadin M.E. and Deeg H.J. (1986) T-cell intestinal lymphoma associated with celiac sprue. Annals of Internal Medicine 104:44–47.

MacCarty W.C. (1924) Excised duodenal ulcers: a report of four hundred and twenty-five specimens. Journal of the American Medical Association 83:1894.

Mackinnon M., Willing R.L. and Whitehead R. (1982) Cimetidine in the management of symptomatic patients with duodenitis: a double-blind controlled trial. Digestive Diseases and Sciences 27:217–219.

Macromichalis J., Brueton M.J., McNeish A.S. and Anderson C.M. (1976) Evaluation of the intraepithelial lymphocyte count in the jejunum in childhood enteropathies. Gut 17:600–603.

McClave S.A., Goldschmid S., Cunningham J.T. and Boyd W.P. (1988) Dieulafoy's cirsoid aneurysm of the duodenum. Digestive Diseases and Sciences 33:801–805.

McDonald G.B., Schuffler M.D., Kadin M.E. and Tytgat G.N.J. (1985) Intestinal pseudo-obstruction caused by diffuse lymphoid infiltration of the small intestine. Gastroenterology 89:882–889.

McLeod R.S., Antonioli D., Cullen J., Dvorak A., Onderdonk A., Silen W., Blair J.E., Monahan-Early R., Cisneros R. and Chen Z. (1994) Histologic and microscopic features of biopsy samples from patients with normal and inflamed pouches. Diseases of the Colon and Rectum 37:26–31.

McNeish A.S. (1980) Coeliac disease: duration of gluten-free diet. Archives of Disease in Childhood 55:110–111.

Madanagopolan N., Shiner M. and Rowe B. (1965) Measurements of small intestinal mucosa obtained by peroral biopsy. American Journal of Medicine 38:42–53.

Magalhaes A.F.N., Trevisan M.A.S. and Pereira A.S. (1975) Jejunal biopsies in protein-calorie malnutrition and intestinal parasitic infestation in Brazil. American Journal of Gastroenterology 64:472–477.

Mahant T.S., Kohli P.K., Mathur J.M., Bhushurmath S.R., Wig J.D. and Kaushik S.P. (1983) Actinomycosis caecum: a case report. Digestion 27:53–55.

Maizel H., Ruffin J.M. and Dobbins W.O. (1970) Whipple's disease: a review of 19 patients from one hospital and a review of the literature since 1950. Medicine 49:175–205.

Major D.A. and Brandt F. (1976) Brunner's gland adenoma associated with high-output congestive heart failure. American Journal of Gastroenterology 66:562–565.

Maluenda C., Phillips A.D., Briddon A. and Walker-Smith J.A. (1984) Quantitative analysis of small intestinal mucosa in cow's milk–sensitive enteropathy. Journal of Pediatric Gastroenterology and Nutrition 3:349–356.

Mangla J.C., Pereira M. and Bhargava A. (1985) Nodular duodenitis in chronic maintenance hemodialysis patients. Gastrointestinal Endoscopy 31:318–321.

Manousos O.N., Economidou J.C., Georgiadou D.E., Pratsika-Ougourloglou K.G., Hadziyannis S.J., Merikas G.E., Henry K. and Doe W.F. (1974) Alpha-chain disease with clinical, immunological and histological recovery. British Medical Journal 2:409–412.

Maratka Z., Kocianova J., Kudrmann J., Jirk P. and Pirk F. (1979) Hyperplasia of Brunner's glands: radiology, endoscopy and biopsy. Acta Hepato-Gastroenterology 26:64–69.

Marcial M.A. and Madara J.L. (1986) Cryptosporidium: cellular localization, structural analysis of absorptive cell-parasite membrane-membrane interactions in guinea pigs, and suggestion of protozoan transport by M cells. Gastroenterology 90:83–94.

Marks J. and Shuster S. (1970) Small intestinal mucosal abnormalities in various skin diseases: fact or fancy? Gut 11:281–291.

Marks R., Whittle M.W., Beard R.J., Robertson W.B. and Gold S.C. (1968) Small bowel abnormalities in dermatitis herpetiformis. British Medical Journal 1:552–555.

Marsh M.N. (1980) Studies of intestinal lymphoid tissue: quantitative analyses of epithelial lymphocytes in the small intestine of human control subjects and of patients with coeliac sprue. Gastroenterology 79:481–492.

Marsh M.N. (1982) Studies of intestinal lymphoid tissue: the predictive value of raised mitotic indices among jejunal epithelial lymphocytes in the diagnosis of gluten-sensitive enteropathy. Journal of Clinical Pathology 35:517–525.

Marsh M.N. (1985) Functional and structural aspects of the epithelial lymphocyte, with implications for coeliac disease and tropical sprue. Scandinavian Journal of Gastroenterology 20 (suppl 114):55–75.

Marsh M.N. and Haeney M.R. (1983) Studies of intestinal lymphoid tissue: proliferative response of small intestinal epithelial lymphocytes distinguishes gluten- from non-gluten–induced enteropathy. Journal of Clinical Pathology 36:149–160.

Marsh M.N. and Hinde J. (1985) Inflammatory component of celiac sprue mucosa: mast cells, basophils, and eosinophils. Gastroenterology 89:92–101.

Marsh M.N., Mathan M. and Mathan V.I. (1983) Studies of intestinal lymphoid tissue: the secondary nature of lymphoid cell "activation" in the jejunal lesion of tropical sprue. American Journal of Pathology 112:302–312.

Marshall A.R., Al-Jumaili I.J., Fenwick G.A., Bint A.J. and Record C.O. (1987) Cryptosporidiosis in patients at a large teaching hospital. Journal of Clinical Microbiology 25:172–173.

Martin I.G. and Aldoori M.I. (1994) Immunoproliferative small intestinal disease: Mediterranean lymphoma and alpha heavy chain disease. British Journal of Surgery 81:20–24.

Martinez-Salmeron J.F., Corral C., Uariachi M., López J., Perales E. and Morales I. (1994) Tropical sprue. Revista Espãnola de Enfermedades Digestivas 85:273–275.

Mathan M., Hughes J. and Whitehead R. (1987) The morphogenesis of the human Paneth cell: an immunocytochemical ultrastructural study. Histochemistry 87:91–96.

Mathan M., Mathan V.I. and Baker S.J. (1975) An electron microscopic study of jejunal mucosal morphology in control subjects and in patients with tropical sprue in Southern India. Gastroenterology 68:17–32.

Mathan M.M., Ponniah J. and Mathan V.I. (1986) Epithelial cell renewal and turnover and relationship to morphologic abnormalities in jejunal mucosa in tropical sprue. Digestive Diseases and Sciences 31:586–592.

Matsui K. and Kitagawa M. (1993) Biopsy study of polyps in the duodenal bulb. American Journal of Gastroenterology 88:253–257.

Matuchansky C., Colin R., Hemet J., Touchard G., Babin P., Eugene C., Bergue A., Zeitoun P. and Barboteau M.A. (1984) Cavitation of mesenteric lymph nodes, splenic atrophy, and a flat small intestinal mucosa. Gastroenterology 87:606–614.

Matuchansky C., Morichau-Beauchant M., Touchard G., Lenormand Y., Bloch P., Tanzer J., Alcalay D. and Babin P. (1980) Nodular lymphoid hyperplasia of the small bowel associated with primary jejunal malignant lymphoma. Gastroenterology 78:1587–1592.

Mauriño E., Capizzano H., Niveloni S., Kogan Z., Valero J., Boerr L. and Bai J.C. (1993) Value of endoscopic markers in celiac disease. Digestive Diseases and Sciences 38:2028–2033.

Mazzanti R. and Jenkins W.J. (1987) Effect of chronic ethanol ingestion on enterocyte turnover in rat small intestine. Gut 28:52–55.

Mead G.M., Whitehouse J.M., Thompson J., Sweetenham J.W., Williams C.J. and Wright D.H. (1987) Clinical features and management of malignant histiocytosis of the intestine. Cancer 60:2791–2796.

Mee A.S., Burke M., Vallon A.G., Newman J. and Cotton P.B. (1985) Small bowel biopsy for malabsorption: comparison of the diagnostic adequacy of endoscopic forceps and capsule biopsy specimens. British Medical Journal 291:769–772.

Meier J., Bergwanger I., Zangana N. and Hellerich O. (1994) Whipple disease with negative duodenal histology: a case report and review of the literature. Zeitschrift für Rheumatologie 53:352–362.

Meisel J.L., Perera D.R., Meligro C. and Rubin C.E. (1976) Overwhelming watery diarrhea associated with a cryptosporidium in an immunosuppressed patient. Gastroenterology 70:1156–1160.

Meyers W.M., Neafie R.C. and Connor D.H. (1976) Ancylostomiasis. In: Pathology of Tropical and Extraordinary Diseases. Volume 2. Edited by C.H. Binford and D.H. Connor. Washington: Armed Forces Institute of Pathology, pp 421–427.

Millan M.S., Morris G.P., Beck I.T. and Henson J.T. (1980) Villous damage induced by suction biopsy and by acute ethanol intake in normal human small intestine. Digestive Diseases and Sciences 25:513–525.

Minford A.M.B., MacDonald A. and Littlewood J.M. (1982) Food intolerance and food allergy in children: a review of 68 cases. Archives of Disease in Childhood 57:742–747.

Mirakian R., Richardson A., Milla P.J., Walker-Smith J.A., Unsworth J., Savage M.O. and Bottazzo G.F. (1986) Protracted diarrhea of infancy: evidence in support of an autoimmune varient. British Medical Journal 293:1132–1136.

Mistilis S.P., Skyring A.P. and Stephen D.D. (1965) Intestinal lymphangiectasia: mechanism of enteric loss of plasma protein and fat. Lancet i:77–79.

Monges H., Aubert L., Chamlian A., Remacle J P., Mathieu B., Cougard A. and Arroyo H. (1975) Maladie des chaines alpha a forme intestinale. Archives francaises du maladie de l'appareil digestif 64:223–231.

Monges H., Aubert L., Remacle J-P., Chamlian A., Mathieu B., Cougard A., Quilichini R. and Chaffanjon P. (1980) Survenue d'une maladie de Hodgkin quatre ans apres remission complete d'une maladie des chaines alpha. Gastroenterologie Clinique et Biologique 4:181–187.

Montero C. and Erlandsen S.L. (1978) Immunocytochemical and histochemical studies on intestinal epithelial cells producing both lysozyme and mucosubstance. Anatomical Record 190:127–141.

Montgomery R.D., Beale D.J., Sammons H.G. and Schneider R. (1973) Postinfective malabsorption: a sprue syndrome. British Medical Journal 2:265–268.

Montgomery R.D. and Shearer A.C.I. (1974) The cell population of the upper jejunal mucosa in tropical sprue and postinfective malabsorption. Gut 15:387–391.

Moon A. and Kleinman R.E. (1995) Allergic gastroenteropathy in children. Annals of Allergy, Asthma, and Immunology 74:5–16.

Moore J.V. (1984) Death of intestinal crypts and of their constituent cells after treatment by chemotherapeutic drugs. British Journal of Cancer 49:25–32.

Moorthy S., Nolley G. and Hermos J.A. (1977) Whipple's disease with minimal intestinal involvement. Gut 18:152–155.

Morecki R. and Parker J.G. (1967) Ultrastructural studies of the human Giardia lamblia and subadjacent jejunal mucosa in a subject with steatorrhea. Gastroenterology 52:151–164.

Morecki R., Paunier L. and Hamilton J.R. (1968) Intestinal mucosa in cystinosis. Archives of Pathology 86:297–307.

Morgensen A.M., Bulow S. and Hage E. (1989) Duodenal adenomas in familial adenomatous polyposis: their structure and cellular composition with particular reference to endocrine hyperplasia. Virchows Archiv A 414:315–319.

Morgensen A.M., Hage E. and Bulow S. (1989) Electron microscopic studies of endocrine hyperplasia in duodenal adenomas in familial adenomatous polyposis. Virchows Archiv A 414:321–324.

Moritz M., Moran J.M. and Patterson J.F. (1971) Chronic ulcerative jejunitis. Gastroenterology 60:96–102.

Muigai R., Gatei D.G., Shaunak S., Wozniak A., and Bryceson A.D.M. (1983) Jejunal function and pathology in visceral leishmaniasis. Lancet ii:476–479.

Nabeyama A. and Leblond C.P. (1974) "Caveolated cells" characterized by deep surface invaginations and abundant filaments in mouse gastro-intestinal epithelia. American Journal of Anatomy 140:147–166.

Nagura H., Kohler P.F. and Brown W.R. (1979) Immunocytochemical characterization of the lymphocytes in nodular lymphoid hyperplasia of the bowel. Laboratory Investigation 40:66–73.

Nakanishi T., Takeuchi T., Hara K. and Sugimoto A. (1984) A great Brunner's gland adenoma of the duodenal bulb. Digestive Diseases and Sciences 29:81–85.

Nakayama M., Kamuro Y., Sagara K., Sato T., Togami K. and Tashiro S. (1983) A case of bleeding duodenal varices located in the third portion. Gastroenterologica Japonica 18:599–602.

Narvaez-Rodriguez I. et al (1993) The brown bowel syndrome. A case report. Revista Espãnola de Enfermedades Digestivas 83:281–283.

Nash J.R.G., Gradwell E. and Day D.W. (1986) Large-cell intestinal lymphoma occurring in coeliac disease: morphological and immunohistochemical features. Histopathology 10:195–205.

Nasr K., Haghighi P., Bakhshandeh K., Abadi P. and Lahimgarzadeh A. (1976) Primary upper small intestinal lymphoma: a report of 40 cases from Iran. Amerian Journal of Digestive Diseases 21:313–323.

Nime F.A., Burek J.D., Page D.L., Holscher M.A. and Yardley J.H. (1976) Acute enterocolitis in a human being infected with the protozoan Cryptosporidium. Gastroenterology 70:592–598.

Noda Y., Watanabe H., Iida M., Narisawa R., Kurosaki I., Iwafuchi M., Satoh M. and Ajioka Y. (1992) Histologic follow-up of ampullary adenomas in patients with familial adenomatous coli. Cancer 70:1847–1856.

Norton A.J. and Isaacson P.G. (1989a) Lymphoma phenotyping in formalin-fixed and paraffin wax–embedded tissues: range of antibodies and staining patterns. Histopathology 14:437–446.

Norton A.J. and Isaacson P.G. (1989b) Lymphoma phenotyping in formalin-fixed and paraffin wax–embedded tissues: range of antibodies and staining patterns. Histopathology 14: 557–579.

Nugent K.P., Spigelman A.D., Williams C.B., Talbot I.C. and Phillips R.K. (1994) Surveillance of duodenal polyps in familial adenomatous polyposis: progress report. Journal of the Royal Society of Medicine 87:704–706.

Obertop H., Nundy S., Malamud D. and Malt R.A. (1977) Onset of cell proliferation in the shortened gut: rapid hyperplasia after jejunal resection. Gastroenterology 72:267–270.

O'Brien B.D., Shnitka T.K., McDougall R., Walker K., Costopoulos L., Lentle B., Anholt L., Freeman H. and Thomson A.B.R. (1982) Pathophysiologic and ultrastructural basis for intestinal symptoms in Fabry's disease. Gastroenterology 82:957–962.

O'Donoghue D.P., Lancaster-Smith M., Laviniere P. and Kumar P.J. (1976) T cell depletion in untreated adult coeliac disease. Gut 17:328–331.

O'Farrelly C., Graeme-Cook F., Hourihane D.O'B., Feighery C. and Weir D.G. (1987) Histological changes associated with wheat protein antibodies in the absence of villous atrophy. Journal of Clinical Pathology 40:1228–1230.

O'Grady J.G., Stevens F.M. and McCarthy C.F. (1985) Celiac disease: does hyposplenism predispose to the development of malignant disease? American Journal of Gastroenterology 80:27–29.

Oliva H., Gonzalez-Campos C., Navarro V. and Mogena H.H. (1972) Two cases of Whipple's disease showing clinical and morphological similarity. Gut 13:430–437.

Olsson R., Kagevi I. and Rydberg L. (1982) On the concurrence of primary biliary cirrhosis and intestinal villous atrophy. Scandinavian Journal of Gastroenterology 17:625–628.

Olubuyide I.O., Williamson R.C.N., Bristol J.B. and Read A.E. (1984) Goblet cell hyperplasia is a feature of the adaptive response to jejunoileal bypass in rats. Gut 25:62–68.

Orchard J.L., Luparello F. and Brunskill D. (1979) Malabsorption syndrome occurring in the course of disseminated histoplasmosis. American Journal of Medicine 60:331–335.

Orenstein S.R. (1986) The small bowel biopsy in intractable diarrhea of infancy. Gastroenterology 90:785–787.

Otto H.F., Bettman I., Weltzien J.V. and Gebbers J-O. (1981) Primary intestinal lymphomas. Virchows Archiv A 391:9–31.

Owen R.L. (1977) Sequential uptake of horseradish peroxidase by lymphoid follicle epithelium of Peyer's patches in the normal unobstructed mouse intestine: an ultrastructural study. Gastroenterology 72:440–451.

Owen R.L., Allen C.L. and Stevens D.P. (1981) Phagocytosis of *Giardia muris* by macrophages in Peyer's patch epithelium in mice. Infection and Immunity 33:591–601.

Owen R.L. and Nemanic P. (1978) Antigen processing structures of the mammalian intestinal tract: an SEM study of lymphoepithelial organs. Scanning Electron Microscopy 2:367–378.

Owen R.L., Nemanic P.C. and Stevens D.P. (1979) Ultrastructural observations on giardiasis in a murine model: intestinal distribution, attachment, and relationship to the immune system of *Giardia muris*. Gastroenterology 76:757–769.

Paerregaard A., Vilien M., Krasilnikoff P.A. and Gudmand-Hoyer E. (1988) Supposed coeliac disease during childhood and its presentation 14–38 years later. Scandinavian Journal of Gastroenterology 23:65–70.

Paimela H., Tallgren L.G., Stenman S., Numers H.v. and Scheinin T.M. (1984) Multiple duodenal polyps in uraemia: a little-known clinical entity. Gut 25:259–263.

Paoluzi P., Pallone F., Palazzesi P., Marcheggiano A. and Iannoni C. (1982) Frequency and extent of bulbar duodenitis in duodenal ulcer: endoscopic and histological study. Endoscopy 14:193–195.

Papadopoulos K.I., Hornblad Y. and Hallengren B. (1994) The occurrence of polyglandular autoimmune syndrome type III associated with coeliac disease in patients with sarcoidosis. Journal of Internal Medicine 236:661–663.

Parrish F.J., Hemming J.D. and Matthewson K. (1994) Endoscopic diagnosis of Waldenstrom's macroglobulinemia. Gastrointestinal Endoscopy 40:102–104.

Partin J.C. and Schubert W.K. (1969) Small intestinal mucosa in cholesterol ester storage disease. Gastroenterology 57:542–558.

Patrick W.J.A., Denham D. and Forrest A.P.M. (1974) Mucous change in the human duodenum: a light and electron microscopic study and correlation with disease and gastric acid secretion. Gut 15:767–776.

Pena A.S., Callender S.T., Truelove S.C. and Whitehead R. (1972) Small intestinal mucosal abnormalities and disaccharidase activity in pernicious anemia. British Journal of Haematology 23:313–321.

Pena A.S., Truelove S.C. and Whitehead R. (1972) Disaccharidase activity and jejunal morphology in coeliac disease. Quarterly Journal of Medicine 41:457–476.

Pena A.S., Truelove S.C. and Whitehead R. (1973) Morphology and disaccharidase levels of jejunal biopsy specimens from healthy British subjects. Digestion 8:317–323.

Penna C., Phillips R.K., Tiret E. and Spigelman A.D. (1993) Surgical polypectomy of duodenal adenomas in familial adenomatous polyposis: experience of two European centres. British Journal of Surgery 80:1027–1029.

Penna F.J., Hill I.D., Kingston D., Robertson K., Slavin G. and Shiner M. (1981) Jejunal mucosal morphometry in children with and without gut symptoms and in normal adults. Journal of Clinical Pathology 34:386–392.

Perlmutter D.H., Leichtner A.M., Goldman H. and Winter H.S. (1985) Chronic diarrhea associated with hypogammaglobulinemia and enteropathy in infants and children. Digestive Diseases and Sciences 30:1149–1155.

Petersen H. (1972) Giardiasis (Lambliasis). Scandinavian Journal of Gastroenterology 7 (suppl 14):4–44.

Phillips A., Fransen J., Hauri H.P. and Sterchi E. (1993) The constitutive exocytotic pathway in microvillous atrophy. Journal of Pediatric Gastroenterology and Nutrition 17:239–246.

Phillips A.D. (1995) The small intestinal mucosa. In: Gastrointestinal and Oesophageal Pathology. Edited by R. Whitehead. Edinburgh: Churchill Livingstone, p 34.

Phillips A.D., Avigad S., Sacks J., Rice S.J., France N.E. and Walker-Smith J.A. (1980) Microvillous surface area in secondary disaccharidase deficiency. Gut 21:44–48.

Phillips A.D., Jenkins P., Raafat F. and Walker-Smith J.A. (1985) Congenital microvillous atrophy: specific diagnostic features. Archives of Disease in Childhood 60:135–140.

Phillips A.D., Rice S.J., France N.E. and Walker-Smith J.A. (1979) Small intestinal intraepithelial lymphocyte levels in cow's milk protein intolerance. Gut 20:509–512.

Pietroletti R., Bishop A.E., Carlei F., Bonamico M., Lloyd R.V., Wilson B.S., Ceccamea A., Lezoche E., Speranza V. and Polak J.M. (1986) Gut endocrine cell population in coeliac disease estimated by immunocytochemistry using a monoclonal antibody to chromogranin. Gut 27:838–843.

Pink I.J. and Creamer B. (1967) Response to gluten-free diet of patients with coeliac syndrome. Lancet i:300–304.

Pink I.J., Croft D.N. and Creamer B. (1970) Cell loss from small intestinal mucosa: a morphological study. Gut 11:217–222.

Pinkerton C.R., Cameron C.H.S., Sloan J.M., Glascow J.F.T. and Gwevava N.J.T. (1982) Jejunal crypt cell abnormalities associated with methotrexate treatment in children with acute lymphoblastic leukaemia. Journal of Clinical Pathology 35:1272–1277.

Polak J.M., Pearse A.G.E., van Noorden S., Bloom S.R. and Rossiter M.A. (1973) Secretin cells in coeliac disease. Gut 14:870–874.

Polanko I., Mearin M.L., Larrauri J., Biemond I., Wipkink-Bakker A. and Pena A.S. (1987) Effect of gluten supplementation in healthy siblings of children with coeliac disease. Gastroenterology 92:678–681.

Pollock D.J., Nagle R.E., Jeejeebhoy K.N. and Coghill N.(1970) The effect on jejunal mucosa of withdrawing and adding dietary gluten in cases of idiopathic steatorrhoea. Gut 11:567–575.

Pomerantz M. and Waldmann T. (1963) Systemic lymphatic abnormalities associated with gastrointestinal protein loss secondary to intestinal lymphangiectasia. Gastroenterology 45:703–711.

Pounder D.J., Ghadially F.N., Mukherjee T.M., Hecker R., Rowland R., Dixon B. and Lalonde J.M.A. (1982) Ultrastructure and electron-probe x-ray analysis of the pigment in melanosis duodeni. Journal of Submicroscopic Cytology 14:389–400.

Prociv P. and Luke R.A. (1995) The changing epidemiology of human hookworm infection in Australia. Medical Journal of Australia 162:150–154.

Pruzanski W., Warren R., Goldie J. and Katz A. (1973) Malabsorption syndrome with infiltration of the intestinal wall by extracellular monoclonal macroglobulin. American Journal of Medicine 54:811–818.

Raizman R.E. (1976) Giardiasis: an overview for the clinician. American Journal of Digestive Diseases 21:1070–1074.

Rambaud J-C., Bognel C., Prost A., Burnier J.J., Le Quintrec Y., Lambling A., Danon F., Hurez D. and Seligmann M. (1968) Clinico-pathological study of a patient with "Mediterranean" type of abdominal lymphoma and a new type of IgA abnormality ("alpha-chain disease"). Digestion 1:321–336.

Rambaud J-C., Galian A., Danon F.G., Preudhomme J-L., Brandtzaeg P., Wassef M., Carrer M.L., Mehaut M.A., Voinchet O.L., Perol R.G. and Chapman A. (1983) Alpha-chain disease without qualitative serum IgA abnormality: report of two cases, including a "nonsecretory" form. Cancer 51:686–693.

Randhawa V.S., Sharma V.K., Malhotra V. and Vij J.C. (1994) Human giardiasis: a morphometric study of duodenal biopsy specimens in relation to the trophozoite count in the duodenal aspirate. Archives of Pathology and Laboratory Medicine 118:891–894.

Rao S.S. and Murthy K.V. (1993) Post-bulbar and coexisting ulceration: unique features of peptic ulcer in Hyberabad. Gut 34:1327–1330.

Rao S.S.C., Dundas S. and Holdsworth C.D. (1987) Intestinal lymphangiectasia secondary to radiotherapy and chemotherapy. Digestive Diseases and Sciences 32:939–942.

Rayford P.L., Miller T.A. and Thompson J.C. (1976a) Secretin, cholecystokinin and newer gastrointestinal hormones: part 1. New England Journal of Medicine 294:1093–1101.

Rayford P.L., Miller T.A. and Thompson J.C. (1976b) Secretin, cholecystokinin and newer gastrointestinal hormones: part 2. New England Journal of Medicine 294:1157–1164.

Reisberg I.R. and Oyakawa S. (1987) Mastocytosis with malabsorption, myelofibrosis, and massive ascites. American Journal of Gastroenterology 82:54–60.

Reunala T., Kosnai I., Karpati S., Kuitunen P., Torok E. and Savilahti E. (1984) Dermatitis herpetiformis: jejunal findings and skin response to gluten-free diet. Archives of Disease in Childhood 59:517–522.

Rex D.K. and Jersild R.A. (1988) Further characterization of the pigment in pseudomelanosis duodeni in three patients. Gastroenterology 95:177–182.

Reynaert H., Debeuckelaere S., De Waele R., Meysman M., Goossens A. and Devis G. (1993) The brown bowel syndrome and gastrointestinal adenocarcinoma: two complications of vitamin E deficiency in celiac sprue and chronic pancreatitis? Journal of Clinical Gastroenterology 16:48–51.

Rhee J.W., Gryboski J.D., Sheahan D.G., Dolan T.F. Jr and Dwyer J.M. (1975) Reversible enteritis and lymphopenia in infantile x-linked agammaglobulinemia. American Journal of Digestive Diseases 20:1071–1075.

Rhodes J. (1964) Experimental production of gastric epithelium in the duodenum. Gut 5:454–458.

Rhodes J., Evans K.T., Lawrie J.H. and Forest A.P.M. (1968) Coarse mucosal folds in the duodenum. Quarterly Journal of Medicine 37:151–169.

Richards W.C.D. (1959) Pigmentation of gastrointestinal muscle. Lancet i:683.

Ridley M.J. and Ridley D.S. (1976) Serum antibodies and jejunal histology in giardiasis associated with malabsorption. Journal of Clinical Pathology 29:30–34.

Riecken E.O. (1970) In: Modern Trends in Gastroenterology. Volume 4. Edited by W.I. Card and B. Creamer. London: Butterworth, p 20.

Riemann J.F. and Schmidt H. (1981) Synopsis of endoscopic and other morphological findings in intestinal lymphangiectasia. Endoscopy 13:60–63.

Rijke R.P.C., Hanson W.R., Plaisier H.M. and Osborne J.W. (1976) The effect of ischemic villus cell damage on crypt cell proliferation in the small intestine: evidence for a feedback control mechanism. Gastroenterology 71:786–792.

Robertson D.A.F., Dixon M.F., Scott B.B., Simpson F.G. and Losowsky M.S. (1983) Small intestinal ulceration: diagnostic difficulties in relation to coeliac disease. Gut 24:565–574.

Robinson J.E., Brown N., Andiman W., Halliday K., Francke U., Robert M.F., Andersson-Anvret M., Horstmann D. and Miller G. (1980) Diffuse polyclonal B-cell lymphoma during primary infection with Epstein-Barr virus. New England Journal of Medicine 302:1293–1297.

Robinson J.W.L. (1972) Intestinal malabsorption in the experimental animal. Gut 13:938–945.

Roca M., Truelove S.C. and Whitehead R. (1975) The histological state of the gastric and duodenal mucosa in healthy volunteers. Gut 16:404.

Rodriguez-Maria R. (1994) A patient with gastrointestinal manifestations and the common variable immunodeficiency syndrome. Revista Espãnola de Enfermedades Digestivas 86:679–681.

Roehrkasse R.L., Roberts I.M., Wald A., Talamo T.S. and Mendelow H. (1986) Celiac sprue complicated by lymphoma presenting with multiple gastric ulcers. Gastroenterology 91:740–745.

Rosch W. and Hoer P.W. (1983) Hyperplasiogenic polyp in the duodenum. Endoscopy 15:117–118.

Rosekrans P.C.M., Lindeman J. and Meijer C.J.L.M. (1981) Quantitative histological and immunohisto-chemical findings in jejunal biopsy specimens in giardiasis. Virchows Archiv A 393:145–151.

Rosekrans P.C.M., Meijer C.J.L.M., Cornelisse C.J., Wal A.M. and Lindeman J. (1980) Use of morphometry and immunohistochemistry of small intestinal biopsy specimens in the diagnosis of food allergy. Journal of Clinical Pathology 33:125–130.

Ross I.N. and Asquith P. (1979) In: Immunology of the Gastrointestinal Tract. Edited by P. Asquith. New York: Churchill Livingstone, pp 152–182.

Rossi T.M., Lebenthal E., Nord K.S. and Fazili R.R. (1980) Extent and duration of small intestinal mucosal injury in intractable diarrhea of infancy. Pediatrics 66:730–735.

Rothenberger D.A. and Wiltz O. (1993) Etiology of pouchitis. Annales de Chirurgie 47:1043–1046.

Roy C.C., Levy E., Green P.H.R., Sniderman A., Letarte J., Buts J-P., Orquin J., Brochu P., Weber A.M., Morin C.L., Marcel Y. and Deckelbaum R.J. (1987) Malabsorption, hypocholesterolemia and fat-filled enterocytes with increased intestinal apoprotein B. Gastroenterology 92:390–399.

Rubin C.E., Brandborg L.L., Phelps P.D., Taylor H.C., Murray C.V., Steinler R., Howry C. and Volwiler W. (1960) Studies of celiac disease: II. Gastroenterology 38:517–535

Rubin C.E. and Dobbins W.O. (1965) Peroral biopsy of the small intestine. Gastroenterology 49:676–697.

Ruchti C., Eisele S. and Kaufmann M. (1990) Fatal intestinal pseudo-obstruction in brown bowel syndrome. Archives of Pathology and Laboratory Medicine 114:76–80.

Rufenacht H., Kasper M., Heitz Ph. U., Streule K. and Harder F. (1986) "Brunneroma": hamartoma or tumor? Pathology, Research and Practice 181:107–109.

Ruseler van Embden J.G., Schouten W.R. and van Lieshout L.M. (1994) Pouchitis: result of microbial imbalance? Gut 35:658–664.

Ryan D.P., Schapiro R.H. and Warshaw A.L. (1986) Villous tumors of the duodenum. Annals of Surgery 203:301–306.

Sadek A. (1965) In: Proceedings of the First National Symposium on Bilharziasis, 1964. Volume 2. Cairo: Ministry of Scientific Research, p 270.

Saha T.K. and Ghosh T.K. (1977) Invasion of small intestinal mucosa by *Giardia lamblia* in man. Gastroen-terology 72:402–405.

Sahn E.E., Salinas C.F., Sens M.A., Key J., Swiger F.K. Jr and Holbrook J.A. (1994) Infantile systemic hyalinosis in a black infant. Pediatric Dermatology 11:52–60.

Salata H.H., Mercader J., Navarro A., Cortes J.M. and Gonzales-Campos C. (1984) Lymphangioma of the duodenum. Endoscopy 16:30–32.

Salem P., El-Hashimi L., Anaissie E., Geha S., Habboubi N., Ibrahim N., Khalyl M. and Allam C. (1987) Primary small intestinal lymphoma in adults. Cancer 59:1670–1676.

Sallon S., Deckelbaum R.J., Schmid I.I., Harlap S., Baras M. and Spira D.T. (1988) Cryptosporidium, malnutrition, and chronic diarrhea in children. American Journal of Diseases in Children 142:312–315.

Salt H.B., Wolff O.H., Lloyd J.K., Fosbrooke A.S., Cameron A.H. and Hubble D.V. (1960) On having no beta-lipoprotein: a syndrome comprising a-beta-lipoprotenaemia, acanthocytosis and steatorrhoea. Lancet ii:325–329.

Sandow M.J. and Whitehead R.(1979) The Paneth cell. Gut 20:420–431.

Sanfilippo G., Pantane R., Fusto A., Passanisi G., Valenti R. and Russo A. (1986) Endoscopic approach to childhood coeliac disease. Acta Gastroenterologica 49:401–408.

Savage M.O., Mirakian R., Wozniak E.R., Jenkins H.R., Malone M., Phillips A.D., Milla P.J., Bottazzo G.F. and Harrie J.T. (1985) Specific autoantibodies to gut epithelium in two infants with severe protracted diarrhea. Journal of Pediatric Gastroenterology and Nutrition 4:187–195.

Schenk E.A., Samloff I.M. and Klipstein F.A. (1965) Morphologic characteristics of jejunal biopsy in celiac disease and tropical sprue. Americal Journal of Pathology 47:765–781.

Schlossberg D., Rudy F.R., Jackson F.W. and Dumalag L.B. (1984) Syphilitic enteritis. Archives of Internal Medicine 144:811–812.

Schmitz-Moormann P., Pittner P.M., Reichmann L. and Massarat S. (1984) Quantitative histological study of duodenitis in biopsies. Pathology, Research and Practice 178:499–507.

Schrander J.J., Dellevoet J.J., Arends J.W., Forget P.P. and Kuijten R. (1993) Small intestinal mucosa IgE plasma cells and specific anti-cow milk IgE in children with cow milk protein intolerance. Annals of Allergy 70:406–409.

Schreibman D., Brenner B., Jacobs R., Ben-Arieh Y., Tatarsky I. and Alroy G. (1988) Small intestinal myeloid metaplasia. Journal of the American Medical Association 259:2580–2582.

Schrenk M. et al (1994) Ocular involvement in Whipple's disease. Klin Monatsbl Augenheilkd 204:538–541.

Schuffler M.D. and Chaffee R.G. (1979) Small intestinal biopsy in a patient with Crohn's disease of the duodenum: the spectrum of abnormal findings in the absence of granulomas. Gastroenterology 76:1009–1014.

Schuger L., Peretz T., Goldin E., Durst A.L. and Okon E. (1988) Duodenal epithelial atypia. Cancer 61:663–666.

Scott B.B., Goodall A., Stephenson P. and Jenkins D. (1985) Duodenal bulb plasma cells in duodenitis and duodenal ulceration. Gut 26:1032–1037.

Scott B.B., Hardy G.J. and Losowsky M.S. (1975) Involvement of the small intestine in systemic mast cell disease. Gut 16:918–924.

Scott B.B. and Losowsky M.S. (1976) Patchiness and duodenal-jejunal variation of the mucosal abnormality in coeliac disease and dermatitis herpetiformis. Gut 17:984–992.

Scott B.B., Miller J.P. and Losowsky M.S. (1979) Hypobetalipoproteinaemia—a variant of the Bassen-Kornzweig syndrome. Gut 20:163–168.

Selby W.S. and Gallagher N.D. (1979) Malignancy in a 19-year experience of adult celiac disease. Digestive Diseases and Sciences 24:684–688.

Selby W.S., Janossy G., Bofill M. and Jewell D.P. (1983) Lymphocyte subpopulations in the human small intestine: the findings in normal small mucosa and in the mucosa of patients with coeliac disease. Clinical and Experimental Immunology 52:219–228.

Selby W.S., Janossy G. and Jewell D.P. (1981) Immunohistological characterisation of intraepithelial lymphocytes of the human gastrointestinal tract. Gut 22:169–176.

Seligmann M., Mihaesco E. and Frangione B. (1971) Alpha chain disease. Annals of the New York Academy of Science 190:487–500.

Setti-Carraro P., Talbot I.C. and Nicholls R.J. (1994) Long-term appraisal of the histological appearances of the ileal reservoir mucosa after restorative proctocolectomy for ulcerative colitis. Gut 35:1721–1727.

Shaw E.B. Jr and Hennigar G.R. (1974) Intestinal lymphoid polyposis. American Journal of Clinical Pathology 61:417–422.

Sheehy T.W., Artenstein M.S. and Green R.W. (1964) Small intestinal mucosa in certain viral diseases. Journal of the American Medical Association 190:1023–1028.

Sheehy T.W., Meroney W.H., Cox R.S. and Soler J.E. (1962) Hookworm disease and malabsorption. Gastroenterology 42:148–156.

Shepherd N.A., Blackshaw A.J., Hall P.A., Bostad L., Coates P.J., Lowe D.C., Levison D.A., Morson B.C. and Stansfeld A.G. (1987) Malignant lymphoma with eosinophilia of the gastrointestinal tract. Histopathology 11:115–130.

Shepherd N.A., Healey C.J., Warren B.F., Richman P.I., Thomson W.H. and Wilkinson S.P. (1993) Distribution of mucosal pathology and an assessment of colonic phenotypic change in the pelvic ileal reservoir. Gut 34:101–105.

Shepherd N.A., Jass J.R., Duval I., Moskowitz R.L., Nicholls R.J. and Morson B.C. (1987) Restorative proctocolectomy with ileal reservoir: pathological and histochemical study of mucosal biopsy specimens. Journal of Clinical Pathology 40:601–607.

Sherif S.M. (1970) Malabsorption and schistosomal involvement of jejunum. British Medical Journal 1:671–672.

Sheth K.J., Werlin S.L., Freeman M.E. and Hodach A.E. (1981) Gastrointestinal structure and function in Fabry's disease. Americal Journal of Gastroenterology 76:246–251.

Shidrawi R.G., Przemioslo R., Davies D.R., Tighe M.R. and Ciclitira P.J. (1994) Pitfalls in diagnosing coeliac disease. Journal of Clinical Pathology 47:693–694.

Shilken K.B., Zerman B.J. and Blackwell J.B. (1968) Lymphangiectatic cysts of the small bowel. Journal of Pathology and Bacteriology 96:353–358.

Shiner M. (1973) Ultrastructural changes suggestive of immune reaction in the jejunal mucosa of coeliac children following gluten challenge. Gut 14:1–12.

Shiner M., Ballard J., Brook C.G.D. and Herman S. (1975) Intestinal biopsy in the diagnosis of cow's milk protein intolerance without acute symptoms. Lancet ii:1060–1063.

Shiner M., Ballard J. and Smith M.E. (1975) The small intestinal mucosa in cow's milk allergy. Lancet i:136–140.

Shiner M. and Pearson J.R. (1981) Abnormalities in the jejunal mucosa in Arab children. Gastroenterologie Clinique et Biologique 5:663–673.

Shiner M., Redmond A.O.B. and Hansen J.D.L. (1973) The jejunal mucosa in protein-energy malnutrition: a clinical, histological, and ultrastructural study. Experimental and Molecular Pathology 19:61–78.

Shiner M. and Shmerling D.H. (1970) The pathogenesis of coeliac disease. (Abstract) Gut 11:1058–1059.

Short R.H.D. (1950) Alveolar epithelium in relation to growth of the lung. Philosophical Transactions B 235:35–86.

Shousha S., Spiller R.C. and Parkins R.A. (1983) The endoscopically abnormal duodenum in patients with dyspepsia: biopsy findings in 60 cases. Histopathology 7:23–34.

Shpilberg O., Shimon I., Bujanover Y. and Ben-Bassat I. (1993) Remission of malabsorption in congenital intestinal lymphangiectasia following chemotherapy for lymphoma. Leukemia and Lymphoma 11:147–148.

Shwachman H., Lloyd-Still J.D., Khaw K-T. and Antonowicz I. (1973) Protracted diarrhea of infancy treated by intravenous alimentation. American Journal of Diseases in Children 125:365–368.

Silva M.T., Macedo P.M. and Nunes J.F.M. (1985) Ultrastructure of bacilli and the bacillary origin of the macrophagic inclusions in Whipple's disease. Journal of General Microbiology 131:1001–1013.

Simmonds J.P. and Rosenthal F.D. (1981) Lymphadenopathy in coeliac disease. Gut 22:756–758.

Singleton J., Kern F. and Waddell W. (1965) Diarrhea and pancreatic islet cell tumor: report of a case with a severe jejunal mucosal lesion. Gastroenterology 49:197–208.

Sircus W. (1985) Duodenitis: a clinical, endoscopic and histopathological study. Quarterly Journal of Medicine 56:593–600.

Sjolund K., Alumets J., Berg N-O., Hakanson R. and Sundler F. (1979) Duodenal endocrine cells in adult coeliac disease. Gut 20:547–552.

Sjolund K., Sanden G., Hakanson R. and Sundler F. (1983) Endocrine cells in human intestine: an immunocytochemical study. Gastroenterology 85:1120–1130.

Skellenger M.E., Kinner B.M. and Jordan P.H. (1983) Brunner's gland hamartomas can mimic carcinoma of the head of the pancreas. Surgery, Gynecology and Obstetrics 156:774–776.

Skinner J.M. and Whitehead R. (1976) Morphological methods in the study of the gut immune system in man. Journal of Clinical Pathology 29:564–567.

Slavin G., Sowter C., Robertson K., McDermott S. and Paton K. (1980) Measurement in jejunal biopsies by computer-aided microscopy. Journal of Clinical Pathology 33:254–261.

Sleisenger M.H., Almy T.P. and Barr D.P. (1953) The sprue syndrome secondary to lymphoma of the small bowel. American Journal of Medicine 15:666–674.

Smallman L.A., Young J.A., Shortland-Webb W.R., Carey M.P. and Michael J. (1986) *Strongyloides stercoralis* hyperinfestation syndrome with *Escherichia coli* meningitis: report of two cases. Journal of Clinical Pathology 39:366–370.

Socinski M.A., Frankel J-P., Morrow P.L. and Krawitt E.L. (1984) Painless diarrhea secondary to intestinal ischemia: diagnosis of atheromatous emboli by jejunal biopsy. Digestive Diseases and Sciences 29:674–677.

Solcia E., Capella C., Buffa R., Fiocca R., Frigerio B. and Usellini L. (1980) Identification, ultrastructure and classification of gut endocrine cells and related growths. Investigative and Cell Pathology 3:37–49.

Solhaug J.H. (1976) Morphometric studies of the small intestine following jejuno-ileal shunt operation. Scandinavian Journal of Gastroenterology 11:155–160.

Solidoro A., Casanova L., Utero J., Santillana S., Carracedo C., Misad O. and Ruiz E. (1993) Lymphomas of the gastrointestinal tract: a neoplastic disease of underdevelopment. Revista de Gastroenterologia del Peru 13:148–159.

Solthoft J. and Soeberg B. (1972a) Immunoglobulin-containing cells in the small intestine in viral hepatitis. Acta Pathologica et Microbiologica Scandinavica 80:379–387.

Solthoft J. and Soeberg B. (1972b) Immunoglobulin-containing cells in the small intestine during acute enteritis. Gut 13:535–538.

Sorensen R.U., Halpin T.C., Abramowsky C.R., Hornick D.L., Miller K.M., Naylor P. and Incefy G.S. (1985) Intestinal lymphangiectasia and thymic hypoplasia. Clinical and Experimental Immunology 59:217–226.

Spencer J., Cerf-Bensussan N., Jarry A., Brousse N., Guy-Grand D., Krajewski A.S. and Isaacson P.G. (1988) Enteropathy-associated T cell lymphoma (malignant histiocytosis of the intestine) is recognized by a monoclonal antibody (HML-1) that defines a membrane molecule on human mucosal lymphocytes. American Journal of Pathology 132:1–5.

Spencer J., MacDonald T.T., Diss T.C., Walker-Smith J.A., Ciclitira P.J. and Isaacson P.G. (1989) Changes in intraepithelial lymphocyte subpopulations in coeliac disease and enteropathy associated T cell lymphoma (malignant histiocytosis of the intestine). Gut 30:339–346.

Sprinz H., Sribhibhadh E.J., Gangarosa E.J., Benyajata C., Kundel D. and Halstead S. (1962) Biopsy of small bowel of Thai people. American Journal of Clinical Pathology 38:43–51.

Stamp G.W.H. and Evans D.J. (1987) Accumulation of ceroid in smooth muscle indicates severe malabsorption and vitamin E deficiency. Journal of Clinical Pathology 40:798–802.

Stern M., Gruttner R. and Krumbach J. (1980) Protracted diarrhoea: secondary monosaccharide malabsorption and zinc deficiency with cutaneous manifestations during total parenteral nutrition. European Journal of Pediatrics 135:175–180.

Stessens L., Van Den Oord J.J., Geboes K., De Wolf-Peeters C. and Desmet V.J. (1986) GI lymphomatous polyposis. Gastroenterology 90:2041–2042.

Stevens F.M., Flanagan R.W., O'Gorman D. and Buchanan K.D. (1984) Glucagonoma syndrome demonstrating giant duodenal villi. Gut 25:784–791.

Stewart J.S., Pollock D.J., Hoffbrand A.V., Mollin D.L. and Booth C.C. (1967) A study of proximal and distal intestinal structure and absorptive function in idiopathic steatorrhoea. Quarterly Journal of Medicine 36:425–444.

Stolte M., Schwabe H. and Prestele H. (1981) Relationship between diseases of the pancreas and hyperplasia of Brunner's glands. Virchows Archiv A 394:75–87.

Strich D., Goldstein R., Phillips A., Shemer R., Goldberg Y., Razin Y. and Freier S. (1993) Anderson's disease: no linkage to the apo B locus. Journal of Pediatric Gastroenterology and Nutrition 16:257–264.

Strobel S., Busuttil A. and Ferguson A. (1983) Human intestinal mucosal mast cells: expanded population in untreated coeliac disease. Gut 24:222–227.

Sukigara M., Koyama I., Komazaki T., Matsuda T., Ishii T. and Omoto R. (1987) Bleeding varices located in the second portion of the duodenum. Japanese Journal of Surgery 17:130–135.

Swanson V.L. and Thomassen R.W. (1965) Pathology of the jejunal mucosa in tropical sprue. American Journal of Pathology 46:511–551.

Swanson V.L., Wheby M.S. and Bayless T.M. (1966) Morphological effects of folic acid and vitamin B_{12} on the jejunal lesion of tropical sprue. American Journal of Pathology 49:167–191.

Swinson C.M., Slavin G., Coles E.C. and Boothe C.C. (1983) Coeliac disease and malignancy. Lancet i:111–115.

Tabaqchali S. and Booth C.C. (1970) In: Modern Trends in Gastroenterology. Volume 4. Edited by W.I. Card and B. Creamer. London: Butterworth, p 143.

Tait R.C., Oogarah P.K., Houghton J.B., Farrand S.E. and Haeney M.R. (1993) Waldenstrom's macroglobulinaemia secreting a paraprotein with lupus anticoagulant activity: possible association with gastrointestinal tract disease and malabsorption. Journal of Clinical Pathology 46:678–680.

Takahashi M. (1994) A study on the fine mucosal pattern in the duodenal bulb. Nippon Ika Daigaku Zasshi 61:405–421.

Talbot I.C., Neoptolemos J.P., Shaw D.E. and Carr-Locke D. (1988) The histopathology and staging of carcinoma of the ampulla of Vater. Histopathology 12:156–165.

Tandon B.N., Tandon R.K., Satpathy B.K. and Shriniwas (1977) Mechanism of malabsorption in giardiasis: a study of bacterial flora and bile salt deconjugation in upper jejunum. Gut 18:176–181.

Tankel H.I., Clark D.H. and Lee F.D. (1965) Radiation enteritis with malabsorption. Gut 6:560–569.

Taylor C.R. (1976) An immunohistological study of follicular lymphoma, reticulum cell sarcoma and Hodgkin's disease. European Journal of Cancer 12:61–75.

Thompson H. (1976) Pathology of coeliac disease. Current Topics in Pathology 63:49–75.

Thomson W.O., Joffe S.N., Robertson A.G., Lee F.D., Imrie C.W. and Blumgart L.H. (1977) Is duodenitis a dyspeptic myth? Lancet i:1197–1198.

Thurlbeck W.M., Benson J.A. and Dudley H.R. (1960) The histopathologic changes of sprue and their significance. American Journal of Clinical Pathology 34:108–117.

Tofler A.H., Hukill P.B. and Spiro H.M. (1963) Brown bowel syndrome. Annals of Internal Medicine 58:872–877.

Tomkins A. (1981) Tropical malabsorption: recent concepts in pathogenesis and nutritional significance. Clinical Science 60:131–137.

Tomkins A.M., Drasar B.S. and James W.P.T. (1975) Bacterial colonisation of jejunal mucosa in acute tropical sprue. Lancet i:59–62.

Touraine J.L., Marseglia G.L., Beteul H., Souilet G. and Gebuhrer L. (1992) The bare lymphocyte syndrome. Bone Marrow Transplant 9 (suppl 1):54–56.

Townley R.R.W., Cass M.H. and Anderson C.M. (1964) Small intestinal mucosal patterns of coeliac disease and idiopathic steatorrhoea seen in other situations. Gut 5:51–55.

Toyoshima M., Sato A., Taniguchi M., Todate A., Nakazawa K., Hayakawa H. and Chida K. (1994) A case of allergic gastroenteropathy provoked by mite inhalation. Arerugi 43:718–720.

Triadafilopoulos G. (1993) Clinical and pathologic features of the nodular duodenum. American Journal of Gastroenterology 88:1058–1064.

Trier J.S. (1962) Morphologic alterations induced by methotrexate in the mucosa of the human proximal intestine. Gastroenterology 42:295–305.

Trier J.S. (1993) Diagnosis and treatment of celiac sprue. Hospital Practice (Office Edition) 28:41–44, 46, 48.

Trier J.S. and Browning T.H. (1966) Morphologic response of the mucosa of human small intestine to x-ray exposure. Journal of Clinical Investigation 45:194–204.

Trier J.S. and Madara J.L. (1981) Functional morphology of the mucosa of the small intestine. In: Johnson L.R. (ed) Physiology of the Gastrointestinal Tract. Edited by L.R. Johnson. New York: Raven Press, pp 925–961.

Tsadilas T. (1984) Duodenal polyp composed of ectopic gastric mucosa. Digestive Diseases and Sciences 29:475–477.

Tsubone M., Kozura S., Taki T., Hoshino M., Yasui A. and Hachisuka K. (1984) Heterotopic gastric mucosa in the small intestine. Acta Pathologica Japonica 34:1425–1431.

Tylki-Szymanska A., Maciejko D., Wozniewicz B. and Muszynska B. (1987) Two cases of cholesteryl ester storage disease (CESD) acid lipase deficiency. Hepato-gastroenterology 34:98–99.

Tytgat G.N., Hoogendijk J.L., Agenant D. and Schellekens P.T. (1977) Etiopathogenetic studies in a patient with Whipple's disease. Digestion 15:309–321.

Tzipori S., Angus K.W., Campbell I. and Gray E.W. (1982) Experimental infection of lambs with cryptosporidium isolated from a human patient with diarrhoea. Gut 23:71–74.

Ulshen M.H. and Rollo J.L. (1980) Pathogenesis of *Escherichia coli* gastroenteritis in man—another mechanism. New England Journal of Medicine 302:99–101.

Unsworth D.J. and Brown D.L. (1994) Serological screening suggests that adult coeliac disease is underdiagnosed in the U.K. and increases the incidence by up to 12%. Gut 35:61–64.

Vanderhoof J.A., Rich K.C., Stiehm E.R. and Ament M.E. (1977) Esophageal ulcers in immunodeficiency with elevated levels of IgM and neutropenia. American Journal of Diseases in Children 131:551–552.

Van Der Valk P., Lindeman J. and Meijer C.J.L.M. (1988) Non-Hodgkin's lymphomas of the gastrointestinal tract: a review with special reference to the gut-associated lymphoid tissue. In: Digestive Disease Pathology. Volume 1. Edited by S. Watanabe, M. Wolff and S.C. Sommers. Philadelphia: Field and Wood Inc, pp 105–119.

Van Spreeuwel J.P., Lindeman J., Van Maanen J. and Meyer C.J.L.M. (1984) Increased numbers of IgE containing cells in gastric and duodenal biopsies: an expression of food allergy secondary to chronic inflammation? Journal of Clinical Pathology 37:601–606.

Variend S., Phillips A.D. and Walker-Smith J.A. (1984) The small intestinal mucosal biopsy in childhood. Perspectives in Pediatric Pathology 1:57–78.

Variend S., Placzek M., Raafat F. and Walker-Smith J.A. (1984) Small intestinal mucosal fat in childhood enteropathies. Journal of Clinical Pathology 37:373–377.

Veloso F.T. and Saleiro J.V. (1982) Mast cells in Whipple's disease. Journal of Submicroscopic Cytology 14:515–520.

Veloso F.T. and Saleiro J.V. (1987) Small bowel changes in recurrent ulceration of the mouth. Hepato-gastroenterology 34:36–37.

Veloso F.T., Saleiro J.V., Baptista F. and Ribeiro E. (1981) Whipple's disease: report of a case with clinical immunological studies. American Journal of Gastroenterology 75:419–425.

Venables C.W. (1985) Duodenitis. Scandinavian Journal of Gastroenterology 20 (suppl 109):91–97.

Vitoria J.C., Camarero C. and Solaguren R.(1979) Cow's milk protein-sensitive enteropathy. Clinical and histological results of the cows' milk provocation test. Helvetica Paediatrica Acta 34:309–318.

Vitoria J.C., Camerero C., Sojo A., Ruiz A. and Rodriguez-Soriano J. (1982) Enteropathy related to fish, rice and chicken. Archives of Disease in Childhood 57:44–48.

Vogelsang H., Genser D., Wyatt J. et al (1995) Screening for celiac disease: a prospective study on the value of noninvasive tests. American Journal of Gastroenterology 90:394–398.

Walan A. (1981) Non-ulcer dyspepsia. Proceedings of a Symposium Held in the Swedish Society of Medical Sciences, Stockholm, November 6, 7. Stockholm: Smith, Kline and French A.B.

Waldmann T.A. (1970) In: Modern Trends in Gastroenterology. Volume 4. Edited by W.I. Card and B. Creamer. London: Butterworth, p 136.

Waldmann T.A., Wochner R.D., Laster L. and Gordon R.S. (1967) Allergic gastroenteropathy. New England Journal of Medicine 276:761–769.

Walker-Smith J.A. (1970) Transient gluten intolerance. Archives of Diseases of Childhood 45:523–526.

Walker-Smith J.A. (1972) Variation of small intestinal morphology with age. Archives of Diseases of Childhood 47:80–83.

Walker-Smith J.A. (1978) Gastrointestinal allergy. The Practitioner 220:562–573.

Walker-Smith J.A. (1994) Intractable diarrhoea in infancy: a continuing challenge for the paediatric gastroenterologist. Acta Paediatrica (suppl) 83:6–9.

Walker-Smith J.A., Unsworth D.J., Hutchins J., Phillips A.D. and Holborow E.G. (1982) Autoantibodies against gut epithelium in child with small intestinal enteropathy. Lancet i:566–567.

Wall A.J., Douglas A.J., Booth C.C. and Pearse A.G.E. (1970) Response of the jejunal mucosa in adult coeliac disease to oral prednisolone. Gut 11:7–14.

Ward H., Jalan K.N., Maitra T.K., Agarwal S.K. and Mahalanabis D. (1983) Small intestinal nodular lymphoid hyperplasia in patients with giardiasis and normal serum immunoglobulins. Gut 24:120–126.

Warnke R., Miller R., Grogan T., Pederson M., Dilley J. and Levy R. (1980) Immunologic phenotype in 30 patients with diffuse large-cell lymphoma. New England Journal of Medicine 303:293–300.

Warren P.M., Pepperman M.A. and Montgomery R.D. (1978) Age changes in the small intestinal mucosa. Lancet ii:849–850.

Watson A.J., Appleton D.R. and Wright N.A. (1982) Adaptive cell-proliferative changes in the small intestinal mucosa in coeliac disease. In: Basic Science in Gastroenterology: Structure of the Gut. Edited by J.M. Polak, S.R. Bloom, N.A. Wright and M.J. Daly. Ware: Glaxo Group Research Ltd, pp 431–443.

Watson A.J. and Parkin J.M. (1970) Jejunal biopsy findings during prodromal stage of measles in a child with coeliac disease. Lancet ii:1134–1135.

Watson J.H.L. and Haubrich W.S. (1969) Bacilli bodies in the lumen and epithelium of the jejunum in Whipple's disease. Laboratory Investigation 21:347–357.

Watt J., Pincott J.R. and Harries J.T. (1983) Combined cow's milk protein and gluten-induced enteropathy: common or rare? Gut 24:165–170.

Webster A.D.B. (1980) Giardiasis and immunodeficiency diseases. Transactions of the Royal Society of Tropical Medicine and Hygiene 74:440–443.

Webster A.D.B., Kenwright S., Ballard J., Shiner M., Slavin G., Levi A.J., Loewi G. and Asherson G.L. (1977) Nodular lymphoid hyperplasia of the bowel in primary hypogammaglobulinaemia: study of in vivo and in vitro lymphocyte function. Gut 18:364–372.

Webster A.D.B., Slavin G., Shiner M., Platts-Mills T.A.E. and Asherson G.L. (1981) Coeliac disease with severe hypogammaglobulinaemia. Gut 22:153–157.

Weibel E.R. (1963) Principles and methods for the morphometric study of the lung and other organs. Laboratory Investigation 12:131–155.

Weinstein L. Edelstein S.M., Madara J.L., Falchuk K.R., McManus B.M. and Trier J.S. (1981) Intestinal cryptosporidiosis complicated by disseminated cytomegalovirus infection. Gastroenterology 81:584–591.

Weinstein W.M., Saunders D.R., Tytgat G.N. and Rubin C.E. (1970) Collagenous sprue—an unrecognized type of malabsorption. New England Journal of Medicine 283:1297–1301.

Weir D.G. and Hourihane D.O'B. (1974) Coeliac disease during the teenage period: the value of serial serum folate estimations. Gut 15:450–457.

Werlin S.L., Chusid M.J., Caya J. and Oechler H.W. (1982) Colitis in chronic granulomatous disease. Gastroenterology 82:328–331.

West B. (1988) Pseudomelanosis duodeni. Journal of Clinical Gastroenterology 10:127–129.

Whalen G.E., Rosenberg E.B., Strickland G.T., Gutman R.A., Cross J.H., Watten R.H., Uylangco C. and Dizou J.J. (1969) Intestinal capillariasis: a new disease in man. Lancet i:13–16.

Wheeler E.E. and Challacombe D.N. (1984) Quantification of enterochromaffin cells with serotonin immuno-reactivity in the duodenal mucosa in coeliac disease. Archives of Disease in Childhood 59:523–527.

Whipple G.H. (1907) A hitherto undescribed disease characterised anatomically by deposits of fat and fatty acids in the intestinal and mesenteric lymphatic tissues: intestinal lipodystrophy. Johns Hopkins Hospital Bulletin 18:382–391.

Whitehead R. (1968a) Primary lymphadenopathy complicating idiopathic steatorrhoea. Gut 9:569–575.

Whitehead R. (1968b) Recent Advances in Clinical Pathology. Series V. Edited by S.C. Dyke. London: Churchill, p 385.

Whitehead R. (1979) Mucosal Biopsy of the Gastrointestinal Tract, 2nd ed. Philadelphia: W.B. Saunders Co., pp 79–87.

Whitehead R. (1996) Mucosal biopsy of the gastrointestinal tract. In: Major Problems in Pathology. Volume 3. London: W.B. Saunders Co.

Whitehead R., Roca M., Meikle D.D., Skinner J. and Truelove S.C. (1975) The histological classification of duodenitis in fibreoptic biopsy specimens. Digestion 13:129–136.

Whitehead R., Roca M. and Truelove S.C. (1972) Antroduodenitis in duodenal ulcers and non-ulcer dyspepsia. In: Chronic Duodenal Ulcer. Edited by C. Wastell. London: Butterworth, pp 17–23.

Wiernik G. (1966) In vivo cell kinetics of a normal human tissue. British Medical Journal ii:385–387.

Wiernik G., Shorter R.G. and Creamer B. (1962) The arrest of intestinal epithelial "turnover" by the use of x-irradiation. Gut 3:26–31.

Wilcox G.M., Tronic B.S., Schecter D.J., Arron M.J., Righi D.F. and Weiner N.J. (1987) Periodic Acid-Schiff-Negative granulomatous lymphadenopathy in patient with Whipple's disease. American Journal of Medicine 83:165–170.

Williamson R.C.N. (1982) Intestinal adaption: factors that influence morphology. In: Basic Science in Gastroenterology: Structure of the Gut. Edited by J.M. Polak, S.R. Bloom, N.A. Wright and M.J. Daly. Ware: Glaxo Group Research Ltd, pp 337–345.

Witham R.R. and Mosser R.S. (1979) An unusual presentation of schistosomiasis duodenitis. Gastroenterology 77:1316–1318.

Won K.C., Jang B.I., Kim T.N., Lee H.W., Chung M.K. and Lee H.W. (1993) A case of primary intestinal lymphangiectasia. Korean Journal of Internal Medicine 8:51–55.

World Health Organisation (1976) Alpha-chain disease and related small intestinal lymphoma. Memorandum Bulletin 54:615–624.

Wright N., Watson A., Morley A., Appleton D., Marks J. and Douglas A. (1973a) The cell cycle time in the flat (avillous) mucosa of the human small intestine. Gut 14:603–606.

Wright N., Watson A., Morley A., Appleton D., Marks J. and Douglas A. (1973b) Cell kinetics in flat (avillous) mucosa of the human small intestine. Gut 14:701–710.

Wright S.G. and Tomkins A.M. (1978) Quantitative histology in giardiasis. Journal of Clinical Pathology 31:712–716.

Yamase H., Norris M. and Gillies C. (1985) Pseudomelanosis duodeni: a clinicopathologic entity. Gastrointestinal Endoscopy 31:83–86.

Zuckerman M.J., Pittman D.L., Boman D. and Farley P.C. (1986) Multiple lymphomatous polyposis of the gastrointestinal tract with immunologic marker studies. Journal of Clinical Gastroenterology 8:295–300.

Zukerman G.R., Mills B.A., Koehler R.E., Siegel A., Harter H.R. and DeSchryver-Kecskemeti K. (1983) Nodular duodenitis: pathologic and clinical characteristics in patients with end-stage renal disease. Digestive Diseases and Sciences 28:1018–1024.

Colonic Biopsy

IV

15

NORMAL APPEARANCES IN COLONIC BIOPSY SPECIMENS

The mucous membrane of the colon (Fig. 15–1) has a comparatively smooth surface because there are no villi. Straight tubular glands extend from the surface down through the entire thickness of the lamina propria to abut the muscularis mucosae. A detailed examination of the epithelium of the human large intestine has been reported by Shamsuddin, Phelps and Trump (1982). They have shown that significant differences occur in the different regions of the large bowel, although the basic structure is the same.

Undifferentiated stem cells occupy the base of the crypts. They are the only cells capable of mitotic division and clearly give rise to the goblet cell population, which is the predominant cell type lining the crypts. They have large supranuclear mucous vacuoles and small apical vesicles. The apical vesicles show variable electron density, which is maximum in the ascending colon and progressively less in the distal direction, to become lucent in the rectum. Histochemically the mucins are predominantly sulphomucins in the lower two thirds of the crypt and sialomucin in the upper crypt and surface epithelium. There are also said to be changes in mucin composition in different parts of the colon. Using a panel of monoclonal antibodies against purified colonic mucins, Podolsky, Fournier and Lynch (1986) have shown that in humans the colonic mucosa contains several subpopulations of goblet cells. It is claimed that they produce distinctive combinations of mucin glycoprotein

Figure 15–1. Rectal biopsy. Normal colonic mucosa; gland tubules cut longitudinally (H&E ×70).

subtypes, but their functional roles have not been elucidated. Interspersed among the goblet or mucous cells, at the surface between the crypt openings, are the occasional columnar cells, which have been equated to the absorptive cells of the small intestine because by light microscopy they have an eosinophilic cytoplasm and by electron microscopy a well defined microvillous border. Shamsuddin, Phelps and Trump (1982) preferred to call them columnar cells and believed them to be a variant of goblet cells that have discharged their large mucous vacuoles. They have all the ultrastructural apparatus for secretion of mucus. Endocrine cells can also be recognised in the lower half of the glands, especially in the rectum where they occur with greater frequency than in the rest of the colon. The increasingly important enterochromaffin system has already been mentioned in the sections concerning the gastric and small intestinal mucosa. In the superficial and crypt epithelium there is an occasional intraepithelial lymphocyte. Paneth's cells may be seen in tissue from the very proximal colon, especially in children, but in rectal or distal colonic biopsy tissues the presence of these cells is invariably abnormal.

Surrounding the crypts is a sheath of cells that have been thought of as fibroblasts. A role in maintaining crypt form and function has been postulated. More recently, these cells have been regarded as myofibroblasts (see also collagenous colitis) on the basis of electron microscopic observations and their reaction with specific monoclonal antibodies (Richman et al 1987).

The lamina propria, which consists of a delicate connective tissue and is richly vascular, contains a few plasma cells and lymphocytes, an occasional mast cell and eosinophil together with a histiocyte, and sometimes a solitary lymphoid follicle (Fig. 15–2). Histiocytes predominate in the more superficial aspects of the lamina propria, as do plasma cells. Leonard and MacLennan (1982) have stressed that this be borne in mind when plasma cells are enumerated so as to arrive at accurate estimations. There is little information concerning the changes in cellularity of the lamina propria along the length of the colon, but a personal subjective observation is that there is a definite increase in the number of lymphocytes and plasma cells in the caecum and neighbouring ascending colon compared with the distal bowel and rectum. On occasion, the density prompts the observer to question the possibility of a colitis, but lack of polymorphs and degenerative epithelial features or architectural distortion allows this to be ruled out. Neutrophil polymorphs are uncommon in the entirely normal biopsy specimen, except inside capillaries, but occasional mast cells occur particularly in the submucosa. Lymphoid follicles are often encountered in

Figure 15–2. Rectal biopsy. Normal colonic mucosa with a lymphoid follicle; gland tubules cut transversely (H&E ×38).

rectal biopsy specimens and, like the Peyer's patches of the small intestine, are most numerous at the time of puberty (Cornes 1965). They become less frequent with increasing age and are rare in elderly persons. They characteristically split the muscularis mucosae, partially extending into the submucosa. Sometimes the lymphoid follicles are accompanied by a few tubular glands, which may extend into the submucosa (Fig. 15–3). It has been claimed that the lymphoglandular complexes (microbursae) constitute weak points in the colonic wall; they have been implicated in the pathogenesis of diverticular disease (Kealy 1976a). This appears highly unlikely, for too frequently diverticula exist in the absence of mural lymphoid tissue. O'Leary and Sweeney (1986) studied these complexes by both immunohistochemistry and electron microscopy and concluded that they are the sites of antigen processing. Indeed, cells that are the equivalent of M cells of the small intestine are found in the epithelium related to these follicles. Jacob, Baker and Swaminathan (1987) believed that these cells have an antigen-sampling function and that their presence may explain the localisation of the early aphthous lesions of Crohn's disease to the lymphoglandular complexes.

Minor changes in the superficial epithelium, consisting of a decrease in goblet cell number and reversion to a flatter and more simple type of epithelium, are seen fairly often (Fig. 15–4). Usually there is an accompanying increase, slight but perceptible, in inflammatory cells in the lamina propria, although invasion of the surface epithelium and that lining the crypts is unusual. Rarely, however, in circumstances such as constipation or more frequently chronic obstruction (e.g., in Hirschsprung's disease) a rather poorly formed crypt abscess may be seen. These minor changes, however, are not usually related to the clinical picture. Nevertheless, whenever colonic biopsy specimen appearances are being assessed, it is always advisable to consider the possibility that factors such as the preparation of the colon for instrumentation, the instrumentation itself, or some other form of trauma or injury may be contributing to the overall picture. Certainly the energetic use of enemas can result in an appreciable although nonspecific acute inflammatory reaction. Acute

Figure 15–3. Lymphoglandular complex (microbursa) in normal rectal mucosa. The superficial epithelium shows a traumatic artefact (H&E ×130).

Figure 15–4. Rectal biopsy. Flattening of the superficial epithelium and a localised increase in the number of round cells in the lamina propria (H&E ×188).

degenerative epithelial changes have been well described after the use of a variety of enemas (Meisel et al 1977, Leriche et al 1978) (Chapter 17). Indeed, in certain societies in which the use of repeated enemas is part of the culture, as in South African black persons, severe inflammation and bowel perforation not uncommonly result (Segal et al 1979). It is clearly extremely helpful for the pathologist to be made aware of any circumstance that could influence the interpretation of a particular biopsy specimen.

Although much has been written about the racial variation in jejunal morphology, there is little in the literature concerning the colon and rectum in this respect. Changes in cellularity of the lamina propria of the colon, however, may even be attributable to differences in the luminal environment of the gut as a whole. Thus, possible racial variations should be borne in mind when rectal biopsy appearances are assessed. Increased cellularity of the lamina propria with more than the usual complement of lymphocytes and plasma cells may have a more specific connotation, for it could reflect a generalised reaction of the gut-associated lymphoid system to a more localised stimulus. When such changes are seen in rectal biopsy specimens, for example, there may be an inflammatory lesion in another part of the gastrointestinal tract. Indeed, Crucioli (1972) has shown that a sigmoidoscopically normal rectum may show an increased lymphoid component in rectal biopsy specimens if Crohn's disease exists in the more proximal parts of the colon. Moreover, Soltoft (1969) found increased numbers of immunoglobulin M and G cells in the lamina propria of jejunal biopsy specimens in patients with ulcerative colitis. Except when rectal biopsy is being used for a specific diagnostic purpose (e.g., in amyloidosis), clinicians have a tendency to biopsy the colonic mucosa only when it appears abnormal to them. There are several instances in which endoscopically normal mucosa will reveal histological abnormalities. It cannot be stressed too strongly that if there is an indication for diagnostic endoscopy, there is also invariably an indication for mucosal biopsy.

This allows the pathologist to gain understanding of rectal biopsy appearances. The pathologist will then be aware of normal variations, age-related changes, and artefactual appearances and thus will be better equipped to diagnose significant abnormalities. For a more detailed consideration of the colonic mucosal dynamics, colonic epithelial cell markers, and cell differentiation the reader is referred to Shamsuddin and Yang (1995) and Goodlad and Wright (1995).

16

ULCERATIVE COLITIS, CROHN'S COLITIS, ISCHAEMIC COLITIS, PSEUDOMEMBRANOUS COLITIS, AND ANTIBIOTIC-ASSOCIATED COLITIS

Rectal and low colonic biopsies have long been employed in the diagnosis and management of neoplasia. However, because of increasing interest in the diagnosis and treatment of inflammatory disease of the large bowel, colonic biopsy has attained a new importance. The clinician faced with the differential diagnosis between ulcerative colitis and other inflammatory conditions of the colon, in particular Crohn's disease, ischaemic colitis, pseudomembranous colitis, amoebic colitis, and the more recently recognized forms of colitis, will increasingly rely on the expert interpretation of colonic biopsy material. With fibreoptic colonoscopes it is possible to obtain tissue as far proximally as the terminal ileum. Although these pieces of mucosa are small and somewhat superficial, when the same principles of interpretation are applied to them as to the larger, more conventional sigmoidoscopic biopsies, useful if sometimes limited information will be revealed. This was particularly well illustrated in the study by Myeren, Serck-Hanssen and Solberg (1976), who not only confirmed the value of fibreoptic colonoscope biopsy examination in ulcerative colitis but also proved the importance of experience in pathological interpretation and the value of biopsy even when endoscopic appearances are normal. The importance of step-wise colonic biopsy in patients being investigated for diarrhoea cannot be stressed too strongly. Microscopic colitis, collagenous colitis, and other less frequent causes of diarrhoea are usually associated with unremarkable endoscopic appearances, which are invariably nondiagnostic (Stolte 1988). Even Crohn's disease may be diagnosed histologically when endoscopic appearances are normal (Sanderson et al 1986).

ULCERATIVE COLITIS

Classic ulcerative colitis is an inflammatory process of the mucosa involving the rectum and a variable length of colon in continuity with the rectum, not infrequently extending as far as the last few inches of the terminal ileum and with associated appendiceal involvement. Indeed, the appendix may show inflammatory changes as a skip lesion just as frequently as when involved in continuity (Groisman, George and Harpaz 1994, Kroft, Stryker and Rao 1994). In view of this, it is a little odd that previous appendectomy seems to have a protective effect against the development of ulcerative colitis (Rutgeerts et al 1994). There is ample evidence (Farmer and Brown 1972, Myers, Humphries and Cox 1976, Das et al 1977, Ritchie, Powell-Tuck and Lennard-Jones 1978) that so-called ulcerative idiopathic or haemorrhagic proctitis is the same disease but a milder form. Sometimes rectal involvement appears minimal or absent sigmoidoscopically when there is evidence of severe disease in the proximal large bowel. Previous local treatment with steroid retention enemas, for example, may account for such a distribution in some cases, but not all. Even in such circumstances, however, the rectal biopsy usually reveals abnormality, but not always. Rectal sparing with normal histological characteristics has been described in children (Markowitz et al 1993) and after therapy with topical 5-aminosalicylic acid (Odze et al 1993). It is not sufficiently recognised that rectal mucosa judged to be normal sigmoidoscopically may reveal marked histological changes in ulcerative colitis. The abnormalities brought to light may be minimal and in some circumstances the mucosa may not differ greatly from normal, but if there have been sequential biopsies, typical changes are almost always seen in previous tissues. In ulcerative colitis, therefore, colonic biopsy is of paramount importance, not only in diagnosis but also in the assessment of therapy.

The course of ulcerative colitis is typically one of remission and exacerbation, and this is reflected in the range of histological appearances in biopsy material. In the acute stage during the first attack (Fig. 16–1), the mucosa shows oedema and prominent vascular congestion of the lamina propria. There is an obvious increase in the number of inflammatory cells; lymphocytes and plasma cells predominate, with conspicuous eosinophils. The lymphocytes and plasma cells are characteristically located in the lamina propria, which is a useful feature when an attempt is made to discriminate between an infective colitis and acute onset ulcerative colitis (Schumacher 1993, Surawicz et al 1994). Polymorphs are most obvious where they show margination on the capillary endothelium, or as they migrate through the glandular epithelium to fill the lumen and thus constitute so-called crypt abscesses. The pus discharges and can often be seen on the surface of the mucosa. The superficial and crypt epithelium loses its goblet cell component as an early feature, sometimes preceding marked inflammatory cell infiltration (Fig. 16–2). It is replaced by a

Figure 16–1. Rectal biopsy. Acute ulcerative colitis in an early stage. Marked inflammatory infiltrate, some crypt abscesses, but only slightly distorted gland pattern (H&E ×84).

Figure 16–2. Rectal biopsy. Acute ulcerative colitis shows early severe goblet cell depletion and replacement by simple columnar epithelium (H&E ×100).

simple basophilic epithelium, and the gland tubular pattern later becomes distorted by the inflammatory exudate and crypt abscess formation (Fig. 16–3). This process is usually limited to the mucosa proper and generally does not extend beyond the muscularis mucosae to any significant degree unless there is ulceration, although in the very acute phase the submucosa may show oedema and vascular dilation (Fig. 16–4). If there is more severe epithelial destruction, ulceration occurs. This varies from superficial erosions to huge areas of total mucosal loss, and in biopsy material this is often manifested by the luminal surface's being represented simply by granulation tissue.

Resolution of the inflammatory process with diminution of the infiltration and with epithelial regeneration and repair can produce a variety of appearances. A mild

Figure 16–3. Rectal biopsy. Acute ulcerative colitis shows distortion of the gland tubular pattern by the inflammatory process (H&E ×72).

Figure 16–4. Rectal biopsy. Acute ulcerative colitis shows oedema and vascular congestion of the submucosa but no significant inflammatory cell infiltration (H&E ×350).

first attack may be followed by complete restoration of the mucosa. More usually, however, there is residual abnormality, even if this is slight, and it is common to find that the bases of the regenerating tubules have fallen short of the muscularis mucosae (Fig. 16–5) despite having regained a relatively normal appearance. Recurrent attacks and their subsequent resolution result in a variety of abnormalities characterised by a relative loss of tubules, and by branching and irregularity of size and orientation of those tubules that remain (Figs. 16–6 to 16–8). As the attack subsides, the simple type of regenerating epithelium is gradually replaced by increasing numbers of goblet cells. Between attacks, therefore, the mucosa may show a variety of appearances that range from normal to one that is distorted, atrophic, and sometimes without significant inflammatory infiltrate. It is of some interest that in a quantitative study of patients with ulcerative colitis in remission the most important feature that

Figure 16–5. Rectal biopsy. Resolution after an acute attack of ulcerative colitis. The gland tubules are irregular, although the goblet cell population is restored, but they fall short of the muscularis mucosae (H&E ×140).

Figure 16–6. Chronic resolving ulcerative colitis reveals progressively more marked tubular loss with abnormalities of shape and size (H&E ×70).

differentiated colitic from noncolitic patients was the diameter of the lumen of the glands of the rectal mucosa (Rubio, Johansson and Kock 1982). Another characteristic appearance in the inactive chronic remitting form is a more or less dense collagenosis of the zone of the lamina propria where successive generations of regenerated tubules have fallen short of the muscularis mucosae (Fig. 16–9).

Instead of having the chronic remitting form, some patients have chronic persistent disease and the mucosa never loses the features of active inflammation. The features are predictably a mixture of those seen in the acute stage, superimposed on an incompletely restored mucosa showing chronic inflammation. Persistent ulceration and attempted healing proceed hand in hand, and it is by this interplay that

Figure 16–7. Chronic resolving ulcerative colitis reveals progressively more marked tubular loss with abnormalities of shape and size (H&E ×70).

Figure 16–8. Chronic resolving ulcerative colitis reveals progressively more marked tubular loss with abnormalities of shape and size (H&E ×70).

inflammatory pseudopolyps are produced. They evolve as areas of granulation tissue and an overexuberant regenerative reaction of the mucosal elements. Sometimes these inflammatory pseudopolyps are so large that they become symptomatic in their own right due to partial obstruction or blood loss (Kelly et al 1986). When biopsied, these lesions not infrequently cause diagnostic difficulties because of pseudomalignant appearances (Fig. 16–10). Beneath the ulcer surface in a zonal distribution one may see a layer of quite bizarre pleomorphic or spindle-shaped cells with large ganglion cell–like nuclei. Immunohistochemistry and electron microscopy prove that they are not epithelial, and although their true nature is not established they are probably mesenchymal (Jessurun et al 1986). A marked reactive hyperplasia of the mucosal lymphoid tissue may also occur (Fig. 16–11), and on occasion this may progress and become so severe that a macroscopically polypoidal state is produced. Flejou et al (1988) have claimed that when lymphoid follicular hyperplasia is associ-

Figure 16–9. Chronic quiescent ulcerative colitis. Goblet cell population is normal but tubular pattern is abnormal. There is a zone of collagen between the tubules and the muscularis mucosae (H&E ×70).

Figure 16–10. Biopsy of inflammatory pseudopolyp. The granulation tissue has a pseudomalignant appearance. Note the large ganglion-like cells with prominant nucleoli *(arrowheads)* (H&E. ×400).

ated with disease limited to the rectum, an absence of ulceration and acute inflammation, and failure to respond to steroid therapy, it constitutes the separate disease entity of chronic follicular proctitis. However, it seems curious that rectal bleeding is said to characterise this disease when it is claimed that ulceration of the mucosa is absent. One must presume that what the authors mean by absence of ulceration is full thickness loss of the mucosa. If bleeding occurs, there must obviously be some breach in the epithelial surface.

There appears to be a somewhat different clinical picture of ulcerative colitis in the elderly. The onset is usually abrupt and severe, but if the acute phase is overcome

Figure 16–11. Chronic active ulcerative colitis. Note that some tubules have a normal goblet cell component; others show crypt abscesses, and there is lymphoid hyperplasia (H&E ×70).

the further course is milder with a lower relapse rate. Brandt et al (1981) have recommended caution in making a diagnosis of ulcerative colitis in patients older than 50 years of age, for in a review of 81 patients, a retrospective diagnosis of ischaemic colitis was made in 75%.

In longstanding ulcerative colitis, Watson and Roy (1960) described Paneth's cell metaplasia, and although this occurs more often in the right side of the colon it can also be seen not infrequently in rectal biopsy tissues. The same authors gained the impression that argentaffin cells were also increased in number, but Skinner, Whitehead and Piris (1971) made a quantitative study in rectal biopsy material and found them to be decreased in number. They also showed that argentaffin cells could be found in all parts of the distorted mucous membrane, not only in the crypts as in a normal mucosa. This has been confirmed by using a glyoxylic acid–induced fluorescence method by Kyosola, Penttila and Salaspuro (1977). Using the Grimelius silver technique, however, Gledhill, Enticott and Howe (1986) claimed that there was an increase in the number of argyrophilic cells in ulcerative colitis, but that there was marked variation from case to case. This apparent discrepancy might well be related to the different techniques used, because the Grimelius method would demonstrate both argyrophilic and argentaffin cells. There are isolated reports of carcinoid tumours arising in the colon in patients with ulcerative colitis. They usually occur in patients with a history of longstanding disease, and it has been supposed that they arise in a background of neuroendocrine cell hyperplasia. Haidar and Dixon (1992), however, described a small carcinoid that developed in a patient with ulcerative colitis of relatively recent onset who did not exhibit an increased neuroendocrine cell population. An increase in eosinophil number occurs in the mucosa in ulcerative colitis (Anthonisen and Riis 1971), and it is claimed that tissue eosinophilia could be used to distinguish between ulcerative colitis and Crohn's colitis. Further work, however, showed that this was true only of longstanding disease, for the eosinophil count was not above normal in a first attack, even if the attack was severe (Willoughby, Piris and Truelove 1979). Heatley and James (1978) claimed, moreover, that a raised eosinophil count occurred in only relatively benign disease, and patients with aggressive disease not responsive to treatment had significantly smaller counts. There is a controversy as to whether or not immunoglobulin E (IgE) plasma cells are also increased in number in ulcerative colitis. This may be partly explained by the fact that some cases of ulcerative proctitis referred to earlier may be quite different from those of ulcerative colitis. Rosekrans et al (1980), for example, showed that whereas in ulcerative colitis IgE cell numbers were normal, in some cases described as allergic proctitis the IgE-containing plasma cells in the lamina propria were increased in number. The patients with this disease responded to the drug disodium cromoglycate, which is known to be beneficial in IgE-mediated immune reactions. Further evidence that IgE plasma cells play no role in ulcerative colitis is provided by Murdoch and Piris (1982). By using a monoclonal antibody in a peroxidase study, they were able to show that IgE plasma cells were rare in the lamina propria in both normal and diseased mucosa. Furthermore, Scott et al (1983) claimed that in a comparison of ulcerative colitis, Crohn's disease, and infective colitis the changes in plasma cell counts of the lamina propria are a nonspecific response to mucosal damage and do not differentiate the type of inflammatory bowel disease. In a more comprehensive immunohistochemical investigation of the lymphoid cells in inflammatory bowel disease, Hirata et al (1986) failed to show specific changes in a variety of lymphoid cell subgroups in ulcerative colitis. Dendritic cells and scavenger macrophages, however, tend to aggregate around ulcers in both ulcerative colitis and Crohn's disease (Seldenrijk et al 1989).

The muscularis mucosae not infrequently shows involvement by the inflammatory infiltrate, and it is common to see it split and disrupted by hyperplastic lymphoid aggregates. Extension of inflammation into the submucosa is unusual, however, except in the region of deep ulceration and in the extremely acute form of the disease known as toxic dilation. Unless the patient has survived such an attack with the aid of intensive medical treatment, fibrosis of the submucosa is not a usual feature of ulcerative colitis. It is associated with clear evidence of deep ulceration that has effaced the muscularis mucosae, which has no capacity for regeneration. In longstanding disease the muscularis mucosae may also show fibromuscular hyperplasia (Fig. 16–12), which, if severe, may result in stricture formation (Goulston and McGovern 1969).

In some patients with severe ulcerative colitis it is necessary to perform total colectomy, but it is common practice to leave a rectal stump in situ while the patients await pelvic ileal reservoir construction. These nonfunctional rectal stumps generally show mucosal disease of usual type, but on occasion they exhibit florid lymphoid hyperplasia, transmural inflammation, fissures, changes similar to those of pseudomembranous colitis, and sometimes granulomas that lead to an erroneous change in diagnosis to Crohn's disease (Warren et al 1993).

Since first proposed by Morson (1966), it is now widely accepted that patients with ulcerative colitis are liable to develop carcinoma of the large intestine (von Herbay et al 1994). Those who seem to be particularly prone to development of carcinoma are patients with total colitis and a history of more than 10 years of disease. It is a traditional concept that patients with an onset of disease in childhood have a higher incidence of carcinoma than patients whose colitis begins in later life, but this idea has been challenged (Sachar and Greenstein 1981). Patients with mild longstanding disease seem especially vulnerable, but there is disagreement about whether those with continuous symptoms (Edwards and Truelove 1964) or quiescent disease (Svartz and Ernberg 1949, Kornman 1971, Sachar and Greenstein 1981) account for the majority. In a critical review, Collins, Feldman and Fordtran (1987) have cast serious doubt on the value of colonoscopic surveillance of colitic patients seemingly at risk of developing colonic cancer, and this view is supported by the results of a study conducted for 12 years involving 160 patients with a history of ulcerative colitis lasting for more than 8 years (Lynch et al 1993). Gyde et al (1988) provided evidence in a large cohort study from three centres that patients with extensive colitis have a genetic predisposition to colorectal cancer and that longstanding inflammation is not of primary importance. Nevertheless, others (Jones, Grogono and Hoare 1988) are convinced that surveillance of even those patients with distal disease is worthwhile. It is probably true that earlier diagnosis and treatment are obtained by those under continuous medical care, and a low incidence is often recorded by centres in which colitic patients are seen regularly. The explanation for this is probably that on the whole more patients in the high-risk group will have a colectomy before any malignant change can occur. Early work in this field by Morson and Pang (1967) provided evidence suggesting that sequential rectal biopsy had value in such cases as

Figure 16–12. Chronic quiescent ulcerative colitis. The muscularis mucosae is hypertrophied and appears as thick as the atrophic gland layer (H&E ×35).

an aid to cancer control. This was disputed by Evans and Pollock (1972) and Cook and Goligher (1975), who described cancer cases in which the rectum was normal, precancer in cases without cancer, and no precancer in the presence of cancer. In common with other epithelial surfaces that undergo precancerous changes, the colonic mucosa may exhibit a wide range of dysplastic features before the stage of frank carcinoma in situ or cancer proper is reached. The difficulty for the pathologist lies in deciding at which stage a firm diagnosis of precancer can be made.

The situation was seemingly clarified by Riddell (1976) who reassessed the available material from St. Mark's Hospital, London, from whence Morson and Pang's original article was published. The importance of clear diagnostic criteria is obvious when one considers that a total colectomy is the only operative procedure that can theoretically offer hope of a cure. However, it seems that there is still much work to be done in this interesting and important field. Certainly Riddell has highlighted the need for a set of working definitions to enable pathologists faced with the problem of diagnosis of precancer in ulcerative colitis to assess each patient. Cases such as those recorded by McGovern (1972) show that precancerous changes may precede the development of invasive cancer by as much as 6 years, and in this interim period diagnosis and subsequent treatment will effect a certain cure. However, the problem is the recognition of the specific pathological criteria on which a decision to advocate colectomy can be based (Riddell et al 1983). Riddell (1984) and Ransohoff, Riddell and Levin (1985) have addressed the problem time and again, and despite their detailed classifications on which clinical decisions can be based, the problem is still current. Dundas et al (1987) have shown, for example, that for some aspects of the assessment for dysplasia that concern columnar mucous cells and dystrophic goblet cells there is poor interobserver agreement. Clearly, the distribution of dysplasia in the colon is also important (Vatn, Elgjo and Bergan 1984), and it may not be visible endoscopically. Thus, biopsy of dysplastic areas may be a hit-and-miss affair, and although patients are under surveillance they may develop a carcinoma that is not discovered. Allen and Biggart (1986) have even drawn attention to the development of invading carcinomas that probably arise from misplaced dysplastic epithelium deep in the colonic wall being covered by nondysplastic mucosa. Despite claims that other markers of dysplasia may be useful, such as those demonstrated by monoclonal antibodies (Olding et al 1985), mucin stains (Ehsanullah et al 1985, Filipe, Edwards and Ehsanullah 1985, Habib et al 1986), lectins (Pihl et al 1985, Ahnen et al 1987, Fozard et al 1987), morphometric analysis (Allen et al 1987, Cuvelier, Morson and Roels 1987), and ploidy studies (Fozard et al 1986, Svendsen et al 1987), none have overcome the central problem that despite the acceptance of a sequence from dysplasia to cancer in ulcerative colitis, cases of cancer still develop undetected. Furthermore, there is still no single criterion on which to base a decision to advocate colectomy for the prevention of cancer in patients with ulcerative colitis. The problem is accentuated by the fact that ostensibly normal asymptomatic people may have active ulcerative colitis (Mayberry et al 1989). On the other hand, there have been claims for successful colonoscopic surveillance programmes that offer an alternative to colectomy in patients with longstanding disease (Leidenius et al 1991).

However, certain macroscopic appearances should lead the endoscopist to the likeliest diagnostic site for biopsy. One is velvet-like mucosa caused by an underlying villous microscopic structure, but this need not be dysplastic (Lee 1987). Polypoidal mucosa is another, despite that this will usually be of the inflammatory type. True adenomatous polyps also occur in ulcerative colitis, and Dawson and Pryse-Davies (1959) have shown that polyps in ulcerative colitis may show a spectrum of features from truly inflammatory through mixed types to those that are truly neoplastic (Figs. 16–13 and 16–14). This was confirmed in a later study by Blackstone et al (1981) who stressed the point that patients with a polyp or plaque showing epithelial dysplasia are more likely to harbour a separate carcinoma than are patients with dysplasia in a flat mucosa. Probably when a mass lesion is found it is chronologically an older one and is more likely to be associated with carcinoma in another part of

Figure 16–13. Polyp removed at sigmoidoscopy from a patient with a 12-year history of ulcerative colitis. The lesion has many of the features of an adenomatous polyp (H&E ×20).

the bowel (Butt and Morson 1981). This notion is at variance, however, with the report by Rubio et al (1982) of relatively nondysplastic villous adenomas described in association with separate invasive carcinomas. The most frequent macroscopic appearance, unfortunately, is less easy to recognise. It is flat and not unlike the usual featureless mucosa of chronic ulcerative colitis. If the underlying vessels are difficult to see, however, biopsy may be rewarding because the overlying mucosa, although flat, is thickened.

Riddell (1976) described two common microscopic changes, namely, adenomatous and basal cell changes. Three others may be seen rarely: in situ anaplasia, clear

Figure 16–14. Detail of Figure 16–13 shows branched and irregular tubules composed of dysplastic epithelium (H&E ×150).

cell change, and pancellular change. The adenomatous change is cytologically the same as that seen in ordinary adenomatous polyps of the colon. It occurs, however, in macroscopically flat, villous, and polypoidal lesions. Increasing nuclear atypia in the form of enlargement, pleomorphism, hyperchromasia, an increased mitotic rate, and loss or modification of goblet cell appearance can be seen (Figs. 16–15 to 16–17). The basal cell change is commonest in flat mucosa and is characterised by tubules formed by intensely hyperchromatic cells arranged in a linear fashion parallel to the basement membrane at the basal pole of the cell. The cell size and shape vary little, and the absence of pleomorphism and of changes in cell polarity is typical, but mitotic figures are increased in number. The cytoplasm is characteristically eosinophilic and the cells occupy most of the tubules, so that goblet cells are often scanty and may be poorly formed (Figs. 16–18 to 16–20).

In situ anaplasia occurs only in flat mucosa, often in the company of basal cell change. It is composed of single malignant cells in sheets, with or without signet ring forms, which are confined by the muscularis mucosae. The appearance is likened to superficial spreading carcinoma of the stomach (see Fig. 8–15). Clear cell change at first glance often appears innocuous. It forms a slightly raised lesion macroscopically and basically has a tubular configuration. The cytoplasm of the cells is clear or has a ground-glass appearance. The tubules nearer the surface have a saw-toothed outline similar to that seen in metaplastic polyps of the colon (Fig. 16–21). In pancellular dysplasia the mucosa is flat and shows enlarged and atypical cells arising from all the normal cell types, i.e., goblet cells, so-called absorptive cells, Paneth's cells, and even argentaffin cells. One or other cell type may predominate, and Riddell (1976) even described an appearance resembling an in situ argentaffinoma. Argyrophilic cell hyperplasia, an atypical carcinoid tumour (Miller and Sumner 1982), and frankly malignant carcinoid complicating chronic ulcerative colitis

Figure 16–15. *A*, Moderate adenomatous dysplasia with retained mucin production (H&E ×120). *B*, Mild dysplasia, but some goblet cells have an "in situ" signet ring appearance (H&E ×120).

Figure 16–16. Adenomatous dysplasia of the villous type (H&E ×48).

Figure 16–17. *A,* Adenomatous dysplasia in a flat area of mucosa. Irregular budding of tubules has produced a back-to-back arrangement of crypts on the right, and all show severe cellular dysplasia (H&E ×190). *B,* Detail of dysplastic epithelium. Note the absence of goblet cells (H&E ×750).

Figure 16–18. *A*, Earliest recognisable basal cell dysplasia. Nuclear hyperchromasia and pleomorphism are apparent. Mucin secretion is still present, but some goblet cells are atypical (H&E ×300). *B*, More severe nuclear changes and atypical mucin production (H&E ×480).

have also been described (Owen et al 1981, Gledhill et al 1986). Rarely, squamous metaplasia of the colonic mucosa occurs in chronic ulcerative colitis, and Adamsen, Ostberg and Norryd (1988) described such a phenomenon, but with superimposed severe squamous dysplasia.

By and large the histological diagnosis of precancer as described should be made only in the absence of significant active inflammation because of the difficulties, even for experienced observers, of evaluating purely reactive epithelial changes, which can appear remarkably bizarre, especially in childhood. Although as illustrated (Figs. 16–19 to 16–21) it is possible to subdivide dysplasia according to the predominant cytological appearance, a mixed appearance is not infrequent. From a practical point of view, until objective methods of assessing increasing dysplasia can be devised the pathologist needs to make a subjective decision. If the dysplasia is severe, i.e., architecturally and cytologically approaching an appearance of carcinoma, a confident diagnosis should make a colectomy the first choice of management. However, this is a clinical decision and is often complex. Even greater difficulty arises when the dysplasia is definite but mild in severity. As many arguments can be raised for follow-up of such patients with regular rebiopsy as can for the recommendation of colectomy.

It is now clear that routine rectal biopsy in the search of precancer will miss a group of cases, not only of precancer elsewhere but also of established cancer in the more proximal colon. With increasing practice of colonoscopy and multiple sampling of the mucosa of the whole colon, some but not all of the problems related to colitis-associated cancer have been solved. In the patient at risk, Lennard-Jones et al (1983) followed the practice of step-wise biopsy of the whole colonic mucosa every 10 cm when it appears flat and also biopsy of any macroscopically abnormal area. Some would recommend that this assessment be performed annually (Yardley et al 1983), but this depends on resources and, as already pointed out, some (Collins, Feldman

Figure 16–19. *A,* Early basal cell dysplasia. The deep aspect of the tubules shows nonspecific pseudopyloric metaplasia, but the upper parts exhibit loss of goblet cells and obvious nuclear enlargement (H&E ×120). *B,* High power of *A* photomicrograph showing abnormal but basally situated nuclei (H&E ×480).

Figure 16–20. *A,* Basal cell dysplasia is obvious, with loss of mucin production and severe nuclear dysplasia but no significant loss of polarity (H&E ×300). *B,* Detail of *A.* Retention of polarity by cells with markedly dysplastic nuclei (H&E ×1,000).

Figure 16–21. Clear cell dysplasia. There is a resemblance to a hyperplastic polyp of the colon. The upper parts of the tubules have a saw-toothed appearance. Most cells have a ground-glass cytoplasmic appearance that contrasts with that of the retained goblet cells (H&E ×75).

and Fordtran 1987) believe that it is not justified. As experience increases in the recognition of earlier stages of precancer, perhaps by objective methodologies, it is possible that the recommendation for total colectomy will be made with confidence. This decision may not be a palatable one for patients without symptoms or with only minor symptoms, however. Nevertheless, it is hoped that eventually no colitic patient in the cancer-prone group will ever come to operation when carcinoma is already present. It may be that for the reasons outlined colonscopic biopsy surveillance will prove not to be the optimum method. Certainly it is less cost-effective than when used for cancer detection in those with positive occult blood tests. Fozard and Dixon (1989), who reviewed the problem, concluded that perhaps the answer lies in the newer molecular biology techniques. These could theoretically be used with good effect in detecting genetic abnormalities in early malignant cells derived from total colonic samples.

Although much less common than adenocarcinoma, non-Hodgkin's colonic lymphoma is now also thought to be a complication of longstanding ulcerative colitis (Shepherd et al 1989, Hill, Mills and Maxwell 1993). Extraintestinal non-Hodgkin's lymphoma also appears to be a complication of ulcerative colitis (Greenstein et al 1992).

CROHN'S COLITIS

Although Crohn's colitis was originally described as a disease of the terminal ileum (Crohn, Ginzburg and Oppenheimer 1932), it was soon realised that any part of the small intestine could be involved. Two years after Crohn's original paper, Colp (1934) stressed that the disease could also involve the colon, and other papers citing colonic involvement followed. There was, however, a general reluctance to accept colonic Crohn's disease as an entity until almost 30 years later, when the criteria for differentiating Crohn's disease of the colon from the more common condition of ulcerative colitis were published (Lockhart-Mummery and Morson 1960). It is now clear that Crohn's disease can involve the mouth, larynx, pharynx, oesophagus, stomach, small and large intestines, anus, musculoskeletal system, and skin (Whitehead 1987). Crohn's disease limited to the colon accounts for 15%–20%

of all cases and is only slightly less common than disease involving both small and large intestines. In the elderly, distal colonic involvement is common (Fabricius et al 1985). However, the very presence of lesions in the small bowel renders the diagnosis of Crohn's disease of the colon easier to make. In a similar way, the diagnosis of Crohn's disease of the skin or mouth can be made with confidence only when there is typical intestinal disease. Crohn's disease confined to the large intestine, therefore, poses a diagnostic challenge to the clinician and pathologist alike.

There is some evidence that Crohn's disease may be linked to the measles virus and that its persistence in bowel tissues is related to a capillary vasculitis, which is the initiating lesion in the pathological process (Sankey et al 1993, Wakefield et al 1993, Ekbom et al 1994, Pounder 1994, Thompson et al 1995).

The importance of colonic biopsy in the diagnosis of this disease cannot be overemphasised (Dyer, Stansfeld and Dawson 1970). When rectal tissue is obtained, whether a suction instrument or forceps is used, every effort should be made to ensure that submucosal tissues are included. If there is obvious sigmoidoscopic inflammation and ulceration, several biopsies should be obtained. Ideally, ulcerative lesions, inflamed but intact mucosa, and mucosa that seems more normal should be sampled when possible. It is claimed that biopsies from ulcers are diagnostically superior (Potzi et al 1989). Rectal biopsy samples should also be taken when the sigmoidoscopic appearances are apparently normal, and multiple colonic biopsies should be done during colonoscopic procedures. One of the fields of greatest difficulty for both clinician and pathologist is the differential diagnosis between Crohn's colitis and ulcerative colitis: if the rectal biopsy is histologically normal, an inflammatory lesion in a more proximal part of the colon is most unlikely to be due to ulcerative colitis and more likely to be due to Crohn's disease or some other segmental lesion. Step-wise colonic biopsy and histological evaluation are the cornerstone in the diagnostic procedure aimed at differentiating between these two serious diseases (Ogorek and Fisher 1994).

The histological features of Crohn's disease as seen in colonic biopsies reflect the pathology of the disease as a whole. It is basically an inflammatory disorder, usually included in the chronic granulomatous group. However, as in tuberculosis, one may rarely observe a more acute inflammatory reaction at one end of the scale and the more common and very chronic hyperplastic fibrous reaction at the other. The fulminating acute onset cases of Crohn's colitis pose extremely difficult problems in differential diagnosis. Early in the course of the disease, tissue reactions may be nonspecific and some of these cases are no doubt similar to the so-called indeterminate colitis to be referred to later. Others with a similar history finally evolve into more histologically typical disease (Linssen and Tytgat 1982). The problem of the relationship of these more acute cases to the more classic cases of colonic disease is in many ways comparable to the relationship of acute terminal ileitis to chronic regional ileitis of the older literature. The evidence seems to point to the fact that when acute terminal ileitis due to other causes such as *Yersinia enterocolitica* infection are excluded, a small proportion of cases of acute disease develop into classic Crohn's disease (Jess 1981).

In typical disease, rectal or colonic biopsy samples of nonulcerated areas situated near ulcers may appear relatively normal but usually show a plasma cell and lymphocytic infiltration of the lamina propria (Fig. 16–22). Polymorphs, either within capillaries or around the basement membranes of tubules, also are not infrequently present, and an occasional collection of polymorphs within the lumen of a gland tubule is not unusual. Rarely, the inflammatory exudate within the crypt is granulomatous (Fig. 16–23). Gross crypt abscess formation and marked epithelial invasion by polymorphs are not seen, however, in nonulcerated mucosa. It is a relatively important diagnostic feature that these inflammatory changes are not usually associated with any significant distortion of gland tubular pattern or goblet cell depletion, and within the biopsy specimen itself they are less evenly distributed than in ulcerative colitis. The inflammation, moreover, is frequently more marked in the submucosa than in the lamina propria and also has a tendency to be perilymphatic. This

Figure 16–22. Rectal biopsy in Crohn's colitis. The tubules retain a good goblet cell component, and their pattern is relatively normal, although they are more widely separated than normal by the inflammatory infiltrate (H&E ×75).

disproportionate inflammation is another useful feature for diagnosis, especially when attended by denser and more clearly demarcated lymphoid aggregates (Fig. 16–24). The submucosal infiltrate may be associated with lymphatic and vascular dilation or, when the reaction is more chronic, with a fibroplasia. These features are less likely to be evaluable in the more superficial colonoscopic biopsies.

Diagnostically the most significant of the more chronic tissue reactions is the presence of epithelioid cell granulomas (Fig. 16–25), which usually contain one or more multinucleate giant cells. They may be seen in the lamina propria but are most common in the submucosa (McGovern and Goulston 1968). With a tendency to

Figure 16–23. Dilated crypt in Crohn's colitis. The exudate contains multinucleate giant cells (H&E ×450).

Figure 16–24. Rectal biopsy in Crohn's colitis. Note the disproportionate inflammation with lymphoid aggregates in the submucosa. Mucosal distortion and goblet cell depletion are minimal (H&E ×38).

Figure 16–25. Rectal biopsy in Crohn's colitis. There is an epithelioid and multinucleate giant cell granuloma splitting the muscularis mucosae (H&E ×180).

form near lymphatics, they sometimes bulge into the lumen. These granulomas are more variable in size and the component cells are less tightly packed together than the usual sarcoid granulomas, although the loose cellular arrangement may simply reflect a generalised tissue oedema. The giant cells (which are not always present) may contain Schaumann's bodies, and the overall appearance of the granulomas is similar to that of granulomas in sarcoidosis. They are particularly diagnostically significant if seen in the submucosa and in areas distant from ulceration. It is important to remember that a giant cell and histiocyte reaction may be of the foreign body type (Figs. 16–26 and 16–27) or may appear as a reaction to mucin (Fig. 16–28) and may be seen occasionally in ulcerative colitis (Figs. 16–29 and 16–30). There is a view that some of the giant cells in the lamina propria in ulcerative colitis may be derived from fibroblasts (Pitt, Knox and Haboubi 1993). However, in Crohn's disease, giant cells and small granulomas also appear to form in relation to degenerating tubules and are associated with a few polymorphs (Figs. 16–31 to 16–34). The importance of these microgranulomas is referred to later. For the significance of granulomas in rectal biopsies, it is necessary to address the question of whether systemic sarcoidosis can involve the gastrointestinal tract. It has been stated in the past that although gastric sarcoidosis occurs occasionally, involvement of the intestine is quite rare. It may be that there is something about the gut-associated lymphoid tissue that makes it resistant to involvement. There are, however, a few cases of sarcoidosis of the small and large bowel that have been described (Macfarlane 1955, Aaronson, Meir and Ulin 1957, Gourevitch and Cunningham 1959, Gould, Handley and Barnardo 1973, Kondo et al 1980, Tobi et al 1982, Bulger et al 1988).

Biopsy specimens from ulcer margins in Crohn's colitis show distortion of gland tubular patterns, crypt abscesses, and epithelial cell degenerative and regenerative changes. As a consequence, the goblet cell population is reduced, but this is rarely as marked a feature as in ulcerative colitis. Many of the ulcers in Crohn's colitis have no special features, but biopsy tissues may reveal evidence of two types of ulceration

Figure 16–26. Rectal biopsy in ulcerative colitis with subepithelial multinucleate giant cells *(arrowheads)* (H&E ×360).

Figure 16–27. Same biopsy as in Figure 16–26 but sectioned serially to locate the foreign body *(arrowhead)* (H&E ×360).

Figure 16–28. Rectal biopsy in ulcerative colitis. This granuloma situated just above the muscularis gave a strong abnormal reaction with mucin stains (H&E ×360).

Figure 16–29. Rectal biopsy in ulcerative colitis in a chronic quiescent stage. A single multinucleate giant cell *(arrow)* is apparent (H&E ×70).

Figure 16–30. Detail of the giant cell in Figure 16–29. On deeper sectioning a birefringent foreign body inclusion was seen in the cytoplasm (H&E ×350).

Figure 16–31. A giant cell with peripheral nuclei in relation to degenerating polymorphs and, to the right, a few epithelioid cells (H&E ×500).

Figure 16–32. Step serial section of a degenerating tubule surrounded by epithelioid histiocytes and containing polymorphs (H&E ×500).

Figure 16–33. Step serial section of a degenerating tubule surrounded by epithelioid histiocytes and containing polymorphs (H&E ×500).

Figure 16–34. A definite microgranuloma composed predominantly of epithelioid histiocytes in relation to an effaced tubule (H&E ×350).

that deserve special mention. The first is the histological equivalent of the aphthoid ulcer seen macroscopically. The early lesion (Fig. 16–35) is composed of a central microabscess, sometimes appearing to occur within a lymphoid aggregate at the mucosal-submucosal junction. The abscess nearly always seems to involve the base of a dilated tubular gland, which shows necrosis of its walls and pus streaming up into the lumen (Fig. 16–36). Focal superficial ulceration is seen in older lesions (Fig. 16–37), and suppuration may thus obliterate any original lymphoid follicle. Biopsy evidence of the fissuring type of ulceration may also be present. These ulcers, which occur at right angles to the long axis of the bowel, often contain pus and are lined by granulation tissue that has a conspicuous histiocytic element. The pale plump cells are quite similar and probably identical to the epithelioid histiocytes that occur in the granulomas. The cells occasionally form multinucleate giant cells of the Langhans type with peripheral nuclei, but in the region of ulcers obvious foreign body giant cells may also be seen. These tend to have more numerous and centrally placed nuclei. It is not always possible to be absolutely certain of the significance of isolated giant cells (Figs. 16–38 and 16–39).

In the absence of endoscopic abnormality, Goodman, Skinner and Truelove (1976) have shown that, although conventional light microscopic examination may reveal no significant abnormality, the volume of lamina propria and the plasma cell per unit length of the muscularis mucosae are quantitatively greater than normal. The mucosal level of glucosamine synthetase is also significantly higher than normal, and these authors concluded that apparently normal rectal mucosa in Crohn's colitis is always abnormal. These subtle abnormalities apparently also exist outside the gastrointestinal tract. Crama-Bohbouth et al (1983) have shown an increase in IgA plasma cells in biopsy samples from the apparently normal lip of patients with Crohn's disease elsewhere. In a much larger series, Korelitz and Sommers (1977), using ordinary light microscopy and subjective assessments of inflammatory cells and features such as granulomas, disproportionate inflammation, and lymphoid aggregates, found evidence of inflammatory involvement of the rectal mucosa when it was sigmoidoscopically normal in 45% of 99 patients with Crohn's disease in another part of the bowel. In 18% of the cases, granulomas were recognised.

In another paper concerning the same cases, Rotterdam, Korelitz and Sommers (1977) drew attention to the importance of superficial, small, and poorly defined

Figure 16–35. Early aphthoid lesion. Central microabscess within a lymphoid aggregate involving the base of a gland. The other glands are relatively normal and have a good goblet cell population (H&E ×75).

Figure 16–36. Later aphthoid lesion. Pus discharges onto the surface (H&E ×75).

Figure 16–37. Established aphthoid ulcer (H&E ×75).

Figure 16–38. Rectal biopsy in Crohn's colitis. A giant cell with centrally placed and abundant nuclei apparently within a gland. Another giant cell is to the right *(arrowhead)* (H&E ×75).

Figure 16–39. A foreign body type of giant cell at the base of a degenerating tubule containing pus (H&E ×200).

collections of histiocytes and lymphocytes with or without giant cells, which they termed microgranulomas. If foreign body or mucin granulomas can be excluded, it is now becoming clear that microgranulomas associated in the same biopsy sample with patchy chronic inflammation can nearly always be regarded as a positive indication of Crohn's disease. They are usually seen in association with other chronic inflammatory cells or a few polymorphs invading a neighbouring tubule and are of greater significance if neighbouring tubules are entirely normal. When present along with other pathological and clinical features, they are clearly of greater diagnostic significance. Microgranulomas are not infrequently found if endoscopists biopsy areas of aphthous ulceration or microerosions (Poulsen, Pedersen and Jarnum 1984). The importance of microgranulomas in colonic biopsies is obvious from the serial sectioning study of colectomy specimens by Kuramoto et al (1987). These workers found that microgranulomas were common in the surface layers of the mucosa, whereas more mature epithelioid and giant cell lesions occurred in deeper tissues. These microgranulomas, which range in size from 80 to 160 μm and contain between 10 and 30 immature macrophages, thus assume great diagnostic importance in superficial colonoscopic biopsy tissues (Fig. 16–40). Because of this, it is growing practice to subject rectal or colonic biopsy samples in patients suspected of having Crohn's disease to serial section. Petri et al (1982) have shown that 30% of single rectal biopsy specimens in patients with colonic Crohn's disease contain granulomas if serial sections are examined. This is certainly a better yield than for a few sections of a rectal biopsy specimen when the figure for detecting granulomas is only 15% (Iliffe and Owen 1981). Schmitz-Moormann et al (1984) have even shown that in Crohn's colitis, if several biopsy samples are examined by serial section, granulomas can be found in 40%–50% of patients.

Figure 16–40. Colonic biopsy with a focally distributed chronic colitis and a central microgranuloma adjacent to a segmental degeneration of a mucosal gland tubule. Note also occasional polymorphs in the infiltrate (H&E ×500).

In a transmission electron microscopic study, Dvorak et al (1980) described an increase in the number of mast cells in the submucosa in Crohn's disease. The claim was entirely subjective and based on relatively minute samples of tissue. Whether or not this finding is substantiated, it has not been found to have diagnostic significance and may be regarded simply as a nonspecific manifestation of the inflammatory response. The lack of diagnostic significance also probably applies to the finding of an increase in chromogranin-positive cells in Crohn's disease (Bishop et al 1987).

In a prospective study of rectal biopsies in patients with Crohn's colitis, Ward and Webb (1977) produced evidence that the severity of histological involvement as revealed by a semiquantitative method is related to the severity and final outcome of the disease. The presence of either fissuring or ulceration suggests a poor prognosis. Whereas the presence of granulomas in the large bowel and anus indicates a good prognosis, this does not hold true for the small bowel (Chambers and Morson 1979).

Differential Diagnosis Between Ulcerative Colitis and Crohn's Colitis

The differential diagnosis between ulcerative colitis and Crohn's colitis is a difficult problem frequently posed. Although there are claims that they may be different manifestations of a basically similar disease (Lewin and Swales 1966, Lewkonia and McConnell 1976), there are well-documented cases of coexistent ulcerative colitis and Crohn's colitis (McDermott et al 1982, White et al 1983). That there is an overlap of features, however, cannot be denied, and this is observed particularly in specimens from patients with a short history of severe disease who undergo surgery for toxic megacolon. This type of disease corresponds to the "colitis indeterminate" of Price (1978), who used the term because the pathological features of deep ulceration and transmural inflammation can occur in fulminant ulcerative colitis as well as in Crohn's disease. However, if previous surgical or biopsy material from such patients is reviewed it is often possible to categorise the patients. Nevertheless, there are cases of idiopathic inflammatory bowel disease that are difficult to classify.

Bonfils et al (1977), for example, described what they claimed to be a distinct form of colitis, often in younger patients, characterised by a discrepancy between the moderate clinical severity and the evidence of total severe colitis obtained by radiological and histiological examination. The colitis resolved spontaneously and did not recur. Except for the course of the disease, the presentation had more the features of Crohn's colitis. The author also has experience of such cases in which there was dramatic recovery, and of others treated surgically because of the evidence of total colitis and the severity of the radiological changes. The striking histological features are deep ulceration of mucosa, which characteristically shows intense vascular dilation and an inflammatory reaction with a relative absence of polymorphonuclear neutrophils and only a slight round cell and histiocyte component. The mucosa bordering the ulcers retains its goblet cell component and features oedema, vascular congestion, and haemorrhage, rather than acute purulent inflammation as in the more typical ulcerative colitis case. There are thus arguable grounds for retaining the term colitis indeterminate for this type of case. In a 25-year incidence study in Sweden (Stewenius et al 1995), the incidence of indeterminate colitis as well as of ulcerative colitis appears to be increasing. This is of interest because at least some cases of indeterminate colitis develop into Crohn's disease (Kangas, Matikainen and Mattila 1994).

The presence of deeply situated granulomas in rectal biopsy tissues makes the diagnosis of Crohn's disease a simple matter, but even in their absence differentiation from ulcerative colitis is often possible. A relative sparing of the mucosa by an inflammatory process that is more obvious in the submucosa is an important sign. The uneven distribution of the inflammation in the same site or in biopsy material from different sites is another. A normal mucosa or one showing goblet cell preservation and a normal gland pattern despite inflammatory infiltration of the lamina propria would favour a diagnosis of Crohn's disease. Lymphoid aggregates may be seen in both Crohn's disease and ulcerative colitis; when they lie in the submucosa and are well separated from the muscularis mucosae, and when there is also submucosal oedema or fibrosis in the presence of an intact mucosa and muscularis mucosae, the diagnosis is Crohn's disease.

Perhaps of greatest practical importance in the differentiation of ulcerative colitis from Crohn's colitis and other forms of colitis is that the pathologist should receive multiple biopsy specimens. Pieces of mucosa should be taken from areas that appear both normal and abnormal by endoscopy. This provides valuable information concerning the focal inflammatory involvement of the mucosa in Crohn's colitis as opposed to a more diffuse involvement in ulcerative colitis. In view of the fact that granulomas may be found in as many as 30% of rectal biopsies in known Crohn's disease of the colon if serial sections are examined, at least three biopsy samples should be taken from different sites. Anthonisen and Riis (1971) have reported that eosinophilia in biopsy smear preparations is indicative of ulcerative colitis rather than Crohn's disease. This author has no personal experience with this method, but in view of the more obvious overall polymorphonuclear nature of the cellular infiltrate in ulcerative colitis this phenomenon might be expected. Nevertheless, in an individual case in the absence of more specific features an eosinophil count of the lamina propria cannot be used by itself as a reliable diagnostic criterion. Eosinophils are also probably seen just as frequently in other forms of colitis, particularly those of infective origin. In a morphometric analysis of 16 variables, Schmitz-Moormann and Himmelmann (1988) claimed an improved rate of discrimination between Crohn's disease and ulcerative colitis. However, it was conceded that the method had no application in daily routine pathology practice.

In addition to rectal biopsy material, tissues for histological examination should be removed from other easily accessible sites (perianal area, skin, mouth, oesophagus, stomach) if these show evidence of disease. They may contain granulomas, and if so a diagnosis of Crohn's disease can be made. This assumes great importance, particularly when a histological diagnosis of a coincident bowel lesion has not been obtained.

There is evidence that patients with longstanding Crohn's colitis are more prone to develop adenocarcinoma than the normal population (Weedon et al 1973, Gyde et al 1980, Gillen et al 1994). In some cases the cancer occurs in an unaffected area, but precancerous changes similar to those in ulcerative colitis have also been described in both colon and small intestine (Craft et al 1981, Simpson, Traube and Riddell 1981, Perzin et al 1984). There is some evidence that colorectal cancer is now equally as common in patients with Crohn's disease and those with ulcerative colitis (Softley et al 1988). However, although dysplastic changes have been described in resection specimens in the region of or separate from the carcinoma, there has been no systematic study to determine the frequency of dysplasia in patients with longstanding Crohn's colitis who do not have adenocarcinoma. This is because patients with widespread longstanding disease are much more likely, because of stenosis or fistulas, for example, to be subjected to surgery. Thus, the identification and characterisation of a sequence of precancer to cancer are much less likely in Crohn's disease than in ulcerative colitis.

ISCHAEMIC COLITIS

If the viability of the tissues of the bowel is in any way endangered, the result is invasion of the wall by the many pathogenic organisms that normally pass through or reside in the lumen. The mechanisms of intestinal ischaemia are complex, and secondary factors modify or accentuate the ordinary ischaemic lesion; as a consequence the range of pathological and clinical entities is extremely wide. There has thus arisen a confusing terminology. As far as the colon is concerned, some of these entities have been better defined (Marston et al 1966, Whitehead 1971, 1972, 1976, Marston 1977).

Ischaemic colitis can be considered in two broad categories. The first is characterised clinically by abdominal pain of sudden onset and the passage of blood and clots per rectum. It is frequently associated with narrowing or occlusion of the mesenteric vessels, although accurate information concerning this is difficult to acquire during life even by use of advanced radiological techniques. Recovery either with or without surgical intervention is usual, and resolution with or without scarring and stricture is the end result. Thromboatheromatous disease of the mesenteric vessels is the usual predisposing cause, and thus it is commonest in the older age group. It is, however, seen occasionally in young adults, when it usually occurs as a single episode with complete resolution. Clarke, Lloyd-Mostyn and Sadler (1972) described 4 such cases and reviewed the previous literature containing 10 others. They commented on the prevalence of right-sided lesions and the low incidence of stricture formation. The precise aetiology in these is not known, although in young women it has been ascribed to the use of oral contraceptive agents (Cotton and Lea Thomas 1971). The most recent work (Deana and Dean, 1995) would tend to support the view that a reversible ischaemic colitis involving the left colon in particular occurs in young women and is associated with the use of exogenous estrogenic agents. Lamy et al (1988) also described a marked intimal hyperplasia and thrombosis of the visceral arteries in a young woman with extensive bowel ischaemia and ascribed it to a combination of oral contraception and smoking. Acute reversible ischaemic colitis in a young female long-distance runner has also been recorded (Heer et al 1987). In addition, the reported incidence of the less severe form of this disease in young men is rising (Neto and Ribeiro 1974, Matsumoto et al 1994, Biaggi and Potet 1995), and the author has personal experience with three typical cases of young men who obtained spontaneous and complete recovery. Archibald et al (1980) were able to demonstrate inferior mesenteric vein thrombosis in their male patient with ischaemic colitis, and additional cases are described by Duffy (1981) and by Heron et al (1981), who referred to the condition as evanescent colitis. It appears to be identical to the colitis that is described in association with the use of oral penicillin derivatives (Moulis and Vender 1994). Despite the prevalence of right-sided lesions in this group, the part of the colon at maximum risk from an ischaemic insult is the watershed area between the superior and inferior mesenteric vessels, and thus the commonest site for ischaemic colitis is the splenic flexure. Surgical interference with the inferior mesenteric vessels, abdominal aorta and iliac arteries, or aortic aneurysms may be associated with colonic lesions (Kim et al 1983, Bayne, Donovan and Henthorne 1994) and rectosigmoid lesions (Stenberg and Risberg 1984, Welling et al 1985), but these also occur spontaneously (Kilpatrick et al 1968). Devroede et al (1982) have shown that faecal incontinence and rectal angina are also part of the spectrum of ischaemic bowel disease and Archibald, Jirsch and Bear (1978) have described an association with renal transplantation. An unusual case of ischaemic proctitis was apparently the result of fibromuscular dysplasia of the superior rectal artery (Quirke, Campbell and Talbot 1984) or all the mesenteric vessels, a condition that may be familial (Meacham and Brantley 1987).

Apart from thromboatheromatous lesions such as may be seen in quite young patients if, for example, they are diabetic (Spotnitz et al 1984), other vascular pathological conditions, in particular the necrotising arteritis group, may on occasion be associated with colonic ischaemia. These conditions include polyarteritis nodosa (Wood et al 1979, Lee et al 1984, Roikjaer 1987, Oosawa and Suzuki 1994), rheumatoid vasculitis (Burt et al 1983), and systemic lupus erythematosus (Gore et al 1983, Helliwell et al 1985, Papa, Shiloni and McDonald 1986, Ho, Teh and Goh 1987, Reissman et al 1994). It is the subject of rare case reports in association with Kawasaki disease (Fan, Lau and Wong 1986), Buerger's disease (Soo et al 1983, Rosen, Sommer and Knobel 1985), blunt abdominal trauma (Davidson and Everson 1987), malignant atrophic papulosis or Degos's disease (Barlow et al 1988), use of ergotamine and oral contraceptives (Rutgeerts et al 1993), amyloidosis (Kyzer et al 1993),

Figure 16–41. Rectal biopsies in mild ischaemic colitis. *A*, Oedema of the lamina propria, capillary dilation, and superficial mucosal necrosis with haemorrhage (H&E ×120). *B*, More extensive ischaemic change, but the bases of the crypts are still intact (H&E ×180).

Figure 16–41 *Continued C,* Early sloughing and ulceration (H&E ×180).

and cocaine abuse (Brown, Rosenholtz and Marshall 1994). Haber, Burrell and West (1993) reported a case due to mesenteric vein endophlebitis. It was apparently unrelated to the use of hydroxyethylrutoside, a drug implicated in similar previously reported cases. Low intestinal flow states also play their part, and colonic obstruction with the attendant decrease in mucosal circulation is a frequent association (Levine and Price 1994). A subgroup of ischaemic colitis occurs specifically in circumstances of colonic obstruction and is thus proximal to the obstructive pathology. It is consequently not seen in biopsy material because the biopsy procedure is not possible. The colitis is basically identical to other forms of ischaemic colitis and is reviewed by Gratama, Smedts and Whitehead (1995). Hunt and Mildenhall (1975) claimed a connection between ischaemic colonic strictures and pancreatitis, but the aetiology of ischaemia in these cases is obscure. It has been described in association with chronic intermittent peritoneal dialysis (Koren et al 1984, Jablonski, Putzki and Heymann 1987) and in renal transplant recipients (Komorowski et al 1986). Occasionally, ischaemic colitis is complicated by significant dilation of the bowel (Carr et al 1986). Focal ischaemia secondary to atheromatous emboli not only can give rise to segmental ischaemic colitis but also can be associated with localised ischaemia resulting in proliferation of ulceration granulation tissue and formation of inflammatory polyps (Grant et al 1993, Pidala, Slezak and Hlivko 1993, Gramlich and Hunter 1994). For a full discussion of the pathology of intestinal ischaemia, the reader is referred to Whitehead (1976).

In biopsy tissues, appearances are characteristic. The mild cases (Fig. 16–41) show an ischaemic necrosis of the superficial epithelium and of a variable extent of the luminal two thirds or so of the mucosa. The surface epithelium and upper parts of the tubules show ischaemic degeneration and sloughing, and the lamina exhibits an oedema, ballooning of capillaries, and sludging of red cells. Rarely does a capillary show a tiny plug of thrombus (Fig. 16–42). Lesions of this severity resolve completely as long as the bases of the crypts are not damaged, and a completely normal mucosa may be seen 5–7 days later (Fig. 16–43). More severe lesions (Fig. 16–44) show ischaemic necrosis of the full thickness of the mucosa and extension into the deeper layers (Fig. 16–45). In these lesions, secondary infection, ulceration (Fig. 16–46), and scarring are usual, and during the healing and healed stages mucosal biopsy tissues reveal a variety of abnormalities. Regenerating gland tubules tend to be

Figure 16–42. Mild ischaemic colitis. There is a tiny fibrin plug in a dilated capillary (H&E ×280).

Figure 16–43. Rectal biopsy from the same patient as in Figure 16–41, taken 1 week later, showing almost perfect resolution of mucosa (H&E ×70).

Figure 16–44. Rectal biopsy in ischaemic colitis with full thickness mucosal necrosis and sloughing ulceration (H&E ×70),

Figure 16–45. Complete ischaemic necrosis of the mucosa and part of the submucosa with secondary inflammatory infiltration. Note the vascular dilation in the submucosa (H&E ×70).

Figure 16–46. Rectal biopsy shows ischaemic ulceration with typical vascular granulation tissue at base and attempted regeneration by marginal epithelium (H&E ×70).

irregular in shape, size, and orientation (Fig. 16–47), and the simple component cells are often a little bizarre and show numerous mitoses (Fig. 16–48). In areas of regenerated mucosa, glandular distortion persists (Fig. 16–49) and there is frequently a fibrosis of the lamina propria, which often extends into the submucosa through the breaches of the muscularis mucosae (Fig. 16–50), which has no capacity for regeneration. The fibrosis is attended by a progressive devascularisation, becoming typically dense and hyaline (Fig. 16–51), and is often associated with collections of haemosiderin-filled histiocytes. Levine et al (1986) described inflammatory polyposis of the colon following ischaemic colitis. As occasional findings in biopsies that also show features of ischaemic colitis, especially in the elderly, one may observe not only severe hyaline sclerosis of small vessels but also atheromatous embolisation (Figs. 16–52 and 16–53).

The second type of ischaemic lesion is described variously as ischaemic enterocolitis (McGovern and Goulston 1965); haemorrhagic enterocolitis (Wilson and Qualheim 1954); necrotising enterocolitis (Killingback and Williams 1961); postoperative enterocolitis, uraemic enterocolitis, or nonocclusive intestinal infarction (Renton

Figure 16–47. Regenerating mucosa in ischaemic colitis. The tubular pattern is abnormal. There is still oedema and vascular congestion (H&E ×75).

Figure 16–48. Detail of Figure 16–47 shows a tubule composed of simple regenerating epithelium and cells in mitoses (H&E ×450).

1972, Byrd, Cunningham and Goldman 1987); and acute intestinal failure (Marston 1977). It is often a terminal condition, presenting with bloody diarrhoea, usually but not always in patients seriously ill owing to some other disease, frequently associated with the postoperative period of an episode of shock. There is no special localisation of lesions in or near the splenic flexure, and sometimes the whole of the large bowel and part of the small bowel are involved. No age group is exempt but it is more common in old age.

In adults the diagnosis is made only at autopsy, and in the usual circumstances of its occurrence it does not pose a diagnostic problem. Rarely, however, it arises without obvious predisposing cause and then must be distinguished from acute onset ulcerative colitis and Crohn's disease. Rectal biopsy is rarely performed but typically shows mucosal necrosis, submucosal haemorrhage and oedema, and a variable

Figure 16–49. Healed ischaemic colitis. Note the glandular distortion (H&E ×75).

Figure 16–50. Healed ischaemic colitis. Fibrosis of the lamina propria extends through the breaches in the muscularis mucosae into the submucosa (H&E ×75).

secondary inflammatory infiltrate depending on the duration of the lesion. The obvious feature is the ballooning of capillaries and venules, which are stuffed with red cells and are invariably occluded by numerous recent fibrin plugs (Fig. 16–54). Gas formation probably due to secondary invasion by bacteria is not evident in biopsy specimens.

The aetiology of this lesion is complex and includes many factors, one or other of which may appear to assume greater importance in any individual case. They include partial or complete blocks of the blood supply and variations in the blood flow controlled by various shunting mechanisms, the intestinal contents including bacterial flora and various intestinal enzymes, the effectiveness of the mucosal barrier to entry of endotoxin or similar agents, and the priming of the mucosal immune mechanism to agents such as endotoxin. The vascular thrombosis already referred to was previously thought to be secondary, but Whitehead (1971) has produced evidence that it may well be primary, the ischaemic necrosis being the local manifes-

Figure 16–51. Ischaemic colitis with persistent ulcer. The fibrosis of the submucosa is characteristically hyaline and dense (H&E ×38).

Figure 16–52. Colonic biopsy with mild ischaemic fibrosis of the lamina propria and submucosa. Note the hyalinised, thickened submucosal vessel (left) and atheromatous cholesterol crystal embolism (right) (H&F. ×350).

Figure 16–53. Atheromatous embolism with foreign body giant cell reaction to the crystals of cholesterol (H&E ×350).

Figure 16–54. Ischaemic enterocolitis. The mucosa is infarcted, and the mucosal and submucosal vessels are occluded by thrombus (fibrin stain ×75).

tation of disseminated intravascular coagulation. It is therefore of some interest that Craner and Burdick (1976) and Dillard (1983) described a colitis in the haemolytic-uraemic syndrome with which disseminated intravascular coagulation is intimately associated. Many cases of so-called clostridial and staphylococcal enterocolitis probably also belong to this group and simply represent primary ischaemia with superimposed massive overgrowth of organisms already within the bowel.

Pseudomembranous lesions that are typical of pseudomembranous enterocolitis (Goulston and McGovern 1965) may also be seen in this condition. Appearances range between predominantly haemorrhagic and predominantly pseudomembranous, and it was postulated by Whitehead (1971) that in the latter cases the process of intravascular coagulation is less severe and evolves much more slowly. Margaretten and McKay (1971), in a paper on thrombotic ulcerations of the gastrointestinal tract, made particular comment of the association of microthrombosis with pseudomembranous enterocolitis. These authors were also able to show evidence not only of widespread microthrombosis at autopsy, but also of alteration in clotting factors indicating an episode of intravascular coagulation occurring during life. The relationship to pseudomembranous enterocolitis is equally as puzzling as the overall aetiology of ischaemic enterocolitis in its normal form, and this is discussed in greater depth by Whitehead (1976), who examined the role of the Shwartzman phenomenon in these disorders. More recent evidence for this is provided by Behan and Mills (1982), who demonstrated complement consumption in four patients with pseudomembranous colitis. Nevertheless, the ways in which these final pathogenetic mechanisms are triggered are far from being understood. That an element of mesenteric vasoconstriction is involved is noted by Bailey et al (1986), who in an experimental study on pigs concluded that nonocclusive ischaemic colitis is mediated by a sensitivity of the colonic vasculature to the renin-angiotensin axis. The association of pseudomembranous colitis and ischaemic enterocolitis is also highlighted by the occurrence of both types of lesions with Hirschsprung's disease, either before or immediately following operation. The toxin of *Clostridium difficile*, which is so frequently demonstrated in association with pseudomembranous colitis, has been recovered from patients with neonatal necrotising colitis (Cashore et al 1981) and patients with Hirschsprung's disease complicated by enterocolitis (Thomas et al 1982). The condition of neonatal necrotising enterocolitis also falls into this category of disease and has been studied more intensely than ischaemic enterocolitis in adults. Not only does the disease affect neonates usually in the setting of an intensive care unit but it is described in older infants and children up to 17 years of age (Takayanagi and Kapila 1981, Moss and Adler 1982). Its aetiology is also obscure, and although clostridial organisms have been implicated in its aetiology (Arseculeratne, Panabokke and Navaratnam 1980, Sturm et al 1980) their precise role is unclear. The fact that it occurs in unfed premature infants (Marchildon, Buck and Abdenour 1982) makes it likely that ischaemia, rather than gut flora, is the most important aetiological factor. On the basis of the examination of so-called intestinal atresia when meconium can be found in the distal part of the intestine, showing that it was once patent, and in the absence of evidence for vascular occlusion, it is believed that nonocclusive ischaemia can occur in utero. Vasoconstrictive agents such as Cafergot ingested by a pregnant mother have been cited as a cause of intestinal atresia in a prematurely born infant (Graham, Marin-Padilla and Hoefnagel 1983). The intestine of infants in utero is, of course, sterile, which makes it likely that gut organisms cannot be wholly implicated in this disease and may indeed be only secondary invaders.

PSEUDOMEMBRANOUS COLITIS AND ANTIBIOTIC-ASSOCIATED COLITIS

Two facts are clear: first, pseudomembranous enterocolitis was an entity before the antibiotic era; and second, the condition has become much more common with increasing antibiotic usage. Its occurrence in patients who have not received antibiotics has been noted in association with colonoscopy (Patterson, Johnson and Schmulen 1984), leukaemia (Panachi et al 1985), paraquat poisoning (Imamura et al 1986), and Hirschsprung's disease (Brearly et al 1987). The list of antibiotics associated with pseudomembranous colitis is now extremely long indeed, and it is perhaps salutory that the very antibiotic that is commonly used to treat the condition (i.e., metronidazole) has also been cited as a cause (Thomson et al 1981, Daly and Chowdary 1983). Bingley and Harding (1987) even described a case following combined therapy with metronidazole and vancomycin, which resolved after treatment with vancomycin alone. An important consequence of the connection with antibiotics has been a greater awareness of the fact that pseudomembranous enterocolitis can present in many clinical settings. It may arise spontaneously in the previously healthy or more commonly after major surgery (Prendergast et al 1994), during or after therapy with broad-spectrum antibiotics, as a complication of colonic obstruction, in the haemolytic-uremic syndrome (Francois et al 1994), and in patients with debilitating diseases such as chronic uraemia or leukaemia. The clinical picture varies from a mild diarrhoeal illness to fulminant colitis with fever, dehydration, and shock. The small intestine, the colon, or both may be involved (Tsutaoka et al 1994), and the characteristic plaques seen endoscopically are strongly suggestive of the disease. It is usually a self-limited disease in its mildest form, and nondebilitated patients improve within a few days. Treatment, therefore, should be medical in the first instance and surgery avoided if feasible. When it is not possible to differentiate between pseudomembranous and ulcerative colitis, the fulminating form usually requires surgery. The mortality in all published series is high but mild forms are being increasingly recognised. These are probably part of the spectrum of antibiotic-associated diarrhoeas. The aetiology is unknown, but as already stated this disease also has a relationship with ischaemic enterocolitis, which may represent the other end of the spectrum. It was postulated that a Shwartzman-like reaction may be the basic pathological process and that absorption of a toxin of bacterial origin with or without a change in intestinal flora, with or without a fall in splanchnic perfusion, could be the triggering mechanism (Whitehead 1971, 1976, Lancet 1977). It was of considerable interest, therefore, when Larson and Price (1977) described a faecal toxin that closely resembled that produced by *Clostridium sordellii* in nine patients with pseudomembranous colitis. The toxin was subsequently shown by Bartlett et al (1978) and Larson, Price and Honour (1978) to be produced by *C. difficile*. In fact, a number of different toxins are now known to be produced by *C. difficile*. Toxin A is an enterotoxin; toxin B is a cytotoxin, which is usually assayed in diagnosis; and toxin C is a motility-altering factor (Taylor, Thorne and Bartlett 1981, Justus et al 1982, Mitchell et al 1986). *C. difficile* also produces a factor that inhibits neutrophil migration and phagocytosis (Bolton et al 1985). The exact relationship of colonisation of the bowel by this anaerobe and production of toxins is not entirely clear in relation to the mechanisms of the colitis, however. Lishman, Al-Jumaili and Record (1981) and George, Rolfe and Finegold (1982) have found that some patients remain clinically well despite high concentrations of faecal toxin. Faecal toxin can be demonstrated in a normal population, particularly in infants (George 1984), even in titres as high as in patients with colitis. Some patients with typical pseudomembranous colitis do not have the toxin or *C. difficile* organisms in their faeces (Dickinson, Rampling and Wight 1985). Moreover, sometimes pseudomembranous colitis is described in association with clostridial infection not of the *difficile* subtype (Chiu and Abraham 1982), and pseudomembranous colitis has progressed and proved fatal even when the organism and toxin have successfully been cleared from the bowel (Hawker et al 1981). *C. difficile* has also been implicated in exacerbation of inflammatory bowel disease (British Medical Journal 1981), but this finding was not substantiated in the study by Hyams and McLaughlin (1985), at least in children. It is becoming clear that *C. difficile*-associated colitis is a disorder with a wide clinicopathological spectrum. It can vary from a mild, short-lived disease associated with diarrhoea to a severe illness associated with toxic dilation (Burke, Wilson and Mehrez 1988). It can present as a localised lesion and mimic carcinoma (Arber et al 1987). *C. difficile* can be responsible for endemic disease in institutions (Bender et al 1986) or epidemic disease with spread to several hospitals (Nolan et al 1987). In essence it seems that the presence of *C. difficile* and its toxin merely reflects the extent to which the ecosystem of the intestine is disturbed by a variety of factors, e.g., the effect of antibiotics or intestinal blood flow. The importance of rectal biopsy in the recognition of pseudomembranous colitis is made plain by Tedesco, Corless and Brownstein (1982), who showed that membranes are noted by flexible sigmoidoscopy in 91% of patients. The fully developed dome-shaped plaque lesion is characteristic, but earlier and later phases also need consideration. Price and Davies (1977) described three lesions. This designation is rather artificial because there is a continuum of appearances, but it serves to characterise the histological features. Type 1, the earliest, consists of focal epithelial necrosis of surface epithelium in the interglandular space (Fig. 16–55). The subjacent lamina propria contains an eosinophilic exudate of polymorphs and nuclear debris. Showers of polymorphs and fibrin erupt into the lumen. Type 2 lesions consist of the typical dome-shaped plaque in which a well-defined group of glands are distended by mucin and polymorphs at their bases and are covered by a plaque of fibrin, mucin, cellular debris, and polymorphs (Fig. 16–56). The intervening mucosa between plaques is normal, but in several cases large areas of "membrane" may be present (Fig. 16–57). Type 3 lesions show complete structured necrosis of the mucosa with few surviving glands and a covering of cellular inflammatory debris, mucin, and fibrin (Fig. 16–58). There is also a series of changes seen in the resolving or healing phase. These consist of regenerative changes and reconstitution of the damaged mucosa from residual crypts in the original lesion or from neighbouring healthy mucosa (Figs. 16–59 to 16–62). Residual glandular irregularity may be seen, but complete restitution of the mucosa also occurs. This may well be accounted for by the fact that only the patients with less severe disease survive, death being the rule for patients with more severe disease, especially if associated with another severe systemic disease. However, occasional cases are seen that are characterised by localised recurrent lesions often without significant systemic illness. The mucosa may then show a marked regenerative reaction, with thickening and a gross polypoidal appearance (Figs. 16–63 and 16–64). There are usually accompanying pseudomembranous lesions at the apex of these excrescences, and it is pertinent that significant hyperplastic reactions of a similar nature occur in the experimental hamster model in which the caecum is affected (Price, Larson and Crow 1979).

Text continued on page 352

Figure 16–55. Early lesion (type 1), which consists of necrosis of interglandular superficial epithelium and an exudate of fibrin and polymorphs into the gut lumen (H&E ×300).

Figure 16–56. Later lesion (type 2), with fusion of exudate covering the necrosed upper part of neighbouring glands (H&E ×150).

Figure 16–57. Extensive type 2 lesion with distended mucin-filled gland bases and a covering layer of fibrin, mucin, and cellular debris. This constitutes the typical membrane (trichrome ×70).

Figure 16–58. Type 3 lesion shows complete structured necrosis of the mucosa with a covering of inflammatory debris, mucin, and fibrin (H&E ×25).

Figure 16–59. Early healing changes in a focal lesion. The residual crypt bases show regenerative changes (H&E ×180).

Figure 16–60. Nearly healed focal lesion with residual architectural abnormality (H&E ×180).

Figure 16–61. Edge of severe lesion from which membrane has sloughed (H&E ×180).

Figure 16–62. Healed deep lesion with a single layer of simple regenerated epithelium (H&E ×180).

Figure 16–63. Marked irregular hyperplastic crypts in relation to a persistent lesion in antibiotic-associated colitis (H&E ×250).

Figure 16–64. Irregular hyperplastic regenerative reaction in persistent antibiotic-associated colitis (H&E ×200).

Figure 16–65. Rectal biopsy in antibiotic-associated colitis. Note the distinctive patchy distribution of the inflammation (H&E ×40).

Another and not infrequent appearance is seen in the clinical situation of mild but significant diarrhoea, usually without blood, in patients who have recently received antibiotics. It is characterised by a nonspecific mild inflammation of the rectal mucosa. The inflammation often tends to be patchy even within the lamina propria of a single biopsy sample (Figs. 16–65 and 16–66). The changes tend to involve the superficial epithelium and the upper quarter or half of the crypts. The lamina shows an increase in the number of inflammatory cells, particularly of the acute type, and this increase is associated with some vascular dilation. There are always changes in

Figure 16–66. Detail of Figure 16–65 shows the variation in intensity of the inflammation (H&E ×180).

Figure 16–67. Antibiotic-associated colitis with superficial vascular dilation and polymorph infiltration of rather degenerative superficial epithelium and upper crypts (H&E ×450).

Figure 16–68. Antibiotic-associated colitis with pronounced syncytial appearance of degenerative epithelial cells between crypt mouths (H&E ×450).

the superficial epithelium, which appears flattened, and occasionally desquamated cells are trapped in adherent mucin. A common appearance is the presence of polymorphs in degenerating and damaged surface and upper crypt epithelium, which often forms syncytial knot-like projections between the crypt mouths (Figs. 16–67 and 16–68).

The polymorphs themselves often show degenerative changes but are not usually present in large numbers, so that classic dilated crypt abscesses are not found, although a few polymorphs may appear in the lumen. Pus overlying a normal mucosa is occasionally seen, but this is a completely nonspecific appearance that may be due to focal sepsis elsewhere in the large bowel, in association with diverticular disease or neoplasm. There is evidence based on the finding of *C. difficile* toxin in the stool that these changes are related to or constitute the earliest lesions of pseudomembranous colitis. Their association was reviewed by Gibson, Rowland and Hecker (1975) and Rocca et al (1984).

Figure 17–3. Colonic mucosa in infective colitis. The infiltrate is mixed with a noticeable neutrophil polymorph component and a poorly developed crypt abscess (H&E ×400).

is the shrinkage and beaded appearance of the mucosal gland profiles that sometimes appear to melt away; this is unusual in other forms of colitis (Figs. 17–4 to 17–6). Kumar, Nostrant and Appelman (1982) stressed that the absence of basal lamina propria plasmacytosis is a feature helpful in differentiating the lesion from ulcerative

Figure 17–4. Colonic mucosa in infective colitis (H&E ×250).

Figure 17–5. Detail of Figure 17–4. Note the thin-walled but not excessively enlarged crypts containing neutrophil polymorphs and the shrinkage and beaded appearance of the glands in longitudinal section (H&E ×350).

Figure 17–6. The glands in infective colitis sometimes appear to "melt away" (H&E ×450).

colitis, but Kelly et al (1990) stressed that plasma cell infiltration is often a feature in advanced lesions of *E. coli* 0157 colitis. Some cases of *Shigella* colitis and more characteristically *Campylobacter* colitis and verotoxin-associated *E. coli* colitis have a distinctive haemorrhagic appearance, and bloody diarrhoea characterises the clinical picture (Chowdhury 1984, Van Spreeuwel et al 1985, Kelly et al 1987). The biopsy appearances reflect this in that the lesion is severe with superficial haemorrhagic necrosis of the mucosa, which is superimposed on a diffuse acute colitis. The paucity of crypt abscesses is also a feature (Figs. 17–7 and 17–8).

Despite assertions that, on the whole, infective colitis and ulcerative colitis have different histopathological appearances, individual cases can pose diagnostic problems (Price, Jewkes and Sanderson 1979, McKendrick, Geddes and Gearty 1982). Loss, Mangla and Pereira (1980) described a case of *Campylobacter* colitis presenting as inflammatory bowel disease with segmental colonic ulceration and colonoscopic appearances suggesting Crohn's disease. A similar case with mucosal giant cells was described by Green et al (1984). Kalkay et al (1983) reported the association of *Campylobacter* colitis and toxic megacolon. The enteroinvasive character of *Campylobacter* infection was confirmed by Van Spreeuwel et al (1985), who demonstrated intramucosal organisms by using specific antiserum in an immunohistochemical study. The increasingly common practice of rectal biopsy in the investigation of patients with diarrhoea has resulted in recognition of surprisingly large numbers of cases with these histological features that resolve completely, but only some of which are proved to be due to a recognised pathogen.

The terminology of transient colitis syndrome (Mandal, Schofield and Morson 1982) has been applied to such cases to highlight the clinicopathological entity. Transient colitis equates to what has also been described as acute self-limited colitis (Holdsworth 1984). Surawicz and Belic (1984), in a retrospective blind study of rectal biopsies, claimed seven histological features that are highly discriminative in favour of idiopathic inflammatory bowel disease; when present, they can virtually rule out acute self-limited colitis as a diagnosis. These features are distorted crypt architecture, increase in round cells and neutrophils in the lamina propria, a villous surface, epithelial granulomas, crypt atrophy, basal lymphoid aggregates, and basally situated isolated giant cells. Similar results were found by Allison et al (1987), who also noted, however, a considerable amount of interobserver error. Basically, the diagnosis of acute self-limited colitis depends on the absence of the criteria usual for

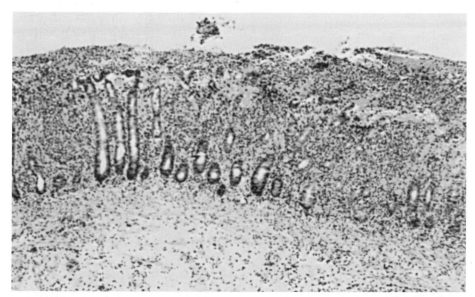

Figure 17–7. Rectal biopsy in *Campylobacter* colitis. It has a distinctive haemorrhagic quality, and the mucosa is superficially necrosed (H&E ×50).

Figure 17–8. Detail of Figure 17–7. The surface exudate is composed largely of blood elements. Note the absence of crypt abscesses (H&E ×250).

ulcerative colitis or Crohn's disease. Although this schema may be helpful in established idiopathic inflammatory bowel disease, it is less useful in first-attack ulcerative colitis and Crohn's disease, especially in ulcerative colitis. Anand et al (1986), for example, showed that in *Shigella* dysentery it is extremely difficult to identify changes recognisably different from inflammatory bowel disease. Nostrant, Kumar and Appelman (1987), in a study similar to but more detailed than that of Surawicz and Belic (1984), found that in first-attack ulcerative colitis the features most helpful in differentiating this from acute self-limited colitis are crypt distortion and plasmacytosis of the lamina propria. Similar findings have been reported in other studies (Schumacher, Kollberg and Sandstedt 1994, Surawicz et al 1994), but as was shown previously, should any doubt remain as to a firm diagnosis, follow-up studies are indicated (*Lancet* 1988, Editorial). Idiopathic inflammatory bowel disease can seemingly be triggered by an infective episode (Dronfield, Fletcher and Langman 1974, Taylor-Robinson et al 1989). *Yersinia enterocolitica* also causes an ileocolitis with a characteristic histopathology in resection specimens (Gleason and Patterson 1982), but there are only occasional reports of the appearance of *Yersinia* colitis in endoscopic biopsies (Vantrappen et al 1977). Basically, these were reported as nonspecific microulcerations. Brown et al (1986), however, described a case originally believed to be antibiotic-associated on the basis of a patchy, mainly superficial, acute colitis. Rarely, *Y. enterocolitica* colitis can cause toxic dilation (Stuart et al 1986).

Tuberculous Colitis

Tuberculosis of the colon is uncommon and likely to be mistaken for Crohn's disease or carcinoma (Knutson and Arosenius 1984) except in certain countries such as India where the disease is generally still prevalent. The primary form is not likely to be diagnosed in biopsy material, and the secondary form usually involves the terminal ileum, appendix, and caecum. Colonoscopies and biopsies have been performed to diagnose ileocaecal disease. Hiatt (1978), Breiter and Hajjar (1981), Medina et al (1990), Bhargava et al (1992), and Shah et al (1992) also described the biopsy diagnosis of the segmental colitic form that radiologically and clinically closely mimics Crohn's disease. In areas where tuberculosis is common, diagnosis of colonic tuberculosis in colonic biopsy is possible when the organisms are demonstrated, but differentiation from Crohn's disease is extremely difficult in their absence and in the absence of caseation (Figs. 17–9 and 17–10). Fujisawa et al (1989) reported three cases in which colonic tuberculosis was due to atypical mycobacteria.

Intestinal Spirochaetosis

Harland and Lee (1967) first described intestinal spirochaetosis as a nontreponemal infestation of the microvilli of rectal mucosal epithelial cells. The organism was categorised as *Brachyspira aalborgi* by Hovind-Hougen et al (1982) but as a treponeme species by others (Cooper et al 1986). The spirochaetes are embedded at right angles to the microvilli, and in ordinary preparations the condition is suspected if a blue haze is recognised at the surface of the epithelial cells (Fig. 17–11). Electron microscopy (Fig. 17–12) shows the spirochaetes measuring 3 µm in length and 0.15 µm in diameter adherent to the epithelium lying parallel to and between the microvilli. There have been other similar observations (Toner, Carr and Wyburn 1971), and it was once generally agreed that the condition was without significance.

Figure 17–9. Colonic biopsy in proven colonic tuberculosis. The differentiation from Crohn's disease in ordinary H&E preparations may not be possible (H&E ×350).

Figure 17–10. Colonic biopsy in proven tuberculosis. There is nothing diagnostic in the absence of caseation about these appearances (H&E ×450).

This has been challenged (Gad et al 1977, Kaplan and Takeuchi 1979, Crucioli and Busuttil 1981, Douglas and Crucioli 1981, Gad 1983), and Rodgers et al (1986) described blunting and destruction of the microvilli seen on electron microscopy. Apparently, an association of heavy infestation and symptoms such as mucus discharge, diarrhoea, and rectal bleeding may occur in the absence of any other pathological problems. The organism has also been reputedly transmitted by homosexual practices (Tompkins, Waugh and Cooke 1981) and is being increasingly reported in patients with acquired immunodeficiency syndrome (AIDS) (Kasbohrer et al 1990, Nathwani et al 1990). Antonakopoulos, Newman and Wilkinson (1982) and Gebbers et al (1987) described cases in which the organism apparently invaded the epithelium. It may be seen in epithelial cells, macrophages, and Schwann's cells, but there was no colitis histologically. Nevertheless, eradication of the organism can

Figure 17–11. Rectal biopsy in intestinal spirochaetosis. The condition is evident as a haematoxophilic border to the surface epithelial cells. Note how it is interrupted by the goblet cells (H&E ×250).

Figure 17–12. Electron micrograph of formalin-fixed tissue showing spirochaetes intimately woven with the surface microvilli. Note their absence in relation to a discharging goblet cell (×66,000).

result in alleviation of concomitant diarrhoea (Cooper et al 1986). It seems that the pathogenicity of the organism is still in doubt; this was reviewed by Lo, Heading and Gilmour (1994). In view of the increasingly reported opportunistic infections in AIDS, which is associated with homosexuals, it is possible that in some circumstances it may prove to be pathogenic. In most instances (Nielsen et al 1983), however, it seems that the elimination of spirochaetes by antibiotic therapy does not affect symptoms, and when they are found in rectal biopsy of patients attending gastroenterology clinics, spirochaetes are of little significance.

VIRAL COLITIS

Although herpesvirus infection is a well-recognised complication, in immunodepressed patients, it usually affects the upper gastrointestinal tract. Boulton, Slater and Hancock (1982), however, described a case of extensive colonic ulceration in a patient with Hodgkin's disease treated with chemotherapy. Occasionally a painful proctitis occurs in otherwise normal people (White, Hanna and Stewart 1984). Colonic ulceration due to cytomegalovirus infection may also occur in renal transplant recipients (Foucar et al 1981) who are immunosuppressed, but it is also occasionally seen when the immune system is ostensibly normal (Bennett, Fine and Hanlon 1985, Buckner and Pomeroy 1993), and cytomegalovirus infection can act as an exacerbating factor in ulcerative colitis (Loftus, Alexander and Carpenter 1994). Berk et al (1985) also drew attention to the possible role of cytomegalovirus infection in the exacerbation of inflammatory bowel disease. In children in particular, rotavirus infection is the most common cause of diarrhoea (Cohen 1991), but the pathological problems revealed by biopsy have not been studied to any great extent.

FUNGAL COLITIS

Histoplasmosis is endemic in many parts of North America, and the clinical features of involvement of the gastrointestinal tract are well documented (Boone and Allison 1969, Smith 1969). Primary infection is probably rare in the gut, and most gastrointestinal lesions result from haematogenous dissemination from the lungs. The pulmonary lesion, however, may be small, asymptomatic, and difficult to identify even at autopsy. Sometimes colonic involvement is the presenting clinical feature (Kinder and Jourdan 1985, Lee et al 1985), and it sometimes mimics Crohn's disease (Alberti-Flor and Granda 1986). Rectal biopsy thus has a role to play in diagnosis in these cases and will show ulceration, inflammation, and characteristic histiocytes in which the intracytoplasmic organisms can be identified. They can be demonstrated best in preparations especially designed to simplify the identification of fungi but are usually obvious in a periodic acid–Schiff (PAS) stain, the capsule of the organism being strongly positive. Kirk, Lough and Warner (1971) used rectal biopsy specimens to study the light and electron microscopic changes that occur in the organism during the course of treatment with amphotericin B. Other fungal infections rarely present as a colitis. Penna (1979) described a case due to *Paracoccidioides brasiliensis* that was confined to the colon and clinically resembled ulcerative colitis. The variable gross features of *Candida* and *Aspergillus* colitis described in an autopsy study by Prescott, Harris and Banerjee (1992) highlights the challenge fungal colitis poses for endoscopists if ante mortem diagnosis is to be achieved. The most characteristic is one that resembles pseudomembranous colitis.

PARASITIC COLITIS

Amoebiasis

In countries where amoebiasis is nonendemic, pathogenic amoebae must be considered as an aetiological agent in all cases of colitis. The histological diagnosis of amoebic colitis in biopsy specimens from ulcerated lesions usually causes little difficulty once the possibility is entertained, but unfortunately it is still far from a rare occurrence for the diagnosis to be made in surgical specimens. Pittman, El-Hashimi and Pittman (1973) described eight cases that were "indistinguishable clinically and sigmoidoscopically from ulcerative or Crohn's colitis." This is further stressed by Pittman and Hennigar (1974), who studied nine cases and commented particularly on the histological similarities to ulcerative and Crohn's colitis in rectal biopsy specimens independent of whether or not amoebae were also seen. Inflammatory pseudopolyposis reverting to normal following specific therapy has also been reported in amoebic colitis (Berkowitz and Bernstein 1975).

The earliest mucosal lesion of amoebic colitis (Fig. 17–13) was described in detail by Prathap and Gilman (1970). Before there is ulceration, the thickness of the mucosa may appear irregular so that the surface outline is wavy. The irregularity is due to focal areas of goblet cell depletion with reversion to a cubical or simple epithelium, and these areas adjoin others showing increased thickness. This latter feature is due to a combination of hyperaemia, oedema, and cellular infiltration. The infiltrate consists of plasma cells, lymphocytes, and a few eosinophils, with polymorphs tending to marginate the capillary endothelium and the basement membrane of the gland tubules. Prathap and Gilman did not see crypt abscesses, but it has been this author's experience to see some polymorphs not only invading the epithelium of glands and surface but also passing into the gland lumen in small numbers so that rather poorly developed crypt abscesses are formed (Fig. 17–14).

When superficial ulceration appears, it tends to occur on the surface between the gland in areas of mucus depletion. A superficial zone of necrosis and an overlying exudate of fibrin, red cells, and mixed inflammatory cells are the first characteristic components. It is in the mucus overlying these zones that amoebae are frequently identified (Figs. 17–15 and 17–16). This can be impressed on the person performing the biopsy so that in early cases overlying mucin is included in the biopsy, and in the laboratory every effort should be made to ensure that any such mucin or mucinous debris is processed and subsequently examined. Deeper ulcers giving rise to the typical flask-shaped lesions (Fig. 17–17) are always characterised by a zone of

Figure 17–13. Amoebic colitis in the preulcerative stage. There is oedema of the lamina propria, dilation of capillaries, and a slight inflammatory infiltrate (H&E ×42).

tissue necrosis at their base that is covered by exudate. The inflammatory exudate by this stage is marked, and the tissue reaction is complicated by secondary infection from faecal organisms. In the submucosa, some of the blood vessels show dilation and others show endothelial swelling, and sometimes there is occlusive thrombosis. At this stage, amoebae are always seen if searched for (Fig. 17–18), particularly in the zone of inflammatory infiltrate, and if found deeper in the tissues, they always appear within a halo of necrosis, sometimes surrounded by an artefactual retraction space.

The amoebae vary in size from 15 to 25 μm and have a single small spherical nucleus, and in ordinary haematoxylin and eosin stained sections, the cytoplasm is faintly granular in appearance and greyish blue. The vegetative forms of *Entamoeba histolytica* are difficult to differentiate from nonpathogenic amoebae in tissue sections and may be present coincidentally in other ulcerative bowel disorders. Important features in the diagnosis of amoebic colitis are engulfed red cells within the cytoplasm of the organisms and organisms within the tissues, where they may rarely be seen within lymphatics or small vessels. They are more easily detected in iron

Figure 17–14. Detail of Figure 17–13 to show goblet cell depletion, degenerating crypt invaded by inflammatory cells *(arrowhead)*, and poorly developed crypt abscess *(arrow)* (H&E ×105).

Figure 17–15. Amoebic colitis at an early stage of ulceration with surface exudate (H&E ×90).

Figure 17–16. Detail of Figure 17–15 with typical vegetative amoebae in the surface exudate (H&E ×500).

Figure 17–17. Amoebic colitis. Edge of flask-shaped ulcer. Vegetative amoebae visible as dark rounded bodies (PAS ×105).

Figure 17–18. Detail of Figure 17–17: vegetative amoebae within the tissues. Note the small single round nucleus and vacuolated cytoplasm (H&E ×280).

haematoxylin and PAS preparations, the latter being widely advocated as the method of choice. However, macrophages that may have phagocytosed mucin are also positive, and because they are frequently found in ulcerative conditions, they can cause some difficulty, especially because they may also contain engulfed red cells. The microscopist is helped in differentiating them from amoebae by their smaller size, a nucleus that is oval or indented with a peripheral condensation of chromatin, and a nucleus that is relatively larger in relation to the overall size of the cell than is the case with a vegetative amoeba. Other PAS-positive cells, such as mast cells, the histiocytes of melanosis coli, cause no diagnostic difficulty. A personal preference for a method that facilitates the easiest recognition of amoebae in tissues is Goldner's modification of Masson's trichrome. However, claims for easier detection by more specific methods such as the indirect immunofluorescent technique described by Parelkar, Stamm and Hill (1971) have been made; in a comparison of six staining methods, including both direct and indirect fluorescent antibody procedures, Gilman et al (1980) showed that ethanol-fixed tissue stained by a fluorescent antibody or by PAS gave the best results.

It is only when amoebae are recognised with certainty in the biopsy specimen that a definite histological diagnosis can be made, but the additional morphological features already outlined are sufficiently characteristic to warrant suspicion of amoebiasis, even if the organisms are not seen. If, therefore, amoebiasis is suspected clinically or on biopsy appearances, a thorough stool examination for both vegetative and encysted organisms should follow; this sometimes proves positive in biopsy-negative cases. Only vegetative forms containing phagocytosed erythrocytes indicate active disease as opposed to a carrier state. Information from stool examination, biopsy, and serological tests (Sodeman and Dowda 1973) enables a diagnosis to be made in virtually all cases, even when amoebiasis is complicating inflammatory bowel disease (Blumencranz et al 1983). The importance of early diagnosis and treatment cannot be overstressed; not only is the likelihood of a liver abscess lessened, but a particularly lethal complication is averted. It is not widely enough appreciated that amoebic colitis is a cause of fulminant toxic dilation and bowel perforation (Kapur and Chopra 1978, Vajrabukka et al 1979, Wig, Talwar and Bushnurmath 1981, Hansen and Louw 1993, Chun, Chandrasoma and Kiyabu 1994). Furthermore, amoebic colitis can seemingly precede the onset of otherwise typical idiopathic ulcerative colitis (Rampton, Salmon and Clark 1983). Sometimes amoebiasis takes on a protracted local form characterised by marked fibrosis and secondary infection. It is usually localised and commonly affects the caecum or rectum (Ruiz-Moreno 1963). The lesion is often referred to as an amoebic granuloma or amoeboma and clinically behaves more like a mass lesion or neoplasm.

Balantidiasis

Balantidium coli is a ciliate and an intestinal commensal of the pig, monkey, and rat that may infest humans when the encysted form is ingested. In a small number of people harbouring the organism, it gives rise to severe diarrhoea, haemorrhage, and sometimes perforation. The common site of involvement is the right half of the colon and caecum, but the rectum and sigmoid are also frequently involved. Histological features are ulceration with coagulative necrosis of ulcer base and margin. Adjacent tissues are oedematous and infiltrated by a mainly chronic inflammatory infiltrate. The characteristic vegetative parasites are oval (Fig. 17–19), 50–100 μm long, and 40–70 μm wide, with a large kidney-shaped macronucleus and a smaller round micronucleus situated at the hilum. The surface is covered with cilia, and the cytoplasm usually contains vacuoles and granules. They are easily identified because of their size, and although they may be seen within venules and lymph nodes, liver involvement does not occur. The largest series described is probably that reported by Arean and Koppisch (1956), who described the pathological condition in detail. Although most descriptions of the organism are in surgical or autopsy tissue (Pin-

Figure 17–19. *Balantidium coli.* Peripheral cilia can be discerned (H&E ×420).

heiro and de Lima 1991), the organism's characteristic morphology lends itself to diagnosis in biopsy material. This is illustrated in the report of two cases by Castro, Vazquez-Iglesias and Arnal-Monreal (1983) (Figs. 17–20 to 17–22). Other single cases have been diagnosed during life (Currie 1990), but unfortunately they frequently prove to be fatal.

Schistosomiasis

In the intestinal form of the disease, *Schistosoma mansoni* and *Schistosoma japonicum* are responsible, and only heavy infestation produces the classic picture.

Figure 17–20. Balantidia organisms in a biopsy from the necrotic base of a colonic ulcer (H&E ×250). (Courtesy of Dr. Francisco Arnal.)

Figure 17–21. Electron micrograph of *Balantidium coli* showing engulfed colonic bacteria (×1600). (Courtesy of Dr. Francisco Arnal.)

Figure 17–22. Detail of cell membrane with cilia arising from the grooved outer surface (×6,000). (Courtesy of Dr. Francisco Arnal.)

The distal part of the intestine, colon, and rectum are the sites of severest involvement. The earliest tissue reaction (Fig. 17–23) around the newly laid eggs consists of plasma cells, lymphocytes, and eosinophils, but later the characteristic inflammatory response involves histiocytes. Most ova produce a histiocytic granulomatous reaction (Fig. 17–24) that subsequently undergoes a concentric fibrosis. Outside the histiocytic granuloma, which may also form giant cells, the zone of mixed inflammatory cells occurs; later this has a conspicuous eosinophil component. Sometimes, especially in the Asian form of the disease, the eosinophil reaction is very pronounced and may delay the histiocytic response. Frequently in this form of reaction, a zone of fibrinoid material is also deposited about the eggs. As the tissue reactions are developing, the shell dissolves slowly or becomes calcified, and the embryo dies. The eggs of *S. mansoni* are oval and about 150 μm long and 50 μm wide, and they have a well-developed lateral spine. The eggs of *S. japonicum* are smaller and less oval, about 85 μm long and 60 μm wide, with a subterminal hooklet, but this is often inconspicuous. Cases occasionally present as a necrotising or pseudomembranous colitis requiring emergency colectomy (Neves et al 1993).

Figure 17–23. Schistosomiasis. *A*, Newly laid eggs in submucosa (H&E ×64). *B*, The earliest signs of tissue reaction to them (H&E ×375).

Figure 17–24. Schistosomiasis. Typical granulomatous reaction to eggs that are dead and calcified (H&E ×35).

In the later stages of the disease, the granulomatous inflammatory fibrosis results in cicatrisation of the bowel wall that is reflected in the biopsy tissues. Inflammatory pseudopolyps also occur, especially in *S. mansoni* infestations. Epithelial and glandular deformity, due to mucosal ulceration and subsequent healing, may also be seen. Gambescia et al (1976) reviewed the colonic manifestations in schistosomiasis in greater detail. According to Nebel et al (1974), there is no hard evidence for an association between schistosomal polyposis and carcinoma of the colon. However, Ming-Chai et al (1965) described 90 cases of large intestinal adenocarcinoma as a complication of schistosomiasis caused by *S. japonicum*. From the description of the lesions, the pathogenesis may well be similar to that responsible for the malignancy occurring in ulcerative colitis in that it arises through a process of progressive dysplasia.

Other helminthic infestation is rarely a cause of mucosal pathology in the colon and rectum. Leoutsakos, Agnadi and Kolisiatis (1977) described a case and reviewed the literature of colonic involvement in infestation with *Oesophagostomum brumpti*. The veins of the submucosa may contain adult worms, and mucosa and deeper tissues reveal an inflammatory and giant cell granulomatous reaction that would be revealed by rectal biopsy. No reports of a diagnosis being reached in biopsy tissues, however, are currently available. The same is true of the occasional case of strongyloidiasis hyperinfection that causes a chronic colitis (Berry et al 1983). The subject of *Cryptosporidium* colitis in patients with AIDS is referred to in detail in Chapter 19. The question of whether cryptosporidiosis is a cause of chronic diarrhoea in normal children or adults, especially in undeveloped countries, is disputed. Some believe it is an important pathogen accounting for a significant proportion of cases of infective diarrhoea (Sallon et al 1988), whereas others find no firm evidence for this either in developed (Biggs et al 1987, Marshall et al 1987) or undeveloped countries (Mathan et al 1985). It seems highly probable that, in common with many other opportunistic infective agents, on occasion it can cause a colitis even in normal people.

IRRADIATION COLITIS

Irradiation-induced lesions of the intestine are becoming less and less frequently encountered as the techniques of radiotherapy become increasingly sophisticated.

The mucosa of the gastrointestinal tract has a susceptibility to irradiation injury comparable to that of lymphoid tissue and the bone marrow. The colon is less susceptible than the stomach and much less so than the small intestine, but it is the one area of the entire gastrointestinal tract that has been most frequently exposed. This is because of the widespread use of radiotherapy in the treatment of malignant disease of the female genital tract.

The early changes are now rarely seen; they come on within a few hours of exposure. There is prompt cessation of mitotic activity, and there may be an initial stage of hypersecretion of mucin, but soon the epithelial cells begin to show signs of degeneration, become swollen with bizarre irregular nuclei, and slough into the lumen with the formation of thin-walled crypt abscesses due to a secondary sparse acute inflammatory response (Figs. 17–25 and 17–26). There are oedema and hyperaemia of the mucosa and submucosa, and in more severe exposure there are hyaline degeneration and necrosis of the collagen. In severe cases, ulcers may form, but gradually the normal crypt-regenerative capacity is regained, and after an interval of weeks or months recovery occurs. Its completeness depends on the initial injury, but a residuum of distortion or irregularity of the gland pattern is usual (Figs. 17–27 and 17–28). Residual hyaline fibrosis of the mucosa and submucosa and hyaline thickening of blood vessels also persist.

Chronic irradiation injuries characterised macroscopically by ulceration and fibrosis may occur from 6 months to several years after the original exposure. The ulcer bed, like radiation ulcers elsewhere, is formed of poorly vascularised connective tissue that has a peculiar hyalinised appearance. Depending on the depth of ulceration, it involves the mucosa, submucosa muscularis, and even the serosa, so that stricture—either actual or functional—results. There is a superimposed nonspecific

Figure 17–25. Earliest stage of irradiation damage to the colonic mucosa. There is swelling and atypia of epithelial cell nuclei and early cytoplasmic degeneration and sloughing, but a mitotic figure is evident *(arrow)* (H&E ×500).

Figure 17–26. Early stage of irradiation injury of the colon. There is degeneration of some crypts that contain degenerate epithelial cells and a few polymorphs. Note the bizarre nuclear profiles and paucity of mitoses (H&E ×350).

Figure 17–27. Rectal biopsy for bleeding 1 year after irradiation to carcinoma of the cervix. The mucosa shows some architectural distortion, and there is a hyalinisation of the lamina propria. There is a central defect in the epithelium (H&E ×80).

Figure 17–28. Detail of Figure 17–27. Polymorphs are included in the cellular infiltrate, but the principal feature is ectatic change in the superficial capillaries. The epithelium of the tubules shows variation in nuclear size and staining (H&E ×450).

inflammatory infiltrate, and the ulcers tend not to heal. A characteristic of the granulation tissue is the bizarre nature of the fibroblast nuclei, which are large and often appear foamy with marginal polypoidal excrescences. New thin-walled and ectatic blood vessels are a feature, but the arterioles and small arteries also exhibit thickening and hyalinisation of their walls and a decrease in lumen size. Fibrin thrombi and fibrinoid necrosis of the walls of vessels are also seen; some believe they are the main cause of the more chronic pathological changes (Hasleton, Carr and Schofield 1985, Haboubi, Schofield and Rowland 1988) and could account for the progressive nature of the disease (Galland and Spencer 1985, Yeoh and Horowitz 1987). Changes such as those described in the connective tissue and blood vessels of the submucosa may occur in areas where the mucosa is intact, but it usually shows some residual deformity of pattern.

The pathology of irradiation damage to the intestine was detailed in great depth by Friedman (1942) and Berthrong and Fajardo (1981). The latter authors also described an unusual late hyperplastic response of the mucosa together with an appearance simulating colitis cystica profunda. Irradiation colitis rarely has a granulomatous component characterised by noncaseating histiocytic collections, mainly within the bowel lymphoid tissues (Mangham et al 1992). There is some evidence that irradiation-induced colonic mucosal damage may predispose to the development of adenocarcinoma (Castro, Rosen and Quan 1973). Shamsuddin and Elias (1981) described the appearance of dysplasia and carcinoma in situ in rectal biopsy tissue of flat nonpolypoidal mucosa similar to that seen in ulcerative colitis. This observation requires confirmation.

COLLAGENOUS COLITIS

Lindstrom (1976) described the first case of this condition in a patient with chronic watery diarrhoea and a thick collagenous deposit under the surface epithelium of the colorectal mucosa. It was proposed that the collagen layer prevented normal reabsorption of water and electrolytes, thus giving rise to the symptoms. A diagnosis of collagenous colitis can be made when the collagen layer measures more than 15 μm and it may reach as much as 60–70 μm. When this is seen in association with an increase in mixed inflammatory cell infiltration of the lamina propria and minor degenerative changes and flattening of the superficial epithelium, there can be no doubt that it is a distinct histological entity (Figs. 17–29 to 17–32). Occasionally, Paneth's cell metaplasia is seen in the base of the colonic tubules. Flejou et al (1984) noted an increase in lamina propria mast cells in their cases, but this was a subjective observation. In some cases intraepithelial lymphocytes are conspicuous. The collagen table is abnormally thick, and it contains an increased number of fibroblasts that are sometimes plump and active and sometimes rather more spindle-shaped. It is possible that the activity of the fibroblasts and collagen production is phasic, which would account for the clinical picture of variation in the severity of symptoms (Palmer et al 1986). Electron microscope observations (Figs. 17–33 to

Figure 17–29. Collagenous colitis. *A*, The subepithelial collagen has a hyalinised appearance (trichrome ×250). *B*, Fibroblast nuclei are thin and elongated. Note the density of inflammatory cells and the degenerative changes in the intercryptal superficial epithelial cells (trichrome ×500).

Figure 17–30. Collagenous colitis. *A,* Thick collagen zone contains numerous plump fibroblasts as well as inflammatory cells and nuclear debris detailed in *B* (*A,* H&E ×250; *B,* H&E ×500).

Figure 17–31. Collagenous colitis. In this case the inflammatory infiltration of tubules and epithelium is more marked, and there are more severe degenerative changes of both crypt and surface epithelium (H&E ×500).

Figure 17–32. Collagenous colitis with a more pronounced neutrophil polymorph component in the lamina propria and in the collagen layer (H&E ×400).

Figure 17–33. Electron micrograph of collagenous colitis. Under the surface epithelium, which depicts two endocrine cells, the basal lamina *(arrows)* is normal. The subepithelial zone is occupied by typical collagen surrounding portions of neutrophils, plasma cells, and a central active fibroblast (×6,637).

Figure 17–34. Electron micrograph of collagenous colitis. Typical collagen surrounds a capillary that is occluded by a platelet thrombus and is indicative of an inflammatory reaction (×6,637).

17–35) have confirmed that basal lamina of the epithelium is in fact normal and the lesion is indeed due to a collagen deposition under the epithelium. The collagen consists of a mixture of types I and III. The author's experience of more than 30 cases and observations on stepwise colonoscopic biopsies of the whole colon have revealed, in addition to the features described in other reports (Bogomoletz et al 1980, Nielsen, Vetner and Harslof 1980, Bamford et al 1982, Galian et al 1982, Grouls, Vogel and Sorger 1982, Pieterse, Hecker and Rowland 1982, Teglbjaerg and Thaysen 1982, Farah et al 1985, Foerster and Fausa 1985, Coverlizza et al 1986, Danzi et al 1988, Tanaka, Mazzoleni and Riddell 1992), that the lesion was not uniform throughout the colon. It was more marked in some areas than in others, the rectum being often less severely affected, and in places collagen occupies a position deeper in the lamina propria (Fig. 17–36). The variability in the collagen band with respect to site was confirmed in a study of 17 patients by Wang et al (1987). A further observation corroborated by Teglbjaerg, Thaysen and Jensen (1984) and Kingham et al (1986) is the development of the collagen band in sequential biopsies being preceded by an inflammatory phase (see the following section on microscopic colitis). The uneven distribution of collagen in some cases could cause problems in the interpretation of reversibility of the lesion in sequential biopsies. Evidence for this was claimed by Bamford et al (1982), Pieterse, Hecker and Rowland (1982), Eaves et al (1983), Debongnie et al (1984), Morgensen, Olsen and Gudmand-Hoyer (1984), and Fausa, Foerster and Hovig (1985). Most authors, however, believe the condition to be progressive and permanent (Kingham et al 1986), although symptoms may be relieved by oral sulfasalazine therapy (Brady and McKee 1993). The collagen layer may be responsible for interference with function of the surface cells and thus impede absorption. However, there is evidence that the diarrhoea is mediated by prostaglandins and is secretory in nature (Rask-Madsen et al 1983, Giardiello et al 1987). The normal colonic crypt of Lieberkuhn is surrounded by a mesenchymal sheath that is a specialised part of the lamina propria.

Figure 17–35. Collagenous colitis. A higher magnification of the dense collagen zone that in this field surrounds a capillary ($\times 15,525$).

Figure 17–36. Collagenous colitis. In this biopsy the collagen layer occurs in the midzone of the lamina propria, but this is unusual (H&E ×400).

It consists of fibroblasts applied to the epithelium and collagen fibres oriented circumferentially to the crypt. Pascal, Kaye and Lane (1968) demonstrated a steady-state renewal of the pericryptal fibroblasts and migration to the upper parts of the crypt in synchronisation with the epithelial migration. The fibroblast stem cells, like the epithelial cells, occupy the lower third of the crypt. The collagen table immediately under the surface epithelium is relatively thicker than elsewhere, and overall the evidence suggests a functional maturation of the pericryptal fibroblast layer as it ascends the crypt. The pericryptal fibroblasts and the epithelium thus act as a unit that maintains the structure and presumably also the function of the crypt. Minor changes in the kinetics involved might easily result in a thicker than normal collagen plate, and we have seen that this can occur in the small intestine in gluten-sensitive enteropathy. Why it should occur in either condition is not clear. It does not seem to be a result of longstanding inflammation, because it does not seem to occur in this site in chronic ulcerative colitis. However, Balazs et al (1988) did find similarities between collagenous and ulcerative colitis, and in both they described an enhanced fibre-forming activity and proliferation of myofibroblasts. In other large series (Steadman et al 1987, Jessurun et al 1987), it has become apparent that this condition is much more common in middle-aged to elderly females and has a predilection to occur in association with thyroid and rheumatoid joint disease and autoimmune disease of other types (Kingsmore et al 1993). Thus, it has been postulated that collagenous colitis itself may be an autoimmune disease. It has been reported (probably coincidentally) in association with colonic adenocarcinoma (Gardiner et al 1984) and Crohn's disease (Chandratre et al 1987). Collagenous colitis has also been reported in association with crypt hyperplastic villous atrophy in two patients, one of whom responded by a return to normal on a gluten-free diet (Hamilton et al 1986); an increasing number of patients with collagenous colitis and coeliac disease have been described (Armes et al 1992, Perisic, Kokai and Pavlovic 1992, Angos et al 1993). These cases appear to be different from that described by Eckstein, Dowsett and Riley (1988), in which in addition to partial villous atrophy the small bowel also showed a thick subepithelial collagen band, which was thought not to be gluten-related. Cases of collagenous colitis with coincidental involvement of the stomach and duodenum (Stolte et al 1990) and terminal ileum (Lewis, Warren and Goff 1991) have been reported. There have also been claims that the use of nonsteroidal anti-inflammatory drugs (NSAIDs) may play a role in aetiology (Giardiello et al 1990, Riddell, Tanaka and Mazzoleni 1992).

MICROSCOPIC COLITIS

Read et al (1980) reported minor histological changes in the colonic biopsies of 8 of 27 patients investigated for intractable watery diarrhoea. The full significance of this was not apparent at that time, but Kingham et al (1982) coined the term microscopic colitis for the same condition that is characterised by a mild total colitis, large-volume watery diarrhoea, and normal endoscopic and radiological appearances. Four of their six patients were female and all were middle-aged. The condition was thought to be quite distinct from ulcerative colitis and Crohn's disease and in particular distinct from the so-called minimal change colitis described by Elliott et al (1982), in which normal sigmoidoscopy and barium enema is associated with histological evidence of overt Crohn's disease in the proximal large bowel or less commonly proves to be due to ulcerative colitis. Bo-Linn et al (1985) put the existence of microscopic colitis on a firmer basis; later the same group (Jessurun et al 1986) examined the evidence that microscopic colitis is the forerunner of collagenous colitis. Microscopic colitis affects the entire colon. It is, however, always characterised by a diffuse increase in lymphocytes and plasma cells in the lamina propria (Fig. 17–37). Eosinophils are usually prominent, and neutrophils vary in number and are commonly seen invading the epithelium of tubules, usually in their upper parts. The surface epithelium tends to be flatter than normal and shows degenerative changes accompanied by an increase in apoptotic bodies. There may also be an impressive increase in intraepithelial lymphocytes throughout the tubules, but this tends to occur later in the disease process (Figs. 17–38 and 17–39). There is no architectural deformity or gross glandular inflammatory destruction such as is seen in ulcerative colitis, Crohn's disease, or the various forms of infective or ischaemic colitis. In some cases, a thin collagen band develops under the epithelium (Fig. 17–40), and there is a tendency for the inflammatory infiltrate to decrease in density, although an increased plasma cell and lymphocyte infiltrate persists. The picture is

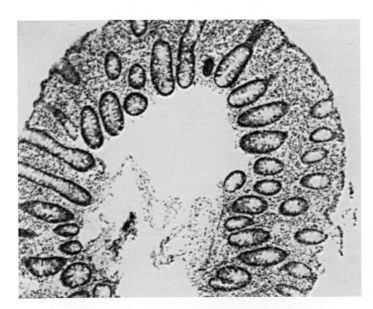

Figure 17–37. Microscopic colitis. A generalised increase in inflammatory cells of the lamina propria is obvious. Note the preservation of the overall mucosal architecture (H&E ×75).

Figure 17–38. Microscopic colitis. In this case the infiltrate has a very prominent neutrophil polymorph infiltrate (H&E ×450).

Figure 17–39. Microscopic colitis. In this case intraepithelial lymphocytes are unusually prominent (H&E ×450).

Figure 17–40. Microscopic colitis. A case in which a thin collagen band is present under the surface epithelium (H&E ×450).

thus arguably identical to some cases of collagenous colitis. Lazenby et al (1989), however, believed that despite the striking similarities between microscopic colitis and collagenous colitis, each has distinctive biopsy appearances. These authors were particularly struck with the intraepithelial lymphocyte component in microscopic colitis and proposed that it be referred to as ''lymphocytic colitis.'' The advantages of this designation at a time when the relationship between microscopic colitis and collagenous colitis is far from clear are doubtful. As in coeliac disease and other lesions of the mucosa in other parts of the gastrointestinal tract, the intraepithelial lymphocytes are probably no more than a manifestation of an underlying pathogenetic mechanism. Nevertheless, there are others, such as Lee et al (1992), who believe there are substantial differences between lymphocytic colitis and collagenous colitis, although increasingly in published reports of both, clinical similarities between the two are stressed (Gebbers and Laissue 1994, Maxson, Klein and Rubin 1994, Zeroogian and Chopra 1994). Lymphocytic colitis has been linked with use of the drug Cyclo 3 Forte (Beaugerie et al 1994); Christ et al (1993) described lymphocytic colitis progressing to collagenous colitis in a patient who also had lymphocytic gastritis. Understanding of these diseases is still evolving.

The cause of microscopic/collagenous colitis is not known, but it is of interest that a similar collagenisation is also seen under the bronchial epithelium in asthma. Contrary to what has long been held, as in collagenous colitis, there is no abnormal thickening of the basement membrane (Roche et al 1989). One might thus postulate that the disease has an allergic basis that would be in keeping with the prominent eosinophil component seen in the lamina propria. Rampton and Baithun (1987) described a case of microscopic colitis that responded to cholestyramine therapy and postulated that at least some of these cases were due to bile salt malabsorption.

COLITIS DUE TO FAECAL DIVERSION

Glotzer, Glick and Goldman (1981) drew attention to the mild focal epithelial degenerative changes and acute and chronic inflammatory infiltration including crypt abscesses that may follow diversion of the faecal stream by ileostomy or colostomy. The condition disappears when continuity is restored and is normally important only because it may be misinterpreted. On occasions, however, it can be severe enough to cause symptoms such as rectal bleeding (Bosshardt and Abel 1984, Ona and Boger 1985) when the inflammation is more severe and associated with ulceration. The ulceration may be aphthoid and mimic Crohn's disease (Lusk, Reichen and Levine 1984, Geraghty and Charles 1994, Whelan et al 1994), which of course has significant implications when diversion of the faecal stream is performed in patients with this disease (Korelitz et al 1984). Diversion colitis is easily mistaken for further manifestations of Crohn's disease in these circumstances. Thorough evaluation of the bypassed colonic mucosa is thus essential. Murray et al (1987) and Warren and Shepherd (1992) described inflammation and erosions, occasional crypt abscesses, and mucin granulomas, and they highlighted the presence of lymphoid hyperplasia in this condition. Paneth's cell metaplasia is described by several observers (Haque, Eisen and West 1993). It has been proposed that faeces contain an essential trophic factor in the form of short-chain fatty acids produced by the anaerobic faecal flora (Korelitz et al 1984, *Lancet* 1989, Editorial). Thus, it is of interest that Harig et al (1989) showed that local administration of these fatty acids to the diverted segment caused the inflammation to disappear. Diversion colitis does not appear to constitute a risk of significant complications following colostomy closure (Orsay et al 1993). Diversion colitis has also been described in neovaginas constructed from sigmoid colon (Toolenaar et al 1993).

COLITIS IN DIVERTICULAR DISEASE

Mucosal biopsy is usually unrewarding in the diagnosis of diverticular disease even if diverticulitis is present, although occasionally a pattern seen is normal mucosa with lumenal pus cells. Cawthorn, Gibbs and Marks (1983) described a segmental inflammation with histological features similar to the changes in solitary rectal ulcer in three patients with diverticular disease. This was probably due to recurrent prolapse of the mucosa lying between diverticula as a result of the abnormal colonic muscular dynamics. The changes of prolapse with marked fibromuscularisation of the lamina propria and architectural gland modification can be extreme. Some of the pathological conditions seen in these circumstances are shared by the condition known as cap polyposis (Campbell et al 1993), in which mucosal prolapse is thought to play a role. It seems, however, that the more usual form of segmental colitis seen in association with diverticular disease is nonspecific, and it is less usual to see fibromuscular obliteration of the lamina propria. Generally, biopsies show moderate patchy acute and chronic inflammation with occasional crypt abscesses and some goblet cell depletion (Sladen and Filipe 1984) (Figs. 17–41 to 17–44).

COLITIS IN INFANTS

Gastrointestinal intolerance to cow's milk protein and soy protein is a well-established cause of enterocolitis in infants younger than the age of 2 or 3 years (Gryboski 1967). In that classic study, sigmoidoscopic evidence of colitis disappeared when cow's milk was removed from the diet. There is more recent evidence for small bowel injury, and the syndrome should properly be regarded as an enterocolitis. Lake, Whitington and Hamilton (1982) described an acute and chronic inflammation with an associated eosinophil infiltration in rectal biopies from babies who developed rectal bleeding in the first month of life. A change from breast milk to soy protein or hydrolysed casein–based milk formula resulted in immediate remission. The problem of proctocolitis in babies and its relationship to milk or other protein intolerance was discussed in an article (*Lancet* 1983, Anonymous), and since that time it has become plain that food allergy is a major cause of infantile colitis

Figure 17–41. Colitis in diverticular disease. An uneven inflammation is associated with considerable architectural distortion of the glands and fibromuscularisation of the lamina propria (H&E ×150).

Figure 17–42. Colitis in diverticular disease has a patchy acute element (H&E ×450).

Figure 17–43. Colitis in diverticular disease. There is fibromuscularisation of the lamina propria as well as architectural distortion (H&E ×450).

(Winter et al 1990, Odze et al 1993, Machida et al 1994, Odze et al 1995). Not only do colonic biopsies show a distinctive eosinophil infiltration and surface erosion, but there are numerous plasma cells containing immunoglobulin E (IgE) in the lamina propria. Other allergic phenomena, increased serum IgE, and blood eosinophilia are also commonly present (Jenkins et al 1984, Goldman and Proujansky 1986, Powell 1986). Clearly, proctocolitis and bloody stools in infants have many causes, and many can be excluded by colonic biopsy. Protein-induced colitis can be suspected by the colonoscopic aphthoid ulceration and biopsy appearances and then confirmed by manipulation of the diet. Food allergy seems to be the most common cause of colitis in this age group (Berezin et al 1989). It is rarely also associated with cholangitis (Schoonbroodt et al 1995).

NEUTROPENIC COLITIS

Neutropenic colitis describes a distinctive caecal or right-sided colonic necrosis due to clostridial infection in association with agranulocytosis. It is also sometimes referred to as the ileocaecal syndrome and typhlitis when only the caecum is involved. It is usually encountered in patients with acute leukaemia, lymphoma, or myeloma but also in association with neutropenia due to aplastic anaemia (Mulholland and Delaney 1983). The diagnosis was seldom made prior to death, and no case, even in the largest series yet reported, has been diagnosed on biopsy (Mower, Hawkins and Nelson 1986). However, with newer imaging techniques and ultrasonography, there has been improved ante mortem diagnosis and treatment (Sloas et al 1993). Although *Clostridium septicum* is the usual organism implicated, other clostridial species are sometimes involved (*Lancet* 1987, Editorial).

Figure 17–44. Colitis in diverticular disease. Note the fibromuscularisation, patchy colitis, and crypt abscess (H&E ×300).

COLITIS DUE TO DRUGS OR CHEMICAL AGENTS

It is estimated that some 10% of newly diagnosed colitis may be due to ingestion of drugs. Rectal biopsies in such patients may show mild nonspecific colitis with a neutrophil polymorph component in the inflammatory infiltrate, and there may be occasional crypt abscesses, but ulceration is unusual. The appearances are similar to an infectious colitis and have been associated with the use of alpha-methyldopa (Bonkowsky and Brisbane 1976) and the vitamin A analogue isotretinoin (Martin et al 1987). The glandular pattern is usually preserved.

A colitis similar to Crohn's disease is described in patients taking oral contraceptives (Rhodes et al 1984), and a proctitis similar to ulcerative colitis has been attributed to salicylates (Pearson et al 1983). Colitis described in association with penicillin and its derivatives usually exhibits ischaemic features (Toffler, Pingoud and Burrell 1978). Innes et al (1988) reported the onset of a total severe colitis in a patient receiving cyclosporine, and toxic megacolon with severe segmental colitis was attributed to methotrexate therapy by Atherton, Leib and Kaye (1984). Drug-induced colitis has also been attributed to the therapeutic use of methyldopa (Graham, Gallagher and Jones 1981) and gold (Martin et al 1981, Wong et al 1993). In the author's experience with the latter in patients treated for rheumatoid arthritis, the colitis is mild, nonulcerative, and histologically nonspecific, except that eosinophilia of the lamina propria and submucosa is often a prominent feature (Figs. 17–45 and 17–46).

The colonic lesions produced by the use of NSAIDs (Kaufmann and Taubin 1987, Tanner and Raghunath 1988) appear to be varied. They can take the form of

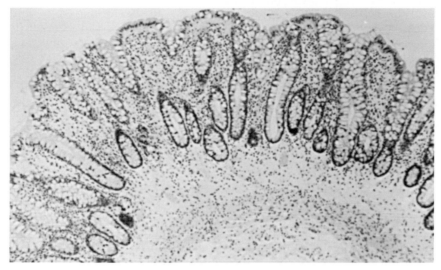

Figure 17–45. Colitis due to gold therapy for rheumatoid arthritis. The infiltrate is slight but definite and tends to involve the submucosa (H&E ×120).

Figure 17–46. Detail of the colitis in Figure 17–45. The infiltrate is rich in eosinophils, which often appear as bilobed polymorphonuclear cells (H&E ×500).

an acute colitis characterised by lymphocyte and neutrophil infiltrates in the lamina propria and within the epithelium (Hall et al 1983, Lee 1993). The relationship between lymphocytic and collagenous colitis has already been referred to, and there is evidence that the use of NSAIDs might be aetiologically involved (Riddell, Tanaka and Mazzoleni 1992). One of the more characteristic features of the colitis associated with the use of NSAIDs, although not in any way specific, is the presence of cryptal apoptotic bodies (Lee 1993 and 1994), which are also a feature of the colonic effects of 5-fluorouracil (Floch and Hellman 1965) and cyclosporine (Murphy et al 1993). Colitis varying from mild to severe with gangrenous change has been associated with the use of various enemas, e.g., soap (Orchard and Lawson 1986), phosphate (Sweeney et al 1986), and sorbitol (Lillemoe et al 1987), and has followed the inadvertent instillation of alcohol (Herrerias et al 1983) or cleaning solutions used for disinfective endoscopy (Jonas et al 1988). The colitis induced by glutaraldehyde contamination of endoscopes can be severe and closely mimic ischaemic colitis in its pathological features (Birnbaum, Gordon and Jacobs 1995, West et al 1995). It should always be suspected when a haemorrhagic acute colitis follows within 24 hours of a normal endoscopy. Strangely, sulfasalazine, the drug used in the treatment of inflammatory bowel disease, has been incriminated as a cause of precipitating attacks of ulcerative colitis (Ruppin and Domschke 1984). Fishel et al (1985) reported an unusual case of colitis associated with the use of cocaine. It had the pathological features of pseudomembranous colitis and was probably of ischaemic origin. An unusual and rare form of distal colitis was reported by Keefe and Girard (1985) in a patient thought to have a self-inflicted abrasive colonic injury secondary to daily consumption of quantities of peanuts while still in their indigestible shells.

COLITIS OF BEHÇET'S SYNDROME

This colitis is characterised by ulceration of the bowel wall, which may mimic Crohn's disease macroscopically very closely (Masugi et al 1994). Usually, the ulcers are more regular in outline and the surrounding mucosa is normal (Jung et al 1991). Proctitis mimicking ulcerative colitis is also described (Hamza 1993). The underlying pathological condition probably has an ischaemic basis, and a vasculitis is implicated. This takes the form in the bowel of a lymphoid venulitis or arteritis, occasionally with thrombosis (Figs. 17–47 to 17–49) (Katoh et al 1985, Lee 1986).

Figure 17–47. Biopsy of ulcer edge in Behçet's disease. The neighbouring mucosa is only slightly abnormal in that it is chronically inflamed (H&E ×400).

Figure 17–48. Behçet's colonic ulceration shows a thrombosed vessel *(arrow)* and oedema of the submucosa (H&E ×350).

Figure 17–49. Detail of thrombosed vessel in Figure 17–48. The inflammatory infiltrate around this vessel is not striking (H&E ×500).

Familial Behçet's syndrome with intestinal involvement has been described and the literature reviewed by Chong and Pathmanathan (1993). In colonic or rectal mucosal biopsies, the appearances are usually not diagnostic, but they confirm a localised inflammation in the mucosa next to the ulcers. However, the presence of entirely normal mucosa a short distance from the ulcers may give an indication of the diagnosis, especially if other manifestations of the disease, such as orogenital ulcers, iritis, arthritis, and skin and nervous system involvement, are present.

COLITIS OF CHRONIC GRANULOMATOUS DISEASE

This colitis may be virtually indistinguishable from Crohn's disease because similar granulomas are seen in association with patchy ulceration and inflammation. A histological clue to the diagnosis, however, is the additional feature of PAS-positive lipofuscin-filled histiocytes in both mucosa and submucosa (Werlin et al 1982, Isaacs et al 1985).

MISCELLANEOUS FORMS OF COLITIS

On rare occasions, other conditions can present as and mimic inflammatory bowel disease. Such diseases as Wegener's granulomatosis (Haworth and Pusey 1984, Sokol, Farrell and McAdams 1984, Wilson et al 1993) and angioimmunoblastic lymphadenopathy (Rosenstein et al 1988) have been reported in this context.

18

MISCELLANEOUS LESIONS

PNEUMATOSIS CYSTOIDES INTESTINALIS

In this condition, air-filled gas cysts occur in the wall of the small or large intestine. On biopsy, the clinician may hear a hissing pop as the gas that is under some pressure escapes. Histological examination reveals cystic spaces in the submucosa. The reaction at the margin of the spaces varies with the age of the lesion. Early cysts have no lining (Fig. 18–1) and at this stage appear not to be dilated lymphatics, as was once thought and for which claims are still made, at least in experimental situations (Sibbons, Spitz and van Velzen 1992). In a histochemical study, evidence was provided by Holl et al (1993) that the lining cells are of histiocytic lineage. The first reaction, thus, is histiocytic, and the spaces come to be lined by macrophages. Later there is a mild collagenisation outside this zone, and the macrophages form multinucleate giant cells (Fig. 18–2). The reaction parallels that seen in subcutaneous tissues after air or its individual component gases are injected (Wright 1930).

The question arises as to how the air finds its way into the bowel wall. Koss (1952) noted a high prevalence (58%) in the reported cases of a coexisting organic lesion of the gut, e.g., ulceration, neoplasm, and obstruction. It has been described in association with diverticular disease (Jorgensen and Wille-Jorgensen 1982) and duodenal ulcer (Fahal, Baraka and el Lider 1994). It seems to complicate the connective tissue diseases more frequently than by chance. Cases occurring in association with mixed connective tissue disease were reported by Lynn et al (1984) and Wilkinson (1992). Lynn et al also reviewed the previous literature. The condition has also been reported as a complication of enteral feeding via catheter jejunostomy (Zern and Clarke-Pearson 1985), after colonoscopy (Heer et al 1983), in Crohn's disease (John et al 1992), and bone marrow (Yeager et al 1987, Day, Ramsay and Letourneau 1988) and renal transplantation (Murphy and Weinfeld 1987). It can complicate chronic idiopathic intestinal pseudo-obstruction (Luks et al 1991). In such cases, a mechanical theory of origin is usually postulated whereby gas is forced into the wall via a breach in the mucosa. Even when it seems reasonable to invoke this mechanism, as, for example, when the condition complicates jejunoileal bypass surgery for obesity (Doolas, Breyer and Franklin 1979), the anatomical site of anastomosis does not necessarily correspond to the location of the pneumatosis, and sometimes the lesions appear many months after operation (Feinberg et al 1977). In many patients, however, no bowel lesion can be demonstrated, and clinical (Doub and Shea 1960) and experimental (Keyting et al 1961) evidence has suggested another origin. Rupture of lung alveoli producing mediastinal emphysema is followed by the movement of gas downward around the aorta. The path upward is blocked by deep fascial attachments at the root of the neck. The gas moves along in the adventitia of branches of the aorta into the mesentery, subsequently entering and disrupting the bowel wall along the vascular planes. Namdaran, Dutz and Ovasepian (1979) were able to produce typical pneumatosis in two cadavers by using

Figure 18–1. Pneumatosis cystoides intestinalis. Early cyst with no definitive lining (H&E ×210).

Figure 18–2. Pneumatosis cystoides intestinalis. Typical macrophage and giant cell lining of later lesion. There is early fibrosis outside the cyst (H&E ×105).

high pressure oxygen insufflation of the lungs. The explanation is therefore tenable in patients with chronic lung diseases, but the claim that all cases can be explained in this way is unfounded. Certainly when pneumatosis is seen in the immediate vicinity of ulcerated lesions and not elsewhere, a local origin is favoured.

In their analysis of 33 cases from the Armed Forces Institute of Pathology, Smith and Welter (1967) drew attention to the age distribution. All cases involved either children younger than 1 year of age or adults. In infants it usually occurs as a complication of necrotising enterocolitis (Chabot, Slovis and Cullen 1992), and there are cases in both children and adults that complicate severe ileocolitis. In this author's experience, these are the result of gas production by clostridial or other gas-forming organisms that are acting as secondary invaders in a primarily ischaemic lesion. It is of some interest in this respect that such cases have a fatal outcome, whereas the condition complicating lung disease or local bowel lesions is benign and self-limiting, although it may recur over several years. This conclusion was also reached in a study of 21 cases by Gruenberg, Grodsinsky and Ponka (1979), who also noted a bad prognosis when the disease process occurred in the setting of severe illness due to other causes. In an ultrastructural study, Haboubi et al (1984) claimed that the cysts were dilated lymphatic channels. On the other hand, Pieterse, Leong and Rowland (1985) claimed that the gas enters from the bowel on the basis of an inflammatory process disrupting the crypts. This is not the experience of most observers; the small spaces they observed are probably related to the lesion known as pseudolipomatosis (referred to later in this chapter). Theegarten and Ruhl (1994) proposed that pneumatosis cystoides intestinalis (PCI) is never a primary disease but a complication sometimes of extraintestinal disorders. They recognised three groups: in group 1 PCI is a complication of lung disease and normal intestinal status; in group 2 it develops on the basis of intestinal disease that is secondary to primary extraintestinal or generalised disease; and in group 3 it develops as a complication of primary gastrointestinal disease.

COLITIS CYSTICA PROFUNDA AND SUPERFICIALIS

Colitis cystica profunda is a benign condition characterised by the presence of mucin-filled epithelial cysts underneath the muscularis mucosae. Rectal biopsy includes part of these structures on occasion (Tedesco, Sumner and Kassens 1976), and awareness of the condition can help prevent unnecessary surgical resections, not only because of histological misinterpretation, but also because clinically it can present as a colonic mass lesion (Schein, Veller and Decker 1987, Kim et al 1992), and it may be misdiagnosed as carcinoma. Rarely does adenocarcinoma coexist (Struyf et al 1995). The wall of the cysts may be incomplete because of lack of depth in biopsy tissues, but the epithelial lining may also be absent because of rupture (Fig. 18–3). The presence of mucin can be verified by appropriate stains, and the condition can thus be easily differentiated from PCI and oil granuloma even if there is a foreign body reaction to the mucin. The condition may be present in localised form more commonly in the rectum, but occasionally elsewhere (Yashiro et al 1985) or as a more diffuse colonic lesion, and is usually associated with a local ulcerative disease process at least sometimes in the course of its development (Zidi et al 1994) (see the section in this chapter on solitary ulcer of the rectum). There seems to be a further strong association with rectal prolapse in the distal form of the disease (Stuart 1984), but sometimes no antecedent bowel pathological condition can be established, and it can be recurrent (Bentley et al 1985). A single case reported by Lifshitz et al (1994) was ascribed to anal masturbation and thought to be self-inflicted. It should be noted that the lesions of colitis cystica profunda are distinct from the colonic lymphoid glandular complexes (microbursae) as described by Kealy (1976b). These structures are a feature in about 10% of normal colons (see Fig. 15–3). It is possible that a colon with numerous microbursae would be more likely to develop colitis cystica profunda lesions than a normal colon if it were subsequently

Figure 18–3. Colitis cystica profunda. This case was the result of an established chronic Crohn's disease. Note the incomplete lining of the submucosal glands, the pus in the lumen, and the calcification *(arrow)* (H&E ×250).

the site of a mucosal inflammatory process associated with regenerative epithelial activity, such as occurs in chronic ulcerative or granulomatous colitis. An association with inflammatory bowel disease is well recognised (Wayte and Helwig 1967, Magidson and Lewin 1981, O'Donnell 1987), and it has complicated radiation-induced colonic stricture (Gardiner, McAuliffe and Murray 1984).

Morson and Dawson (1979) referred to a rare condition in children dying from leukaemia, pellagra, and tropical sprue called colitis cystica superficialis. The mucous membrane of the colon is atrophic and exhibits numerous small cysts due to ectasia of the glands. There is no record in the literature that the condition has been encountered in rectal biopsy specimens. However, it is not unusual occasionally to see thin-walled cystic glands in follow-up biopsies of patients with infective colitis. This is probably a transient architectural abnormality, secondary to obstruction of the gland opening due to the healing process (Fig. 18–4).

AMYLOIDOSIS

Primary amyloidosis must be advanced before results of the Congo red test are positive; the test is thus of little diagnostic value in early cases. Diagnosis by other means, especially by histological examination of biopsy tissues, has gradually become popular. Aspiration of tissues from internal organs carries a small but nevertheless real risk, and gingival biopsy (Calkins and Cohen 1960) or small intestinal biopsy (Green et al 1961) gives a high false-negative rate. With rectal biopsy (Figs. 18–5 and 18–6), the diagnosis is achieved in 78% of cases (Gafni and Sohar 1960), results that compare well with those obtained by renal biopsy and that are better than those for liver biopsy. It is optimum for the rectal biopsy to include the submucosa because

Figure 18–4. Cystic crypt in a follow-up biopsy from a case of infective colitis (H&E ×500).

amyloid may be present at this site when absent from the lamina propria (Kyle, Spencer and Dahlin 1966). Amyloid deposits may be seen in the small arterioles of the lamina propria and submucosa, in the basement membrane of the surface epithelium and glands, and between fibres of the muscularis mucosae. Blood vessel involvement may be so marked that amyloid deposition may precipitate severe ischaemic lesions with gross secondary inflammatory disease (Perarnau et al 1982, Vernon 1982, Kumar et al 1983, Maher et al 1988, Kawaguchi et al 1993), and it can mimic ulcerative colitis (Herrera et al 1991). A great deal has been learned about the chemical composition of amyloid and its subtypes; for practical purposes, mate-

Figure 18–5. Rectal biopsy in severe amyloidosis. Even in H&E preparations the material is clearly visible under the superficial epithelium and in the upper third of the lamina (H&E ×70).

Figure 18–6. Rectal biopsy in severe amyloidosis. Distribution in lower lamina propria and submucosal vessels (H&E ×140).

rial that gives green birefringence in the polarising microscope when Congo red–stained sections are examined and an orange-red fluorescence in ultraviolet light can be regarded as amyloid (Zucker-Franklin, Pras and Franklin 1969). In such circumstances, the more conventional methods will also be positive, but when there is serious doubt, it may prove necessary to resort to more sophisticated methods that employ amyloid-specific fluorescein-conjugated antisera immunohistochemistry (Tada et al 1994) and electron microscopy (Zucker-Franklin and Franklin 1970). Goldblum, Beals and Weiss (1992) described elastofibromatous change in the rectum and how this variety can be differentiated from amyloid by appropriate staining procedures and electron microscopy.

MUCOVISCIDOSIS

There is a decrease in the diagnostic specificity of the sweat test with increasing age (Anderson and Freeman 1960, McKendrick 1962); even in children it is sometimes false-negative (Schwachman and Antonowicz 1962). All glandular epithelia may show abnormalities in this disorder, and this applies to the intestinal mucosa (Parkins et al 1963). A meconium ileus equivalent occurs in postneonatal children and young adults (Matseshe, Go and Dimagno 1977), and rectal biopsy therefore assumes increasing diagnostic importance. The goblet cells are conspicuous, the mouths of the colonic glands tend to gape, and the crypts are widely dilated, being filled with lamellated mucin (Fig. 18–7). In some cases, a mild inflammatory infiltrate is present in the lamina propria. Similar but less marked changes may occur normally in the region just above the mucocutaneous junction and occasionally also in healed inflammatory lesions of the colon, but they are then patchy; if marked changes are present in several biopsy specimens, the diagnosis of mucoviscidosis is certain. A mucoviscidosis-like syndrome can rarely occur in the absence of cystic fibrosis; in a series of nine cases Toyosaka et al (1994) ascribed this condition to immaturity of the myenteric plexus in the ileum and colon.

SOLITARY ULCER OF THE RECTUM

This condition classically affects young adults of either sex who present with constipation and a combination of the following symptoms: difficulty in defaecation, sensations of incomplete evacuation, rectal prolapse, and rectal bleeding (Malhotra

Figure 18–7. Mucoviscidosis in rectal biopsy of a child. The glands contain thick inspissated secretion (H&E ×375).

et al 1992). It is being recognised more frequently in older age groups, and there are claims that it is underdiagnosed (Saul and Sollenberger 1985). Despite the name of the disease, in about a third of cases there is more than one ulcer; uncommonly, there are several. Conversely, in the solitary rectal ulcer syndrome, ulceration, especially in the early stages, is not always ulcerated (Knoepp and Davis 1992). Healing may occur, but reulceration is usual, and the condition is chronic. A rectal biopsy from the healed area or the ulcer edge shows typical features (Madigan and Morson 1969). Apart from the expected changes due to ulceration and attempted healing, a characteristic feature is obliteration of the lamina propria by a fibromuscular proliferation (Figs. 18–8 and 18–9) continuous with the muscularis mucosae,

Figure 18–8. Rectal biopsy of mucosa at the edge of a solitary rectal ulcer. The muscularis mucosae is splayed, fibrotic, and hypertrophied, and it merges with the lamina propria (H&E ×70).

Figure 18–9. Detail of Figure 18–8 shows fibromuscular obliteration of the lamina propria (H&E ×210).

Figure 18–10. Deep biopsy from a case of solitary ulcer showing deep glandular elements embedded in hypertrophied muscularis (H&E ×350).

Figure 18–11. Detail of Figure 18–10 shows the intimate relationship between glandular elements and muscle (H&E ×500).

which is hypertrophied and splayed. This can be shown to great effect in a connective tissue trichrome stain. In deep biopsies, a further feature sometimes seen is glandular epithelium and related lamina propria in the submucosa (Figs. 18–10 and 18–11). These are prone to cystic dilation of the epithelial elements, which by virtue of their position are sometimes erroneously regarded as malignant. The lesion is a localised form of colitis cystica profunda and, like the diffuse condition, probably represents a regenerative reactive phenomenon. It is analogous to the lesions described in Chapter 8 as gastritis cystica profunda. Its importance lies in the fact that it appears grossly as a mass lesion and may be misdiagnosed as carcinoma (Nagasako et al 1977).

Rectal biopsy carried out in the investigation of a variety of colorectal-associated symptoms occasionally reveals fibrous obliteration of the lamina propria and mild degenerate changes in the superficial epithelium (Fig. 18–12). It seems possible that these are the morphological consequences of repeated minimal mucosal trauma or ischaemia accompanying disorders of defaecation, either real or otherwise, which result in straining at stool. Fibromuscular obliteration of the lamina propria is also seen in prolapsed rectal mucosa, in prolapsed colostomy stomas, and in the mucosa of chronically recurrent intussusception. Levine et al (1988) drew particular attention to this histological feature in differentiating the solitary ulcer syndrome from Crohn's disease and ulcerative colitis in biopsy tissues. If this is a manifestation of the low-grade mucosal trauma in these situations, similar but more severe trauma may be implicated in the mucosa, producing a solitary rectal ulcer. Parks, Porter and Hardcastle (1966) described the syndrome of the descending perineum, in which chronic

Figure 18–12. Slight architectural disturbance of glands and flattening of superficial epithelium in a mucosa from a patient with a long history of difficulty with defaecation (H&E ×175).

straining at stool results in a prolapse of the anterior rectal wall, further sensation of fullness, and further straining. That a similar mechanism is involved in the aetiology of solitary ulcer seems likely. Martin, Parks and Biggart (1981) and Ford et al (1983) showed that there is a spectrum of histological, gross, and clinical abnormalities that culminate in frank ulceration in patients with abnormal rectal descent on straining. This has been further substantiated in the studies of Mackle and Parks (1986), Levine (1987), and Womack et al (1987). The regenerative and hyperplastic reactive changes that follow the repeated ischaemic trauma have been analysed histochemically (Ehsanullah, Filipe and Gazzard 1982, Franzin et al 1982), and it has been shown that a change from mainly sulfomucin to mainly sialomucin accompanies the histological abnormalities in the rectal mucosa (Khan and Pandey 1993). Similar changes in mucins and histological appearances are found in so-called cloacogenic polyps; some if not all of these are due to mucosal prolapse (Saul 1987).

CATHARTIC COLON

The excessive and chronic use of purgatives may lead to either intractable diarrhoea with hypokalaemia (Houghton and Pears 1958) or protein-losing enteropathy (Heizer et al 1968). Reversible cachexia, hypogammaglobulinaemia, and finger clubbing have also been described (Levine, Goode and Wingate 1981). It can also lead to increasing constipation, which in turn results in increased drug dosage, so that a vicious circle is set up. The large bowel wall is thin and loses its haustra, its mobility is impaired, and there is melanosis coli if the anthracene group of drugs (aloe, senna, cascara, rhubarb) is used. The lesion is most marked in the right side, and it progresses distally. With increased awareness of the consequences over the years, the incidence of cathartic colon has decreased significantly and is now quite rare (Muller-Lissner 1992). Rectal biopsy (Figs. 18–13 and 18–14) is therefore valuable in diagnosis, because it indicates a severe form due to long and significant exposure, which apparently increases the risk of developing colorectal adenomatous polyps and adenocarcinoma (Siegers et al 1993). Whether this increase in neoplasia is the cause or an effect of mechanical obstruction due to the lesions has not been proved. Its presence also indicates recent exposure, because the amount of pigmentation varies when the use of purgatives is periodic. The exact nature of the pigment is the subject of doubt. It gives a positive periodic acid–Schiff (PAS) reaction and is autofluorescent. Lillee and Geer (1965) showed that it has a protein component and a more or less closely bound glycolipid with free fatty acid residues. Rarely is it claimed that the pigment gives a reaction with Perls's stain for iron, but this author has not seen this phenomenon. The pigment is more or less similar to lipofuscin. The superficial cells of the mucosa may be flattened, but there are no destructive epithelial changes. The lamina propria may also contain an excess of chronic inflammatory cells, the muscularis mucosae is often markedly hypertrophied, and the submucosa shows fatty infiltration (Fig. 18–15). There are also changes in the myenteric neurones (Smith 1972), which cannot be appreciated in mucosal biopsy tissues. The use of anthracene purgatives is so common that the finding of melanosis alone in colonic biopsies is not sufficient ground to make a diagnosis of cathartic colon (Badiali et al 1985). Balazs (1986) claimed that in patients with melanosis, motility disorders are better correlated with electron microscopic evidence of ballooning and degeneration of autonomic neural elements in the mucosa. There

Figure 18–13. Rectal biopsy in cathartic colon. There is slight excess of chronic inflammatory cells and melanosis pigment-filled macrophages (H&E ×150).

Figure 18–14. Melanosis coli pigmentation of a severe extent involving deeply situated macrophages in the submucosa and the submucosal neurones (H&E ×500).

Figure 18–15. Cathartic colon shows hypertrophy of the muscularis mucosae and fatty infiltration of the submucosa (H&E ×38).

is experimental evidence that the pigment itself is due to anthraquinone epithelial cell damage that results in increased apoptosis. The apoptotic bodies are then phagocytosed by intraepithelial macrophages that migrate into the lamina propria where the bodies are converted in heterolysosomes to lipofuscin (Walker, Bennett and Axelsen 1988, Geboes et al 1993). In early melanosis coli changes in humans, apoptotic bodies are a prominent feature in the overlying superficial epithelium (Fig. 18–16). Involvement of the ileum is also said to occur in association with melanosis coli, but another form of ileal melanosis has been described in which the pigment shares features with similar brown pigment found in pulmonary macrophages (Ghadially, Boone and Walley 1993). The topic of melanosis of the gastrointestinal tract was reviewed extensively by Ghadially and Walley (1994).

NEUROLOGICAL DISORDERS

In the past, there was a great deal of controversy over the place of suction biopsy in the diagnosis of Hirschsprung's disease. Although the disease occurs in adolescents and adults (Parc, Douvin and Loygue 1979, Lefebvre et al 1984, Barnes et al 1986, Pescatori, Mattana and Castiglioni 1986, Starling, Croom and Thomas 1986) and has a familial occurrence (Russell et al 1994), possibly with an autoimmune basis (Hirobe et al 1992), it is in the very young patient that precise diagnosis is a problem. This centres on the adequacy of examination of only the submucosal plexus instead of both the submucosal and myenteric plexuses as in full thickness biopsies. However, experienced observers became satisfied that histological examination of suction rectal and colonic biopsies has an established place in the diagnosis and treatment of this disease (Kurer, Lawson and Pambakian 1986). The tissue provided must include the submucosa where, in the normal biopsy, ganglion cells are easily recognised if sufficient sections are examined, and the biopsy sample must be taken at least 1 cm above the anorectal junction. Below this, ganglion cells are absent. As a rough guide, any specimen that includes squamous epithelium and less submucosa than mucosa should be regarded as inadequate. In the usual case, the involved segment of bowel exhibits not only an absence of ganglion cells but also nonmyelinated nerve trunks (Figs. 18–17 and 18–18), which are not present in the normal condition (Bodian 1960). A transitional zone often separates the aganglionic segment from the normal bowel, which may be considerably dilated and hypertro-

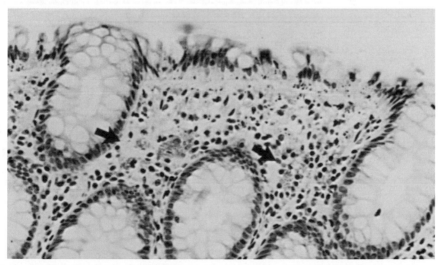

Figure 18–16. Early melanosis coli. Note occasional pigment macrophages *(arrows)* and the numerous apoptotic bodies in the epithelium and upper lamina propria (H&E ×500).

Figure 18–17. Rectal biopsy shows normal submuco-sal ganglion cells *(arrow)* (H&E ×225).

Figure 18–18. Rectal biopsy in Hirschsprung's disease. Absence of ganglion cells is associated with the presence of abnormal nerve trunks *(arrowheads)* (H&E ×113).

phied. In the transition zone, ganglion cells are fewer and smaller than normal. Total colonic (Fekete et al 1986) and total intestinal aganglionosis occur but are less common (Caniano et al 1985, Fekete et al 1986, Rudin et al 1986). Total colonic aganglionosis may lack hypertrophic nerves and increased cholinergic nerve endings and certain zonal areas with ganglion cells. These can prove to be a diagnostic pitfall (Qualman and Murray 1994).

The diagnosis of Hirschsprung's aganglionosis is very difficult in the neonate and in patients up to 6 months of age because of the immaturity of the submucosal neural elements (Smith 1968). With experience, however, these are easy to recognise; Yunis, Dibbins and Sherman (1976) have described them in some detail.

Rather than as ganglion cells with obvious cytoplasm and prominent nucleoli, the neural units appear as small bare nuclei often set in a horseshoe pattern around central fibrillary neural tissue (Fig. 18–19). Their form varies depending on the plane of sectioning, and sometimes stages in mature neurone development among one or more of the primitive cells are seen. When they are recognised, the diagnosis of Hirschsprung's disease is excluded. As seems likely, a group of clinically classic cases of this disease has only immature ganglia at a time when they would normally have matured. These and others with short distal segments showing an appearance characteristic of the transition zone, i.e., few ganglion cells but no abnormal nerve trunks, probably represent a less severe form of Hirschsprung's disease. Occasional cases with short incomplete distal aganglionosis and abnormal nerve trunks were described by MacMahon, Moore and Cussen (1981). In the past, methods based on demonstration of acetylcholinesterase, either by quantitative biochemical assay (Boston, Dale and Riley 1975, Dale et al 1979) or a histochemical procedure, were used as adjuncts to the diagnosis of Hirschsprung's disease (Trigg et al 1974, Patrick, Besley and Smith 1980, Barr et al 1985, Schofield, Devine and Yunis 1990, Park et al

Figure 18–19. Neonatal rectal biopsy shows usual appearance of relatively immature ganglion cells *(between arrows)* that are not unlike the neighbouring inflammatory cells but have a distinctive horseshoe-like configuration and sometimes central fibrils (H&E ×500).

1992). More recently, immunohistochemical demonstration of neuronal microtubule proteins (Tam and Owen 1993), synaptic vesicles (Yamataka et al 1992), and nerve growth factor receptor (Kobayashi et al 1994) has been used. In expert hands these are useful, but the value of these methods is often measured against the results of an examination by an expert observer of serial sections of the tissue stained by ordinary haematoxylin and eosin (H&E) (Challa et al 1987). If doubt persists, a reappraisal of the clinical situation is undertaken. These histochemical methods proved useful in situations in which biopsy material was limited to the mucosa by demonstrating an excessive permeation of nerve fibres throughout the lamina propria and muscularis mucosae in aganglionosis and positive ganglion cells in the lamina propria in neuronal dysplasia (Lake, Nixon and Claireaux 1978, Ziegler et al 1984).

Huntley et al (1982) described two types of acetylcholinesterase nerve fibres. In type A the fibres are prominent in both the muscularis and the lamina, but in type B they are present mainly in the muscularis mucosae. Type B tends to be seen in infants 1 month of age or younger, and the diagnosis of Hirschsprung's disease then needs to be substantiated by conventional routine histology. It has become apparent that the ganglion cells and nerve fibres in the rectal mucosa and submucosa can be much more easily visualised in immunohistochemical preparations using antibodies to neuron-specific enolase and S100 protein (Hall and Lampert 1985, Vinores and May 1985, Blisard and Kleinman 1986, Tam 1986) (Figs. 18–20 and 18–21). Nevertheless they need to be used in conjunction with routine serial sections stained by H&E, particularly because although the location of ganglion cells is facilitated, the delineation of mucosal nerve fibres is said not to be as good as with the acetylcholinesterase method, and both are liable to be misinterpreted and produce false-positive and false-negative results (Robey, Kuhajda and Yardley 1988). There are conflicting reports concerning changes in endocrine polypeptide cells in the excised bowel in Hirschsprung's disease. Cristina et al (1978) found no abnormalities in enteroglucagon and somatostatin cells, whereas Bishop et al (1981) found them increased, together with a vasoactive intestinal peptide content. There are no reports of the value of demonstrating changes in these cell types in rectal biopsies for the diagnosis of the disease.

McIver and Whitehead (1972) drew attention to a disease characterised by zonal aganglionosis in which a rectal biopsy may be normal. Rarely, therefore, in otherwise

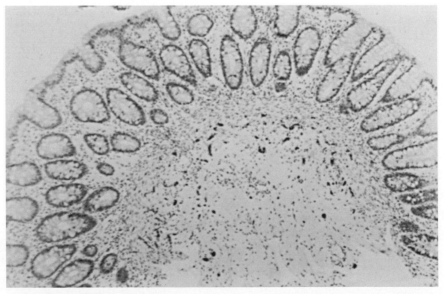

Figure 18–20. Hirschsprung's disease. A rectal biopsy shows abnormal nerve trunks (S100 ×150).

Figure 18–21. Detail of Figure 18–20 shows proliferation of nerve fibres in the submucosa and involving the muscularis mucosae (S100 ×500).

typical cases of Hirschsprung's disease is a normal low rectal biopsy seen, but this does not exclude the possibility of an aganglionic segment at a higher level. It is possible that this entity has a different aetiology, and zonal aganglionosis is described in the terminal ileum. A different and temporary intrauterine insult could be involved. The neural elements migrate into the bowel in a craniocaudal direction from the neural crest, and it could be postulated that whereas in Hirschsprung's disease the migration is terminated more or less abruptly and permanently, in zonal aganglionosis the interference is relatively brief. De Chadarevian, Slim and Akel (1982) and Seldenrijk et al (1986) reported further cases of double zonal aganglionosis and reviewed the literature on this curious variant. Another subtype or related disorder is segmental hypoganglionosis (Matsui et al 1987) and hypoganglionosis of the myenteric plexus with normal Meissner's plexus (Ariel et al 1985).

NEURONAL DYSPLASIA

Since its earliest use to describe a condition akin to Hirschsprung's disease, neuronal dysplasia has been the subject of considerable controversy. Nezelov, Guygrand and Thomine (1970) and Meier-Ruge (1971) first drew attention to this Hirschsprung-like disease, which was defined later by Meier-Ruge (1974) in mucosal biopsy samples as showing giant ganglia in the submucosa, nerve fibre proliferation in the submucosa, and ectopic ganglion cells and sometimes scattered islands of ectopic smooth muscle in the lamina propria. In full-thickness biopsies the muscle layer is said to contain giant ganglia of neurones that form an almost continuous layer, and the circular muscle also contains an excess of nerve fibres. There have been many publications describing this variant of Hirschsprung's disease (Scharli and Meier-Ruge 1981, Fadda et al 1983, Ziegler et al 1984, Kessler and Campbell 1985, Munakata et al 1985, Athow, Filipe and Drake 1991). Two forms were identified: type A with absent adrenergic innervation and an acute early onset, and type B with a later onset and megacolic obstruction, a clinical situation more like classic Hirschsprung's disease. Neuronal dysplasia may accompany Hirschsprung's disease. Some researchers found it almost as common as true Hirschsprung's disease, and others denied its existence as a separate entity (Schofield and Yunis 1990). Large series continued to be published (Martucciello et al 1994, Qualman and Murray

1994, Ure, Holschneider and Meier-Ruge 1994). However, even Meier-Ruge et al (1994) claimed neuronal dysplasia type B is the mildest form of a developmental abnormality of the autonomic nervous system that shows in most cases a spontaneous normalisation of gut motility. They added that isolated neuronal dysplasia is no different from that which is proximal to aganglionosis in Hirschsprung's disease. After applying rigid criteria to the diagnosis, Smith (1992) was unable to confirm the existence of neuronal dysplasia, except in association with Hirschsprung's disease where, in the transition zone, there is a marked increase in fine acetylcholinesterase-positive nerve fibres in the lamina propria, a hyperplasia of the myenteric plexus (hyperganglionosis) with up to three times the number of ganglion cells, and an increase in nerves in the circular muscle coat shown by acetylcholinesterase staining. The ganglia in the myenteric plexus may be large and form a continuous band with numerous neurones.

Intestinal neuronal dysplasia with ganglioneuromatosis and hyperplasia of nerve trunks is also seen in the multiple endocrine neoplasia syndrome type 2B and may occur in type 1 neurofibromatosis. Hyperplasia of the myenteric plexus with an excess of glial cells and fibres usually accompanied by hypoganglionosis is also a recognised finding in pseudo–Hirschsprung's disease. The changes may be diffuse or confined to the rectum. A detailed account of Hirschsprung's disease and related disorders is given by Lake (1995).

Early researchers (Bodian and Lake 1963, Brett and Berry 1967) showed that rectal biopsy examination was helpful in the diagnosis of some central nervous system disorders. In neurolipidosis, metachromatic leukodystrophy, and Hunter's syndrome, changes similar to those in the brain were found in the ganglion cells of the myenteric plexus. Jager, Den Hartog and Bethlem (1960) also reported Lewy's body inclusions of Parkinson's disease, not only in the pigment-containing neurones within the brain but also in neurones of the autonomic ganglia. To be of maximum value, a biopsy should include the muscularis proper, and the technique for providing such a biopsy via the rectum is not without risk.

With the refinement of biochemical procedures and advances in enzymology, the need for biopsy procedures in the diagnosis of the storage disorders has decreased. Brett and Lake (1975) reviewed the situation and concluded that although rectal neuronal involvement is present in many of these syndromes, easier, more reliable, and safer methods are preferred. They suggested that, except in the case of Batten's disease, which is really a group of diseases associated with the storage of ceroid-like pigment lipofuscin in which rectal biopsy is still used (Rapola, Santavuori and Savilahti 1984), it has been superseded as a diagnostic method. Nevertheless, rectal involvement has been described in gangliosidoses, mucopolysaccharidoses, mucolipidoses, fucosidosis, monosidosis, Fabry's disease, Gaucher's disease, Niemann-Pick disease, Wolman's disease, Batten's disease, Tangier disease (Dechelotte et al 1985), and metachromatic leukodystrophy. An ultrastructural study of the rectal mucosa in a variety of storage diseases was reported by Yamano et al (1982). In addition to neuronal storage material, dense bodies and membrane-bound vacuoles were seen in a variety of other cell types, including plasma cells.

Colonic involvement is also described in systemic histiocytosis X and may cause ulceration (Moroz et al 1984, Hyams et al 1985).

In megacolon due to Chagas's disease the myenteric plexus shows a depletion of ganglion cells with an associated inflammatory cell infiltration of variable intensity that seems to be less marked the longer the history of the disease.

Smith (1972 and 1982) pointed out that many of the powerful drugs in everyday use are neurotoxic. Central neurones are usually protected by the blood-brain barrier, but the neurones of the autonomic nervous system are not. She described in detail changes in myenteric neurones of the gut produced in experimental animals by a variety of therapeutic agents and in pseudo-obstruction of the intestine in the child and adult, but whether these results will have an application in detecting drug-induced or congenital neurone abnormality in human rectal biopsy material remains to be seen.

MALACOPLAKIA

Although more commonly found as a rare lesion of the bladder, malacoplakia can occur as a colonic lesion (Terner and Lattes 1963, González-Angulo et al 1965). Even in the colon, it occurs most frequently in association with an obvious focus of suppuration, e.g., an abscess, carcinoma (Sandmeier and Guillou 1993), diverticular disease, and, very rarely, ulcerative colitis (MacKay 1978, Ng and Ng 1993). Sometimes it mimics tumour (Pattnaik et al 1991) and presents as lobulated masses in the mucosa, but occasionally it occurs as a diffuse lesion of the bowel, and it can present as a massive haemorrhage (Arenas-Marquez et al 1994). Lewin et al (1974) reviewed the literature on intestinal malacoplakia; they stressed the particularly aggressive nature of the disease when it involves this site. Histological examination of biopsy specimens reveals typical sheets of histiocytes (Fig. 18–22), some of which contain the rounded, laminated, and calcified Michaelis-Gutmann bodies. The histiocytes have been shown to contain alpha$_1$-antitrypsin (Callea, Van Damme and Desmet 1982).

Electron microscopic studies (Lewin et al 1976, MacKay 1978, Chaudhry et al 1979, Chaudhry et al 1980) have revealed intact bacteria or bacteria showing various stages of destruction in macrophage lysosomes. The organisms show characteristics of *Escherichia coli,* and the lysosomes are gradually filled with amorphous aggregates that become encrusted by calcium phosphate to form the typical Michaelis-Gutmann bodies. They sometimes also contain iron. Stevens and McClure (1982) conducted a comprehensive histochemical study of these curious inclusions. The unusual reponse may represent the result of inadequate macrophage function. El Mouzan et al (1988) reported colonic disease in two children of the same family and proposed that there may be a genetic predisposition.

HISTIOCYTOSIS AND OIL GRANULOMA

Macrophages containing mucoprotein (Azzopardi and Evans 1966) that stain positively with mucicarmine, Alcian blue, and aldehyde fuchsin are commonly seen in the lamina propria of the colon. They occur in otherwise normal biopsy specimens and more commonly in association with other mucosal abnormalities such as might

Figure 18–22. Malacoplakia of the colon. Typical histiocytes with their inclusions *(arrowheads)* (H&E ×460).

be produced by previous inflammatory disruption (Fig. 18–23). They may be scattered throughout the lamina propria, but they tend to be more frequent on the mucosal aspect of the muscularis mucosae. This is invariably the site where muciphages are found in otherwise normal mucosae (Fig. 18–24). These staining reactions, which are probably due to the ingested mucin, serve to differentiate so-called muciphages from Whipple's cells, which can occur in rectal mucosa. Both are PAS-positive.

There is some confusion in the literature on the subject of colonic histiocytosis, and this is in part related to the fact that muciphages, macrophages containing lipofuscin (as seen in the brown bowel syndrome), and melanosis coli macrophages share one or more histochemical properties. In addition, these different types of macrophages may occur in the same biopsy material. Furthermore, in some cases of systemic storage diseases, histiocytes of the lamina propria may be involved in addition to the neural elements. This happens, for example, in that rare disorder of congenital absence of high-density lipoproteins (Tangier disease) and the deposition in histiocytes throughout the reticuloendothelial system of cholesterol esters. The colon and rectum are also involved by histiocytosis; this may be seen in the rectal biopsy tissues (Fig. 18–25). Cholesterol and other lipids are also involved in Wolman's disease, a much more severe type of histiocytosis that also affects the small intestine. It produces a malabsorption syndrome with diarrhoea and is usually fatal in the first 6 months of life. The histiocytes of the reticuloendothelial system in all areas outside the central nervous system are affected. In gangliosidosis the lamina propria histiocytes contain a metachromatic water-soluble acid mucosubstance, some in an insoluble form (Fig. 18–26). Histiocytic involvement is also said to occur in Niemann-Pick disease and Gaucher's disease.

A local histiocytic and giant cell reaction also characterise the established lesion

Figure 18–23. Rectal biopsy after resolution of a first mild attack of ulcerative colitis. Muciphages in the lamina propria stain in a manner identical to that of goblet cells (Alcian blue ×140).

Figure 18–24. Normal rectal biopsy shows numerous muciphages next to muscularis mucosae below (H&E ×522).

of oil granuloma that may follow the injection of oily sclerosants or the use of local ointments or lubricants or oral intake of paraffin oil associated with trauma or ulceration (Greaney and Jackson 1977, Mazier, Sun and Robertson 1978). It is sometimes an incidental finding, but it can present as a local rectal or anal canal tumefaction with or without ulceration. The severity of the histiocytic reaction probably varies with different oils and the time that the oil is in the tissues, but in some biopsy specimens it appears to be minimal and superficial and needs to be distinguished from so-called pseudolipomatosis (see later) (Figs. 18–27 and 18–28). Histologically typical, the histiocytic and giant cell reaction surrounds circular spaces

Figure 18–25. Rectal biopsy in Tangier disease. Pale histiocytes occupy the lamina propria (H&E ×510).

Figure 18–26. Rectal biopsy in GM$_1$ gangliosidosis. The histiocytes have been made more obvious because of the PAS method (PAS ×500).

that before tissue processing contain the oil. Both mucosa and submucosa may be involved (Figs. 18–29 and 18–30).

Another form of colonic histiocyte accumulation is so-called colonic xanthomatosis or lipid islands (Figs. 18–31 and 18–32). They appear to be the colonic counterpart of gastric xanthomas or xanthelasmas. The light and electron microscopic appearances are similar (Remmele, Beck and Kaiserling 1988, Schaefer 1988). Scheiman et al (1988), however, in reporting two cases made a claim that xanthomatosis is associated with colonic dysmotility.

DIABETIC ANGIOPATHY AND VASCULITIS

Biopsy has been used to detect microangiopathy in the capillaries of the rectal mucosa in patients with diabetes mellitus (Missmahl and Riemann 1968). Frank

Figure 18–27. Incidental finding in rectal biopsy. The lamina propria shows numerous oil globule spaces (H&E ×70).

Figure 18–28. Detail of Figure 18–27. Note the minimal histiocytic reaction (H&E ×210).

necrotising arteritis may also be seen in the biopsy tissues of patients with systemic autoimmune diseases (Fig. 18–33). A low posterior rectal biopsy, as a very safe procedure, has actually been used for the diagnosis of arteritis in patients with rheumatoid arthritis and related disorders (Schneider and Dobbins 1968). In rheumatoid arthritis patients, Tribe, Scott and Bacon (1981) found that an adequate biopsy is positive in 40% of patients with a clinical vasculitis. They advocated, however, the necessity to examine step serial sections. The problem of classifying necrotising vasculitis is exemplified by its occurrence in the gut. Kalla, Lee and Voss (1980) highlighted this in a case of necrotising and granulomatous arteritis with giant cells that was confined to the vessels of the right colon. The presence of arteritis in rectal biopsy tissues need not be associated with ischaemic lesions of the

Figure 18–29. Oil granuloma in rectal biopsy. There is involvement of the mucosa and submucosa (H&E ×38).

Figure 18–30. Detail of Figure 18–29. The histiocytic reaction is much more pronounced than in Figure 18–28 (H&E ×113).

gut, and this is simply a reflection of its very good anastomotic blood supply. Many of the systemic autoimmune disorders, however, can be associated with a vasculitis so widespread and severe that it causes ischaemic colitis; this was mentioned earlier. Diffuse colitis has been described as the result of vasculitis in the Churg-Strauss syndrome (Malaval et al 1993).

BARIUM GRANULOMA

Rarely, following x-ray procedures and usually in association with inflammatory bowel disease, barium is forced into or through the bowel wall. Small leaks are

Figure 18–31. Colonic biopsy of a pale raised mucosal patch (H&E ×150).

Figure 18–32. Detail of Figure 18–31. The collection of lipid-filled histiocytes is typical of colonic xanthoma or xanthelasma (H&E ×500).

probably more common than is generally appreciated (Fielding and Lumsden 1973), and it occurs in 0.2%–0.4% of patients. Serious perforations are more likely when the bowel is diseased (Williams and Harned 1991). The medium excites a histiocytic reaction (Figs. 18–34 and 18–35) that may subsequently be seen in rectal biopsy specimens. Barium can also be responsible for some unusual histological appearances

Figure 18–33. Rectal biopsy from a patient with rheumatoid arthritis. There is a necrotising vasculitis in the submucosa (H&E ×85).

Figure 18–34. Rectal biopsy some months after a barium enema examination. There is a histiocytic reaction involving the muscularis mucosae and submucosa (H&E ×75).

Figure 18–35. Detail of Figure 18–34. Histiocytes filled with slightly birefringent barium (H&E ×240).

that take the form of birefringent rhomboidal crystals (Womack 1984) or smaller birefringent particles within histiocytes (Levison et al 1984, Mayorga et al 1992).

CRONKHITE-CANADA SYNDROME

This is referred to in Chapter 8. The entire intestine is involved to a greater or lesser extent. Nonetheless, even when there are no frankly polypoidal lesions, abnormality in size, shape, and components of goblet cells can be seen in mucosal biopsies from regions of the gastrointestinal tract other than the stomach (Fig. 18–36). Peart et al (1984), Freeman (1985), Aanestad et al (1987), and Casalnuovo et al (1991) described polypoid colonic lesions. There are reports (Katayama, Kimura and Konn 1985, Malhotra and Sheffield 1988, Murai et al 1993, Harned, Buck and Sobin 1995) that describe adenomatous change in the polyps and coexisting adenocarcinoma. It is rarely recorded in infants (Kucukaydin et al 1992).

PELVIC LIPOMATOSIS

This unusual condition consists of a nontumoural, adipose infiltration of the pelvis that may cause visceral compression and interference with bladder and rectal function (Henriksson, Liljeholm and Lonnerholm 1984). Chen et al (1991) described a case associated with cystitis glandularis. Goldfain et al (1981) described a further case in which a rectal biopsy showed submucosal and mucosal adipocyte infiltration, which, taken in conjunction with the clinical features and radiology, allowed the diagnosis to be made, but this is unusual. Rarely, a few adipocytes may normally be seen in the rectal mucosa, especially in the aged, and often at the site of atrophic lymphoid follicles, but they have no significance. It is usually an easy

Figure 18–36. Rectal biopsy in Cronkhite-Canada syndrome. There is glandular enlargement, distortion, branching, and variation in size. The individual goblet cells are also larger and more varied in shape than normal (H&E ×100).

Figure 18–37. Rectal biopsy shows adipocyte infiltration (H&E ×500).

matter to differentiate this lesion from oil granuloma because there is no reactive histiocyte component (Figs. 18–37 and 18–38). An appearance referred to as pseudo-lipomatosis (Snover, Sandstad and Hutton 1985) is similar, but apparently these authors found no evidence that fat was present in these small clear spaces. It is possible that this lesion is an artefact whereby luminal gas is introduced into the tissues during the biopsy procedure. Another biopsy artefact of interest is the appearance described by Dankwa and Davies (1988) of smooth muscle pseudotu-mours due to forceps pinching and rounding up a portion of muscularis propria so that it appears as a small tumour nodule arising in the submucosa.

Figure 18–38. Adipocyte infiltration involves a lymphoid follicle (H&E ×500).

Figure 18–39. Rectal biopsy from a child with graft-versus-host disease following marrow transplantation. There is an obvious mild colitis and patchy tubular abnormalities with focal atrophy (H&E ×150).

GRAFT-VERSUS-HOST DISEASE

Sale et al (1979) and Epstein et al (1980) performed a rectal biopsy in the evaluation of graft-versus-host disease (GVHD) in humans. Patients undergoing marrow transplantation were shown to have crypt epithelial degenerative changes and occasional crypt abscesses. This is independent of any intestinal infection that might affect up to 20% of cases (Cox et al 1994). The changes proved to be a good indication of GVHD if the biopsy was performed after resolution of radiation or chemotherapeutic effects. Sviland et al (1988) showed that rectal mucosa is a sensitive indicator of GVHD, with single-cell necrosis, degeneration of crypts, and crypt abscesses all being seen. In the author's observations the most sensitive indicator is the appearance of apoptotic bodies in the crypt bases (Figs. 18–39 and 18–40). Sometimes gross changes with epithelium denudation (Beschorner 1984, Thorning

Figure 18–40. Detail of Figure 18–39. There is prominent apoptosis of crypt epithelial cells and cellular apoptotic debris in the dilated glands. A mild coincident colitis is present (H&E ×500).

and Howard 1986) or widespread ulceration (Spencer et al 1986) are described. Lampert et al (1985) and Bryan et al (1991) described a selective sparing of enterochromaffin cells so that small groups of these cells occupied crypt bases at the sites of destroyed crypt epithelium. Cytotoxic drug therapy or irradiation may produce similar changes, however (Fig. 18–41). A GVHD-like colitis has been reported as a complication in a patient with a malignant thymoma (Kornacki, Hansen and Lazenby 1995).

SARCOIDOSIS

Rectal involvement in sarcoidosis has already been referred to. Although it is apparently a rare finding, it is possible that it may be seen more frequently if rectal biopsy were performed routinely in known cases. Sometimes colonic sarcoid can present as a tumour (Zissiadis et al 1994). The question arises as to its differential diagnosis from other noncaseating granulomatous lesions, in particular Crohn's disease. Apart from the fact that in sarcoidosis ulceration does not occur and the clinical picture will be different, in sarcoidosis there is a tendency for granulomas to be localised to colonic mucosal lymphoid aggregates (Figs. 18–42 and 18–43).

HETEROTOPIC GASTRIC MUCOSA AND SALIVARY GLAND OF THE RECTUM

Gastric heterotopia may be the cause of fresh rectal bleeding and usually presents in childhood. The abnormally located mucosa may be polypoidal or present as ulceration. Histologically, biopsies reveal a body-type mucosa of usual histological appearance (Picard et al 1978, Edouard et al 1983, Pistoia et al 1987, Murray et al 1988, Devereaux and Devereaux 1994). Sometimes gastric mucosa lines a rectal duplication (Schwarzenberg and Whitington 1983). Ectopic gastric mucosa sometimes presents in early adult life (Castellanos et al 1984). Weitzner (1983) described ectopic salivary gland tissue in the rectum. In previous cases on record it has usually been accompanied by gastric mucosa.

Figure 18–41. Colonic mucosa in cytotoxic drug therapy. The appearances are like those of graft-versus-host disease, but the crypts contain more obvious collections of pus cells (H&E ×125).

Figure 18–42. Rectal biopsy in sarcoidosis. Epithelioid granulomas are characteristically localised to mucosal lymphoid tissue (H&E ×200).

Figure 18–43. Detail of a typical epithelioid histiocyte granuloma in rectal sarcoidosis (H&E ×500).

Figure 18–44. Colonic endometriosis. The abnormal tissue lies at the base of the mucosa (H&E ×250).

Figure 18–45. Detail of Figure 18–44. Note the subtle but distinct difference between colonic and endometrial glands, the surrounding lamina propria, and the endometrial stroma (H&E ×500).

ALCOHOL-INDUCED CHANGES

Brozinsky et al (1978) studied 11 patients with a history of recent heavy drinking. A decrease in goblet cells, whose number returned to normal after 2 weeks' abstinence, was seen in rectal biopsy specimens by light microscopy. These changes were accompanied by loss of microvilli, swollen mitochondria with distorted cristae, dilation of the endoplasmic reticulum and Golgi's complex and an increase in multivesicular bodies in an electron microscopic evaluation.

COLONIC ENDOMETRIOSIS

The sigmoid colon is the most common site of endometriosis, where it may give rise to obstruction and bleeding (Petros, Spirito and Gosshein 1992). It used to be uncommon for a diagnosis to be made in biopsy tissues (Croom, Donovan and Schwesinger 1984, Samper, Slagle and Hand 1984), but this is no longer the case (Bozdech 1992). Sometimes endometriosis masquerades as colitis (Langlois, Park and Keenan 1994) (Figs. 18–44 and 18–45).

REFERENCES—SECTION FOUR: COLONIC BIOPSY

Aanestad O., Raknerud N., Aase S.T. and Narverud G. (1987) The Cronkhite-Canada syndrome. Acta Chirurgica Scandinavica 153:143–145.

Aaronson H.G., Meir J.H. and Ulin A.W. (1957) A case of sarcoidosis of the colon. Journal of the Albert Einstein Medical Center 6:14–16.

Adamsen S., Ostberg G. and Norryd C. (1988) Squamous-cell metaplasia with severe dysplasia of the colonic mucosa in ulcerative colitis. Diseases of the Colon and Rectum 31:558–562.

Ahnen D.J., Warren G.H., Greene L.J., Singleton J.W. and Brown W.R. (1987) Search for a specific marker of mucosal dysplasia in chronic ulcerative colitis. Gastroenterology 93:1346–1355.

Alberti-Flor J.J. and Granda A. (1986) Ileocecal histoplasmosis mimicking Crohn's disease in a patient with Job's syndrome. Digestion 33:176–180.

Allen D.C. and Biggart J.D. (1986) Misplaced epithelium in ulcerative colitis and Crohn's disease of the colon and its relationship to malignant mucosal changes. Histopathology 10:37–52.

Allen D.C., Hamilton P.W., Watt P.C.H. and Biggart J.D. (1987) Morphological analysis in ulcerative colitis with dysplasia and carcinoma. Histopathology 11:913–926.

Allison M.C., Hamilton-Dutoit S.J., Dhillon A.P. and Pounder R.E. (1987) The value of rectal biopsy in distinguishing self-limited colitis from early inflammatory bowel disease. Quarterly Journal of Medicine 65:985–995.

Anand B.S., Malhotra V., Bhattacharya S.K., Datta P., Datta D., Sen D., Bhattacharya M.K., Mukherjee P.P. and Pal S.C. (1986) Rectal histology in acute bacillary dysentery. Gastroenterology 90:654–660.

Anderson C.M. and Freeman M. (1960) "Sweat test" results in normal persons of different ages compared with families with fibrocystic disease of the pancreas. Archives of Disease in Childhood 35:581–587.

Angos R., Idoate M.A., Zozaya J.M., Munoz M. and Conchillo F. (1993) Collagenous colitis: clinicopathologic study of 6 new cases. Revista Española de Enfermedades Digestivas 83:161–167.

Anonymous (1977) Pseudomembranous enterocolitis. Lancet i:839–840.

Anonymous (1981) Antibiotic-associated colitis: the continuing saga. British Medical Journal 282:1913–1914.

Anonymous (1983) Colitis in term babies. Lancet i:1083–1084.

Anonymous (1988) Which type of colitis? Lancet i:336.

Anthonisen P. and Riis P. (1971) Eosinophilic granulocytes in the rectal mucus of patients with ulcerative colitis and Crohn's disease of the ileum and colon. Scandinavian Journal of Gastroenterology 6:731–734.

Antonakopoulos G., Newman J. and Wilkinson M. (1982) Intestinal spirochaetosis: an electron microscopic study of an unusual case. Histopathology 6:477–488.

Arber N., Udassin R., Amir G., Zamir O. and Nissan S. (1987) Localized pseudomembranous colitis simulating carcinoma of the cecum. American Journal of Gastroenterology 82:1193–1195.

Archibald R.B., Burnstein A.V., Knackstedt V.E., Tolman K.G. and Holbrook J.H. (1980) Ischemic colitis in a young adult due to inferior mesenteric vein thrombosis. Endoscopy 12:140–143.

Archibald S.D., Jirsch D.W. and Bear R.A. (1978) Gastrointestinal complications of renal transplantation: the colon. Canadian Medical Association Journal 119:1301–1314.

Arean V.M. and Koppisch E. (1956) Balantidiasis. American Journal of Pathology 32:1089–1115.

Arenas-Marquez H., Lopez-Neblina F., Barrera-Torres H. and Flores-Marquez M.R. (1994) Massive hemorrhage of the digestive system secondary to ulcerated colonic malacoplakia. Revista de Gastroenterologia de Mexico 59:49–51.

Ariel I., Hershlag A., Lernau O.Z., Nissan S. and Rosenmann E. (1985) Hypoganglionosis of the myenteric plexus with normal Meissner's plexus: a new variant of colonic ganglion cell disorders. Journal of Pediatric Surgery 20:90–92.

Armes J., Gee D.C., Macrae F.A., Schroeder W. and Bhathal P.S. (1992) Collagenous colitis: jejunal and colorectal pathology. Journal of Clinical Pathology 45:784–787.

Arseculeratne S.N., Panabokke R.G. and Navaratnam C. (1980) Pathogenesis of necrotising enteritis with special reference to intestinal hypersensitivity reactions. Gut 21:265–278.

Atherton L.D., Leib E.S. and Kaye M.D. (1984) Toxic megacolon associated with methotrexate therapy. Gastroenterology 86:1583–1588.

Athow A.C., Filipe M.I. and Drake D.P. (1991) Hyperganglionosis mimicking Hirschsprung's disease. Archives of Diseases of Childhood 66:1300–1303.

Azzopardi J.G. and Evans D.J. (1966) Mucoprotein-containing histiocytes (muciphages) in the rectum. Journal of Clinical Pathology 19:368–374.

Badiali D., Marcheggiano A., Pallone F., Paoluzi P., Bausano G., Iannoni C., Materia E., Anzini F. and Corazziari E. (1985) Melanosis of the rectum in patients with chronic constipation. Diseases of the Colon and Rectum 28:241–245.

Bailey R.W., Hamilton S.R., Morris J.B., Bulkley G.B. and Smith G.W. (1986) Pathogenesis of nonocclusive ischaemic colitis. Annals of Surgery 203:590–599.

Bamford M.J., Matz L.R., Armstrong J.A. and Harris A.R.C. (1982) Collagenous colitis: a case report and review of the literature. Pathology 14:481–484.

Balazs M. (1986) Melanosis coli: ultrastructural study of 45 patients. Diseases of the Colon and Rectum 29:839–844.

Balazs M., Egerszegi P., Vadasz G. and Kovacs A. (1988) Collagenous colitis: an electron microscopic study including comparison with the chronic fibrotic stage of ulcerative colitis. Histopathology 13:319–328.

Barlow R.J., Heyl T., Simson I.W. and Schulz E.J. (1988) Malignant atrophic papulosis (Degos' disease):

diffuse involvement of brain and bowel in an African patient. British Journal of Dermatology 118:117–123.

Barnes P.R.H., Lennard-Jones J.E., Hawley P.R. and Todd I.P. (1986) Hirschsprung's disease and idiopathic megacolon in adults and adolescents. Gut 27:534–541.

Barr L.C., Booth J., Filipe M.I. and Lawson J.O.N. (1985) Clinical evaluation of the histochemical diagnosis of Hirschsprung's disease. Gut 26:393–399.

Bartlett J.G., Chang T.W., Curwith M., Gorbach S.L. and Onderdonk A.B. (1978) Antibiotic-associated pseudomembranous colitis due to toxin-producing clostridia. New England Journal of Medicine 298:531–534.

Bayne S.R., Donovan D.L. and Henthorne W.A. (1994) A rare complication in elective repair of an abdominal aortic aneurysm: multiple transmural colonic infarcts secondary to atheroemboli. Annals of Vascular Surgery 8:290–295.

Beaugerie L., Luboinski J., Brousse N., Cosnes J., Chatelet F.P., Gendre J.P. and Le Quintrec Y. (1994) Drug induced lymphocytic colitis. Gut 35:426–428.

Behan W.M.H. and Mills P.R. (1982) Possible evidence for a Shwartzman reaction in pseudomembranous colitis. Digestion 23:141–150.

Bender B.S., Bennett R., Laughon B.E., Greenough W.B. III, Gaydos C., Sears S.D., Forman M.S. and Bartlett J.G. (1986) Is *Clostridium difficile* endemic in chronic-care facilities? Lancet ii:11–13.

Bennett M.R., Fine A.P. and Hanlon J.T. (1985) Cytomegalovirus hemorrhagic colitis in a nontransplant patient. Postgraduate Medicine 77:227–230.

Bentley E., Chandrasoma P., Cohen H., Radin R. and Ray M. (1985) Colitis cystica profunda, presenting with complete intestinal obstruction and recurrence. Gastroenterology 89:1157–1161.

Berezin S., Schwarz S.M., Glassman M., Davidian M. and Newman L.J. (1989) Gastrointestinal milk intolerance of infancy. American Journal of Disease in Children 143:361–362.

Berk T., Gordon S.J., Choi H.Y. and Cooper H.S. (1985) Cytomegalovirus infection of the colon: a possible role in exacerbations of inflammatory bowel disease. American Journal of Gastroenterology 80:355–360.

Berkowitz D. and Bernstein L.H. (1975) Colonic pseudopolyps in association with amoebic colitis. Gastroenterology 68:786–789.

Berry A.J., Long E.G., Smith J.H., Gourley W.K. and Fine D.P. (1983) Chronic relapsing colitis due to *Strongyloides stercoralis*. American Journal of Tropical Medicine and Hygiene 32:1289–1293.

Berthrong M. and Fajardo L.F. (1981) Radiation injury in surgical pathology: alimentary tract. American Journal of Surgical Pathology 5:153–178.

Beschorner W.E. (1984) Destruction of the intestinal mucosa after bone marrow transplantation and graft-versus-host disease. Survey and Synthesis of Pathology Research 3:264–274.

Bhargava D.K., Kushwaha A.K., Dasarathy S., Shriniwas, and Chopra P. (1992) Endoscopic diagnosis of segmental colonic tuberculosis. Gastrointestinal Endoscopy 38:571–574.

Biaggi A.M. and Potet F. (1995) Ischaemic colitis in the young person. Annales de Pathologie 15:45–49.

Biggs B.A., Megna R., Wickremesinghe S. and Dwyer B. (1987) Human infection with *Cryptosporidium* spp.: results of a 24-month survey. Medical Journal of Australia 147:175–177.

Bingley P.J. and Harding G.M. (1987) *Clostridium difficile* colitis following treatment with metronidazole and vancomycin. Postgraduate Medical Journal 63:993–994.

Birnbaum B.A., Gordon R.B. and Jacobs J.E. (1995) Glutaraldehyde colitis; radiologic findings. Radiology 195:131–134.

Bishop A.E., Pietroletti R., Taat C.W., Brummelkamp W.H. and Polak J.M. (1987) Increased populations of endocrine cells in Crohn's ileitis. Virchows Archiv A 410:391–396.

Bishop A.E., Polak J.M., Lake B.D., Bryant M.G. and Bloom S.R. (1981) Abnormalities of the colonic regulatory peptides in Hirschsprung's disease. Histopathology 5:679–688.

Blackstone M.O., Riddell R.H., Rogers B.H.G. and Levin B. (1981) Dysplasia-associated lesion or mass (DALM) detected by colonoscopy in long-standing ulcerative colitis: an indication for colectomy. Gastroenterology 80:366–374.

Blaser M.J., Parsons R.B. and Wang W-L.L. (1980) Acute colitis caused by *Campylobacter fetus* ss. jejuni. Gastroenterology 78:448–453.

Blisard K.S. and Kleinman R. (1986) Hirschsprung's disease: a clinical and pathologic overview. Human Pathology 17:1189–1191.

Blumencranz H., Kasen L., Romeu J., Waye J.D. and LeLeiko N.S. (1983) The role of endoscopy in suspected amebiasis. American Journal of Gastroenterology 78:15–18.

Bodian M. (1960) Hirschsprung's Disease. In: Recent Advances in Clinical Pathology. Series III. Edited by S.C. Dyke. London: Churchill, p 384.

Bodian M. and Lake B.D. (1963) The rectal approach to neuropathology. British Journal of Surgery 50:702–714.

Bogomoletz W.V., Adnet J.J., Birembaut P., Feydy P. and Dupont P. (1980) Collagenous colitis: an unrecognised entity. Gut 21:164–168.

Bo-Linn G.W., Vendrell D.D., Lee E. and Fordtran J.S. (1985) An evaluation of the significance of microscopic colitis in patients with chronic diarrhea. Journal of Clinical Investigation 75:1559–1569.

Bolton R.P., Cotter K.L. and Losowsky M.S. (1985) Inhibition of neutrophil chemotaxis and phagocytosis by *Clostridium difficile*. Clinical Science 68:53.

Bonfils S., Hervoir P., Girodet J., le Quintrec Y., Bader J.P. and Gastard J. (1977) Acute spontaneously recovering ulcerating colitis (ARUC): report of 6 cases. American Journal of Digestive Diseases 22:429–436.

Bonkowsky H.L. and Brisbane J. (1976) Colitis and hepatitis caused by methyldopa. Journal of the American Medical Association 236:1602–1603.

Boone W.T. and Allison F. Jr (1969) Histoplasmosis. American Journal of Medicine 46:818–826.

Bosshardt R.T. and Abel M.E. (1984) Proctitis following fecal diversion. Diseases of the Colon and Rectum 27:605–607.

Boston V.E., Dale G. and Riley K.W.A. (1975) Diagnosis of Hirschsprung's disease by quantitative biochemical assay of acetylcholinesterase in rectal tissue. Lancet ii:951–953.

Boulton A.J.M., Slater D.N. and Hancock B.W. (1982) Herpesvirus colitis: a new cause of diarrhoea in a patient with Hodgkin's disease. Gut 23:247–249.

Boyd J.F. (1985) Pathology of the alimentary tract in Salmonella typhimurium food poisoning. Gut 26:935–944.

Bozdech J.M. (1992) Endoscopic diagnosis of colonic endometriosis. Gastrointestinal Endoscopy 38:568–570.

Brady S.K. and McKee D.D. (1993) Collagenous colitis: a cause of chronic diarrhea. American Family Physician 48:1081–1084.

Brandt L., Boley S., Goldberg L., Mitsudo S. and Berman A. (1981) Colitis in the elderly: a reappraisal. American Journal of Gastroenterology 76:239–245.

Brearly S., Armstrong G.R., Nairn R., Gornall P., Currie A.B.M., Buick R.G. and Corkery J.J. (1987) Pseudomembranous colitis: a lethal complication of Hirschsprung's disease unrelated to antibiotic usage. Journal of Pediatric Surgery 22:257–259.

Breiter J.R. and Hajjar J.J. (1981) Segmental tuberculosis of the colon diagnosed by colonoscopy. American Journal of Gastroenterology 76:369–373.

Brett E.M. and Berry C.L. (1967) Value of rectal biopsy in paediatric neurology: report of 165 biopsies. British Medical Journal 3:400–403.

Brett E.M. and Lake B.D. (1975) Reassessment of rectal approach to neuropathology in childhood: review of 307 biopsies over 11 years. Archives of Disease in Childhood 50:753–762.

Brown D.N., Rosenholtz M.J. and Marshall J.B. (1994) Ischemic colitis related to cocaine abuse. American Journal of Gastroenterology 89:1558–1561.

Brown R., Tedesco F.J., Assad R.T. and Rao R. (1986) Yersinia colitis masquerading as pseudomembranous colitis. Digestive Diseases and Sciences 31:548–551.

Brozinsky S., Fani K., Grosberg S.J. and Wapnick S. (1978) Alcohol ingestion–induced changes in the human rectal mucosa: light and electron microscopic studies. Diseases of the Colon and Rectum 21:329–335.

Bryan R.L., Antonakopoulos G.N., Newman J. and Milligan D.W. (1991) Intestinal graft-versus-host disease. Journal of Clinical Pathology 44:866–867.

Buckner F.S. and Pomeroy C. (1993) Cytomegalovirus disease of the gastrointestinal tract in patients without AIDS. Clinical Infectious Diseases 17:644–656.

Bulger K., O'Riordan M., Purdy S., O'Brien M. and Lennon J. (1988) Gastrointestinal sarcoidosis resembling Crohn's disease. American Journal of Gastroenterology 83:1415–1417.

Burke G.W., Wilson M.E. and Mehrez I.O. (1988) Absence of diarrhea in toxic megacolon complicating Clostridium difficile pseudomembranous colitis. American Journal of Gastroenterology 83:304–307.

Burt R.W., Berenson M.M., Samuelson C.O. and Cathey W.J. (1983) Rheumatoid vasculitis of the colon presenting as pancolitis. Digestive Diseases and Sciences 28:183–188.

Butt J.H. and Morson B. (1981) Dysplasia and cancer in inflammatory bowel disease. Gastroenterology 80:865–868.

Byrd R.L., Cunningham M.W. and Goldman L.I. (1987) Nonocclusive ischemic colitis secondary to hemorrhagic shock. Diseases of the Colon and Rectum 30:116–118.

Calkins E. and Cohen A.S. (1960) Diagnosis of amyloidosis. Bulletin of Rheumatic Diseases 10:215–218.

Callea F., Van Damme B. and Desmet V.J. (1982) Alpha-1-antitrypsin in malakoplakia. Virchows Archiv A 395:1–9.

Campbell A.P., Cobb C.A., Chapman R.W., Kettlewell M., Hoang P., Haot B.J. and Jewell D.P. (1993) Cap polyposis: an unusual cause of diarrhoea. Gut 34:562–564.

Caniano D.A., Ormsbee H.S., Polito W., Sun C-C., Barone F.C. and Hill J.L. (1985) Total intestinal aganglionosis. Journal of Pediatric Surgery 20:456–460.

Carr N.D., Wells S., Haboubi N.Y., Salem R.J. and Schofield P.F. (1986) Ischaemic dilatation of the colon. Annals of the Royal College of Surgeons of England 68:264–266.

Casalnuovo C., Ghigliani M., Avagnina A., Elsner B. and Palau G. (1991) Cronkhite-Canada syndrome: report of a case. Medicina 51:155–160.

Cashore W.J., Peter G., Lauermann M., Stonestreet B.S. and Oh W. (1981) Clostridia colonization and clostridial toxin in neonatal necrotizing enterocolitis. Journal of Pediatrics 98:308–311.

Castellanos D., Menchen P., de la Riva M.P., Clemente G., Senen M., Rabago L., Garcia Andrade M. and Alcala-Santaella R. (1984) Heterotopic gastric mucosa in the rectum. Endoscopy 16:197–199.

Castro E.B., Rosen P.P. and Quan S.H.Q. (1973) Carcinoma of large intestine in patients irradiated for carcinoma of cervix and uterus. Cancer 31:45–52.

Castro J., Vazquez-Iglesias J.L. and Arnal-Monreal F. (1983) Dysentery caused by Balantidium coli: report of two cases. Endoscopy 15:272–274.

Cawthorn S.J., Gibbs N.M. and Marks C.G. (1983) Segmental colitis: a new complication of diverticular disease. Gut 24:500.

Chabot V.H., Slovis T.L. and Cullen M. (1992) Recurrent pneumatosis intestinalis in young infants. Pediatric Radiology 22:120–122.

Challa V.R., Moran J.R., Turner C.S. and Lyerly A.D. (1987) Histologic diagnosis of Hirschsprung's disease: the value of concurrent hematoxylin and eosin and cholinesterase staining in rectal biopsies. American Journal of Clinical Pathology 88:324–328.

Chambers T.J. and Morson B.C. (1979) The granuloma in Crohn's disease. Gut 20:269–274.

Chandratre S., Bramble M.G., Cooke W.M. and Jones R.A. (1987) Simultaneous occurrence of collagenous colitis and Crohn's disease. Digestion 36:55–60.

Chaudhry A.P., Saigal K.P., Intengan M. and Nickerson P.A. (1979) Malakoplakia of the large intestine found incidentally at necropsy: light and electron microscopic features. Diseases of the Colon and Rectum 22:73–81.

Chaudhry A.P., Satchidanand S.K., Anthone R., Baumler R.A. and Gaeta J.F. (1980) An unusual case of supraclavicular and colonic malakoplakia: a light and ultrastructural study. Pathology 131:193–208.

Chen S.L., Wong C.M., Lin B.H., Hong J.G. and Kue H.T. (1991) Pelvic lipomatosis associated with cystitis glandularis: case report. Chung-Hua I Hsueh Tsa Chih 48:76–79.

Chiu A.O. and Abraham A.A. (1982) Pseudomembranous colitis associated with an unidentified species of clostridium. American Journal of Clinical Pathology 78:398–402.

Chong V.F. and Pathmanathan R. (1993) Familial Behçet's syndrome with intestinal involvement: case reports and a review of the literature. Annals of the Academy of Medicine, Singapore 22:807–810.

Chowdhury M.N.H. (1984) *Campylobacter jejuni* enteritis: a review. Tropical and Geographical Medicine 36:215–222.

Christ A.D., Meier R., Bauerfeind P., Wegmann W. and Gyr K. (1993) Simultaneous occurrence of lymphocytic gastritis and lymphocytic colitis with transition to collagenous colitis. Schweizerische Medizinische Wochenschrift 123:1487–1490.

Chun D., Chandrasoma P. and Kiyabu M. (1994) Fulminant amebic colitis: a morphologic study of four cases. Diseases of the Colon and Rectum 37:535–539.

Clarke A.W., Lloyd-Mostyn R.H. and Sadler M.R. de C. (1972) Ischaemic colitis in young adults. British Medical Journal 4:70–72.

Cohen M.B. (1991) Etiology and mechanisms of acute infectious diarrhea in infants in the United States. Journal of Pediatrics (suppl):118:s34–s39.

Colgan T., Lambert J.R., Newman A. and Luk S.C. (1980) *Campylobacter jejuni* enterocolitis: a clinicopathologic study. Archives of Pathology and Laboratory Medicine 104:571–574.

Collins R.H., Feldman M. and Fordtran J.S. (1987) Colon cancer, dysplasia, and surveillance in patients with ulcerative colitis. New England Journal of Medicine 316:1654–1658.

Colp R. (1934) A case of non-specific granuloma of the terminal ileum and cecum. Surgical Clinics of North America 14:443–449.

Cook M.G. and Goligher J.C. (1975) Carcinoma and epithelial dysplasia complicating ulcerative colitis. Gastroenterology 68:1127–1136.

Cooper C., Cotton D.W.K., Hudson M.J., Kirkham N. and Wilmott F.E.W. (1986) Rectal spirochaetosis in homosexual men: characterisation of the organism and pathophysiology. Genitourinary Medicine 62:47–52.

Cornes J.S. (1965) Number, size and distribution of Peyer's patches in the human small intestine. Gut 6:225–233.

Cotton P.B. and Lea Thomas M. (1971) Ischaemic colitis and the contraceptive pill. British Medical Journal 3:27–28.

Coverlizza S., Ferrari A., Scevola F., Gemme C., Cavallero M., Spandre M., Risio M. and Rossini F.P. (1986) Clinico-pathological features of collagenous colitis: case report and literature review. American Journal of Gastroenterology 81:1098–1103.

Cox G.J., Matsui S.M., Lo R.S. et al (1994) Etiology and outcome of diarrhea after marrow transplantation: a prospective study. Gastroenterology 107:1398–1407.

Craft C.F., Mendelsohn G., Cooper H.S. and Yardley J.H. (1981) Colonic ''precancer'' in Crohn's disease. Gastroenterology 80:578–584.

Crama-Bohbouth G., Bosman F.T., Vermeer B.J., van der Wal A.M., Biemond I., Weterman I.T. and Pena A.S. (1983) Immunohistological findings in lip biopsy specimens from patients with Crohn's disease and healthy subjects. Gut 24:202–205.

Craner G.E. and Burdick G.E. (1976) Acute colitis resembling ulcerative colitis in the hemolytic-uremic syndrome. American Journal of Digestive Diseases 21:74–76.

Cristina M.L., Lehy T., Voillemot N., Arhan P., Pellerin D. and Bonfils S. (1978) Endocrine cells of the colon in Hirschsprung's and control children. Virchows Archiv A 377:287–300.

Crohn B.B., Ginzburg L. and Oppenheimer G.D. (1932) Regional ileitis: a pathological and clinical entity. Journal of the American Medical Association 99:1323–1328.

Croom R.D., Donovan M.L. and Schwesinger W.H. (1984) Intestinal endometriosis. American Journal of Surgery 148:660-667.

Crucioli V. (1972) Rectal biopsy in Crohn's disease. Rendiconti di Gastroenterologia 4:73–80.

Crucioli V. and Busuttil A. (1981) Human intestinal spirochaetosis. Scandinavian Journal of Gastroenterology 16 (suppl 70):177–179.

Currie A.R. (1990) Human balantidiasis: a case report. South African Journal of Surgery 28:23–25.

Cuvelier C.A., Morson B.C. and Roels H.J. (1987) The DNA content in cancer and dysplasia in chronic ulcerative colitis. Histopathology 11:927–939.

Dale G., Bonham J.R., Lowdon P., Wagget J., Rangecroft L. and Scott D.J. (1979) Diagnostic value of rectal mucosal acetylcholinesterase levels in Hirschsprung's disease. Lancet i:347–349.

Daly J.J. and Chowdary K.V.S. (1983) Pseudomembranous colitis secondary to metronidazole. Digestive Diseases and Sciences 28:573–574.

Dankwa E.K. and Davies J.D. (1988) Smooth muscle pseudotumours: a potentially confusing artefact of rectal biopsy. Journal of Clinical Pathology 41:737–741.

Danzi J.T., McDonald T.J. and King J. (1988) Collagenous colitis. American Journal of Gastroenterology 83:83–85.

Das K.M., Morecki R., Nair P. and Berkowitz J.M. (1977) Idiopathic proctitis: the morphology of proximal colonic mucosa and its clinical significance. American Journal of Digestive Diseases 22:524–528.

Davidson B.R. and Everson N.W. (1987) Colonic stricture secondary to blunt abdominal trauma: report of a case and review of the aetiology. Postgraduate Medical Journal 63:911–913.

Dawson I.M.P. and Pryse-Davies J. (1959) The development of carcinoma of the large intestine in ulcerative colitis. British Journal of Surgery 47:113–128.

Day D.L., Ramsay N.K.C. and Letourneau J.G. (1988) Pneumatosis intestinalis after bone marrow transplantation. American Journal of Radiology 151:85–87.

Deana D.G. and Dean P.J. (1995) Reversible ischemic colitis in young women. American Journal of Surgical Pathology 19:454–462.

Debongnie J.C., De Galocsy C., Caholessur M.O. and Haot J. (1984) Collagenous colitis: a transient condition? Diseases of the Colon and Rectum 27:672–676.

De Chadarevian J-P., Slim M. and Akel S. (1982) Double zonal aganglionosis in long segment Hirschsprung's disease with a "skip area" in transverse colon. Journal of Pediatric Surgery 17:195–197.

Dechelotte P., Kantelip B., de Laguillaumie B.V., Labbe A. and Meyer M. (1985) Tangier disease: a histological and ultrastructural study. Pathology, Research and Practice 180:424-430.

Devereaux C.E. and Devereaux R.G. (1994) Heterotopic gastric mucosa of the rectum with a review of the literature. Journal of Clinical Gastroenterology 19:41–45.

Devroede G., Vobecky S., Masse S., Arhan P., Leger C., Duguay C. and Hemond M. (1982) Ischemic fecal incontinence and rectal angina. Gastroenterology 83:970–980.

Dickinson R.J., Rampling A. and Wight D.G.D. (1985) Spontaneous pseudomembranous colitis not associated with *Clostridium difficile*. Journal of Infection 10:252–255.

Dillard R.P. (1983) Hemolytic-uremic syndrome mimicking ulcerative colitis: lack of early diagnostic laboratory findings. Clinical Pediatrics 22:66–67.

Doman D.B., Golding M.I., Goldberg H.J. and Doyle R.B. (1989) *Aeromonas hydrophila* colitis presenting as medically refractory inflammatory bowel disease. American Journal of Gastroenterology 84:83–85.

Doolas A., Breyer R.H. and Franklin J.L. (1979) Pneumatosis cystoides intestinalis following jejunoileal by-pass. American Journal of Gastroenterology 72:271–275.

Doub H.P. and Shea J.J. (1960) Pneumatosis cystoides intestinalis. Journal of American Medical Association 172:1328–1342.

Douglas J.G. and Crucioli V. (1981) Spirochaetosis: a remediable cause of diarrhoea and rectal bleeding? British Medical Journal 283:1362.

Dronfield M.W., Fletcher J. and Langman M.J.S. (1974) Coincident salmonella infections and ulcerative colitis: problems of recognition and management. British Medical Journal 19:99–100.

Duffy T.J. (1981) Reversible ischaemic colitis in young adults. British Journal of Surgery 68:34–37.

Dundas S.A.C., Kay R., Beck S., Cotton D.W.K., Coup A.J., Slater D.N. and Underwood J.C.E. (1987) Can histopathologists reliably assess dysplasia in chronic inflammatory bowel disease? Journal of Clinical Pathology 40:1282–1286.

Dvorak A.M., Monahan R.A., Osage J.E. and Dickersin G.R. (1980) Crohn's disease: transmission electron microscopic studies. Human Pathology 11:606–619.

Dyer N.H., Stansfeld A.G. and Dawson A.M. (1970) The value of rectal biopsy in the diagnosis of Crohn's disease. Scandinavian Journal of Gastroenterology 5:491–496.

Eaves E.R., McIntyre R.L.E., Wallis P.L. and Korman M.G. (1983) Collagenous colitis: a recently recognised reversible clinico-pathological entity. Australian and New Zealand Journal of Medicine 13:630–632.

Eckstein R.P., Dowsett J.F. and Riley J.W. (1988) Collagenous enterocolitis: a case of collagenous colitis with involvement of the small intestine. American Journal of Gastroenterology 83:767–771.

Editorial (1987) *Clostridium septicum* and neutropenic enterocolitis. Lancet ii:608.

Editorial (1988) Which type of colitis? Lancet i:336.

Editorial (1989) Diversion colitis. Lancet i:764.

Edouard A., Jouannelle A., Amar A., Doutone P., Maurice P. and Galand A. (1983) Heterotopie de muqueuse gastrique dans le rectum avec ulceration. Gastroenterology and Clinical Biology 7:39–42.

Edwards F.C. and Truelove S.C. (1964) The course and prognosis of ulcerative colitis. Gut 5:15–22.

Ehsanullah M., Filipe M.I. and Gazzard B. (1982) Morphological and mucus secretion criteria for differential diagnosis of solitary ulcer syndrome and non-specific proctitis. Journal of Clinical Pathology 35:26–30.

Ehsanullah M., Morgan M.N., Filipe M.I. and Gazzard B. (1985) Sialomucins in the assessment of dysplasia and cancer-risk patients with ulcerative colitis treated with colectomy and ileorectal anastomosis. Histopathology 9:223–235.

Ekbom A., Wakefield A.J., Zack M. and Adami H.O. (1994) Perinatal measles infection and subsequent Crohn's disease. Lancet 344:508–510.

Elliott P.R., Williams C.B., Lennard-Jones J.E., Dawson A.M., Bartram C.I., Thomas B.M., Swarbrick E.T. and Morson B.C. (1982) Colonoscopic diagnosis of minimal change colitis in patients with a normal sigmoidoscopy and normal air-contrast barium enema. Lancet i:650–651.

El-Mouzan M.I., Satti M.B., Al-Quorain A.A. and El-Ageb A. (1988) Colonic malacoplakia: occurrence in a family: report of cases. Diseases of the Colon and Rectum 31:390–393.

Epstein R.J., McDonald G.B., Sale G.E., Shulman H.M. and Thomas E.D. (1980) The diagnostic accuracy of the rectal biopsy in acute graft-versus-host disease: a prospective study of thirteen patients. Gastroenterology 78:764–771.

Evans D.J. and Pollock D.J. (1972) In-situ and invasive carcinoma of the colon in patients with ulcerative colitis. Gut 13:566–570.

Fabricious P.J., Gyde S.N., Shouler P., Keighley M.R.B., Alexander-Williams J. and Allan R.N. (1985) Crohn's disease in the elderly. Gut 26:461–465.

Fadda B., Maier W.A., Meier-Ruge W., Scharli A. and Daum R. (1983) Neuronale intestinale dysplasie: eine kritische 10-Jahres-analyse klinischer und bioptischer diagnostick. Zeitschrift für Kinderchirurgie 38:305–311.

Fahal A.H., Baraka O.Z. and el Lider A.M. (1994) Pneumatosis cystoid intestinalis: a case report. East African Medical Journal 71:401–402.

Fan S.T., Lau W.Y. and Wong K.K. (1986) Ischemic colitis in Kawasaki disease. Journal of Pediatric Surgery 21:964–965.

Farah D.A., Mills P.R., Lee F.D., McLay A. and Russell R.I. (1985) Collagenous colitis: possible response to sulfasalazine and local steroid therapy. Gastroenterology 88:792–797.

Farmer R.G. and Brown C.H. (1972) Emerging concepts of proctosigmoiditis. Diseases of the Colon and Rectum 15:142–146.

Fausa O., Foerster A. and Hovig T. (1985) Collagenous colitis: a clinical, histological and ultrastructural study. Scandinavian Journal of Gastroenterology 20 (suppl 107):8–23.

Feinberg S.B., Schwartz M.Z., Clifford S., Buchwald H. and Varco R.L. (1977) Significance of pneumatosis cystoides intestinalis after jejunoileal bypass. American Journal of Surgery 133:149–152.

Fekete C.N., Ricour C., Martelli H., Jacob S.L. and Pellerin D. (1986) Total colonic aganglionosis (with or without ileal involvement): a review of 27 cases. Journal of Pediatric Surgery 21:251–254.

Fielding J.F. and Lumsden K. (1973) Large-bowel perforations in patients undergoing sigmoidoscopy and barium enema. British Medical Journal 1:471–473.

Figueroa-Colon R., Grunow J.E., Torres-Pinedo R. and Rettig P.J. (1984) Group A streptococcal proctitis and vulvovaginitis in a prepubertal girl. Pediatric Infectious Disease 3:439–441.

Filipe M.I., Edwards M.R. and Ehsanullah M (1985) A prospective study of dysplasia and carcinoma in the rectal biopsies and rectal stump of eight patients following ileorectal anastomosis in ulcerative colitis. Histopathology 9:1139–1153.

Fishel R., Hamamoto G., Barbul A., Jiji V. and Efron G. (1985) Cocaine colitis: is this a new syndrome? Diseases of the Colon and Rectum 28:264–266.

Flejou J.F., Grimaud J.A., Molas G., Baviera E. and Potet F. (1984) Collagenous colitis: ultrastructural study and collagen immunotyping of four cases. Archives of Pathology and Laboratory Medicine 108:977–982.

Flejou J.F., Potet F., Bogomoletz W.V., Rigaud C., Fenzy A., Le Quintrec Y., Goldfain D. and Brousse N. (1988) Lymphoid follicular proctitis: a condition different from ulcerative proctitis? Digestive Diseases and Sciences 33:314–320.

Floch M.H. and Hellman L. (1965) The effect of 5-fluorouracil on rectal mucosa. Gastroenterology 48:430–437.

Foerster A. and Fausa O. (1985) Collagenous colitis. Pathology, Research and Practice 180:99–104.

Ford M.J., Anderson J.R., Gilmour H.M., Holt S., Sircus W. and Heading R.C. (1983) Clinical spectrum of "solitary ulcer" of the rectum. Gastroenterology 84:1533–1540.

Foucar E., Mukai K., Foucar K., Sutherland D.E.R. and Van Buren C.T. (1981) Colon ulceration in lethal cytomegalovirus infection. American Journal of Clinical Pathology 76:788–801.

Fozard J.B.J. and Dixon M.F. (1989) Colonoscopic surveillance in ulcerative colitis: dysplasia through the looking glass. Gut 30:285–292.

Fozard J.B.J., Dixon M.F., Axon A.T.R. and Giles G.R. (1987) Lectin and mucin histochemistry as an aid to cancer surveillance in ulcerative colitis. Histopathology 11:385–394.

Fozard J.B.J., Quirke P., Dixon M.F., Giles G.R. and Bird C.C. (1986) DNA aneuploidy in ulcerative colitis. Gut 27:1414–1418.

Francois A., Dhib M., Eustache M.L., Etienne I., Scotte M., Lemoine F., Godin M. and Hemet J. (1994) Pseudomembranous colitis revealing adult hemolytic-uremic syndrome. Annales de Pathologie 14:182–185.

Franzin G., Dina R., Scarpa A. and Fratton A. (1982) "The evolution of the solitary ulcer of the rectum": an endoscopic and histopathological study. Endoscopy 14:131–134.

Freeman K., Anthony P.P., Miller D.S. and Warin A.P. (1985) Cronkhite-Canada syndrome: a new hypothesis. Gut 26:531–536.

Friedman N.B. (1942) Effects of radiation on the gastrointestinal tract including the salivary glands, the liver and the pancreas. Archives of Pathology 34:748–787.

Fujisawa K., Watanabe H., Yamamoto K., Nasu T., Kitahara Y. and Nakano M. (1989) Primary atypical mycobacteriosis of the intestine: a report of three cases. Gut 30:541–545.

Gad A. (1983) The pathogenicity of intestinal spirochaetosis. Histopathology 7:140–141.

Gad A., Willen R., Furugard K., Forbes B. and Hradsky M. (1977) Intestinal spirochaetosis as a cause of longstanding diarrhoea. Upsala Journal of Medical Sciences 82:49–54.

Gafni J. and Sohar E. (1960) Rectal biopsy for the diagnosis of amyloidosis. Americal Journal of Medical Science 240:332–336.

Galian A., Le Charpentier Y., Goldfain D. and Chauveinc L. (1982) La colite collagene: a propos d'un nouveau cas avec etude ultrastructurale. Gastroenterology and Clinical Biology 6:365–370.

Galland R.B. and Spencer J. (1985) The natural history of clinically established radiation enteritis. Lancet i:1257–1258.

Gambescia R.A., Kaufman B., Noy J., Young J. and Tedesco F.J. (1976) *Schistosoma mansoni* infection of the colon: a case report and review of the late colonic manifestations. American Journal of Digestive Diseases 21:988–991.

Gardiner G.W., Goldberg R., Currie D. and Murray D. (1984) Colonic carcinoma associated with an abnormal collagen table. Cancer 54:2973–2977.

Gardiner G.W., McAuliffe N., and Murray D. (1984) Colitis cystica profunda occurring in a radiation-induced colonic stricture. Human Pathology 15:295–298.

Gebbers J-O., Ferguson D.J.P., Mason C., Kelly P. and Jewell D.P. (1987) Spirochaetosis of the human rectum associated with an intraepithelial mast cell and IgE plasma cell response. Gut 28:588–593.

Gebbers J-O. and Laissue J.A. (1994) Diarrhea due to rare forms of colitis: microscopic colitis and spirochetosis. Schweizerische Medizinische Wochenschrift 124:1852–1861.

Geboes K., Spiessens C., Nijs G. and de Witte P. (1993) Anthranoids and the mucosal immune system of the colon. Pharmacology 47 (suppl 1):49–57.

George W.L. (1984) Antimicrobial agent–associated colitis and diarrhea: historical background and clinical aspects. Reviews of Infectious Diseases 6:s208–s213.

George W.L., Nakata M.M., Thompson J. and White M.L. (1985) *Aeromonas*-related diarrhea in adults. Archives of Internal Medicine 145:2207–2211.

George W.L., Rolfe R.D., and Finegold S.M. (1982) *Clostridium difficile* and its cytotoxin in feces of patients with antimicrobial agent–associated diarrhea and miscellaneous conditions. Journal of Clinical Microbiology 15:1049–1053.

Geraghty J.M. and Charles A.K. (1994). Aphthoid ulceration in diversion colitis. Histopathology 24:395–397.

Ghadially F.N., Boone S.A. and Walley V.M. (1993) A comparison of the ultrastructure of pigment granules in melanosis ilei and pulmonary lymph nodes. Histopathology 23:167–172.

Ghadially F.N. and Walley V.M. (1994) Melanoses of the gastrointestinal tract. Histopathology 25:197–207.

Giardiello F.M., Bayless T.M., Jessurun J., Hamilton S.R. and Yardley J.H. (1987) Collagenous colitis: physiologic and histopathologic studies in seven patients. Annals of Internal Medicine 106:46–49.

Giardiello F.M., Hansen F.C. III, Lazenby A.J., Hellman D.B., Milligan F.D., Bayless T.M. and Yardley J.H. (1990) Collagenous colitis in setting of nonsteroidal antiinflammatory drugs and antibiotics. Digestive Diseases and Sciences 35:257–260.

Gibson G.E., Rowland R., and Hecker R. (1975) Diarrhoea and colitis associated with antibiotic treatment: a report of 16 cases. Australian and New Zealand Journal of Medicine 5:340–347.

Gillen C.D., Andrews H.A., Prior P. and Allan R.N. (1994) Crohn's disease and colorectal cancer. Gut 35:651–655.

Gilman R., Islam M., Paschi S., Goleburn J. and Ahmad F. (1980) Comparison of conventional and immunofluorescent techniques for the detection of *Entamoeba histolytica* in rectal biopsies. Gastroenterology 78:435–439.

Gleason T.H. and Patterson S.D. (1982) The pathology of *Yersinia enterocolitica* ileocolitis. American Journal of Surgical Pathology 6:347–355.

Gledhill A., Enticott M.E. and Howe S. (1986) Variation in the argyrophil cell population of the rectum in ulcerative colitis and adenocarcinoma. Journal of Pathology 149:287–291.

Gledhill A., Hall P.A., Cruse J.P. and Pollock D.J. (1986) Enteroendocrine cell hyperplasia, carcinoid tumours and adenocarcinoma in long-standing ulcerative colitis. Histopathology 10:501–508.

Glotzer D.J., Glick M.E. and Goldman H. (1981) Proctitis and colitis following diversion of the fecal stream. Gastroenterology 80:438–441.

Goldblum J.R., Beals T. and Weiss S.W. (1992) Elastofibromatous change of the rectum: a lesion mimicking amyloidosis. American Journal of Surgical Pathology 16:793–795.

Goldfain D., Potet F., Chauveinc L. and Rozenberg H. (1981) Lipomatose rectale: association a une lipomatose pelvienne. Gastroenterology and Clinical Biology 5:884–891.

Goldman H. and Proujansky R. (1986) Allergic proctitis and gastroenteritis in children. American Journal of Surgical Pathology 10:75–86.

Gonzalez-Angulo A., Corral E., Garcia-Torres R. and Quijano M. (1965) Malakoplakia of the colon. Gastroenterology 48:383–387.

Goodlad R.A. and Wright N.A. (1995) Epithelial kinetics, control and consequences of alteration in disease. In: Gastrointestinal and Oesophageal Pathology. Edited by R. Whitehead. Edinburgh: Churchill Livingstone, pp 97–115.

Goodman M.J., Skinner J.M. and Truelove S.C. (1976) Abnormalities in the apparently normal bowel mucosa in Crohn's disease. Lancet i:275–278.

Gore R.M. (1982) Acute colitis and the hemolytic-uremic syndrome. Diseases of the Colon and Rectum 25:589–591.

Gore R.M., Marn C.S., Ujiki G.T., Craig R.M., and Marquardt J. (1983) Ischemic colitis associated with systemic lupus erythematosus. Diseases of the Colon and Rectum 26:449–451.

Gould S.R., Handley A.J. and Barnardo D.E. (1973) Rectal and gastric involvement in a case of sarcoidosis. Gut 14:971–973.

Goulston S.J.M. and McGovern V.J. (1965) Pseudo-membranous colitis. Gut 6:207–212.

Goulston S.J.M. and McGovern V.J. (1969) The nature of benign strictures in ulcerative colitis. New England Journal of Medicine 281: 290-295.

Gourevitch A. and Cunningham I.J. (1959) Sarcoidosis of the sigmoid colon. Postgraduate Medical Journal 35:689–691.

Graham C.F., Gallagher K. and Jones J.K. (1981) Acute colitis with methyldopa. New England Journal of Medicine 304:1044–1045.

Graham J.M., Marin-Padilla M. and Hoefnagel D. (1983) Jejunal atresia associated with Cafergot ingestion during pregnancy. Clinical Pediatrics 22:226–228.

Gramlich T.L. and Hunter S.B. (1994). Focal polypoid ischemia of the colon: atheroemboli presenting as a colonic polyp. Archives of Pathology and Laboratory Medicine 118:308–309.

Grant D.J., Sanders D.S., McMurdo M.E. and Lyall M.H. (1993) Recurrent anaemia due to ischaemic colonic ulceration caused by cholesterol embolism. Postgraduate Medical Journal 69:320–322.

Gratama S., Smedts F. and Whitehead R. (1995) Obstructive colitis: an analysis of 50 cases and a review of the literature. Pathology 27:324–329.

Greaney M.G. and Jackson P.R. (1977) Oleogranuloma of the rectum produced by Lasonil ointment. British Medical Journal 2:997–998.

Green E.S., Parker N.E., Gellert A.R. and Beck E.R. (1984) *Campylobacter* infection mimicking Crohn's disease in an immunodeficient patient. British Journal of Medicine 289:159–160.

Green P.A., Higgins J.A., Brown A.L. Jr, Hoffman H.N. and Sommerville R.L. (1961) Amyloidosis: appraisal of intubation biopsy of the small intestine in diagnosis. Gastroenterology 41:452–456.

Greenstein A.J., Mullin G.E., Strauchen J.A., Heimann T., Janowitz H.D., Aufses A.H. Jr and Sachar D.B. (1992) Lymphoma in inflammatory bowel disease. Cancer 69:1119–1123.

Groisman G.M., George J. and Harpaz N. (1994) Ulcerative appendicitis in universal and nonuniversal ulcerative colitis. Modern Pathology 7:322–325.

Grouls V., Vogel J. and Sorger M. (1982) Collagenous colitis. Endoscopy 14:31–33.

Gruenberg J.C., Grodsinsky C. and Ponka J.L. (1979) Pneumatosis intestinalis: a clinical classification. Diseases of the Colon and Rectum 22:5–9.

Gryboski J.D. (1967) Gastrointestinal mild allergy in infants. Pediatrics 40:354–362.

Guss C. and Larsen J.G. (1984) Group A beta-hemolytic streptococcal proctocolitis. Pediatric Infectious Disease 3:442–443.

Gyde S.N., Prior P., Allan R.N., Stevens A., Jewell D.P., Truelove S.C., Lofberg R., Brostrom O. and Hellers G. (1988) Colorectal cancer in ulcerative colitis: a cohort study of primary referrals from three centres. Gut 29:206–217.

Gyde S.N., Prior P., Macartney J.C. and Thompson H. (1980) Malignancy in Crohn's disease. Gut 21:1024–1029.

Haber M.M., Burrell M. and West A.B. (1993) Enterocolic lymphocytic phlebitis: clinical, radiologic, and pathologic features. Journal of Gastroenterology 17:327–332.

Habib N.A., Dawson P.M., Krausz T., Blount M.A., Kersten D. and Wood C.B. (1986) A study of histochemical changes in mucus from patients with ulcerative colitis, Crohn's disease, and diverticular disease of the colon. Diseases of the Colon and Rectum 29:15–17.

Haboubi N.Y., Honan R.P., Hasleton P.S., Ali H.H., Anfield C., Hobbiss J. and Schofield P.F. (1984) Pneumatosis coli: a case report with ultrastructural study. Histopathology 8:145–155.

Haboubi N.Y., Schofield P.F. and Rowland P.L. (1988) The light and electron microscopic features of early and late phase radiation-induced proctitis. American Journal of Gastroenterology 83:1140–1144.

Haidar A. and Dixon M.F. (1992) Solitary microcarcinoid in ulcerative colitis. Histopathology 21:487–488.

Hall C.L. and Lampert P.W. (1985) Immunohistochemistry as an aid in the diagnosis of Hirschsprung's disease. American Journal of Clinical Pathology 83:177–181.

Hall R.I., Pehy A.H., Cobden I. and Lendrum R. (1983) Enteritis and colitis associated with mefenamic acid. British Medical Journal 287:1182.

Hamilton I., Sanders S., Hopwood D. and Bouchier I.A.D. (1986) Collagenous colitis associated with small intestinal villous atrophy. Gut 27:1394–1398.

Hamza M. (1993) Proctitis in Behçet disease: study of 6 cases. Revue du Rhumatisme, Edition Française 60:925–927.

Hansen C.R. and Louw P. (1993) Fatal transmural colitis caused by *Entamoeba histolytica*: differential diagnosis of chronic inflammatory bowel disease and colon cancer. Ugeskrift for Laeger 155:2901–2902.

Haque S., Eisen R.N. and West A.B. (1993) The morphologic features of diversion colitis: studies of a pediatric population with no other diseases of the intestinal mucosa. Human Pathology 24:211–219.

Harig J.M., Soergel K.H., Komorowski R.A. and Wood C.M. (1989) Treatment of diversion colitis and short-chain fatty acid irrigation. New England Journal of Medicine 320:23–28.

Harland W.A. and Lee F.D. (1967) Intestinal spirochaetosis. British Medical Journal 3:718–719.

Harned R.K., Buck J.L. and Sobin L.H. (1995) The hamartomatous polyposis syndromes: clinical and radiologic features. American Journal of Roentgenology 164:565–571.

Hasleton P.S., Carr N. and Schofield P.F. (1985) Vascular changes in radiation bowel disease. Histopathology 9:517–534.

Hawker P.C., Hine K.R., Burdon D.W., Thompson H. and Keighley M.R.B. (1981) Fatal pseudomembranous colitis despite eradication of *Clostridium difficile*. British Medical Journal 282:109–110.

Haworth S.J. and Pusey C.D. (1984) Severe intestinal involvement in Wegener's granulomatosis. Gut 25:1296–1300.

Heatley R.V. and James P.D. (1978) Eosinophils in the rectal mucosa. Gut 20:787–791.

Heer M., Altorfer J., Pirovino M. and Schmid M. (1983) Pneumatosis cystoides coli: a rare complication of colonoscopy. Endoscopy 15:119–120.

Heer M., Repond F., Hany A., Sulser H., Kehl O. and Jager K. (1987) Acute ischaemic colitis in a female long-distance runner. Gut 28:896–899.

Heizer W.D., Warshaw A.L., Waldmann T.A. and Laster L. (1968) Protein-losing gastroenteropathy and malabsorption associated with factitious diarrhoea. Annals of Internal Medicine 68:839–852.

Helliwell T.R., Flook D., Whitworth J. and Day D.W. (1985) Arteritis and venulitis in systemic lupus erythematosus resulting in massive lower intestinal haemorrhage. Histopathology 9:1103–1113.

Henriksson L., Liljeholm H. and Lonnerholm T. (1984) Pelvic lipomatosis causing constriction of the lower urinary tract and the rectum. Scandinavian Journal of Urology and Nephrology 18:249–252.

Heron H.C., Khubchandani I.T., Trimpi H.D., Sheets J.A. and Stasik J.J. (1981) Evanescent colitis. Diseases of the Colon and Rectum 24:555–561.

Herrera J.M., Vega P., Caravaca F., Soria A., Sáenz de Santa María J., Pascasio J.M., Márquez J.L. and Pabón M (1991) Amyloid colitis. Revista Española de Enfermedades Digestivas 80:120–122.

Herrerias J.M., Muniain M.A., Sanchez S. and Garrido M. (1983) Alcohol induced colitis. Endoscopy 15:121–122.

Hiatt G.A. (1978) Miliary tuberculosis with ileocecal involvement diagnosed by colonoscopy. Journal of the American Medical Association 240:561–563.

Hill D.H., Mills J.O. and Maxwell R.J. (1993) Metachronous colonic lymphomas complicating chronic ulcerative colitis. Abdominal Imaging 18:369–370.

Hirata I., Berrebi G., Austin L.L., Keren D.F. and Dobbins W.O. (1986) Immunohistological characterization of intraepithelial and lamina propria lymphocytes in control ileum and colon and in inflammatory bowel disease. Digestive Diseases and Sciences 31:593–603.

Hirobe S., Doody D.P., Ryan D.P., Kim S.H. and Donahoe P.K. (1992) Ectopic class II major histocompatibility antigens in Hirschsprung's disease and neuronal intestinal dysplasia. Journal of Pediatric Surgery 27:357–362.

Ho M.S., Teh L.B. and Goh H.S. (1987) Ischaemic colitis in systemic lupus erythematosus: report of a case and review of the literature. Annals of the Academy of Medicine 16:501–503.

Holdsworth C.D. (1984) Acute self-limited colitis. British Medical Journal 289:270–271.

Holl K., Nolte H., Zornig C. and Schroder S. (1993) Pneumatosis intestinalis: histology, immunocytochemistry and new theory of morphogenesis. Pathologe 14:199–204.

Houghton B.J. and Pears M.A. (1958) Chronic potassium depletion due to purgation with cascara. British Medical Journal 1:1328–1330.

Hovind-Hougen K., Birch-Andersen A., Henrik-Nielsen R., Orholm M., Pedersen J.O., Teglbjaerg P.S. and Thaysen E.H. (1982) Intestinal spirochetosis: morphological characterization and cultivation of the spirochete *Brachyspira aalborgi* gen. nov., sp. nov. Journal of Clinical Microbiology 16:1127–1136.

Hunt D.R. and Mildenhall P. (1975) Etiology of strictures of the colon associated with pancreatitis. American Journal of Digestive Diseases 20:941–946.

Huntley C.C., Shaffner L. de S., Challa V.R. and Lyerly A.D. (1982) Histochemical diagnosis of Hirschsprung disease. Pediatrics 69:755–761.

Hyams J.S., Haswell J.E., Gerber M.A. and Berman M.M. (1985) Colonic ulceration in histiocytosis X. Journal of Pediatric Gastroenterology and Nutrition 4:286–290.

Hyams J.S. and McLaughlin J.C. (1985) Lack of relationship between *Clostridium difficile* toxin and inflammatory bowel disease in children. Journal of Clinical Gastroenterology 7:387–390.

Iliffe G.D. and Owen D.A. (1981) Rectal biopsy in Crohn's disease. Digestive Diseases and Sciences 26:321–324.

Imamura T., Tsuruta J., Kambara T. and Maki S. (1986) Pseudomembranous colitis in a patient of paraquat intoxication. Acta Pathologica Japonica 36:309–316.

Innes A., Rowe P.A., Foster M.C., Steiger M.J. and Morgan A.G. (1988) Cyclosporin toxicity and colitis. Lancet ii:957.

Isaacs D., Wright V.M., Shaw D.G., Raafat F. and Walker-Smith J.A. (1985) Chronic granulomatous disease mimicking Crohn's disease. Journal of Pediatric Gastroenterology and Nutrition 4:498–501.

Islam M.M., Azad A.K., Bardhan P.K., Raqib R. and Islam D. (1994) Pathology of shigellosis and its complications. Histopathology 24:65–71.

Jablonski M., Putzki H. and Heymann H. (1987) Necrosis of the ascending colon in chronic hemodialysis patients. Diseases of the Colon and Rectum 30:623–625.

Jacob E., Baker S.J. and Swaminathan S.P. (1987) ''M'' cells in the follicle-associated epithelium of the human colon. Histopathology 11:941–952.

Jager W.A., Den Hartog and Bethlem J. (1960) The distribution of Lewy bodies in the central and autonomic nervous system in idiopathic paralysis agitans. Journal of Neurology, Neurosurgery and Psychiatry 23:283–290.

Jenkins H.R., Pincott J.R., Soothill J.F., Milla P.J. and Harries J.T. (1984) Food allergy: the major cause of infantile colitis. Archives of Disease in Childhood 59:326–329.

Jess P. (1981) Acute terminal ileitis: a review of recent literature on the relationship to Crohn's disease. Scandinavian Journal of Gastroenterology 16:321–324.

Jessurun J., Paplanus S.H., Nagle R.B., Hamilton S.R., Yardley J.H. and Tripp M. (1986) Pseudosarcomatous changes in inflammatory pseudopolyps of the colon. Archives of Pathology and Laboratory Medicine 110:833–836.

Jessurun J., Yardley J.H., Giardiello F.M., Hamilton S.R. and Bayless T.M. (1987) Chronic colitis with thickening of the subepithelial collagen layer: collagenous colitis. Human Pathology 18:839–848.

Jessurun J., Yardley J.H., Lee E.L., Vendrell D.D., Schiller L.R. and Fordtran J.S. (1986) Microscopic and collagenous colitis: different names for the same condition? Gastroenterology 91:1583–1584.

John A., Dickey K., Fenwick J., Sussman B. and Beeken W. (1992) Pneumatosis intestinalis in patients with Crohn's disease. Digestive Diseases and Sciences 37:813–817.

Jonas G., Mahoney A., Murray J. and Gertler S. (1988) Chemical colitis due to endoscope cleaning solutions: a mimic of pseudomembranous colitis. Gastroenterology 95:1403–1408.

Jones H.W., Grogono J. and Hoare A.M. (1988) Surveillance in ulcerative colitis: burdens and benefit. Gut 29:325–331.

Jorgensen A. and Wille-Jorgensen P. (1982) Pneumatosis intestinalis and pncumopcritoncum duc to a solitary sigmoid diverticulum. Acta Chirurgica Scandinavica 148:625–626.

Jung H.C., Rhee P.L., Song I.S., Choi K.W. and Kim C.Y. (1991) Temporal changes in the clinical type or diagnosis of colonic ulcerations. Journal of Korean Medical Science 6:313–318.

Justus P.G., Martin J.L., Goldberg D.A., Taylor N.S., Bartlett J.G., Alexander R.W. and Mathias J.R. (1982) Myoelectric effects of *Clostridium difficile:* motility-altering factors distinct from its cytotoxin and enterotoxin in rabbits. Gastroenterology 83:836–843.

Kalkay M.N., Ayanian Z.S., Lehaf E.A. and Baldi A. (1983) *Campylobacter*-induced toxic megacolon. American Journal of Gastroenterology 78:557–559.

Kalla A.H., Lee K.U. and Voss E.C. Jr. (1980) The dilemma of colonic vasculitis: report of a unique case. Diseases of the Colon and Rectum 23:590–596.

Kangas E., Matikainen M. and Mattila J. (1994) Is "indeterminate colitis" Crohn's disease in the long-term follow-up? International Surgery 79:120–123.

Kaplan L.R. and Takeuchi A. (1979) Purulent rectal discharge associated wih a nontreponemal spirochete. Journal of the American Medical Association 241:52–53.

Kapur B.M.L. and Chopra P. (1978) Necrotizing amebic colitis: report of five cases. Diseases of the Colon and Rectum 21:447–449.

Kasbohrer A., Gelderblom H.R., Arasteh K., Heise W., Grosse G., L'age M., Schoenberg A, Koch M.A. and Pauli G. (1990) Intestinal spirochetosis in HIV infection: prevalence, isolation and morphology of spirochetes. Deutsche Medizinische Wochenschrift 115:1499–1506.

Katayama Y., Kimura M. and Konn M. (1985) Cronkhite-Canada syndrome associated with a rectal cancer and adenomatous changes in colonic polyps. American Journal of Surgical Pathology 9:65–71.

Katoh K., Matsunaga K., Ishigatsubo Y., Chiba J., Tani K., Kitamura H., Tani S. and Handwerger B.S. (1985) Pathologically defined neuro-, vasculo-, entero-Behçet's disease. Journal of Rheumatology 12:1186–1190.

Kaufmann H.J. and Taubin H.L. (1987) Nonsteroidal anti-inflammatory drugs activate quiescent inflammatory bowel disease. Annals of Internal Medicine 107:513–516.

Kawaguchi M., Koizumi F., Shimao M. and Hirose S. (1993) Protein-losing enteropathy due to secondary amyloidosis of the gastrointestinal tract. Acta Pathologica Japonica 43:333–339.

Kealy W.F. (1976a) Colonic lymphoid glandular complex (microbursa) nature and morphology. Journal of Clinical Pathology 29:241–244.

Kealy W.F. (1976b) Lymphoid tissue and lymphoid-glandular complexes of the colon: relation to diverticulosis. Journal of Clinical Pathology, 29:245–249.

Keefe E.B. and Girard D.E. (1985) Peanut shell colitis. Archives of Internal Medicine 145:1314–1315.

Kelly J., Oryshak A., Wenetsek M., Grabiec J. and Handy S. (1990) The colonic pathology of *Escherichia coli* 0157:H7 infection. American Journal of Surgical Pathology 14:87–92.

Kelly J.K., Langevin J.M., Price L.M., Hershfield N.B., Share S. and Blustein P. (1986) Giant and symptomatic inflammatory polyps of the colon in idiopathic inflammatory bowel disease. American Journal of Surgical Pathology 10:420–428.

Kelly J.K., Pai C.H., Jadusingh I.H., Macinnis M.L., Shaffer E.A. and Hershfield N.B. (1987) The histopathology of rectosigmoid biopsies from adults with bloody diarrhea due to verotoxin-producing *Escherichia coli.* American Journal of Clinical Pathology 88:78–82.

Kessler S. and Campbell J.R. (1985) Neuronal colonic dysplasia associated with short-segment Hirschsprung's disease. Archives of Pathology and Laboratory Medicine 109:532–533.

Keyting W.S., McCarver R.R., Kovarik J.L. and Daywitt A.I. (1961) Pneumatosis intestinalis: a new concept. Radiology 76:733–741.

Khan E.M. and Pandey R. (1993) Histological and mucin secretion patterns in solitary rectal ulcer syndrome. Indian Journal of Gastroenterology 12:47–48.

Killingback M.J. and Williams K.L. (1961) Necrotising colitis. British Journal of Surgery 49:175–185.

Kilpatrick Z.M., Farman J., Yesner R. and Spiro H.M. (1968) Ischemic proctitis. Journal of the American Medical Association 205:74–80.

Kim M.W., Hundahl S.A., Dang C.R., McNamara J.J., Straehley C.J. and Whelan T.J. (1983) Ischemic colitis after aortic aneurysmectomy. American Journal of Surgery 145:392–394.

Kim W.H., Choe G.Y., Kim Y.I. and Kim J.P. (1992) Localized form of colitis cystica profunda: a case of occurrence in the descending colon. Journal of Korean Medical Science 7:76–78.

Kinder R.B. and Jourdan M.H. (1985) Disseminated aspergillosis and bleeding colonic ulcers in renal transplant patient. Journal of the Royal Society of Medicine 78:338–339.

Kingham J.G.C., Levison D.A., Ball J.A. and Dawson A.M. (1982) Microscopic colitis: a cause of chronic watery diarrhoea. British Medical Journal 285:1601–1604.

Kingham J.G.C., Levison D.A., Morson B.C. and Dawson A.M. (1986) Collagenous colitis. Gut 27:570–577.

Kingsmore S.F., Kingsmore D.B., Hall B.D., Wilson J.A., Gottfried M.R. and Allen N.B. (1993) Co-occurrence of collagenous colitis with seronegative spondyloarthropathy: report of a case and literature review. Journal of Rheumatology 20:2153–2157.

Kirk M.E., Lough J. and Warner H.A. (1971) Histoplasma colitis: an electron microscopic study. Gastroenterology 61:46–54.

Knoepp L.F. Jr and Davis W.M. (1992) Solitary rectal ulcer syndrome: not always ulcerated. Southern Medical Journal 85:1033–1034.

Knutson L. and Arosenius K-E. (1984) Tuberculosis of the large bowel. Acta Chirurgica Scandinavica 150:345–348.

Kobayashi H., Hirakawa H., O'Briain D.S. and Puri P. (1994) Nerve growth factor receptor staining of suction biopsies in the diagnosis of Hirschsprung's disease. Journal of Pediatric Surgery 29:1224–1227.

Komorowski R.A., Cohen E.B., Kauffman H.M. and Adams M.B. (1986) Gastrointestinal complications in renal transplant recipients. American Journal of Clinical Pathology 86:161–167.

Kondo J., Ruth M., Sassaris M. and Hunter F.M. (1980) Sarcoidosis of the stomach and rectum. American Journal of Gastroenterology 73:516–518.

Korelitz B.I., Cheskin L.J., Sohn N. and Sommers S.C. (1984) Proctitis after fecal diversion in Crohn's disease and its elimination with reanastomosis: implications for surgical management: report of four cases. Gastroenterology 87:710–713.

Korelitz B.I. and Sommers S.C. (1977) Rectal biopsy in patients with Crohn's disease. Normal mucosa on sigmoidoscopic examination. Journal of the American Medical Association 237:2742–2744.

Koren G., Aladjem M., Militiano J., Seegal B., Jonash A. and Boichis H. (1984) Ischemic colitis in chronic intermittent peritoneal dialysis. Nephron 36:272–274.

Kornacki S., Hansen F.C. and Lazenby A. (1995) Graft-versus-host–like colitis associated with malignant thymoma. American Journal of Surgical Pathology 19:224–228.

Kornman B.S. (1971) Ulcerative colitis, autoimmune epiphenomena and colonic cancer. Cancer 28:82–88.

Koss L.G. (1952) Abdominal gas cysts (pneumatosis cystoides intestinorum hominis): analysis with report of case and critical review of literature. Archives of Pathology 53:523–549.

Kroft S.H., Stryker S.J. and Rao M.S. (1994) Appendiceal involvement as a skip lesion in ulcerative colitis. Modern Pathology 7:912–914.

Kucukaydin M., Patiroglu T.E., Okur H. and Icer M. (1992) Infantile Cronkhite-Canada syndrome? Case report. European Journal of Pediatric Surgery 2:295–297.

Kumar N.B., Nostrant T.T. and Appelman H.D. (1982) The histopathologic spectrum of acute self-limited colitis: acute infectious-type colitis. American Journal of Surgical Pathology 6:523–529.

Kumar S.S., Appavu S.S., Abcarian H. and Barreta T. (1983) Amyloidosis of the colon: report of a case and review of the literature. Diseases of the Colon and Rectum 26:541–544.

Kuramoto S., Oohara T., Ihara O., Shimazu R. and Kondo Y. (1987) Granulomas of the gut in Crohn's disease. Diseases of the Colon and Rectum 30:6–11.

Kurer M.H.J., Lawson J.O.N. and Pambakian H. (1986) Suction biopsy in Hirschsprung's disease. Archives of Disease in Childhood 61:83–84.

Kyle R.A., Spencer R.J. and Dahlin D.C. (1966) Value of rectal biopsy in the diagnosis of primary systemic amyloidosis. American Journal of Medical Science 251:501–506.

Kyosola K., Penttila O. and Salaspuro M. (1977) Rectal mucosal adrenergic innervation and enterochromaffin cells in ulcerative colitis and irritable colon. Scandinavian Journal of Gastroenterology 12:363–367.

Kyzer S., Korzets A., Zevin D., Rath-Wolfson L., Chagnac A., Chaimoff C. and Levi J. (1993) Ischemic colitis complicating AA amyloidosis and familial Mediterranean fever. Israel Journal of Medical Sciences 29:212–214.

Lake A.M., Whitington P.F. and Hamilton S.R. (1982) Dietary protein–induced colitis in breast-fed infants. Journal of Pediatrics 101:906–910.

Lake B.D. (1995) Hirschsprung's disease and related disorders. In: Gastrointestinal and Oesophageal Pathology. Edited by R. Whitehead. Edinburgh: Churchill Livingstone, pp 327–341.

Lake B.D., Nixon H.H. and Claireaux A.E. (1978) Hirschsprung's disease: an appraisal of histochemically demonstrated acetylcholinesterase activity in suction rectal biopsy specimens as an aid to diagnosis. Archives of Pathology and Laboratory Medicine 102:244–247.

Lambert M.E., Schofield P.F., Ironside A.G. and Mandal B.K. (1979) Campylobacter colitis. British Medical Journal 1:857–859.

Lampert I.A., Thorpe P., Van Noorden S., Marsh J., Goldman J.M., Gordon-Smith E.C. and Evans D.J. (1985) Selective sparing of enterochromaffin cells in graft versus host disease affecting the colonic mucosa. Histopathology 9:875–886.

Lamy A.L., Roy P.H., Morisette J-J. and Cantin R. (1988) Intimal hyperplasia and thrombosis of the visceral arteries in a young woman: possible relation with oral contraceptives and smoking. Surgery 103:706–710.

Langlois N.E., Park K.G. and Keenan R.A. (1994) Mucosal changes in the large bowel with endometriosis: a possible cause of misdiagnosis of colitis? Human Pathology 25:1030–1034.

Larson H.E. and Price A.B. (1977) Pseudomembranous colitis: presence of clostridial toxin. Lancet ii:1312–1314.

Larson H.E., Price A.B. and Honour P. (1978) *Clostridium difficile* and the aetiology of pseudomembranous colitis. Lancet i:1063–1066.

Lazenby A.J., Yardley J.H., Giardiello F.M., Jessurun J. and Bayless T.M. (1989) Lymphocytic ("microscopic") colitis: a comparative histopathologic study with particular reference to collagenous colitis. Human Pathology 20:18–28.

Lee E., Schiller L.R., Vendrell D., Santa-Ana C.A. and Fordtran J.S. (1992) Subepithelial collagen table thickness in colon specimens from patients with microscopic colitis and collagenous colitis. Gastroenterology 103:1790–1796.

Lee E.L., Smith H.J., Miller G.L., Burns D.K. and Weiner H. (1984) Ischemic pseudomembranous colitis with perforation due to polyarteritis nodosa. American Journal of Gastroenterology 79:35–38.

Lee F.D. (1993) Importance of apoptosis in the histopathology of drug-related lesions in the large intestine. Journal of Clinical Pathology 46:118–122.

Lee F.D. (1994) Drug-related pathological lesions of the intestinal tract. Histopathology 25:303–308.

Lee R.G. (1986) The colitis of Behçet's syndrome. American Journal of Surgical Pathology 10.888–893.

Lee R.G. (1987) Villous regeneration in ulcerative colitis. Archives of Pathology and Laboratory Medicine 111:276–278.

Lee S.H., Barnes W.G., Hodges G.R. and Dixon A. (1985) Perforated granulomatous colitis caused by *Histoplasma capsulatum*. Diseases of the Colon and Rectum 28:171–176.

Lefebvre M.P., Leape L.L., Pohl D.A., Safaii H. and Grand R.J. (1984) Total colonic aganglionosis initially diagnosed in an adolescent. Gastroenterology 87:1364–1366.

Leidenius M., Kellokumpu I., Husa A., Riihela M. and Sipponen P. (1991) Dysplasia and carcinoma in longstanding ulcerative colitis: an endoscopic and histological surveillance programme. Gut 32:1521–1525.

Lennard-Jones J.E., Morson B.C., Ritchie J.K. and Williams C.B. (1983) Cancer surveillance in ulcerative colitis. Lancet ii:149–152.

Leonard R.C.F. and MacLennan I.C.M. (1982) Distribution of plasma cells in normal rectal mucosa. Journal of Clinical Pathology 35:820–823.

Leoutsakos B., Agnadi N. and Kolisiatis S. (1977) Rectal bleeding due to *Esophagostomum brumpti*: report of a case. Diseases of the Colon and Rectum 20:632–634.

Leriche M., Devroede G., Sanchez G. and Rossano J. (1978) Changes in the rectal mucosa induced by hypertonic enemas. Diseases of the Colon and Rectum 21:227–236.

Levine D., Goode A.W. and Wingate D.L. (1981) Purgative abuse associated with reversible cachexia, hypogammaglobulinaemia, and finger clubbing. Lancet i:919–920.

Levine D.S. (1987) "Solitary" rectal ulcer syndrome: are "solitary" rectal ulcer syndrome and "localized" colitis cystica profunda analogous syndromes caused by rectal prolapse? Gastroenterology 92:243–253.

Levine D.S., Surawicz C.M., Ajer T.N., Dean P.J. and Rubin C.E. (1988) Diffuse excess mucosal collagen in rectal biopsies facilitates differential diagnosis of solitary rectal ulcer syndrome from other inflammatory bowel diseases. Digestive Diseases and Sciences 33:1345–1352.

Levine D.S., Surawicz C.M., Spencer G.D., Rohrmann C.A. and Silverstein F.E. (1986) Inflammatory polyposis two years after ischemic colon injury. Digestive Diseases and Sciences 31:1159–1167.

Levine M.M. (1987) *Escherichia coli* that cause diarrhea: enterotoxigenic, enteropathogenic, enteroinvasive, enterohemorrhagic, and enteroadherent. Journal of Infectious Diseases 155:377–389.

Levine T.S. and Price A.B. (1994) Obstructive enterocolitis: a clinico-pathological discussion. Histopathology 25.57–64.

Levison D.A., Crocker P.R., Smith A., Blackshaw A.J. and Bartram C.I. (1984) Varied light and scanning electron microscopic appearances of barium sulphate in smears and histological sections. Journal of Clinical Pathology 37:481–487.

Lewin K. and Swales J.D. (1966) Granulomatous colitis and atypical ulcerative colitis: histological features, behaviour, and prognosis. Gastroenterology 50:211–223.

Lewin K.J., Fair W.R., Steigbigel R.T., Winberg C.D. and Droller M.J. (1976) Clinical and laboratory studies into the pathogenesis of malacoplakia. Journal of Clinical Pathology 29:354–363.

Lewin K.J., Harell G.S., Lee A.S. and Crowley L.G. (1974) Malacoplakia: an electron-microscopic study: demonstration of bacilliform organisms in malacoplakic macrophages. Gastroenterology 66:28–45.

Lewis F.W., Warren G.H. and Goff J.S. (1991) Collagenous colitis with involvement of terminal ileum. Digestive Diseases and Sciences 36:1161–1163.

Lewkonia R.M. and McConnell R.B. (1976) Progress report: familial inflammatory bowel disease. Gut 17:235–243.

Lifshitz D., Cytron S., Yossiphov J., Lelcuk S. and Rabau M. (1994) Colitis cystica profunda: self-inflicted by rectal trauma? Report of a case. Digestive Diseases 12:318–320.

Lillee R.D. and Geer J.C. (1965) On the relation of enterosiderosis pigments of man and guinea pig: melanosis and pseudomelanosis of colon and villi and the intestinal iron uptake and storage mechanism: histochemical and experimental studies. American Journal of Pathology 47:965–1009.

Lillemoe K.D., Romolo J.L., Hamilton S.R., Pennington L.R., Burdick J.F. and Williams G.M. (1987) Intestinal necrosis due to sodium polystyrene (Kayexalate) in sorbitol enemas: clinical and experimental support for the hypothesis. Surgery 101:267–272.

Lindstrom C.G. (1976) "Collagenous colitis" with watery diarrhoea: a new entity? Pathologia Europaea 11:87–89.

Linssen A. and Tytgat G.N. (1982) Fulminant onset of Crohn's disease of the colon (CDC): an observation of six cases. Digestive Diseases and Sciences 27:731–736.

Lishman A.H., Al-Jumaili I.J. and Record C.O. (1981) Spectrum of antibiotic-associated diarrhoea. Gut 22:34–37.

Lo T.C., Heading R.C. and Gilmour H.M. (1994) Intestinal spirochaetosis. Postgraduate Medical Journal 70:134–137.

Lockhart-Mummery H.E. and Morson B.C. (1960) Crohn's disease (regional enteritis) of the large intestine and its distinction from ulcerative colitis. Gut 1:87–105.

Loftus E.V. Jr, Alexander G.L. and Carpenter H.A. (1994) Cytomegalovirus as an exacerbating factor in ulcerative colitis. Journal of Clinical Gastroenterology 19:306–309.

Longfield R., O'Donnell J., Yudt W., Lissner C. and Burns T. (1979) Acute colitis and bacteremia due to *Campylobacter fetus*. Digestive Diseases and Sciences 24:950–953.

Loss R.W. Jr, Mangla J.C. and Pereira M. (1980) *Campylobacter* colitis presenting as inflammatory bowel disease with segmental colonic ulcerations. Gastroenterology 79:138–140.

Luks F.I., Chung M.A., Brandt M.L., Hertecant J., Roy C.C., Blanchard H. and Bensoussan A.L. (1991) Pneumatosis and pneumoperitoneum in chronic idiopathic intestinal pseudoobstruction. Journal of Pediatric Surgery 26:1384–1386.

Lusk L.B., Reichen J. and Levine J.S. (1984) Aphthous ulceration in diversion colitis: clinical implications. Gastroenterology 87:1171–1173.

Lynch D.A., Lobo A.J., Sobala G.M., Dixon M.F. and Axon A.T. (1993) Failure of colonoscopic surveillance in ulcerative colitis. Gut 34:1075–1080.

Lynn J.T., Gossen G., Miller A. and Russell I.J. (1984) Pneumatosis intestinalis in mixed connective tissue disease: two case reports and literature review. Arthritis and Rheumatism 27:1186–1189.

MacKay E.H. (1978) Malakoplakia in ulcerative colitis. Archives of Pathology and Laboratory Medicine 102:140–145.

MacMahon R.A., Moore C.C.M. and Cussen L.J. (1981) Hirschsprung-like syndromes in patients with normal ganglion cells on suction rectal biopsy. Journal of Pediatric Surgery 16:835–839.

McDermott F.T., Pihl E.A., Kemp D.R. and Polglase A.L. (1982) Co-existing Crohn's disease and ulcerative colitis. Diseases of the Colon and Rectum 25:600–602.

McGovern V.J. (1972) Rectal biopsy in the differential diagnosis of colitis: Rendiconti di Gastroenterologia 4:94–102.

McGovern V.J. and Goulston S.J.M. (1965) Ischaemic enterocolitis. Gut 6:213–220.

McGovern V.J. and Goulston S.J.M. (1968) Crohn's disease of the colon. Gut 9:164–176.

McIver A.G. and Whitehead R. (1972) Zonal colonic aganglionosis, a variant of Hirschsprung's disease. Archives of Disease in Childhood 47:233–237.

McKendrick M.W., Geddes A.M. and Gearty J. (1982) *Campylobacter* enteritis: a study of clinical features and rectal mucosal changes. Scandinavian Journal of Infectious Diseases 14:35–38.

McKendrick T. (1962) Sweat sodium levels in normal subjects, in fibrocystic patients and their relatives, and in chronic bronchitic patients. Lancet i:183–186.

Macfarlane D.A. (1955) Intestinal sarcoidosis. British Journal of Surgery 42:639–642.

Machida H.M., Catto-Smith A.G., Gall D.G., Trevenen C. and Scott R.B. (1994) Allergic colitis in infancy: clinical and pathologic aspects. Journal of Pediatric Gastroenterology and Nutrition 19:22–26.

Mackle E.J. and Parks T.G. (1986) The pathogenesis and pathophysiology of rectal prolapse and solitary rectal ulcer syndrome. Clinics in Gastroenterology 15:985–1002.

Madigan M.R. and Morson B.C. (1969) Solitary ulcer of the rectum. Gut 10:871–881.

Magidson J.G. and Lewin K.J. (1981) Diffuse colitis cystica profunda: report of a case. American Journal of Surgical Pathology 5:393–399.

Maher E.R., Dutoit S.H., Baillod R.A., Sweny P. and Moorhead J.F. (1988) Gastrointestinal complications of dialysis-related amyloidosis. British Medical Journal 297:265–266.

Malaval T., Li V., Jang G., Martins Ramos J., Mézin P., Fournet J. and Hostein J. (1993) Churg-Strauss syndrome with rectal localization and exudative enteropathy. Gastroenterologie Clinique et Biologique 17:386–390.

Malhotra R. and Sheffield A. (1988) Cronkhite-Canada syndrome associated with colon carcinoma and adenomatous changes in C-C polyps. American Journal of Gastroenterology 83:772–776.

Malhotra V., Tatke M., Gondal R., Jain R. and Kumar N. (1992) Solitary rectal ulcer syndrome. Journal of the Association of Physicians of India 40:231–233.

Mandal B.K., Schofield P.F. and Morson B.C. (1982) A clinicopathological study of acute colitis: the dilemma of transient colitis syndrome. Scandinavian Journal of Gastroenterology 17:865–869.

Mangham D.C., Newbold K.M., Dover S. and Fielding J.W. (1992) Granulomatous enterocolitis associated with therapeutic irradiation. Histopathology 20:444–446.

Marchildon M.B., Buck B.E. and Abdenour G. (1982) Necrotizing enterocolitis in the unfed infant. Journal of Pediatric Surgery 17:620–624.

Margaretten W. and McKay D.G. (1971) Thrombotic ulcerations of the gastrointestinal tract. Archives of Internal Medicine 127:250–253.

Markowitz J., Kahn E., Grancher K., Hyams J., Treem W. and Daum F. (1993) Atypical rectosigmoid histology in children with newly diagnosed ulcerative colitis. American Journal of Gastroenterology 88:2034–2037.

Marsh P.K. and Gorbach S.L. (1982) Invasive enterocolitis caused by *Edwardsiella tarda*. Gastroenterology 82:336–338.

Marshall A.R., Al-Jumaili I.J., Fenwick G.A., Bint A.J. and Record C.O. (1987) Cryptosporidiosis in patients at a large teaching hospital. Journal of Clinical Microbiology 25:172–173.

Marston A. (1977) In: Intestinal Ischaemia. London: Edward Arnold.

Marston A., Pheils M.T., Lea Thomas M. and Morson B.C. (1966) Ischaemic colitis. Gut 7:1–15.

Martin C.J., Parks T.G. and Biggart J.D. (1981) Solitary rectal ulcer syndrome in Northern Ireland, 1971–1980. British Journal of Surgery 68:744–747.

Martin D.M., Goldman J.A., Gilliam J. and Nasrallah S.M. (1981) Gold-induced eosinophilic enterocolitis: response to oral cromolyn sodium. Gastroenterology 80:1567–1570.

Martin P., Manley P.N., Depew W.T. and Blakeman J.H. (1987) Isotretinoin-associated proctosigmoiditis. Gastroenterology 93:605–609.

Martucciello G., Caffarena P.E., Lerone M., Mattioli G., Baradino A., Bisio G. and Jasonni V. (1994) Neuronal intestinal dysplasia: clinical experience in Italian patients. European Journal of Pediatric Surgery 4:287–292.

Masugi J., Matsui T., Fujimori T. and Maeda S. (1994) A case of Behçet's disease with multiple longitudinal ulcers all over the colon. American Journal of Gastroenterology 89:778–780.

Mathan M.M., Venkatesan S., George R., Mathew M. and Mathan V.I. (1985) *Cryptosporidium* and diarrhoea in Southern Indian children. Lancet ii:1172–1175.

Matseshe J.W., Go V.L.W. and Dimagno E.P. (1977) Meconium ileus equivalent complicating cystic fibrosis in postneonatal children and young adults: report of 12 cases. Gastroenterology 72:732–736.

Matsui T., Iwashita A., Iida M., Kume K. and Fujishima M. (1987) Acquired pseudoobstruction of the colon due to segmental hypoganglionosis. Gastrointestinal Radiology 12:262–264.

Matsumoto T., Iida M., Kimura Y., Nanbu T. and Fujishima M. (1994) Clinical features in young adult patients with ischaemic colitis. Journal of Gastroenterology and Hepatology 9:572–575.

Maxson C.J., Klein H.D. and Rubin W. (1994) Atypical forms of inflammatory bowel disease. Medical Clinics of North America 78:1259–1273.

Mayberry J.F., Ballantyne K.C., Hardcastle J.D., Mangham C. and Pye G. (1989) Epidemiological study of asymptomatic inflammatory bowel disease: the identification of cases during a screening programme for colorectal cancer. Gut 30:481–483.

Mayorga M., Castro F., Fernandez F., Val Bernal F. and Arribas V. (1992) Radiohistology and histochemistry of barium granuloma of the colon and rectum. Histology and Histopathology 7:625–628.

Mazier W.P., Sun K.M. and Robertson W.G. (1978) Oil-induced granuloma (eleoma) of the rectum: report of four cases. Diseases of the Colon and Rectum 21:292–294.

Meacham P.W. and Brantley B. (1987) Familial fibromuscular dysplasia of the mesenteric arteries. Southern Medical Journal 80:1311–1316.

Medina E., Orti E., Tome A., Quiles F., Canelles P. and Martinez A. (1990) Segmental tuberculosis of the colon diagnosed by colonoscopy. Endoscopy 22:188–190.

Meier-Ruge W. (1971) Über eine erkränksbildung des colon mit Hirschsprung's-symptomatik. Verhandlungen der deutschen Gesellschaft für Pathologie 55:506–510.

Meier-Ruge W. (1974) Hirschsprung's disease: its aetiology, pathogenesis and differential diagnosis. In: Current Topics in Pathology. Volume 59. Berlin: Springer, pp 131–179.

Meier-Ruge W., Gambazzi F., Kaufeler R.E., Schmid P. and Schmidt C.P. (1994) The neuropathological diagnosis of neuronal intestinal dysplasia (NID B). European Journal of Pediatric Surgery 4:267–273.

Meisel J.L., Bergman D., Grancy D., Saunders D.R. and Rubin C.E. (1977) Human rectal mucosa: proctoscopic and morphological changes caused by laxatives. Gastroenterology 72:1274–1279.

Miller R.R. and Sumner H.W. (1982) Argyrophilic cell hyperplasia and an atypical carcinoid tumor in chronic ulcerative colitis. Cancer 50:2920–2925.

Ming-Chai C., Jen-Chun H., P'ei-Yu C., Ch'i-Yuan C., P'eng-Fei T., Shen-Hsing C., Fu-P'an W., Ts'u-Ling C. and Shun-Ch'uan C. (1965) Pathogenesis of carcinoma of the colon and rectum in Schistosomiasis japonica: a study of 90 cases. Chinese Medical Journal 84:513–525.

Missmahl H.P. and Riemann J. (1968) Einfacher nachweis der mikroangiopathie an den capillaren der rectumschleimhaut bei diabetikern. Klinische Wochenschrift 46:374–376.

Mitchell T.J., Ketley J.M., Haslam S.C., Stephen J., Burdon D.W., Candy D.C.A. and Daniel R. (1986) Effect of toxin A and B of *Clostridium difficile* on rabbit ileum and colon. Gut 27:78–85.

Morgensen A.M., Olsen J.H. and Gudmand-Hoyer E. (1984) Collagenous colitis. Acta Medica Scandinavica 216:535–540.

Moroz S.P., Schroeder M., Trevenen C.L. and Cross H. (1984) Systemic histiocytosis: an unusual cause of perianal disease in a child. Journal of Pediatric Gastroenterology and Nutrition 3:309–311.

Morson B.C. (1966) Factors influencing the prognosis of early cancer of the rectum. Proceedings of the Royal Society of Medicine 59:607–608.

Morson B.C. and Dawson I.M.P. (1979) Gastrointestinal Pathology. 2nd Edition. London: Blackwells, p 514.

Morson B.C. and Pang L.S. (1967) Rectal biopsy as an aid to cancer control in ulcerative colitis. Gut 8:423–434.

Moss T.J. and Adler R. (1982) Necrotizing enterocolitis in older infants, children, and adolescents. Journal of Pediatrics 100:764–768.

Moulis H. and Vender R.J. (1994) Antibiotic-associated hemorrhagic colitis. Journal of Clinical Gastroenterology 18:227–231.

Mower W.J., Hawkins J.A. and Nelson E.W. (1986) Neutropenic enterocolitis in adults with acute leukemia. Archives of Surgery 121:571–574.

Mulholland M.W. and Delaney J.P. (1983) Neutropenic colitis and aplastic anemia. Annals of Surgery 197:84–90.

Muller-Lissner S. (1992) Side effects of laxatives. Zeitschrift für Gastroenterologie 30:418–427.

Munakata K., Morita K., Okabe I. and Sueoka H. (1985) Clinical and histologic studies of neuronal intestinal dysplasia. Journal of Pediatric Surgery 20:231–235.

Murai N., Fukuzaki T., Nakamura T., Hayashida H., Okazaki M., Fujimoto K. and Hirai T. (1993) Cronkhite-Canada syndrome associated with colon cancer: report of a case. Surgery Today 23:825–829.

Murdoch D.L. and Piris J. (1982) Immunoglobulin E in non-specific proctitis and ulcerative colitis: studies with a monoclonal antibody. Digestion 25:201–204.

Murphy B.J. and Weinfeld A. (1987) Innocuous pneumatosis intestinalis of the right colon in renal transplant recipients. Diseases of the Colon and Rectum 30:816–819.

Murphy E.A., Morris J., Walker E., Lee F.D. and Sturrock R.D. (1993) Cyclosporine A–induced colitis and acquired selective IgA deficiency in a patient with juvenile chronic arthritis. Journal of Rheumatology 20:1397–1398.

Murray F.E., Lombard M., Dervan P., Fitzgerald R.J. and Crowe J. (1988) Bleeding from multifocal heterotopic gastric mucosa in the colon controlled by an H2 antagonist. Gut 29:848–851.

Murray F.E., O'Brien M.J., Birkett D.H., Kennedy S.M. and LaMont J.T. (1987) Diversion colitis: pathologic findings in a resected sigmoid colon and rectum. Gastroenterology 93:1404–1408.

Myeren J., Serck-Hanssen A. and Solberg L. (1976) Routine and blind histological diagnoses on colonoscopic biopsies compared to clinical-colonoscopic observations in patients without and with colitis. Scandinavian Journal of Gastroenterology 11:135–140.

Myers A., Humphries D.M. and Cox E.V. (1976) A ten year follow-up of haemorrhagic proctitis. Postgraduate Medical Journal 52:224–228.

Nagasako K., Nakae Y., Kitao Y. and Aoki G. (1977) Colitis cystica profunda: report of a case in which differentiation from rectal cancer was difficult. Diseases of the Colon and Rectum 20:618–624.

Namdaran F., Dutz W. and Ovasepian A. (1979) Pneumatosis cystoides intestinalis in Iran. Gut 20:16–21.

Nathwani D., McWhinney P.H., Green S.T. and Boyd J.D. (1990) Intestinal spirochaetosis in a man with the acquired immune deficiency syndrome (AIDS). Journal of Infection 21:318–319.

Nebel O.T., El-Masry N.A., Castell D.O., Farid Z., Fornes M.F. and Sparks H.A. (1974) Schistosomal colonic polyposis. Gastrointestinal Endoscopy 20:99–101.

Neto J.A.R. and Ribeiro A.P. (1974) Trombose mesenterica inferior. Revista da Associacao Medica Brasileira 20:180–190

Neves J., Raso P., Pinto D. de M., da Silva S.P. and Alvarenga R.J. (1993) Ischaemic colitis (necrotizing colitis, pseudomembranous colitis) in acute schistosomiasis mansoni: report of two cases. Transactions of the Royal Society of Tropical Medicine and Hygiene 87:449–452.

Nezelov C., Guygrand D. and Thomine E. (1970) Les megacolons avec hyperplasie du plexus myenterique. Nouveau Presse Medicale 78:1501–1506.

Ng I.O. and Ng M. (1993) Colonic malacoplakia: unusual association with ulcerative colitis. Journal of Gastroenterology and Hepatology 8:110–115.

Nielsen R.H., Orholm M., Pedersen J.O., Hovind-Hougen K., Teglbjaerg P.S. and Thaysen E.H. (1983) Colorectal spirochetosis: clinical significance of the infestation. Gastroenterology 85:62–67.

Nielsen V.T., Vetner M. and Harslof E. (1980) Collagenous colitis. Histopathology 4:83–86.

Nolan N.P.M., Kelly C.P., Humphreys J.F.H., Cooney C., O'Connor R., Walsh T.N., Weir D.G. and O'Briain D.S. (1987) An epidemic of pseudomembranous colitis: importance of person to person spread. Gut 28:1467–1473.

Nostrant T.T., Kumar N.B. and Appelman H.D. (1987) Histopathology differentiates acute self-limited colitis from ulcerative colitis. Gastroenterology 92:318–328.

O'Donnell N. (1987) Enteritis cystica profunda: revisited. Human Pathology 18:1300–1301.

Odze R., Antonioli D., Peppercorn M. and Goldman H. (1993). Effect of topical 5-aminosalicylic acid (5-ASA) therapy on rectal mucosal biopsy morphology in chronic ulcerative colitis. American Journal of Surgical Pathology 17:869–875.

Odze R.D., Bines J., Leichtner A.M., Goldman H. and Antonioli D.A. (1993) Allergic proctocolitis in infants: a prospective clinicopathologic biopsy study. Human Pathology 24:668–674.

Odze R.D., Wershil B.K., Leichtner A.M. and Antonioli D.A. (1995) Allergic colitis in infants. Journal of Pediatrics 126:163–170.

Ogorek C.P. and Fisher R.S. (1994) Differentiation between Crohn's disease and ulcerative colitis. Medical Clinics of North America 78:1249–1258.

Olding L.B., Ahren C., Thurin J., Karlsson K-A., Svalander C. and Koprowski H. (1985) Gastrointestinal carcinoma–associated antigen detected by a monoclonal antibody in dysplasia and adenocarcinoma associated with chronic ulcerative colitis. International Journal of Cancer 36:131–136.

O'Leary A.D. and Sweeney E.C. (1986) Lymphoglandular complexes of the colon: structure and distribution. Histopathology 10:267–283.

Ona F.V. and Boger J.N. (1985) Rectal bleeding due to diversion colitis. American Journal of Gastroenterology 80:40–41.

Oosawa H. and Suzuki T. (1994) A case of ischemic colitis due to polyarteritis nodosa. Nippon Ronen Igakkai Zasshi 31:472–476.

Orchard J.L. and Lawson R. (1986) Severe colitis induced by soap enemas. Southern Medical Journal 79:1459–1460.

Orsay C.P., Kim D.O., Pearl R.K. and Abcarian H. (1993) Diversion colitis in patients scheduled for colostomy closure. Diseases of the Colon and Rectum 36:366–367.

Owen D.A., Hwang W.S., Thorlakson R.H. and Walli E. (1981) Malignant carcinoid tumor complicating chronic ulcerative colitis. American Journal of Clinical Pathology 76:333–338.

Pai C.H., Gordon R., Sims H.V. and Bryan L.E. (1984) Sporadic cases of hemorrhagic colitis associated with *Escherichia coli* 0157:H7. Annals of Internal Medicine 101:738–742.

Palmer K.R., Berry H., Wheeler P.J., Williams C.B., Fairclough P., Morson B.C. and Silk D.B.A. (1986) Collagenous colitis: a relapsing and remitting disease. Gut 27:578–580.

Panachi G., Pantosti A., Gentile G., Testore G.P., Venditti M., Martinos P. and Serra P. (1985) *Clostridium difficile* colitis in leukemia patients. European Journal of Cancer and Clinical Oncology 21:1159–1163.

Papa M.Z., Shiloni E. and McDonald H.D. (1986) Total colonic necrosis: a catastrophic complication of systemic lupus erythematosus. Diseases of the Colon and Rectum 29:576–578.

Parc R., Douvin D. and Loygue J. (1979) Le megacolon congenital de l'adulte: etude de 15 cas. Gastroenterologie Clinique et Biologique 3:321–328.

Parelkar S.N., Stamm W.P. and Hill K.R. (1971) Indirect immunofluorescent staining of *Entamoeba histolytica* in tissues. Lancet i:212–213.

Park W.H., Choi S.O., Kwon K.Y. and Chang E.S. (1992) Acetyl-cholinesterase histochemistry of rectal suction biopsies in the diagnosis of Hirschsprung's disease. Journal of Korean Medical Science 7:353–359.

Parkins R.A., Eidelman S., Rubin C.E., Dobbins W.O. and Phelps P.C. (1963) The diagnosis of cystic fibrosis by rectal suction biopsy. Lancet ii:851–856.

Parks A.G., Porter N.H. and Hardcastle J. (1966) The syndrome of the descending perineum. Proceedings of the Royal Society of Medicine 59:477–482.

Pascal R.R., Kaye G.I. and Lane N. (1968) Colonic pericryptal fibroblast sheath: replication, migration, and cytodifferentiation of a mesenchymal cell system in adult tissue: autoradiographic studies of normal rabbit colon. Gastroenterology 54:835–851.

Patrick W.J.A., Besley G.T.N. and Smith I.I. (1980) Histochemical diagnosis of Hirschsprung's disease and a comparison of the histochemical and biochemical activity of acetylcholinesterase in rectal mucosal biopsies. Journal of Clinical Pathology 33:336–343.

Patterson D.J., Johnson E.H. and Schmulen A.C. (1984) Fulminant pseudomembranous colitis occurring after colonoscopy. Gastrointestinal Endoscopy 30:249–253.

Pattnaik S., Banerjee M., Jalan R., Mathew P.J., Ghosh S., Agarwal S.K. and Maitra T.K. (1991) Malakoplakia simulating rectal carcinoma. Indian Journal of Pathology and Microbiology 34:52–56.

Pearson D.J., Stones N.A., Bentley S.J. and Reid H. (1983) Proctocolitis induced by salicylate and associated with asthma and recurrent nasal polyps. British Medical Journal 287:1675.

Peart A.G., Sivak M.V., Rankin G.B., Kish L.S. and Steck W.D. (1984) Spontaneous improvement of Cronkhite-Canada syndrome in a postpartum female. Digestive Diseases and Sciences 29:470–474.

Penna F.J. (1979) Blastomycosis of the colon resembling clinically ulcerative colitis. Gut 20:896–899.

Perarnau J.M., Raabe J.J., Courrier A., Peiffer G., Hennequin J.P., Bene M.C. and Arbogast J. (1982) A rare etiology of ischemic colitis: amyloid colitis. Endoscopy 14:107–109.

Perisic V.N., Kokai G. and Pavlovic M. (1992) Coeliac disease and collagenous colitis. Italian Journal of Gastroenterology 24:418–420.

Perzin K.H., Peterson M., Castiglione C.L., Fenoglio C.M. and Wolff M. (1984) Intramucosal carcinoma of the small intestine arising in regional enteritis (Crohn's disease). Cancer 54:151–162.

Pescatori M., Mattana C. and Castiglioni G.C. (1986) Adult megacolon due to total hypoganglionosis. British Journal of Surgery 73:765.

Petri M., Poulsen S.S., Christensen K. and Jarnum S. (1982) The incidence of granulomas in serial sections of rectal biopsies from patients with Crohn's disease. Acta Pathologica et Microbiologica Immunologica Scandinavica 90:145–147.

Petros J.G., Spirito N. and Gosshein R. (1992) Endometriosis causing colon obstruction in two postmenopausal women. Mt Sinai Journal of Medicine 59:362–365.

Picard E.J., Picard J.J., Jorissen J. and Jardon M. (1978) Heterotopic gastric mucosa in the epiglottis and rectum. American Journal of Digestive Diseases 23:217–221.

Pidala M.J., Slezak F.A. and Hlivko T.J. (1993) Delayed presentation of an inflammatory polyp following colonic ischemia. American Surgeon 59:315–318.

Pieterse A.S., Hecker R. and Rowland R. (1982) Collagenous colitis: a distinctive and potentially reversible disorder. Journal of Clinical Pathology 35:338–340.

Pieterse A.S., Leong A.S.Y. and Rowland R. (1985) The mucosal changes and pathogenesis of pneumatosis cystoides intestinalis. Human Pathology 16:683–688.

Pihl E., Peura A., Johnson W.R., McDermott F.T. and Hughes E.R.S. (1985) T-antigen expression by peanut agglutinin staining relates to mucosal dysplasia in ulcerative colitis. Diseases of the Colon and Rectum 28:11–17.

Pinheiro M.C. and de Lima M.A. (1991) A fatal case of intestinal balantidiasis. Revista da Sociedade Brasileira de Medicina Tropical 24:173–176.

Pistoia M.A., Guardagni S., Tuscano D., Negro P., Pistoia F. and Carboni M. (1987) Ulcerated ectopic gastric mucosa of the rectum. Gastrointestinal Endoscopy 33:41–43.

Pitt M.A., Knox W.F. and Haboubi N.Y. (1993) Multinucleated stromal giant cells of the colonic lamina propria in ulcerative colitis. Journal of Clinical Pathology 46:874–875.

Pittman F.E., El-Hashimi W.K. and Pittman J.C. (1973) Studies of human amebiasis: clinical and laboratory findings in eight cases of acute amebic colitis. Gastroenterology 65:581–587.

Pittman F.E. and Hennigar G.R. (1974) Sigmoidoscopic and colonic mucosal biopsy findings in amebic colitis. Archives of Pathology 97:155–158.

Podolsky D.K., Fournier D.A. and Lynch K.E. (1986) Human colonic goblet cells. Journal of Clinical Investigation 77:1263–1271.

Potzi R., Walgram M., Lochs H., Holzner H. and Gangl A. (1989) Diagnostic significance of endoscopic biopsy in Crohn's disease. Endoscopy 21:60–62.

Poulsen S.S., Pedersen N.T. and Jarnum S. (1984) "Microerosions" in rectal biopsies in Crohn's disease. Scandinavian Journal of Gastroenterology 19:607–612.

Pounder R.E. (1994) The pathogenesis of Crohn's disease. Journal of Gastroenterology 29 (suppl 7):11–15.

Powell G.K. (1986) Food protein–induced enterocolitis of infancy: differential diagnosis and management. Comprehensive Therapy 12:28–37.

Prathap K. and Gilman R. (1970) The histopathology of acute intestinal amebiasis: a rectal biopsy study. American Journal of Pathology 60:229–246.

Prendergast T.M., Marini C.P., D'Angelo A.J., Sher M.E. and Cohen J.R. (1994) Surgical patients with pseudomembranous colitis: factors affecting prognosis. Surgery 116:768–775.

Prescott R.J., Harris M. and Banerjee S.S. (1992) Fungal infections of the small and large intestine. Journal of Clinical Pathology 45:806–811.

Price A.B. (1978) Overlap in the spectrum of non-specific inflammatory bowel disease: "colitis indeterminate". Journal of Clinical Pathology 31:567–577.

Price A.B. and Davies D.R. (1977) Pseudomembranous colitis. Journal of Clinical Pathology 30:1–12.

Price A.B., Jewkes J. and Sanderson P.J. (1979) Acute diarrhoea: *Campylobacter* colitis and the role of rectal biopsy. Journal of Clinical Pathology 32:990–997.

Price A.B., Larson H.E. and Crow J. (1979) Morphology of experimental antibiotic-associated enterocolitis in the hamster: a model for human pseudomembranous colitis and antibiotic-associated diarrhoea. Gut 20:467–475.

Qualman S.J. and Murray R. (1994) Aganglionosis and related disorders. Human Pathology 25:1141–1149.

Quirke P., Campbell I. and Talbot I.C. (1984) Ischaemic proctitis and adventitial fibromuscular dysplasia of the superior rectal artery. British Journal of Surgery 71:33–38.

Rampton D.S. and Baithun S.I. (1987) Is microscopic colitis due to bile-salt malabsorption? Diseases of the Colon and Rectum 30:950–952.

Rampton D.S., Salmon P.R. and Clark C.G. (1983) Nonspecific ulcerative colitis as a sequel to amebic dysentery. Journal of Clinical Gastroenterology 5:217–219.

Ransohoff D.F., Riddell R.H. and Levin B. (1985) Ulcerative colitis and colonic cancer. Diseases of the Colon and Rectum 28:383–388.

Rapola J., Santavuori P. and Savilahti E. (1984) Suction biopsy of rectal mucosa in the diagnosis of infantile and juvenile types of neuronal ceroid lipofuscinoses. Human Pathology 15:352–360.

Rask-Madsen J., Grove O., Hansen M.G.J., Bukhave K., Scient C. and Henrik-Nielsen R. (1983) Colonic transport of water and electrolytes in a patient with secretory diarrhea due to collagenous colitis. Digestive Diseases and Sciences 28:1141–1146.

Read N.W., Krejs G.J., Read M.G., Santa Ana C.A., Morawski S.G. and Fordtran J.S. (1980) Chronic diarrhoea of unknown origin. Gastroenterology 78:264–271.

Reissman P., Weiss E.G., Teoh T.A., Lucas F.V. and Wexner S.D. (1994) Gangrenous ischemic colitis of the rectum: a rare complication of systemic lupus erythematosus. American Journal of Gastroenterology 89:2234–2236.

Remis R.S., MacDonald K.L., Riley L.W., Puhr N.D., Wells J.G., Davis B.R., Blake P.A. and Cohen M.L. (1984) Sporadic cases of hemorrhagic colitis associated with *Escherichia coli* 0157.H7. Annals of Internal Medicine 101:624–626.

Remmele W., Beck K. and Kaiserling E. (1988) Multiple lipid islands of the colonic mucosa: a light and electron microscopic study. Pathology, Research and Practice 183:336–342.

Renton C.J.C. (1972) Non-occlusive intestinal infarction. Clinics in Gastroenterology 1:655–671.

Rhodes J.M., Cockel R., Allan R.N., Hawker P.C., Dawson J. and Elias E. (1984) Colonic Crohn's disease and use of oral contraception. British Medical Journal 288:595–596.

Richman P.I., Tilly R., Jass J.R. and Bodmer W.F. (1987) Colonic pericrypt sheath cells: characterisation of cell type with new monoclonal antibody. Journal of Clinical Pathology 40:593–600.

Ricotti G.C., Buonomini M.I., Merlitti A., Karch H., Luzzi I. and Caprioli A. (1994) A fatal case of hemorrhagic colitis, thrombocytopenia, and renal failure associated with verocytotoxin-producing non-0157 *Escherichia coli*. Clinical Infectious Diseases 19:815–816.

Riddell R.H. (1976) The precarcinomatous phase of ulcerative colitis. In: Current Topics in Pathology: Pathology of the Gastrointestinal Tract. Edited by B.C. Morson. Berlin, Heidelberg, New York: Springer-Verlag, p 179.

Riddell R.H. (1984) Dysplasia and cancer in ulcerative colitis: a soluble problem? Scandinavian Journal of Gastroenterology 19 (suppl 104):137–149.

Riddell R.H., Goldman H., Ransohoff D.F., Appelman H.D., Fenoglio C.M., Haggitt R.C., Ahren C., Correa P., Hamilton S.R., Morson B.C., Sommers S.C. and Yardley J.H. (1983) Dysplasia in inflammatory bowel disease: standardized classification with provisional clinical applications. Human Pathology 14:931–968.

Riddell R.H., Tanaka M. and Mazzoleni G. (1992) Non-steroidal anti-inflammatory drugs as a possible cause of collagenous colitis: a case control study. Gut 33:683–687.

Ritchie J.K., Powell-Tuck J. and Lennard-Jones J.E. (1978) Clinical outcome of the first ten years of ulcerative colitis and proctitis. Lancet i:1140–1143.

Robey S.S., Kuhajda F.P. and Yardley J.H. (1988) Immunoperoxidase stains of ganglion cells and abnormal mucosal nerve proliferations in Hirschsprung's disease. Human Pathology 19:432–437.

Rocca J.M., Hecker R., Pieterse A.S., Rich G.E. and Rowland R. (1984) *Clostridium difficile* colitis. Australian and New Zealand Journal of Medicine 14:606–610.

Roche W.R., Beasley R., Williams J.H. and Holgate S.T. (1989) Subepithelial fibrosis in the bronchi of asthmatics. Lancet i:520–523.

Rodgers F.G., Rodgers C., Shelton A.P. and Hawkey C.J. (1986) Proposed pathogenic mechanism for the diarrhea associated with human intestinal spirochetes. American Journal of Clinical Pathology 86:679–682.

Roikjaer O. (1987) Perforation and necrosis of the colon complicating polyarteritis nodosa. Acta Chirurgica Scandinavica 153:385–386.

Rosekrans P.C.M., Meijer C.J.L.M., van der Wal A.M. and Lindeman J. (1980) Allergic proctitis, a clinical and immunopathological entity. Gut 21:1017–1023.

Rosen N., Sommer I. and Knobel B. (1985) Intestinal Buerger's disease. Archives of Pathology and Laboratory Medicine 109:962–963.

Rosenstein E.D., Rickert R.R., Gutkin M., Bacay A. and Kramer N. (1988) Colonic involvement in angioimmunoblastic lymphadenopathy resembling inflammatory bowel disease. Cancer 61:2244–2250.

Rotterdam H., Korelitz B.I. and Sommers S.C. (1977) Microgranulomas in grossly normal rectal mucosa in Crohn's disease. American Journal of Clinical Pathology 67:550–554.

Rubio C.A., Johansson C. and Kock Y. (1982) A quantitative method of estimating inflammation in the rectal mucosa. Scandinavian Journal of Gastroenterology 17:1083–1087.

Rubio C.A., Nylander G., Johansson C. and Slezak P. (1982) Non-dysplastic villous changes in endoscopic biopsies in ulcerative colitis with carcinoma. Acta Pathologica Microbiologica Immunologica Scandinavica 90:277–282.

Rudin C., Jenny P., Ohnacker H. and Heitz P.U. (1986) Absence of the enteric nervous system in the newborn: presentation of three patients and review of the literature. Journal of Pediatric Surgery 21:313–318.

Ruiz-Moreno F. (1963) Amoebic granuloma of the colon and rectum. Diseases of the Colon and Rectum 6:201.

Ruppin H. and Domschke S. (1984) Acute ulcerative colitis: a rare complication of sulfasalazine therapy. Hepato-gastroenterology 31:192–193.

Russell M.B., Russell C.A., Fenger K. and Niebuhr E. (1994) Familial occurrence of Hirschsprung's disease. Clinical Genetics 45:231–235.

Rutgeerts L., Ghillebert G., Drognee W., Tanghe W., Vuylsteke P. and Decoster M. (1993) Ischemic colitis in a patient with Crohn's disease taking oral contraceptive and an ergotamine alkaloid. Acta Clinica Belgica 48:48–51.

Rutgeerts P., D'Haens G., Hiele M., Geboes K. and Vantrappen G. (1994) Appendectomy protects against ulcerative colitis. Gastroenterology 106:1251–1253.

Sachar D.B. and Greenstein A.J. (1981) Cancer in ulcerative colitis: good news and bad news. Annals of Internal Medicine 95:642–644.

Sachdev H.P., Chadha V., Malhotra V., Verghese A. and Puri R.K. (1993) Rectal histopathology in endemic Shigella and Salmonella diarrhea. Journal of Pediatric Gastroenterology and Nutrition 16:33–38.

Sack R.B. (1981) Escherichia coli and acute diarrheal disease. Annals of Internal Medicine 94:129–130.

Sale G.E., McDonald G.B., Shulman H.M. and Thomas E.D. (1979) Gastrointestinal graft-versus-host disease in man. American Journal of Surgical Pathology 3:291–299.

Sallon S., Deckelbaum R.J., Schmid I.I., Harlap S., Baras M. and Spira D.T. (1988) Cryptosporidium, malnutrition, and chronic diarrhea in children. American Journal of Diseases of Children 142:312–315.

Samper E.R., Slagle G.W. and Hand A.M. (1984) Colonic endometriosis: its clinical spectrum. Southern Medical Journal 77:912–914.

Sanderson I.R., Boyle S., Williams C.B. and Walker-Smith J.A. (1986) Histological abnormalities in biopsies from macroscopically normal colonoscopies. Archives of Disease in Childhood 61:274–277.

Sandmeier D. and Guillou L. (1993) Malakoplakia and adenocarcinoma of the caecum: a rare association. Journal of Clinical Pathology 46:959–960.

Sankey E.A., Dhillon A.P., Anthony A., Wakefield A.J., Sim R., More L., Hudson M., Sawyer A.M. and Pounder R.E. (1993) Early mucosal changes in Crohn's disease. Gut 34:375–381.

Saul S.H. (1987) Inflammatory cloacogenic polyp: relationship to solitary rectal ulcer syndrome/mucosal prolapse and other bowel disorders. Human Pathology 18:1120–1125.

Saul S.H. and Sollenberger L.C. (1985) Solitary rectal ulcer syndrome. American Journal of Surgical Pathology 9:411–421.

Schaefer H.E. (1988) Multiple lipid islands of the colonic mucosa: a light and electron microscopic study. Pathology, Research and Practice 183:343–346.

Scharli A.F. and Meier-Ruge W. (1981) Localized and disseminated forms of neuronal intestinal dysplasia mimicking Hirschsprung's disease. Journal of Pediatric Surgery 16:164–170.

Scheiman J., Elta G., Colturi T. and Nostrant T. (1988) Colonic xanthomatosis: relationship to disorder motility and review of the literature. Digestive Diseases and Sciences 33:1491–1494.

Schein M., Veller M. and Decker G.A.G. (1987) Colitis cystica profunda simulating rectal carcinoma. South African Medical Journal 72:289–290.

Schmitz-Moorman P. and Himmelmann G.W. (1988) Does quantitative histology of rectal biopsy improve the differential diagnosis of Crohn's disease and ulcerative colitis in adults? Pathology, Research and Practice 183:481–488.

Schmitz-Moormann P., Pittner P.M., Malchow H. and Brandes J.W. (1984) The granuloma in Crohn's disease. Pathology, Research and Practice 178:467–476.

Schneider R.E. and Dobbins W.O. (1968) Suction biopsy of the rectal mucosa for diagnosis of arteritis in rheumatoid arthritis and related diseases. Annals of Internal Medicine 68:561–568.

Schofield D.E., Devine W. and Yunis E.J. (1990) Acetylcholinesterase-stained suction rectal biopsies in the diagnosis of Hirschsprung's disease. Journal of Pediatric Gastroenterology and Nutrition 11:221–228.

Schofield D.E. and Yunis E.J. (1990) Intestinal neuronal dysplasia. Journal of Pediatric Gastroenterology and Nutrition 12:182–189.

Schoonbroodt D., Horsmans Y., Laka A., Geubel A.P. and Hoang P. (1995) Eosinophilic gastroenteritis presenting with colitis and cholangitis. Digestive Diseases and Sciences 40:308–314.

Schumacher G. (1993) First attack of inflammatory bowel disease and infectious colitis: a clinical, histological and microbiological study with special reference to early diagnosis. Scandinavian Journal of Gastroenterology 198 (suppl):1–24.

Schumacher G., Kollberg B. and Sandstedt B. (1994) A prospective study of first attacks of inflammatory bowel disease and infectious colitis: histologic course during the first year after presentation. Scandinavian Journal of Gastroenterology 29:318–332.

Schwachman H. and Antonowicz I. (1962) The sweat test in cystic fibrosis. Annals of the New York Academy of Science 93:600–620

Schwarzenberg S.J. and Whitington P.F. (1983) Rectal gastric mucosa heterotopia as a cause of hematochezia in an infant. Digestive Diseases and Sciences 28:470–472.

Scott B.B., Goodall A., Stephenson P. and Jenkins D. (1983) Rectal mucosal plasma cells in inflammatory bowel disease. Gut 24:519–524.

Segal I., Tim L.O., Hamilton D.G., Lawson H.H., Solomon A., Kalk F. and Cooke S.A.R. (1979) Ritual-enema–induced colitis. Diseases of the Colon and Rectum 22:195–199.

Seldenrijk C.A., Drexhage H.A., Meuwissen S.G.M., Pals S.T. and Meijer C.J.L.M. (1989) Dendritic cells and scavenger macrophages in chronic inflammatory bowel disease. Gut 30:484–491.

Seldenrijk C.A., van der Harten H., Kluck P., Tibboel D., Moorman-Voestermans K. and Meijer C.J.L.M. (1986) Zonal aganglionosis: an enzyme and immunohistochemical study of two cases. Virchows Archiv A 410:75–81.

Shah S., Thomas V., Mathan M., Chacko A., Chandy G., Ramakrishna B.S. and Rolston D.D. (1992) Colonoscopic study of 50 patients with colonic tuberculosis. Gut 33:347–351.

Shalygina N.B., Tikhomirov D.E., Zhukhovitskii V.G. and Voronin V.I. (1994) Acute *Campylobacter* colitis. Arkhiv Patologii 56:27–30.

Shamsuddin A.K.M. and Elias E.G. (1981) Rectal mucosa: malignant and premalignant changes after radiation therapy. Archives of Pathology and Laboratory Medicine 105:150–151.

Shamsuddin A.K.M. and Yang G.Y. (1995) The large intestinal mucosa. In: Gastrointestinal and Oesophageal Pathology. Edited by R. Whitehead. Edinburgh: Churchill Livingstone pp 45–56.

Shamsuddin A.M., Phelps P.C. and Trump B.F. (1982) Human large intestinal epithelium: light microscopy, histochemistry and ultrastructure. Human Pathology 13:790–803.

Shepherd N.A., Hall P.A., Williams G.T., Codling B.W., Jones E.L., Levison D.A. and Morson B.C. (1989) Primary malignant lymphoma of the large intestine complicating chronic inflammatory bowel disease. Histopathology 15:325–337.

Sibbons P., Spitz L. and van Velzen D. (1992) The role of lymphatics in the pathogenesis of pneumatosis in experimental bowel ischaemia. Journal of Pediatric Surgery 27:339–342.

Siegers C.P., von Hertzberg-Lottin E., Otte M. and Schneider B. (1993) Anthranoid laxative abuse: a risk for colorectal cancer? Gut 34:1099–1101.

Simpson S., Traube J. and Riddell R.H. (1981) The histologic appearance of dysplasia (precarcinomatous change) in Crohn's disease of the small and large intestine. Gastroenterology 81:492–501.

Skinner J.M., Whitehead R. and Piris J. (1971) Argentaffin cells in ulcerative colitis. Gut 12:636–638.

Skirrow M.B. (1977) *Campylobacter* enteritis: a "new" disease. British Medical Journal 2:9–11.

Sladen G.E. and Filipe M.I. (1984) Is segmental colitis a complication of diverticular disease? Diseases of the Colon and Rectum 27:513–514.

Sloas M.M., Flynn P.M., Kaste S.C. and Patrick C.C. (1993) Typhlitis in children with cancer: a 30-year experience. Clinical Infectious Diseases 17:484–490.

Smith B. (1968) Pre- and postnatal development of the ganglion cells of the rectum and its surgical implications. Journal of Pediatric Surgery 3:386–391.

Smith B. (1972) The Neuropathology of the Alimentary Tract. London: Edward Arnold, p 80.

Smith B. (1982) The neuropathology of pseudo-obstruction of the intestine. Scandinavian Journal of Gastroenterology 17:103–109.

Smith B.H. and Welter L.H. (1967) Pneumatosis intestinalis. American Journal of Clinical Pathology 48:455–465.

Smith H.R., Rowe B., Gross R.J., Fry N.K. and Scotland S.M. (1987) Haemorrhagic colitis and verocytotoxin–producing *Escherichia coli* in England and Wales. Lancet i:1062–1065.

Smith J.M.B. (1969) Mycoses of the alimentary tract. Gut 10:1035–1040.

Smith V.V. (1992) Isolated intestinal neuronal dysplasia: a descriptive histological pattern or a distinct clinicopathological entity? In: Paediatric Gastroenterology. Inflammatory Bowel Diseases and Morbus Hirschsprung. Edited by F. Hadziselimovic and B.K. Herzog. Dordrecht: pp 203–214.

Snover D.C., Sandstad J. and Hutton S. (1985) Mucosal pseudolipomatosis of the colon. American Journal of Clinical Pathology 84:575–580.

Sodeman W.A. Jr and Dowda M.C. (1973) Rapid serological methods for the demonstration of *Entamoeba histolytica* activity. Gastroenterology 65:604–607.

Softley A., Clamp S.E., Watkinson G., Bouchier I.A.D., Myren J. and De Dombal F.T. (1988) The natural history of inflammatory bowel disease: has there been a change in the last 20 years? Scandinavian Journal of Gastroenterology 23 (suppl 144):20–23.

Sokol R.J., Farrell M.K. and McAdams A.J. (1984) An unusual presentation of Wegener's granulomatosis mimicking inflammatory bowel disease. Gastroenterology 87:426–432.

Soltoft J. (1969) Immunoglobulin-containing cells in normal jejunal mucosa and in ulcerative colitis and regional enteritis. Scandinavian Journal of Gastroenterology 4:353–360.

Soo K.C., Hollinger-Vernea S., Miller G., Pritchard G. and Frawley J. (1983) Buerger's disease of the sigmoid colon. Australian and New Zealand Journal of Surgery 53:111–112.

Spencer G.D., Shulman H.M., Myerson D., Thomas E.D. and McDonald G.B. (1986) Diffuse intestinal ulceration after marrow transplantation: a clinicopathologic study of 13 patients. Human Pathology 17:621–633.

Spotnitz W.D., Van Natta F.C., Bashist B., Wolff M., Green P. and Weber C.J. (1984) Localized ischemic colitis in a young woman with diabetes. Diseases of the Colon and Rectum 27:481–484.

Starling J.R., Croom R.D. and Thomas C.G. (1986) Hirschsprung's disease in young adults. American Journal of Surgery 151:104–109.

Steadman C., Teague C., Kerlin P., Harris O., Hourigan K. and Sampson J. (1987) Collagenous colitis: clinical and histological spectrum in ten patients. Journal of Gastroenterology and Hepatology 2:459–466.

Stenberg B. and Risberg B. (1984) Abdominal aortic aneurysm complicated by rectal necrosis. Acta Chirurgica Scandinavica 150:497–498.

Stevens S. and McClure J. (1982) The histochemical features of the Michaelis-Gutmann body and a consideration of the pathophysiological mechanisms of its formation. Journal of Pathology 137:119–127.

Stewenius J., Adnerhill I., Ekelund G,. Floren C.H., Fork F.T., Janzon L., Lindstrom C., Mars I., Nyman M. and Rosengren J.E. (1995). Ulcerative colitis and indeterminate colitis in the city of Malmo, Sweden: a 25-year incidence study. Scandinavian Journal of Gastroenterology 30:38–43.

Stolte M. (1988) "Normal" endoscopic findings in the gastrointestinal tract: when should a biopsy be taken? Endoscopy 20:111–113.

Stolte M., Ritter M., Borchard F. and Koch-Scherrer G. (1990) Collagenous gastroduodenitis on collagenous colitis. Endoscopy 22:186–187.

Struyf N.J., Verbist L.M., Colemont I.J., Vallaeys J. and van Moer E.M. (1995) Colitis cystica profunda. Nederlands Tijdschrift voor Geneeskunde 139:238–240.

Stuart M. (1984) Proctitis cystica profunda: incidence, etiology and treatment. Diseases of the Colon and Rectum 27:153–156.

Stuart R.C., Leahy A.L., Cafferkey M.T. and Stephens R.B. (1986) *Yersinia enterocolitica* infection and toxic megacolon. British Journal of Surgery 73:590.

Sturm R., Staneck J.L., Stauffer L.R. and Neblett W.W. III (1980) Neonatal necrotizing enterocolitis associated with penicillin-resistant, toxigenic *Clostridium butyricum*. Pediatrics 66:928–931.

Surawicz C.M. and Belic L. (1984) Rectal biopsy helps to distinguish acute self-limited colitis from idiopathic inflammatory bowel disease. Gastroenterology 86:104–113.

Surawicz C.M., Haggitt R.C., Husseman M. and McFarland L.V. (1994) Mucosal biopsy diagnosis of colitis: acute self-limited colitis and idiopathic inflammatory bowel disease. Gastroenterology 107:755–763.

Svartz N. and Ernberg T. (1949) Cancer coli in cases of colitis ulcerosa. Acta Medica Scandinavica 135:444.

Svendsen L.B., Sondergaard J.O., Hegnhoj J., Hojgard L., Lauritsen K.B., Bulow S., Horn T. and Danes B.S. (1987) In vitro tetraploidy in patients with ulcerative colitis. Scandinavian Journal of Gastroenterology 22:601–605.

Sviland L., Pearson A.D.J., Eastham E.J., Hamilton P.J., Proctor S.J., Malcolm A.J. and the Newcastle Upon Tyne Bone Marrow Transplant Group. (1988) Histological features of skin and rectal biopsy specimens after autologous and allogeneic bone marrow transplantation. Journal of Clinical Pathology 41:148–154.

Sweeney J.L., Hewett P., Riddell P. and Hoffmann D.C. (1986) Rectal gangrene: a complication of phosphate enema. Medical Journal of Australia 144:374–375.

Symonds J. (1988) Haemorrhagic colitis and *Escherichia coli* 0157: a pathogen unmasked. British Medical Journal 296:875–876.

Tada S., Iida M., Yao T., Kawabuko K., Yao T., Okada M. and Fujishima M. (1994) Endoscopic features in amyloidosis of the small intestine: clinical and morphological differences between chemical types of amyloid protein. Gastrointestinal Endoscopy 40:45–50.

Takayanagi K. and Kapila L. (1981) Necrotising enterocolitis in older infants. Archives of Diseases in Childhood 56:468–471.

Tam P.K.H. (1986) An immunochemical study with neuron-specific enolase and substance P of human enteric innervation: the normal developmental pattern and abnormal deviations in Hirschsprung's disease and pyloric stenosis. Journal of Pediatric Surgery 21:227–232.

Tam P.K.H. and Owen G. (1993) An immunohistochemical study of neuronal microtubule–associated proteins in Hirschsprung's disease. Human Pathology 24:424–431.

Tanaka M., Mazzoleni G. and Riddell R.H. (1992) Distribution of collagenous colitis: utility of flexible sigmoidoscopy. Gut 33:65–70.

Tanner A.R. and Raghunath A.S. (1988) Colonic inflammation and nonsteroidal anti-inflammatory drug administration. Digestion 41:116–120.

Taylor N.S., Thorne G. and Bartlett J.G. (1981) Comparison of two toxins produced by *Clostridium difficile*. Infection and Immunity 34:1036–1043.

Taylor-Robinson S., Miles R., Whitehead A. and Dickinson R.J. (1989) *Salmonella* infection and ulcerative colitis. Lancet i:1145.

Tedesco F.J., Corless J.K. and Brownstein R.E. (1982) Rectal sparing in antibiotic-associated pseudomembranous colitis: a prospective study. Gastroenterology 83:1259–1260.

Tedesco F.J., Hardin R.D., Harper R.N. and Edwards B.H. (1983) Infectious colitis endoscopically simulating inflammatory bowel disease: a prospective evaluation. Gastrointestinal Endoscopy 29:195–197.

Tedesco F.J., Sumner H.W. and Kassens W.D. Jr (1976) Colitis cystica profunda. American Journal of Gastroenterology 65:339–343.

Teglbjaerg P.S. and Thaysen E.H. (1982) Collagenous colitis: an ultrastructural study of a case. Gastroenterology 82:561–563.

Teglbjaerg P.S., Thaysen E.H. and Jensen H.H. (1984) Development of collagenous colitis in sequential biopsy specimens. Gastroenterology 87:703–709.

Terner J. and Lattes R. (1963) Malacoplakia of the colon. Federation Proceedings 22. Abstract 2103, p 512.

Theegarten D. and Ruhl G.H. (1994). Pneumatosis cystoides intestinalis: associated diseases, morphology and presumed pathogenesis. Leber Magen Darm 24:123–124, 127–130.

Thomas D.F.M., Fernie D.S., Malone M., Bayston R. and Spitz L. (1982) Association between _Clostridium difficile_ and enterocolitis in Hirschsprung's disease. Lancet i:78–79

Thompson N.P., Montgomery S.M., Pounder R.E. and Wakefield A.J. (1995) Is measles vaccination a risk factor for inflammatory bowel disease? Lancet 345:1071–1074.

Thomson G., Clark A.H., Hare K. and Spilg W.G.S. (1981) Tea consumption: a cause of constipation. British Medical Journal 282:864–865.

Thorning D. and Howard J.D. (1986) Epithelial denudement in the gastrointestinal tracts of two bone marrow transplant recipients. Human Pathology 17:560–566.

Tobi M., Kobrin I. and Ariel I. (1982) Rectal involvement in sarcoidosis. Diseases of the Colon and Rectum 25:491–493.

Toffler R.B., Pingoud E.G. and Burrell M.I. (1978) Acute colitis related to penicillin and penicillin derivatives. Lancet ii:707–709.

Tompkins D.S., Waugh M.A. and Cooke E.M. (1981) Isolation of intestinal spirochaetes from homosexuals. Journal of Clinical Pathology 34:1385–1387.

Toner P.G., Carr K.E. and Wyburn G.M. (1971) The Digestive System: An Ultrastructural Atlas and Review. London: Butterworths, p 114.

Toolenaar T.A.M., Freundt I., Huikeshoven F.J.M., Drogendijk A.A.T.C., Jeekel H. and Chadha-Ajwani S. (1993) The occurrence of diversion colitis in patients with a sigmoid neovagina. Human Pathology 24:846–849.

Toyosaka A., Tomimoto Y., Nose K., Seki Y. and Okamoto E. (1994) Immaturity of the myenteric plexus in the aetiology of meconium ileus without mucoviscidosis: a histopathologic study. Clinical Autonomic Research 4:175–184.

Tribe C.R., Scott D.G.I. and Bacon P.A. (1981) Rectal biopsy in the diagnosis of systemic vasculitis. Journal of Clinical Pathology 34:843–850.

Trigg P.H., Belin R., Haberkorn S., Long W.J., Nixon H.H., Plaschkes J., Spitz L. and Willital G.H. (1974) Experience with a cholinesterase histochemical technique for rectal suction biopsies in the diagnosis of Hirschsprung's disease. Journal of Clinical Pathology 27:207–213.

Tsutaoka B., Hansen J., Johnson D. and Holodniy M. (1994) Antibiotic-associated pseudomembranous enteritis due to _Clostridium difficile_. Clinical Infectious Diseases 18:982–984.

Ure B.M., Holschneider A.M. and Meier-Ruge W. (1994) Neuronal intestinal malformations: a retro- and prospective study on 203 patients. European Journal of Pediatric Surgery 4:279–286.

Vajrabukka T., Dhitavat A., Kichananta B., Sukonthamand Y., Tanphiphat C. and Vongviriyatham S. (1979) Fulminating amoebic colitis: a clinical evaluation. British Journal of Surgery 66:630–632.

Van Spreeuwel J.P., Duursma G.C., Meijer C.J.L.M., Bax R., Rosekrans P.C.M. and Lindeman J. (1985) _Campylobacter_ colitis: histological, immunohistochemical and ultrastructural findings. Gut 26:945–951.

Vantrappen G., Ponette E., Geboes K. and Bertrand P. (1977) _Yersinia_ enteritis and enterocolitis: gastroenterological aspects. Gastroenterology 72:220–227.

Vatn M.H., Elgjo K. and Bergan A. (1984) Distribution of dysplasia in ulcerative colitis. Scandinavian Journal of Gastroenterology 19:893–895.

Vernon S.E. (1982) Amyloid colitis. Diseases of the Colon and Rectum 25:728–730.

Vinores S.A. and May E. (1985) Neuron-specific enolase as an immunohistochemical tool for the diagnosis of Hirschsprung's disease. American Journal of Surgical Pathology 9:281–285.

Von Herbay A., Herfarth C. and Otto H.F. (1994) Cancer and dysplasia in ulcerative colitis: a histologic study of 301 surgical specimens. Zeitschrift für Gastroenterologie 32:382–388.

Wakefield A.J., Pittilo R.M., Sim R., Cosby S.L., Stephenson J.R., Dhillon A.P. and Pounder R.E. (1993) Evidence of persistent measles virus infection in Crohn's disease. Journal of Medical Virology 39:345–353.

Walker N.I., Bennett R.E. and Axelsen R.A. (1988) Melanosis coli: a consequence of anthraquinone-induced apoptosis of colonic epithelial cells. American Journal of Pathology 131:465–476.

Wang K.K., Perrault J., Carpenter H.A., Schroeder K.W. and Tremaine W.J. (1987) Collagenous colitis: a clinicopathologic correlation. Mayo Clinic Proceedings 62:665–671.

Ward M. and Webb J.N. (1977) Rectal biopsy as a prognostic guide in Crohn's colitis. Journal of Clinical Pathology 30:126–131.

Warren B.F. and Shepherd N.A. (1992) Diversion proctocolitis. Histopathology 21:91–93.

Warren B.F., Shepherd N.A., Bartolo D.C. and Bradfield J.W. (1993) Pathology of the defunctioned rectum in ulcerative colitis. Gut 34:514–516.

Watson A.J. and Roy A.D. (1960) Paneth cells in the large intestine in ulcerative colitis. Journal of Pathology and Bacteriology 80:309–316.

Wayte D.M. and Helwig E.B. (1967) Colitis cystica profunda. American Journal of Clinical Pathology 48:159–169.

Weedon D.D., Shorter R.G., Ilstrup D.M., Huizenga K.A. and Taylor W.F. (1973) Crohn's disease and cancer. New England Journal of Medicine 289:1099–1103.

Weitzner S. (1983) Ectopic salivary gland tissue in submucosa of rectum. Diseases of the Colon and Rectum 26:814–817.

Welling R.E., Roedersheimer L.R., Arbaugh J.J. and Cranley J.J. (1985) Ischemic colitis following repair of ruptured abdominal aortic aneurysm. Archives of Surgery 120:1368–1370.

Werlin S.L., Chusid M.J., Caya J. and Oechler H.W. (1982) Colitis in chronic granulomatous disease. Gastroenterology 82:328–331.

West A.B., Kuan S.F., Bennick M. and Lagarde S. (1995) Glutaraldehyde colitis following endoscopy: clinical and pathological features and investigation of an outbreak. Gastroenterology 108:1250–1255.

Whelan R.L., Abramson D., Kim D.S. and Hashmi H.F. (1994) Diversion colitis: a prospective study. Surgical Endoscopy 8:19–24.

White C.L., Hamilton S.R., Diamond M.P. and Cameron J.L. (1983) Crohn's disease and ulcerative colitis in the same patient. Gut 24:857–862.

White W.B., Hanna M. and Stewart J.A. (1984) Systemic herpes simplex virus type 2 infection: proctitis, urinary retention, arthralgias, and meningitis in the absence of primary mucocutaneous lesions. Archives of Internal Medicine 144:826–827.

Whitehead R. (1971) Ischaemic enterocolitis: an expression of the intravascular coagulation syndrome. Gut 12:912–917.

Whitehead R. (1972) The pathology of intestinal ischaemia. Clinics in Gastroenterology 1:613–637.

Whitehead R. (1976) The pathology of ischaemia of the intestines. In: Pathology Annual. Edited by S.C. Sommers. Norwalk, Conn.: Appleton-Century-Crofts, pp 1–52.

Whitehead R. (1987) Extra-intestinal Crohn's disease: does it exist? In: Surgery of Inflammatory Bowel Disease. Clinical Surgery International Volume 14. Edited by E.C.G. Lee and D.J. Nolan. London: Churchill Livingstone, pp 197–201.

Wig J.D., Talwar B.L. and Bushnurmath S.R. (1981) Toxic dilatation complicating fulminant amoebic colitis. British Journal of Surgery 68:135–136.

Wilkinson M.M. (1992) Small intestinal complications in progressive systemic sclerosis. Gastroenterological Nursing 15:50–53.

Williams S.M. and Harned R.K. (1991) Recognition and prevention of barium enema complications. Current Problems in Diagnostic Radiology 20:123–151.

Willoughby C.P., Piris J. and Truelove S.C. (1979) Tissue eosinophils in ulcerative colitis. Scandinavian Journal of Gastroenterology 14:395–399.

Wilson R. and Qualheim R.E. (1954) A form of acute hemorrhagic colitis affecting chronically ill individuals. Gastroenterology 27:431–444.

Wilson R.H., Kerr P.P., McLoughlin J. and Gormley M. (1993) Symptomatic colitis as the initial presentation of Wegener's granulomatosis. British Journal of Clinical Practice 47:315–318.

Winter H.S., Antonioli D.A., Fukagawa N., Marcial M. and Goldman H. (1990) Allergy-related proctocolitis in infants: diagnostic usefulness of rectal biopsy. Modern Pathology 3:5–10.

Womack C. (1984) Unusual histological appearances of barium sulphate: a case report with scanning electron microscopy and energy dispersive X-ray analysis. Journal of Clinical Pathology 37:488–493.

Womack N.R., Williams N.S., Holmfield J.H.M. and Morrison J.F.B. (1987) Pressure and prolapse: the cause of solitary rectal ulceration. Gut 28:1228–1233.

Wong V., Wyatt J., Lewis F. and Howdle P. (1993) Gold-induced enterocolitis complicated by cytomegalovirus infection: a previously unrecognised association. Gut 34:1002–1005.

Wood M.K., Read D.R., Kraft A.R. and Barreta T.M. (1979) A rare cause of ischemic colitis: polyarteritis nodosa. Diseases of the Colon and Rectum 22:428–433.

Wright A.W. (1930) Local effect of injection of gases into the subcutaneous tissues. American Journal of Pathology 6:87–124.

Yamano T., Shimada M., Okada S., Yutaka T., Kato T. and Yabuucki H. (1982) Ultrastructural study of biopsy specimens of rectal mucosa. Archives of Pathology and Laboratory Medicine 106:673–677.

Yamataka A., Miyano T., Urao M. and Nishiye H. (1992) Hirschsprung's disease: diagnosis using monoclonal antibody 171B5. Journal of Pediatric Surgery 27:820–822.

Yardley J.H., Ransohoff D.F., Riddell R.H. and Goldman H. (1983) Cancer in inflammatory bowel disease: how serious is the problem and what should be done about it? Gastroenterology 85:197–200.

Yashiro K., Murakami Y., Iizuka B., Hasegawa K., Nagasako K. and Yamada A. (1985) Localized colitis cystica profunda of the sigmoid colon. Endoscopy 17:198–199.

Yeager A.M., Kanof M.E., Kramer S.S., Jones B., Saral R., Lake A.M. and Santos G.W. (1987) Pneumatosis intestinalis in children after allogeneic bone marrow transplantation. Pediatric Radiology 17:18–22.

Yeoh E.K. and Horowitz M. (1987) Radiation enteritis. Surgery, Gynaecology and Obstetrics 165:373–379.

Yunis E.J., Dibbins A.W. and Sherman F.E. (1976) Rectal suction biopsy in the diagnosis of Hirschsprung disease in infants. Archives of Pathology and Laboratory Medicine 100:329–333.

Zern R.T. and Clarke-Pearson D.L. (1985) Pneumatosis intestinalis associated with enteral feeding by catheter jejunostomy. Obstetrics and Gynecology (suppl) 65:81s–83s.

Zeroogian J.M. and Chopra S. (1994) Collagenous colitis and lymphocytic colitis. Annual Review of Medicine 45:105–118.

Zidi S.H., Marteau P., Piard F., Coffin B., Favre J.P. and Rambaud J.C. (1994) Enterocolitis cystica profunda lesions in a patient with unclassified ulcerative enterocolitis. Digestive Diseases and Sciences 39:426–432.

Ziegler H.W., Heitz Ph.U., Kasper M., Spichtin H-P. and Ulrich J. (1984) Aganglionosis of the colon: morphologic investigations in 524 patients. Pathology, Research and Practice 178:543–547.

Zissiadis A., Papageorgiou A., Meyer-Papageorgiou S., Christoforidou B. and Aletras H. (1994) Sarcoidosis of the large intestine. Chirurg 65:646–648.

Zucker-Franklin D. and Franklin E.C. (1970) Intracellular localization of human amyloid by fluorescence and electron microscopy. American Journal of Pathology 59:23–41.

Zucker-Franklin D., Pras M. and Franklin E.C. (1969) Studies on human amyloid. Journal of Clinical Investigation 48:93–94.

V

Human Immunodeficiency Virus Infection and Mucosal Biopsy

19

ACQUIRED IMMUNODEFICIENCY SYNDROME, OESOPHAGEAL AND GASTROINTESTINAL MANIFESTATIONS

In the late 1970s and early 1980s it was realised that an increasing range of gastroenterological conditions were being described in the homosexual population. Thus it was that these became collectively known as the "gay bowel syndrome" (Kazal et al 1976), which was arguably bad terminology for a list of different disease states. Following the identification of the human immunodeficiency virus (HIV) and its association with the acquired immunodeficiency syndrome (AIDS), the pathological processes underlying these conditions are now better understood, and it is now recognised that AIDS is not confined to the homosexual population. Some 50% of AIDS victims will have gastroenterological clinical presentations, and virtually 100% develop gut lesions during the course of their disease (Chui and Owen 1994, Elshazly, Serwadda and Freers 1994, Rotterdam and Tsang 1994). For ease of description these lesions are best considered on a regional basis, but often more than one region of the gastrointestinal tract is involved by the same pathological process. There are several review articles concerning the gastrointestinal tract and AIDS, several of which detail the various biopsy appearances (Weller 1985, Surawicz et al 1986, Boylston et al 1987, Gazzard 1988, Stamm and Grant 1988).

AIDS AND THE OESOPHAGUS

The most common manifestation is oesophageal candidiasis, which may or may not be symptomatic. Candidiasis is the second most common infection in AIDS patients (Macher 1984). Cytomegaloviral (CMV) infection is generally the most common and can also cause oesophageal ulceration, as can herpes simplex virus (HSV) (Agha, Lee and Nostrant 1986). CMV ulceration is most often located in the middle or distal oesophagus and varies widely in macroscopic appearance (Wilcox, Straub and Schwartz 1994). Diagnosis using the polymerase chain reaction vastly increases the diagnostic positivity rate in biopsy tissues (Goodgame et al 1993). Rabeneck et al (1986) described oesophageal ulceration, which on light microscopy was nonspecific but on electron microscopy showed viral particles consistent with the morphology of a retrovirus and quite different from CMV or HSV. There is some evidence from studies in other immunocompromised patients (Walsh, Belitsos and Hamilton 1986) that bacterial oesophagitis is more common than has been recognised in the past in such patients. Involvement of the oesophagus by *Pneumocystis carinii* organisms (Grimes et al 1987, Dieterich et al 1992) and by histoplasmosis (Cappell et al 1988, Boulard et al 1994) has also been described.

Other oesophageal lesions in AIDS patients include Kaposi's sarcoma (Friedman, Wright and Altman 1985) and malignant lymphoma (Bernal and del Junco 1986).

AIDS AND THE STOMACH

In addition to the conditions listed for the oesophagus, other unusual lesions described in the stomach include phlegmonous gastritis (Mittleman and Suarez 1985) and invasion of the mucosa by *Helicobacter pylori* (Meiselman et al 1988). *H. pylori* and its relationship to gastritis and peptic ulcer were discussed earlier, in Chapter 7, when it was noted that normally it is seen in the superficial mucous layer and is noninvasive. Marano, Smith and Bonanno (1993) were unable to confirm Meiselman's findings and showed that the prevalence of *H. pylori* in AIDS patients with chronic active gastritis is much lower than that usually reported for HIV-negative patients with similar pathological conditions.

AIDS AND THE SMALL INTESTINE

Diarrhoea of small bowel origin is a frequent symptom in AIDS, and endoscopic biopsies often contribute to identifying the cause. Sometimes, abnormalities revealed by light microscopy are minimal, and a firm diagnosis may be reached only by electron microscopy (Yi and Powell 1994). Such is the case with infection by some protozoa, of which *Cryptosporidium* is the most common (Chiampi et al 1983, Current et al 1983, Guarda et al 1983, Ma and Soave 1983, Pitlik et al 1983, Cohen et al 1984, Gerstoft et al 1984, Weber et al 1992, Cotte et al 1993, Field et al 1993, Genta et al 1993, Goodgame et al 1995). The identification of microsporidia such as *Enterocytozoon bieneusi, Isospora belli,* as well as *Cryptosporidium* species, is also described in AIDS patients with diarrhoea and malabsorption whose small bowel mucosa was morphologically only minimally abnormal on light microscopy (Forthal and Guest 1984, Dobbins and Weinstein 1985, Modigliani et al 1985, Curry et al 1988, Miro et al 1995). Biopsies often show only partial villous atrophy and a mild inflammation of the lamina propria. Developmental stages of microsporidia and *Isospora* may be visible in Giemsa-stained sections, actually within the enterocytes, whereas *Cryptosporidium* organisms are typically seen attached to the brush border. In a significant number of cases, similar small intestinal inflammation and villous abnormality are associated with diarrhoea without the recognition of an infective agent. It is possible that patients with AIDS are predisposed to unidentified enteric pathogens (Gillin et al 1983), but enterocyte dysfunction is postulated (Heise et al 1991, Patterson, Ehrenpreis and Yokoo 1993, Carlson, Yokoo and Craig 1994). Benhamou et al (1994) have described lipid accumulation in enterocytes and the lamina propria. On the other hand, damage to the small bowel mucosa has been ascribed to the HIV infection itself and compared with graft-versus-host disease (Batman et al 1989); there may be a direct HIV infective role in altering the function of the intestinal immune system (Trajman et al 1994) or enterocyte function (Carlson, Yokoo and Craig 1994).

A Whipple-like small bowel lesion due to infection with *Mycobacterium avium-intracellulare* has also been described (Gillin et al 1983, Strom and Gruninger 1983,

Kooijman and Poen 1984, Roth et al 1985). The histiocytes that occupy the bloated villi, in addition to being positive on periodic acid–Schiff stain, contain large numbers of tubercle bacilli that are positive on Ziehl-Neelsen stain.

Although *P. carinii* infection usually involves the lungs in AIDS patients, it is occasionally described in the small intestine (Carter et al 1988). Confluent lakes of eosinophilic foamy material in vessels and submucosa occur, and cysts and trophozoites can be demonstrated in them.

AIDS AND THE COLORECTUM

Anorectal infections in homosexual males have been studied by sigmoidoscopy and rectal biopsy (McMillan and Lee 1981, Quinn et al 1981a, Goodell et al 1983). There can be no doubt that these infections can mimic ulcerative colitis and Crohn's disease grossly and microscopically. Whereas in the majority of cases the histological lesions mimic ulcerative colitis, as does infective colitis acquired by usual routes, in chlamydial proctitis and syphilis the presence of granulomas or giant cells introduces the possibility of Crohn's disease (Geller, Zimmerman and Cohen 1980, Quinn et al 1982).

The polymicrobial origin of colorectal infections in homosexual men is well recognised (Quinn et al 1983). Acute proctitis in biopsy specimens due to gonococci and meningococci has been described (McMillan et al 1983a). Similar appearances are produced by *Campylobacter jejuni* and other *Campylobacter*-like organisms (Quinn et al 1984). Proctocolitis has also been ascribed to *Chlamydia, Salmonella, Shigella* species, *Treponema,* and *Aeromonas hydrophila,* in addition to amoebae and *Penicillium marneffei* (Quinn et al 1982, Klotz et al 1983, Mindel 1983, Quinn et al 1983, Owen 1986, Roberts, Parenti and Albert 1987, Antony et al 1988, Smith et al 1988, Connolly et al 1989, Tsui, Ma and Tsang 1992). In an electron microscopic study, Orenstein and Kotler (1995) believed that *Escherichia* coliform organisms are more important as a cause of diarrhoea in AIDS patients than hitherto appreciated. A colitis grossly resembling Crohn's disease due to tuberculosis may occur (Lax et al 1988, Gutberlet and Rosch 1992), and rectal leishmaniasis is described (Rosenthal et al 1988, Jablonowski et al 1994, Laguna et al 1994). HSV (Guttman et al 1983, McMillan et al 1983b) and CMV (Meiselman, Cello and Margaretten 1985, Reyes and Gamboa-Dominguez 1993, De Rodriguez, Fuhrer and Lake-Bakaar 1994) frequently cause a proctitis or a colitis; in CMV colitis it can be so severe as to cause toxic dilation (Rene et al 1988). The inflamed mucosa may be ulcerated, but it has a nonspecific appearance in herpes proctocolitis, although Guttman et al (1983) described ground glass nuclei in endothelial and stromal cells. Likewise, in CMV colitis typical intranuclear inclusions are seen (Figs. 19–1 and 19–2). As in the small intestine, *Mycobacterium avium-intracellulare* infection can occur and present as an ulcerating inflammation with typical histiocytes occupying the mucosa (Wolke et al 1984). Similarly, cryptosporidiosis occurs and occasionally causes toxic dilation (Connolly and Gazzard 1987).

An interesting phenomenon was described by James (1988), who reported a patient with an 18-year history of Crohn's disease of the colon and whose disease remitted completely on contracting AIDS. This suggests that CD4 T lymphocytes play a role in the pathogenesis of Crohn's disease. There are several studies describing an increase in the incidence of colorectal spirochaetosis in homosexuals (Surawicz et al 1987), but there is as yet no firm evidence that even in AIDS patients the organism is a confirmed pathogen. There are also recorded cases of recurrent pseudomembranous colitis (Churchill et al 1994). Also, pseudomembranous colitis complicated by pneumatosis intestinalis has been recorded (Collins et al 1992, Burton, Mercado-Deane and Patel 1994).

Homosexuals are also known to show lymphoid hyperplasia of the rectal mucosa.

Figure 19–1. Cytomegalovirus colitis in an AIDS patient. The inflammation is nonspecific but involves the submucosa, where typical inclusions are present *(arrowheads)* (H&E ×250).

In AIDS patients, follicular dendritic cell processes are shortened and fragmented (Bishop, McMillan and Gilmour 1987). In an electron microscopy biopsy study, intraepithelial lymphocytes in AIDS patients appear activated in that they possess more than the usual number of lysosomes and surface projections. It is postulated that these cells play a role in the autoimmune injury of the intestinal mucosa that has been proposed in AIDS patients (Weber and Dobbins 1986). Kaposi's sarcoma can affect the whole gastrointestinal tract, including the colon, in AIDS patients (Friedman, Wright and Altman 1985, Zoller et al 1994). There is also an increased incidence of other malignancy, including lymphoma (Ziegler et al 1984, Ioachim and Cooper 1986).

Finally, there is every possibility that even in the absence of a microbiological cause, a low-grade proctitis with or without superficial ulcers may result in passive homosexuals as the result of trauma or the use of enemas or lubricants and so on. It is also suggested that a chronic colitis can occur as the direct result of HIV infection (Hing et al 1992). Colonic biopsies were characterised by a mixed inflammatory infiltrate and a preserved crypt architecture after histological follow-up at 6 to 39 months. HIV DNA was identified in the colonic mucosa. A similar claim has been made by Kotler, Reka and Clayton (1993).

AIDS AND THE ANAL CANAL

Homosexual men and AIDS patients are at high risk for anal condyloma, epithelial dysplasia, and anal carcinoma (Sohn and Robilotti 1977, Gottlieb et al

Figure 19–2. Detail of cytomegalovirus inclusions in Figure 19–1 (H&E ×500).

1981, Nash, Allen and Nash 1986, Schofield, Lindley and Harcourt-Webster 1989). Using an immunohistochemical method, Gal, Meyer and Taylor (1987) showed a high incidence of human papillomavirus (HPV) in the lesions. In a large study of homosexual men, Surawicz et al (1993) showed that 87% had HPV-associated abnormalities, including warts, white perianal epithelium, and dysplasia.

REFERENCES—SECTION FIVE: HUMAN IMMUNODEFICIENCY VIRUS INFECTION AND MUCOSAL BIOPSY

Agha F.P., Lee H.H. and Nostrant T.T. (1986) Herpetic esophagitis: a diagnostic challenge in immuno-compromised patients. American Journal of Gastroenterology 81:246–253.

Antony M.A., Brandt L.J., Klein R.S. and Bernstein L.H. (1988) Infectious diarrhea in patients with AIDS. Digestive Diseases and Sciences 33:1141–1146.

Batman P.A., Miller A.R.O., Forster S.M., Harris J.R.W., Pinching A.J. and Griffin G.E. (1989) Jejunal enteropathy associated with human immunodeficiency virus infection: quantitative histology. Journal of Clinical Pathology 42:275–281.

Benhamou Y., Hilmarsdottir I., Desportes-Livage I., Hoang C., Datry A., Danis M., Gentilini M. and Opolon P. (1994) Association of lipid accumulation in small intestinal mucosa with decreased serum triglyceride and cholesterol levels in AIDS. Digestive Diseases and Sciences 39:2163–2169.

Bernal A. and del Junco G.W. (1986) Endoscopic and pathologic features of esophageal lymphoma: a report of four cases in patients with acquired immune deficiency syndrome. Gastrointestinal Endoscopy 32:96–99.

Bishop P.E., McMillan A. and Gilmour H.M. (1987) A histological and immunocytochemical study of lymphoid tissue in rectal biopsies from homosexual men. Histopathology 11:1133–1147.

Boulard F., Cnudde F., Teron-Aboud B., Kermanac'h P., Nicolas M. and Juminer B. (1994) Digestive histoplasmosis in a patient with AIDS from Guadeloupe. Annales de Gastroenterologie et d'Hepatologie 30:97–100.

Boylston A.W., Cook H.T., Francis N.D. and Goldin R.D. (1987) Biopsy pathology of acquired immune deficiency syndrome (AIDS). Journal of Clinical Pathology 40:1–8.

Burton E.M., Mercado-Deane M.G. and Patel K. (1994) Pneumatosis intestinalis in a child with AIDS and pseudomembranous colitis. Pediatric Radiology 24:609–610.

Cappell M.S., Mandell W., Grimes M.M. and Neu H.C. (1988) Gastrointestinal histoplasmosis. Digestive Diseases and Sciences 33:353–360.

Carlson S., Yokoo H. and Craig R.M. (1994) Small intestinal HIV-associated enteropathy: evidence for panintestinal enterocyte dysfunction. Journal of Laboratory and Clinical Medicine 124:652–659.

Carter T.R., Cooper P.H., Petri W.A., Kim C.K., Walzer P.D. and Guerrant R.L. (1988) *Pneumocystis carinii* infection of the small intestine in a patient with acquired immune deficiency syndrome. American Journal of Clinical Pathology 89:679–683.

Chiampi N.P., Sundberg R.D., Klompus J.P. and Wilson A.J. (1983) Cryptosporidial enteritis and *pneumocystis* pneumonia in a homosexual man. Human Pathology 14:734–737.

Chui D.W. and Owen R.L. (1994) AIDS and the gut. Journal of Gastroenterology and Hepatology 9:291–303.

Churchill D.R., Lucas S.B., Williams I., Foley N.M. and Miller R.F. (1994) Recurrent pseudomembranous colitis due to *Clostridium difficile* in AIDS (clinical conference). Genitourinary Medicine 70:51–55.

Cohen J.D., Ruhlig L., Jayich S.A., Tong M.J., Lechago J. and Snape W.J. (1984) *Cryptosporidium* in acquired immunodeficiency syndrome. Digestive Diseases and Sciences 29:773–777.

Collins C.D., Blanshard C., Cramp M., Gazzard B. and Gleeson J.A. (1992) Case report: pneumatosis intestinalis occurring in association with cryptosporidiosis and HIV infection. Clinical Radiology 46:410–411.

Connolly G.M. and Gazzard B.G. (1987) Toxic megacolon in cryptosporidiosis. Postgraduate Medical Journal 63:1103–1104.

Connolly G.M., Shanson D., Hawkins D.A., Webster J.N.H. and Gazzard B.G. (1989) Non-cryptosporidial diarrhoea in human immunodeficiency virus (HIV)–infected patients. Gut 30:195–200.

Cotte L., Rabodonirina M., Piens M.A., Perreard M., Mojon M. and Trepo C. (1993) Prevalence of intestinal protozoans in French patients infected with HIV. Journal of Acquired Immune Deficiency Syndromes 6:1024–1029.

Current W.L., Reese N.C., Ernst J.V., Bailey W.S., Heyman M.B. and Weinstein W.M. (1983) Human cryptosporidiosis in immunocompetent and immunodeficient persons. New England Journal of Medicine 308:1252–1257.

Curry A., McWilliam L.J., Haboubi N.Y. and Mandal B.K. (1988) Microsporidiosis in a British patient with AIDS. Journal of Clinical Pathology 41:477–478.

De Rodriguez C.V., Fuhrer J. and Lake-Bakaar G. (1994) Cytomegalovirus colitis in patients with acquired immunodeficiency syndrome. Journal of the Royal Society of Medicine 87:203–205.

Dieterich D.T., Lew E.A., Bacon D.J., Pearlman K.I. and Scholes J.V. (1992) Gastrointestinal pneumo-cystosis in HIV-infected patients on aerosolized pentamidine: report of five cases and literature review. American Journal of Gastroenterology 87:1763–1770.

Dobbins W.O. and Weinstein W.M. (1985) Electron microscopy of the intestine and rectum in acquired immunodeficiency syndrome. Gastroenterology 88:738–749.

Elshazly M.A., Serwadda D.M. and Freers J. (1994) Endoscopic study of African AIDS patients with upper gastrointestinal symptoms. East African Medical Journal 71:496–500.

Field A.S., Hing M.C., Milliken S.T. and Marriott D.J. (1993) Microsporidia in the small intestine of HIV-infected patients: a new diagnostic technique and a new species. Medical Journal of Australia 158:390–394.

Forthal D.N. and Guest S.S. (1984) *Isospora belli* enteritis in three homosexual men. American Journal of Tropical Medicine and Hygiene 33:1060–1064.

Friedman S.L., Wright T.L. and Altman D.F. (1985) Gastrointestinal Kaposi's sarcoma in patients with acquired immunodeficiency syndrome. Gastroenterology 89:102–108.

Gal A.A., Meyer P.R. and Taylor C.R. (1987) Papillomavirus antigens in anorectal condyloma and carcinoma in homosexual men. Journal of the American Medical Association 257:337–340.

Gazzard B.G. (1988) HIV disease and the gastroenterologist. Gut 29:1497–1505.

Geller S.A., Zimmerman M.J. and Cohen A. (1980) Rectal biopsy in early lymphogranuloma venereum proctitis. American Journal of Gastroenterology 74:433–435.

Genta R.M., Chappell C.L., White A.C. Jr, Kimball K.T. and Goodgame R.W. (1993) Duodenal morphology and intensity of infection in AIDS-related intestinal cryptosporidiosis. Gastroenterology 105:1769–1775.

Gerstoft J., Holten-Andersen W., Blom J. and Nielsen J.O. (1984) *Cryptosporidium* enterocolitis in homosexual men with AIDS. Scandinavian Journal of Infectious Diseases 16:385–388.

Gillin J.S., Urmacher C., West R. and Shike M. (1983) Disseminated *Mycobacterium avium-intracellulare* infection in acquired immuno-deficiency syndrome mimicking Whipple's disease. Gastroenterology 85:1187–1191.

Goodell S.E., Quinn T.C., Mkrtichian E., Schuffler M.D., Holmes K.K. and Corey L. (1983) Herpes simplex virus proctitis in homosexual men: clinical, sigmoidoscopic, and histopathological features. New England Journal of Medicine 308:868–871.

Goodgame R.W., Genta R.M., Estrada R., Demmler G. and Buffone G. (1993) Frequency of positive tests for cytomegalovirus in AIDS patients: endoscopic lesions compared with normal mucosa. American Journal of Gastroenterology 88:338–343.

Goodgame R.W., Kimball K., Ov C.N., White A.C. Jr, Genta R.M., Lifschitz C.H. and Chappell C.L. (1995) Intestinal function and injury in acquired immunodeficiency syndrome–related cryptosporidiosis. Gastroenterology 108:1075–1082.

Gottlieb M.S., Schroff R., Schanker H.M., Weisman J.D., Fan P.T., Wolf R.A. and Saxon A. (1981) *Pneumocystis carinii* pneumonia and mucosal candidiasis in previously healthy homosexual men: evidence of a new acquired cellular immunodeficiency. New England Journal of Medicine 305:1425–1431.

Grimes M.M., LaPook J.D., Bar M.H., Wasserman II.S. and Dwork A. (1987) Disseminated *Pneumocystis carinii* infection in a patient with acquired immunodeficiency syndrome. Human Pathology 18:307–308.

Guarda L.A., Stein S.A., Cleary K.A. and Ordonez N.G. (1983) Human cryptosporidiosis in the acquired immune deficiency syndrome. Archives of Pathology and Laboratory Medicine 107:562–566.

Gutberlet H. and Rosch W. (1992) Primary intestinal tuberculosis in AIDS. Zeitschrift für Gastroenterologie 30:869–872.

Guttman D., Raymond A., Gelb A., Ehya H., Mather U., Mildvan D. and Spigland I. (1983) Virus-associated colitis in homosexual men: two case reports. American Journal of Gastroenterology 78:167–169.

Heise C., Dandekar S., Kumar P., Duplantier R., Donovan R.M. and Halsted C.H. (1991) Human immunodeficiency virus infection of enterocytes and mononuclear cells in human jejunal mucosa. Gastroenterology 100:1521–1527.

Hing M.C., Goldschmidt C., Mathijs J.M., Cunningham A.L. and Cooper D.A. (1992) Chronic colitis associated with human immunodeficiency virus infection. Medical Journal of Australia 156:683–687.

Ioachim H.L. and Cooper M.C. (1986) Lymphomas of AIDS. Lancet i:96–97.

Jablonowski H., Szelenyi H., Borchard F., Dohring-Schwerdtfeger E. and Hengels K.J. (1994) Visceral leishmaniasis with gastrointestinal involvement in a 30-year-old HIV infected patient. Zeitschrift für Gastroenterologie 32:405–407.

James S.P. (1988) Remission of Crohn's disease after human immunodeficiency virus infection. Gastroenterology 95:1667–1669.

Kazal H.L., Sohn N., Carrasco J.I., Robilotti J.G. and Delaney W.E. (1976) The gay bowel syndrome: clinico-pathologic correlation in 260 cases. Annals of Clinical Laboratory Science 6:184–192.

Klotz S.A., Drutz D.J., Tam M.R. and Reed K.H. (1983) Hemorrhagic proctitis due to lymphogranuloma venereum serogroup L2. New England Journal of Medicine 308:1563–1565.

Kooijman C.D. and Poen H. (1984) Whipple-like disease in AIDS. Histopathology 8:705–707.

Kotler D.P., Reka S. and Clayton F. (1993) Intestinal mucosal inflammation associated with human immunodeficiency virus infection. Digestive Diseases and Sciences 38:1119–1127.

Laguna F., Garcia-Samaniego J., Soriano V., Valencia E., Redondo C., Alonso M.J. and Gonzalez-Lahoz J.M. (1994) Gastrointestinal leishmaniasis in human immunodeficiency virus–infected patients: report of five cases and review. Clinics of Infective Diseases 19:48–53.

Lax J.D., Haroutiounian G., Attia A., Rodriguez R., Thayaparan R. and Bashist B. (1988) Tuberculosis of the rectum in a patient with acquired immune deficiency syndrome. Diseases of the Colon and Rectum 31:394–397.

McMillan A., Gilmour H.M., Slatford K. and McNeillage G.J.C. (1983a) Proctitis in homosexual men. British Journal of Venereal Diseases 59:260–264.

McMillan A. and Lee F.D. (1981) Sigmoidoscopic and microscopic appearance of the rectal mucosa in homosexual men. Gut 22:1035–1041.

McMillan A., McNeillage G., Gilmour H.M. and Lee F.D. (1983b) Histology of rectal gonorrhoea in men, with a note on anorectal infection with *Neisseria* meningitidis. Journal of Clinical Pathology 36:511–514.

Ma P. and Soave R. (1983) Three-step stool examination for cryptosporidiosis in 10 homosexual men with protracted watery diarrhea. Journal of Infectious Diseases 147:824–828.

Macher A.M. (1984) In: Fauci A.S. (moderator) Acquired immunodeficiency syndrome: epidemiologic, clinical, immunologic and therapeutic considerations. Annals of Internal Medicine 100:92–106.

Marano B.J. Jr, Smith F. and Bonanno C.A. (1993) *Helicobacter pylori* prevalence in acquired immunodeficiency syndrome. American Journal of Gastroenterology 88:687–690.

Meiselman M.S., Cello J.P. and Margaretten W. (1985) Cytomegalovirus colitis: report of the clinical, endoscopic and pathologic findings in two patients with the acquired immune deficiency syndrome. Gastroenterology 88:171–175.

Meiselman M.S., Miller-Catchpole R., Christ M. and Randall E. (1988) *Campylobacter pylori* gastritis in the acquired immuno-deficiency syndrome. Gastroenterology 95:209–212.

Mindel A. (1983) Lymphogranuloma venereum of the rectum in a homosexual man. British Journal of Venereal Diseases 59:196–197.

Miro O., Moreno A., Valls M.E., Miro J.M., Pique J.M., Bordas J.M., Moreno-Martinez A., Bombi J.A. and Gatell J.M. (1995) Intestinal microsporidiosis in patients with AIDS: study of 3 cases. Medicina Clinica 104:96–99.

Mittleman R.E. and Suarez R.V. (1985) Phlegmonous gastritis associated with the acquired immunodeficiency syndrome/pre-acquired immunodeficiency syndrome. Archives of Pathology and Laboratory Medicine 109:765–767.

Modigliani R., Bories C., Le Charpentier Y., Salmeron M., Messing B., Galian A., Rambaud J.C., Lavergne A., Cochand-Priollet B. and Desportes I. (1985) Diarrhoea and malabsorption in acquired immune deficiency syndrome: a study of four cases with special emphasis on opportunistic protozoan infestations. Gut 26:179–187.

Nash G., Allen W. and Nash S. (1986) Atypical lesions of the anal mucosa in homosexual men. Journal of the American Medical Association 256:873–876.

Orenstein J.M. and Kotler D.P. (1995) Diarrheogenic bacterial enteritis in acquired immune deficiency syndrome. Human Pathology 26:481–492.

Owen R.L. (1986) Role of biopsy in diagnosis of rectal infections. Gastroenterology 91:770–772.

Patterson B.K., Ehrenpreis E.D. and Yokoo H. (1993) Focal enterocyte vacuolization: a new microscopic finding in the acquired immune deficiency wasting syndrome. American Journal of Clinical Pathology 99:24–27.

Pitlik S.D., Fainstein V., Garza D., Guarda L., Bolivar R., Rios A., Hopfer R.L. and Mansell P.A. (1983) Human cryptosporidiosis: spectrum of disease. Archives of Internal Medicine 143:2269–2275.

Quinn T.C., Corey L., Chaffee R.G., Schuffler M.D., Brancato F.P. and Holmes K.K. (1981a) The etiology of anorectal infections in homosexual men. American Journal of Medicine 71:395–406.

Quinn T.C., Goodell S.E., Fennell C., Wang S-P., Schuffler M.D., Holmes K.K. and Stamm W.E. (1984) Infections with *Campylobacter jejuni* and *Campylobacter*-like organisms in homosexual men. Annals of Internal Medicine 101:187–192.

Quinn T.C., Goodell S.E., Mkrtichian E., Schuffler M.D., Wang S-P., Stamm W.E. and Holmes K.K. (1981) *Chlamydia* trachomatis proctitis. New England Journal of Medicine 305:195–200.

Quinn T.C., Lukehart S.A., Goodell S., Mkrtichian E., Schuffler M.D. and Holmes K.K. (1982) Rectal mass caused by *Treponema pallidum:* confirmation by immunofluorescent staining. Gastroenterology 82:135–139.

Quinn T.C., Stamm W.E., Goodell S.E., Mkrtichian E., Benedetti J., Corey L., Schuffler M.D. and Holmes K.K. (1983) The polymicrobial origin of intestinal infections in homosexual men. New England Journal of Medicine 309:576–582.

Rabeneck L., Boyko W.J., McLean D.M., McLeod W.A. and Wong K.K. (1986) Unusual esophageal ulcers containing enveloped viruslike particles in homosexual men. Gastroenterology 90:1882–1889.

Rene E., Marche C., Chevalier T., Rouzioux C., Regnier B., Saimot A.G., Negesse Y., Matheron S., Leport C., Wolff B., Moriniere B., Katlama C., Godeberge B., Vittecoq B., Bricaire F., Brun-Vesinet C., Pangon B., Deluol A.M., Coulaud J.P., Modai J., Frottier J., Vilde J.L., Vachon F., Mignon M. and Bonfils S. (1988) Cytomegalovirus colitis in patients with acquired immunodeficiency syndrome. Digestive Diseases and Sciences 33:741–750.

Reyes E. and Gamboa-Dominguez A. (1993) Cytomegalovirus colitis in patients with acquired immunodeficiency syndrome. Histopathologic, endoscopic and clinical correlation. Revista de Gastroenterologia de Mexico 58:214–219.

Roberts I.M., Parenti D.M. and Albert M.B. (1987) *Aeromonas hydrophila*–associated colitis in a male homosexual. Archives of Internal Medicine 147:1502–1503.

Rosenthal P.J., Chaisson R.E., Hadley W.K. and Leech J.H. (1988) Rectal leishmaniasis in a patient with acquired immunodeficiency syndrome. American Journal of Medicine 84:307–309.

Roth R.I., Owen R.L., Keren D.F. and Volberding P.A. (1985) Intestinal infection with *Mycobacterium avium* in acquired immune deficiency syndrome (AIDS): histological and clinical comparison with Whipple's disease. Digestive Diseases and Sciences 30:497–504.

Rotterdam H. and Tsang P. (1994) Gastrointestinal disease in the immunocompromised patient. Human Pathology 25:1123–1140.

Schofield J.B., Lindley R.P. and Harcourt-Webster J.N. (1989) Biopsy pathology of HIV infection: experience at St. Stephen's Hospital, London. Histopathology 14:277–288.

Smith P.D., Lane H.C., Gill V.J., Manischewitz J.F., Quinnan G.V., Fauci A.S. and Masur H. (1988) Intestinal infections in patients with the acquired immunodeficiency syndrome (AIDS). Annals of Internal Medicine 108:328–333.

Sohn N. and Robilotti J.G. (1977) The gay bowel syndrome: a review of colonic and rectal conditions in 200 male homosexuals. American Journal of Gastroenterology 67:478–484.

Stamm B. and Grant J.W. (1988) Biopsy pathology of the gastrointestinal tract in human immunodeficiency virus–associated disease: a 5 year experience in Zurich. Histopathology 13:531–540.

Strom R.L. and Gruninger R.P. (1983) AIDS with *Mycobacterium avium-intracellulare* lesions resembling those of Whipple's disease. New England Journal of Medicine 309:1323–1334.

Surawicz C.M., Goodell S.E., Quinn T.C., Roberts P.L., Corey L., Holmes K.K., Schuffler M.D. and Stamm W.E. (1986) Spectrum of rectal biopsy abnormalities in homosexual men with intestinal symptoms. Gastroenterology 91:651–659.

Surawicz C.M., Kirby P., Critchlow C., Sayer J., Dunphy C. and Kiviat N. (1993) Anal dysplasia in homosexual men: role of anoscopy and biopsy. Gastroenterology 105:658–666.

Surawicz C.M., Roberts P.L., Rompalo A., Quinn T.C., Holmes K.K. and Stamm W.E. (1987) Intestinal spirochetosis in homosexual men. American Journal of Medicine 82:587–592.

Trajman A., Belo M., Oliveira A., Madi K. and Elia C. (1994) Quantitative and qualitative changes in intestinal immunoglobulin-bearing plasma cells in jejunal mucosa of 52 HIV-infected patients. Brazilian Journal of Medical and Biological Research 27:1215–1224.

Tsui W.M.S., Ma K.F. and Tsang D.N.C. (1992) Disseminated *Penicillium marneffei* infection in HIV-infected patients. Histopathology 20:287–293.

Walsh T.J., Belitsos N.J. and Hamilton S.R. (1986) Bacterial esophagitis in immunocompromised patients. Archives of Internal Medicine 146:1345–1348.

Weber J.R. and Dobbins W.O. (1986) The intestinal and rectal epithelial lymphocyte in AIDS. American Journal of Surgical Pathology 10:627–639.

Weber R., Muller A., Spycher M.A., Opravil M., Ammann R. and Briner J. (1992) Intestinal *Enterocytozoon bieneusi* microsporidiosis in an HIV-infected patient: diagnosis by ileo-colonoscopic biopsies and long-term follow up. Clinical Investigations 70:1019–1023.

Weller I.V.D. (1985) AIDS and the gut. Scandinavian Journal of Gastroenterology 20 (suppl 114):77–89.

Wilcox C.M., Straub R.F. and Schwartz D.A. (1994) Prospective endoscopic characterization of cytomegalovirus esophagitis in AIDS. Gastrointestinal Endoscopy 40:481–484.

Wolke A., Meyers S., Adelsberg B.R., Bottone E.J., Damsker B., Schwartz I.S. and Janowitz H.D. (1984) *Mycobacterium avium-intracellulare*-associated colitis in a patient with the acquired immunodeficiency syndrome. Journal of Clinical Gastroenterology 6:225–229.

Yi E.S. and Powell H.C. (1994) Adenovirus infection of the duodenum in an AIDS patient: an ultrastructural study. Ultrastructural Pathology 18:549–551.

Ziegler J.L., Beckstead J.A., Volberding P.A., Abrams D.I., Levine A.M. and Lukes R.J. et al (1984) Non-Hodgkin's lymphoma in 90 homosexual men: relationship to generalized lymphadenopathy and acquired immunodeficiency syndrome (AIDS). New England Journal of Medicine 311:565–570.

Zoller W.G., Bogner J.R., Liess H., Powitz F. and Goebel F.D. (1994) Diagnosis and therapy of gastrointestinal Kaposi's sarcoma in AIDS. Bildgebung 46 (suppl):52.

Index

Note: Page numbers in *italics* refer to illustrations; numbers followed by *t* indicate tables.